湖南省教育委员会湖南省高水平研究生
教材建设项目资助　编号 2019~34

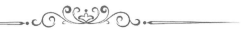

双语医学
影像学

（第二版）

主　编◎肖恩华　尚全良　袁友红　颜荣华　谭　艳

副主编◎陈　柱　梁　斌　肖运平　陈翔宇　马　聪

主　审◎刘　军　张子曙　谭长连　谭利华　刘　辉　罗建光

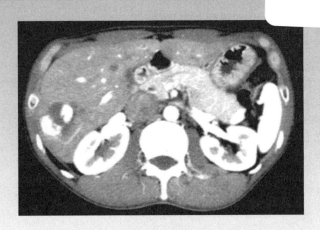

中南大学出版社
www.csupress.com.cn
·长沙·

内容提要

本书英汉双语共7篇29章,将医学影像学分为总论、骨骼系统、胸部、腹部与盆腔、中枢神经系统、头颈部、介入放射学七大部分。详细介绍了 X 线、CT、MRI 等成像技术,在各系统的诊断、检查方法、正常表现、基本病变、常见疾病诊断和介入放射学,以及常用的、较成熟的血管性和非血管性介入治疗方法。

图书在版编目(CIP)数据

双语医学影像学:英汉对照 / 肖恩华等主编.
—2 版. —长沙:中南大学出版社,2022.11
ISBN 978-7-5487-5171-7

Ⅰ. ①双… Ⅱ. ①肖… Ⅲ. ①医学摄影—英、汉
Ⅳ. ①R445

中国版本图书馆 CIP 数据核字(2022)第 212196 号

双语医学影像学(第二版)
SHUANGYU YIXUE YINGXIANG XUE(DI-ER BAN)

肖恩华　尚全良　袁友红　颜荣华　谭　艳　主编

□出 版 人	吴湘华
□责任编辑	谢新元
□责任印制	唐　曦
□出版发行	中南大学出版社
	社址:长沙市麓山南路　　　　邮编:410083
	发行科电话:0731-88876770　　传真:0731-88710482
□印　　装	长沙市宏发印刷有限公司

□开　　本	889 mm×1194 mm 1/16	□印张 41	□字数 1718 千字
□版　　次	2022 年 11 月第 2 版	□印次 2022 年 11 月第 1 次印刷	
□书　　号	ISBN 978-7-5487-5171-7		
□定　　价	110.00 元		

编 者
List of Contributors

主 编

肖恩华，中南大学湘雅二医院放射科，医学博士后，主任医师，教授

Xiao Enhua, Department of Radiology, The Second Xiangya Hospital, Central South University, Postdoctoral Fellowship, Chief Physician, Professor

尚全良，中南大学湘雅二医院放射科，医学博士，副主任医师，副教授

Shang Quanliang, Department of Radiology, The Second Xiangya Hospital, Central South University, Doctor's Degree of Medicine, Associate Chief Physician, Associate Professor

袁友红，湖南省人民医院(湖南师范大学第一附属医院)放射科，医学博士，主任医师，研究员，副教授

Yuan Youhong, Department of Radiology, Hunan Provincial People's Hospital (The First Affiliated Hospital of Hunan Normal University), Doctor's Degree of Medicine , Chief physician, Researcher, Associate Professor

颜荣华，北京大学深圳医院医学影像科，医学博士，副主任医师，副教授

Yan Ronghua, Department of Medical Imging, Peking University Shenzhen Hospital, Doctor's Degree of Medicine, Associate Chief Physician, Associate Professor

谭艳，山西医科大学第一医院磁共振室，医学博士，主任医师，教授

Tan Yan, Depart of Magnetic Resonance Imaging, The First Hospital of Shanxi Medical University, Doctor's Degree of Medicine, Chief Physician, Professor

副主编

陈柱，中南大学湘雅二医院放射科，医学博士后，副主任医师，副教授

Chen Zhu, Department of Radiology, The Second Xiangya Hospital, Central South University, Postdoctoral Fellowship, Associate Chief Physician, Associate Professor

梁斌，华中科技大学同济医学院附属协和医院放射科，医学博士，主任医师，教授

Liang Bin, Department of Radiology, Union Hospital, Tongji Medical College, Huazhong University of Science and Technology, Doctor's Degree of Medicine, Chief Physician, Professor

肖运平，广西医科大学附属柳州市人民医院放射科，医学硕士，主任医师，教授

Xiao Yunping, Department of Radiology, The Affiliated Liuzhou People's Hospital of Guangxi Medical University, Master's Degree of Medicine, Chief Physician, Professor

陈翔宇，中南大学湘雅二医院放射科，医学博士，副主任医师，副教授

Chen Xiangyu, Department of Radiology, The Second Xiangya Hospital, Central South University, Doctor's Degree of Medicine, Associate Chief Physician, Associate Professor

马聪，中南大学湘雅二医院放射科，医学博士，副主任医师，副教授

Ma Cong, Department of Radiology, The Second Xiangya Hospital, Central South University, Doctor's Degree of Medicine, Associate Chief Physician, Associate Professor

主审

刘军，中南大学湘雅二医院放射科，医学博士后，主任医师，教授

Liu Jun, Department of Radiology, The Second Xiangya Hospital, Central South University, Postdoctoral Fellowship, Chief Physician, Professor

张子曙，中南大学湘雅二医院放射科，医学博士后，主任医师，教授

Zhang Zixu, Department of Radiology, The Second Xiangya Hospital, Central South University, Postdoctoral Fellowship, Chief Physician, Professor

谭长连，中南大学湘雅二医院放射科，医学博士，主任医师，教授

Tan Changlian, Department of Radiology, The Second Xiangya Hospital, Central South University, Doctor's Degree of Medicine, Chief Physician, Professor

谭利华，中南大学湘雅二医院放射科，医学硕士，主任医师，教授

Tan Lihua, Department of Radiology, The Second Xiangya Hospital, Central South University, Master's Degree of Medicine, Chief Physician, Professor

刘辉，中南大学湘雅二医院放射科，医学硕士，副主任医师，副教授

Liu Hui, Department of Radiology, The Second Xiangya Hospital, Central South University, Master's Degree of Medicine, Associate Chief Physician, Associate Professor

罗建光，中南大学湘雅二医院放射科，医学硕士，副主任医师，副教授

Luo Jiangguan, Department of Radiology, The Second Xiangya Hospital, Central South University, Master's Degree of Medicine, Associate Chief Physician, Associate Professor

编委：(按章节顺序排列)

肖恩华，中南大学湘雅二医院放射科，医学博士后，主任医师，教授

Xiao Enhua, Department of Radiology, The Second Xiangya Hospital, Central South University, Postdoctoral Fellowship, Chief Physician, Professor

张洁湖南省常德市第一人民医院放射科　医学硕士，医师

Zhang Jie, Department of Radiology, The first people's Hospital of Changde City, Hunan Province, Master's Degree of Medicine, Physician

禹成，中南大学湘雅二医院放射科　医学博士生

Yu Cheng, Department of Radiology, The Second Xiangya Hospital, Central South University, Doctor of Medicine

郭建伟，邵阳学院附属第一医院放射科，医学硕士，副主任医师

Guo Jianwei, Department of Radiology, The First Affiliated Hospital of Shaoyang University, Master's Degree of Medicine, Associate Chief Physician

谭长连，中南大学湘雅二医院放射科，医学博士，主任医师，教授

Tan Changlian, Department of Radiology, The Second Xiangya Hospital, Central South University, Doctor's Degree of Medicine, Chief Physician, Professor

康振，华中科技大学同济医学院附属同济医院放射科，医学博士，主治医师，讲师

Kang Zhen, Department of Radiology, Tongji Hospital, Tongji Medical College, Huazhong University of Technology and Science, Doctor's Degree of Medicine, Attending Physician, Lecturer

梅习龙，中南大学湘雅二医院放射科，医学硕士，副主任技师

Mei Xilong, Department of Radiology, The Second Xiangya Hospital, Central South University, Master's Degree of Medicine, Deputy Chief Technician

2

罗志凌，长沙市第三医院放射科，医学硕士，副主任医师

Luo Zhiling, Department of Radiology, The Third Hospital of Changsha, Master's Degree of Medicine, Associate Chief Physician

卞读军，中南大学湘雅二医院放射科，医学博士，副主任技师

Bian Dujun, Department of Radiology, The Second Xiangya Hospital, Central South University, Doctor's Degree of Medicine, Deputy Chief Technician

李华兵，中南大学湘雅二医院放射科，医学硕士，副主任技师

Li Huabing, Department of Radiology, The Second Xiangya Hospital, Central South University, Master's Degree of Medicine, Deputy Chief Technician

刘宁远，中南大学湘雅二医院放射科，医学博士生

Liu Ningyuan, Department of Radiology, The Second Xiangya Hospital, Central South University, Doctor of Medicine

韦小芳，浏阳市骨伤科医院放射科，医学硕士，医师

Wei Xiaofang, Department of Radiology, Liuyang Orthopedic Hospital, Master's Degree of Medicine, Physician

陈柱，中南大学湘雅二医院放射科，医学博士后，副主任医师，副教授

Chen Zhu, Department of Radiology, The Second Xiangya Hospital, Central South University, Postdoctoral Fellowship, Associate Chief Physician, Associate Professor

罗涛，中南大学湘雅二医院放射科，医学硕士生

Luo Tao, Department of Radiology, The Second Xiangya Hospital, Central South University, Master of Medicine

吴海军，广东省人民医院放射科，医学博士，副主任医师，副教授

Wu Haijun, Department of Radiology, Guangdong Provincial People's Hospital, Guangdong Academy of Medical Sciences. Doctor's Degree of Medicine, Associate Chief physician, Associate Professor

蔡晔雨，中南大学湘雅二医院放射科，医学博士生

Cai Yanyu, Department of Radiology, The Second Xiangya Hospital, Central South University, Doctor of Medicine

彭书慧，中南大学湘雅二医院放射科，医学博士生

Peng Shuhui, Department of Radiology, The Second Xiangya Hospital, Central South University, Doctor of Medicine

孙双婧，香港大学深圳医院放射科，医学硕士，医师

Sun Shanjin, Department of Radiology, The University of Hong Kong-Shenzhen Hospital, Master's Degree of Medicine, Physician

谭利华，中南大学湘雅二医院放射科，医学硕士，主任医师，教授

Tan Lihua, Department of Radiology, The Second Xiangya Hospital, Central South University, Master's Degree of Medicine, Chief Physician, Professor

尚全良，中南大学湘雅二医院放射科，医学博士，副主任医师，副教授

Shang Quanliang, Department of Radiology, The Second Xiangya Hospital, Central South University, Doctor's Degree of Medicine, Associate Chief Physician, Associate Professor

尹芝兰，中南大学湘雅二医院放射科，医学博士，主治医师，讲师

Yin Zhilan. Department of Radiology, The Second Xiangya Hospital, Central South University, Doctor's Degree of Medicine, Attending Physician, Lecturer

陈娟，中南大学湘雅二医院放射科，医学博士，主治医师，讲师

Chen Juan, Department of Radiology, The Second Xiangya Hospital, Central South University, Doctor's Degree of Medicine, Attending Physician, Lecturer

郭茜，中南大学湘雅二医院放射科，医学硕士生

Guo Qian, Department of Radiology, The Second Xiangya Hospital, Central South University, Master of Medicine

曾牧，中南大学湘雅二医院放射科，医学博士，主治医师，讲师

Zeng Mao, Department of Radiology, The Second Xiangya Hospital, Central South University, Doctor's Degree of Medicine, Attending Physician, Lecturer

刘佳易，中南大学湘雅二医院放射科，医学博士生

LiuJiayi, Department of Radiology, The Second Xiangya Hospital, Central South University, Doctor of Medicine

李艳辉，中南大学湘雅二医院放射科，医学博士，主治医师，讲师

Li Yanhui, Department of Radiology, The Second Xiangya Hospital, Central South University, Doctor's Degree of Medicine, Attending Physician, Lecturer

龙孟平，北京大学肿瘤医院病理科，医学博士，医师

Long Mengping, Department of Pathology, Peking University Cancer Hospital, Doctor's Degree of Medicine, Physician

肖曼君，中南大学湘雅二医院放射科，医学博士，主治医师，讲师

Xiao Manjun, Department of Radiology, The Second Xiangya Hospital, Central South University, Doctor's Degree of Medicine, Attending Physician, Lecturer

陈珊珊，中南大学湘雅二医院放射科，医学博士，主治医师，讲师

Chen Shanshan, Department of Radiology, The Second Xiangya Hospital, Central South University, Doctor's Degree of Medicine, Attending Physician, Lecturer

罗建光，中南大学湘雅二医院放射科，医学硕士，副主任医师，副教授

Luo Jiangguan, Department of Radiology, The Second Xiangya Hospital, Central South University, Master's Degree of Medicine, Associate Chief Physician, Associate Professor

颜荣华，北京大学深圳医院医学影像科，医学博士，副主任医师，副教授

Yan Ronghua, Department of Medical Imaging, Peking University Shenzhen Hospital, Doctor's Degree of Medicine, Associate Chief physician, Associate Professor

郭焯欣，中山大学附属第三医院放射科　医学硕士，医师

Guo Zhuoxin, Department of Radiology, The Third Affiliated Hospital, Sun Yat－sen University, Master's Degree of Medicine, Physician

王宾，海南医学院第二附属医院放射科，医学硕士，副主任医师，副教授

Wang Bin, Department of Radiology, The Second Affiliated Hospital of Hainan Medical College, Master's Degree of Medicine, Associate Chief Physician, Associate Professor

周子懿，中南大学湘雅二医院放射科，医学硕士生

Zhou Ziyi, Department of Radiology, The Second Xiangya Hospital, Central South University, Master of Medicine

丁竹远，中南大学湘雅二医院放射科，医学硕士生

Ding Zhuyuan, Department of Radiology, The Second Xiangya Hospital, Central South University, Master of Medicine

周广，湖南省人民医院(湖南师范大学附属第一医院)放射科，医学硕士，主治医师，讲师

Zhou Guang, Department of Radiology, Hunan Provincial People's Hospital(The First Affiliated Hospital of Hunan Normal University), Master's Degree of Medicine, Attending Physician, Lecturer

邓志奇，邵阳学院附属第二医院放射科，医学硕士，副主任医师，副教授

Deng Zhiqi, Department of Radiology, The Second Affiliated Hospital of Shaoyang University, Master's Degree of Medicine, Associate Chief Physician, Associate Professor

袁友红, 湖南省人民医院(湖南师范大学附属第一医院)放射科, 医学博士, 主任医师, 研究员, 副教授

Yuan Youhong, Department of Radiology, Hunan Provincial People's Hospital (The First Affiliated Hospital of Hunan Normal University), Doctor's Degree of Medicine, Chief Physician, Researcher, Associate Professor

罗伟, 南华大学附属长沙中心医院放射科, 医学硕士, 副主任医师, 副教授

Luo Wei, Department of Radiology, The Affiliated Changsha Central Hospital of University of South China, Master's Degree of Medicine, Associate Chief Physician, Associate Professor

李秀梅, 福建医科大学附属第一医院医学影像科, 医学博士, 副主任医师, 副教授

Li Xiumei, Department of Medical Imaging, The First Affiliated Hospital of Fujian Medical University, Doctor's Degree of Medicine, Associate Chief Physician, Associate Professor

蒋洪涛, 邵阳学院附属第一医院放射科, 医学硕士, 副主任医师, 副教授

Jiang Hongtao, Department of Radiology, The First Affiliated Hospital of Shaoyang University, Master's Degree of Medicine, Associate chief physician, Associate Professor

毛志群, 湖南省人民医院(湖南师范大学附属第一医院)放射科, 医学硕士, 主任医师

Mao Zhiqun, Department of Radiology, Hunan Provincial People's Hospital (The First Affiliated Hospital of Hunan Normal University), Master's Degree of Medicine, Chief physician

刘辉, 中南大学湘雅二医院放射科, 医学硕士, 副主任医师, 副教授

Liu Hui, Department of Radiology, The Second Xiangya Hospital, Central South University, Master's Degree of Medicine, Associate Chief Physician, Associate Professor

陈翔宇, 中南大学湘雅二医院放射科, 医学博士, 副主任医师, 副教授

Chen Xiangyu, Department of Radiology, The Second Xiangya Hospital, Central South University, Doctor's Degree of Medicine, Associate Chief Physician, Associate Professor

柴甜, 中南大学湘雅二医院放射科, 医学硕士生

Chai Tian, Department of Radiology, The Second Xiangya Hospital, Central South University, Master of Medicine

李亚, 中南大学湘雅二医院放射科, 医学硕士生

Li Ya, Department of Radiology, The Second Xiangya Hospital, Central South University, Master of Medicine

刘梅桃, 中南大学湘雅二医院放射科, 医学硕士生

Liu Meitao, Department of Radiology, The Second Xiangya Hospital, Central South University, Master of Medicine

肖运平, 广西医科大学附属柳州市人民医院放射科, 医学硕士, 主任医师

Xiao Yunping, Department of Radiology, The Affiliated Liuzhou People's Hospital of Guangxi Medical University, Master's Degree of Medicine, Chief Physician

欧幼宽, 晋江市医院影像科, 医学硕士, 副主任医师

OU Youkuan, Department of Radiololgy, Jinjiang City Hospital, Master's Degree of Medicine, Deputy Chief Physician

王小业, 中南大学湘雅二医院放射科, 医学硕士, 技师

Wang Xiaoye, Department of Radiology, The Second Xiangya Hospital, Central South University, Master's Degree of Medicine, Technician

张敏萍, 中南大学湘雅二医院超声诊断科, 医学博士, 助理研究员

Zhang Minping, Department of Ultrasound Diagnosis, The Second Xiangya Hospital, Central South University, Doctor's Degree of Medicine, Assistant Research Fellow

廖秋玲, 中南大学湘雅二医院放射科, 医学博士生

Liao Qiuling, Department of Radiology, The Second Xiangya Hospital, Central South University, Doctor of Medicine

张邢，长沙市第三医院放射科，医学硕士，主治医师

Zhang Xing, Department of Radiology, The Third Hospital of Changsha, Master's Degree of Medicine, Attending Doctor

戴生珍，海南省人民医院放射科，医学硕士，医师

Dai Shengzhen, Department of Radiology, Hainan General Hospital, Master's Degree of Medicine, Physician

吕敏，中南大学湘雅二医院放射科，医学硕士生

Lv Min, Department of Radiology, The Second Xiangya Hospital, Central South University, Master of Medicine

谭艳，山西医科大学第一医院磁共振室，医学博士，教授，主任医师

Tan Yan, Depart of Magnetic Resonance Imaging, The First Hospital of Shanxi Medical University, Doctor's Degree of Medicine, Chief Physician, Professor

胡瑟，坦桑尼亚 Ifakara 卫生研究所，研究士(放射科医生-研究科学家)，医生

Hussein Said Mbarak, Ifakara Health Institute Tanzania, MMed[Radiologist - Research Scientist], MD, Physician

孙祥茹，山西医科大学第一医院磁共振室，医学硕士生

Sun Xiangru, Depart of Magnetic Resonance Imaging, The First Hospital of Shanxi Medical University, Master of Medicine

江浩茹，山西医科大学第一医院磁共振室，医学硕士生

Jiang Haoru, Depart of Magnetic Resonance Imaging, The First Hospital of Shanxi Medical University, Master of Medicine

田大伟，山西医科大学第一医院磁共振室，医学硕士生

Tian Dawei, Depart of Magnetic Resonance Imaging, The First Hospital of Shanxi Medical University, Master of Medicine

刘泽亮，山西医科大学第一医院磁共振室，医学硕士生

Liu Zeliang, Depart of Magnetic Resonance Imaging, The First Hospital of Shanxi Medical University, Master of Medicine

昌倩，北京京煤集团总医院医学影像科，医学硕士，主治医师

Chang Qian, Department of Medical lmaging, Beijing Jingmei Group General Hospital, Master's Degree of Medicine, Attending Physician

刘军，中南大学湘雅二医院放射科，医学博士后，主任医师，教授

Liu Jun, Department of Radiology, The Second Xiangya Hospital, Central South University, Postdoctoral Fellowship, Chief Physician, Professor

李秋云，湖南省第二人民医院放射科，医学博士，副主任医师

Li Qiuyun, Department of Radiology, The Second People's Hospital of Hunan Province, Doctor's Degree of Medicine, Associate Chief Physician

骆永恒，中南大学湘雅二医院放射科，医学博士后，主治医师，讲师

Luo Yongheng, Department of Radiology, The Second Xiangya Hospital, Central South University, Postdoctoral Fellowship, Attending Physician, Lecturer

刘欢，中南大学湘雅二医院放射科　医学硕士生

Liu Huan, Department of Radiology, The Second Xiangya Hospital, Central South University, Master of Medicine

韦勇，海南省妇女儿童医学中心放射科，医学硕士，主任医师

Wei Yong, Department of Radiology, Women and Children Medical Center of Hainan Province, Master's Degree of Medicine, Chief Physician

梁斌，华中科技大学同济医学院附属协和医院放射科，医学博士，主任医师，教授

Liang Bin, Department of Radiology, Union Hospital, Tongji Medical College, Huazhong University of Science and Technology, Doctor's Degree of Medicine, Chief Physician, Professor

张利捷，华中科技大学同济医学院附属协和医院放射科，医学硕士生

Zhang Lijie, The Department of Radiology, Union Hospital, Tongji Medical College, Huazhong University of Science and Technology, Master of Medicine

黄炜，中南大学湘雅二医院放射科　医学博士生

Huang Wei, Department of Radiology, The Second Xiangya Hospital, Central South University, Doctor of Medicine

王耀恒，湖南省益阳市中心医院医学影像中心，医学硕士，主任医师

Wang Yaoheng, The Medical Imaging Center, Central Hospital of YiYang City, Hunan Province, Master's Degree of Medicine, Chief physician,

熊付，华中科技大学同济医学院附属协和医院放射科，医学博士后，主治医师，讲师

Xiong Fu, Department of Radiology, Union Hospital, Tongji Medical College, Huazhong University of Science and Technology, Postdoctoral Fellowship, Attending Physician, Lecturer

郭栋，郑州大学第一附属医院介入科，医学博士，副主任医师，副教授

Guo Dong, Depatment of Interventional Radiology, The First Affiliated Hospital of Zhengzhou University, Doctor's Degree of Medicine, Associate Chief Physician, Associate Professor

张子曙，中南大学湘雅二医院放射科，医学博士后，主任医师，教授

Zhang Zixu, Department of Radiology, The Second Xiangya Hospital, Central South University, Postdoctoral Fellowship, Chief Physician, Professor

马聪，中南大学湘雅二医院放射科，医学博士，副主任医师，副教授

Ma Cong, Department of Radiology, The Second Xiangya Hospital, Central South University, Doctor's Degree of Medicine, Associate Chief Physician, Associate Professor

王福安，江苏省苏北人民医院介入放射科，医学博士，副主任医师。

Wang Fuan, Department of Interventional Radiology, Subei People's Hospital of Jiangsu Province（Clinical Medical College of Yangzhou University）, Doctor's Degree of Medicine, Associate Chief Physician

胡李男，湖南省株洲市中心医院放射介入科，医学博士，副主任医师

Hu Linan, Department of Interventional Radiology, Zhuzhou Central Hospital, Hunan Province, Dopctor's Degree of Medicine, Associate Chief Physician

王天明，中南大学湘雅医院放射介入科，医学博士，医师

Wang Tianmin, Department of Interventional Radiology, The Xiangya Hospital, Central South University, Dopctor's Degree of Medicine, Physician

前　言

　　《双语医学影像学》第一版于 2005 年随着我国医学影像学教学改革诞生的，为适应我国医学影像学的快速发展及教学改革的深入进行了第二版修正，对全书内容进行了调整，分设了总论、骨骼系统、胸部、腹部与盆腔、中枢神经系统、头颈部、介入放射学七大部分，主要介绍了 X 线、CT、MRI 等成像技术以及检查方法、常见疾病诊断和介入放射学。

　　本书的出版，我们感谢编辑委员会所有成员，我们也感谢在本书写作、编辑和出版过程中作出贡献的所有人员！

　　我们期望此书再版后，能对国内广大从事医学影像学双语教学的教师和学生们起到一定的指导和参考作用。但由于我们的水平有限，缺点和错误在所难免，我们真诚欢迎与感谢各位前辈、同道多提宝贵意见，以便日后修正。

肖恩华，尚全良，袁友红，颜荣华，谭艳

2022.4

Preface

The first edition of Bilingual Medical Imaging was born in 2005 with the reform of medical imaging teaching in our country. In order to adapt to the rapid development of medical imaging and the deepening of teaching reform in our country, the second edition of Bilingual Medical Imaging was revised, the contents of the book have been adjusted to include seven sections: the general introduction, skeletal system, chest, abdomen and pelvis, central nervous system, head and neck, interventional radiology, the imaging techniques such as X-ray, CT, MRI, examination methods, diagnosis of common diseases and interventional radiology were introduced.

We thank all members of the editorial board for the publication of this book, and we also thank all those who contributed to the writing, editing and publishing of this book.

We hope that this book will play a guiding and referential role to the teachers and students who are engaged in bilingual teaching of medical imaging. However, due to our limited skills, shortcomings and mistakes are inevitable. We sincerely welcome and thank fellow seniors and colleagues for your valuable comments so that we can correct them in the future.

Xiao Enhua, Shang Quanliang, Yuan Youhong, Yan Ronghua, Tan Yan

2022.4

目 录

Contents

总 论

　　像人类历史上许多具有记念意义的发现一样，X线是在完全偶然的情况下被发现的。1895 年，一名叫威海尔姆·伦琴的德国物理学家在一个真空放电管中用电子束做实验时发现了这一现象。伦琴注意到，当电子束运行时，实验室里一个荧光屏开始发光。这个反应本身并不奇怪，因为正常情况下荧光物质可对电磁辐射产生反应而发光，但是伦琴所用的真空放电管却被厚的黑纸板包围，认为这应当阻挡大部分的电磁辐射。当他在放电管和荧光屏之间放上各种物体时，荧光屏仍然熠熠发光。最后当他把他的手放到放电管的前面时，却发现他的手部骨骼轮廓影投射在荧光屏上。因此，伦琴认为一定存在某种未知的不可见的射线能够传过厚厚的黑纸板及人体的组织器官后激发荧光屏发光，因而命名为 X线。在 X线本身被发现后不久，就得到了广泛的应用。

　　伦琴的这一不平凡的发现是人类历史上最重要的医学成就之一。6 年后伦琴因这一发现而被授予第一个诺贝尔物理学奖。X线可以让医生非常容易地透过人体组织检查骨折、观察腔道以及吞下的物体。对其作恰当的调整，可用来检查诸如肺、血管和肠道等软组织。

　　X射线被发现后不久，就被用于人类疾病的诊断，并且形成了诊断放射学和奠定了医学影像学的基础。今天它仍然在医学影像学领域占有重要的地位，在保护人民健康方面发挥越来越重要的作用。随着计算机和相关高科技技术的发展，1971 年通过把传统的 X 射线和计算机技术结合起来，第一台计算机断层扫描仪（CT）诞生了，这使得我们比传统 X 射线更清楚地看到人体内部的结构。目前，CT 已经发展到了超快速 CT 和多层螺旋 CT 阶段。20 世纪 80 年代初核磁共振或磁共振（MRI）技术开始应用于临床诊断以来，诸如磁共振血管成像（MRA）、磁共振波谱成像（MRS）等 MRI 新技术逐渐变得成熟。MRI 的未来只是受限于我们的想像能力，比较来说，这种技术仍然处于婴儿期，它的广泛应用只有 20 年的历史（与 X 线 100 多年的历史相比）。对 MRI 的未来作出预测充其量是推断性的，但毫无疑问，它对我们这一领域中的那些人来讲是令人激动的，对我们所关怀的患者是非常有益的。MRI 是一个有着无限前途的领域。CT 和 MRI 的临床应用开创了影像诊断的一个新纪元。20 世纪 70 年代后迅速兴起的介入放射学正在日新月异迅猛发展，使放射学由单纯的影像诊断功能转变到了诊断与治疗并重的发展阶段，打开了医学影像学更多的应用领域。此外，超声成像和 γ 闪烁成像从 50—60 年代开始用于人体扫描，70 年代单光子发射计算机断层成像（SPECT）与正电子发射体层成像（PET）用于临床了解器官和组织的功能、代谢和进行受体显像。

　　因此，在仅仅 100 年的时间内形成了包括 X 线在内的诊断影像学，尽管在各种成像技术之间，其成像原理和方法及其诊断价值、局限性不同，但是这些成像技术都能显示人体内部的结构和器官，从而使我们能够在活体情况下观察人体解剖、生理功能和病理变化来诊断人类疾病。综上所述，现代医学影像学包括传统 X 线、CT、MRI、超声和核医学，这里我们仅仅介绍前三者。

Part 1

General introduction

As with many of mankind's monumental discoveries, X-ray was invented completely by accident. In 1895, a German physicist named Wilhelm Roentgen made the discovery while experimenting with electron beams in a vacuum discharge tube. Roentgen noticed that a fluorescent screen in his lab started to glow when the electron beam was turned on. This response in itself wasn't so surprising — fluorescent material normally glows in reaction to electromagnetic radiation — but Roentgen's tube was surrounded by heavy black cardboard. Roentgen assumed this would have blocked most of the radiation. Roentgen placed various objects between the tube and the screen, and the screen still glowed. Finally, he put his hand in front of the tube, and saw the silhouette of his bones projected onto the fluorescent screen. Therefore, he concluded that an unknown invisible ray can penetrate heavy black cardboard and his hand to arrive at the fluorescent screen and cause the fluorescent screen to glow. Immediately after discovering X-ray, its most beneficial applications had been discouered.

Roentgen's remarkable discovery precipitated one of the most important medical advancements in human history. Six years later the first Nobel Prize in physics was awarded to Roentgen for his discovery. X-ray technology lets doctors see straight through human tissue to examine broken bones, cavities and swallowed objects with extraordinary ease. Modified X-ray procedures can be used to examine softer tissue, such as the lung, blood vessels or the intestines.

Soon after the discovery of x-rays, it was used in diagnosis of human diseases and formed diagnositic radiology and established the basis of medical imageology. Today it is still important in the field of medical imageology and plays more and more important roles in safeguarding people's health. With the advent of computer and development of relative high science and technology, the first computerized tomographic scanner was born in 1971 by the combination of traditional X-rays with the computer technology and made us to see structures inside human body more clearly than traditional X-rays. At present, CT has been developed into ultrafast CT and multi-slice spiral CT. Since Magnetic Resonance Imaging (MRI) was used in clinic diagnosis from the beginning of 1980's, new MRI techniques, such MR angiography (MRA), MR spectroscopy(MRS) and so on, are gradually mature. The future of MRI seems limited only by our imagination. This technology is still in its infancy, comparatively speaking. It has been in widespread use for less than 20 years (compared with over 100 years for X-rays). Predicting the future of MRI is speculative at best, but I have no doubt it will be exciting for those of us in the field, and very beneficial to the patients we care for. MRI is a field with a virtually limitless future. The clinic application of CT and MRI opened a new era of imagiological diagnosis. Interventional radiology springing up after 1970's has being rapidly developed and changed with each passing day, thus it made radiology from simply imageological diagnosis into imageological diagnosis co-existing with imageological treatment, and opened up much more applying areas of medical imageology. In addition, Ultrasonography and γ-scintigraphy were used in scanning human body from the beginning of 1950's ~ 1960's. Single photon emission computed tomography (SPECT) and positron emission tomography (PET) was born in 1970's.

Thus, Diagnostic imaging including X-rays formed within only 100 years. Although the imaging principles and methods, as well as its diagnostic value and limitations, are different between all kinds of imaging techniques, these imaging techniques can mapping the inner structures and organs inside human body, and therefore make us obserre human anatomy, physiological function and pathological changes to diagnose disease in vivo in human body. In general, modern medical imageology includes traditional X-rays, CT, MRI, Ultrasonography and Nuclear medicine.

第一章

X 线成像

X 线成像包括普通 X 线成像、数字化 X 线成像和数字减影血管成像，它们将在以下各节中详细描述。

第一节　普通 X 线成像

1. X 线成像的原理和设备

（1）X 线的产生：X 线是波长范围为 0.0006 nm 至 50 nm 的电磁波，是快速运动的电子撞击固体钨靶时产生的且它们的能量转变为辐射能。如果所用物质是具有高原子序数的金属，而电子具有足够的能量（速度），那么 X 线就可产生。因此，产生 X 线的装置包括 X 线管、高压变压器和操作台。

产生 X 线最有效的工具是一个 X 线球管，而一个球管最简单的形状是一个固定的阳极位于一个密闭的玻璃真空管内。球管两个最重要的部分是阴极和阳极。在一个 X 线球管内，钨灯丝产生电子云并被阴极负电荷排斥，聚焦杯使电子流成形并以高速度被吸引到阳极的正电荷靶区和原子相互作用。阳极和阴极之间的电压差特别高，因而电子流能以相当大的能量飞越球管。当高速运行的电子与钨原子撞击时，可导致处于原子低轨道之一的电子被冲撞脱落，而高轨道上的电子以一个光子的形式释放能量则回到低能态。能态大，则释放的光子具有较高的能量状态，即它是一个 X 线光子。换句话说，当电子与钨靶原子相互作用时，电子以热的形式释放大多数的能量。在医学 X 线成像中，只有大约 1% 的能量以 X 线辐射的形式释放出来。

（2）X 线的特性：X 线具有许多与光线共同的特性。然而，X 线的独有特性使得它在影像诊断中具有无可衡量的价值。与 X 线成像相关的特性有：

1）穿透效应：X 线能够穿透吸收或反射可见光的物质。

2）荧光效应：当 X 线被吸收时，可导致某些物质发出荧光，也就是说，发出低能量的辐射（例如可见光和紫外光）。

3）感光效应：像光线一样，X 线可在感光胶片上产生影像，如照相胶卷或 X 线胶片，通过冲洗能够显影。

4）电离效应：由于能量较高，因此 X 线能产生离子，也就是说，能使电子从原子逃逸出来形成正离子和负离子。以可控制的方式形成和收集时，这些离子也许用来测量和控制 X 线成像曝光。在活体组织中形成这些离子时，就有机会产生生物学变化。当有意使用高辐射剂量时，这些生物学变化在放射治疗中便可用来治疗肿瘤。在影像诊断中实际使用的低剂量对人体的损害可能性远低得多。然而，也不是零风险，谨慎和小心是使用 X 线辐射的关键措施。

X 线的这些特性应用于医学和工业 X 线摄影、放射治疗和研究。

2. X 线摄影的原理

X 线使人体内部的结构在荧光屏上或胶片上显影可归结为这两个原因：①X 线的特性，即穿透效应、荧光效应和感光效应；②在人体组织中存在密度和厚度的差异。当 X 线穿过人体内部，X 线吸收程度有差异的不同组织和结构时，到达荧光屏或胶片的 X 线光子总量存在着差异，因此 X 线吸收的体现产生在一张 X 线片或荧光屏中包含信息的灰度影。

所以，产生一张 X 线片有三个基本条件。第一，X 线必须具备能够穿透人体内部组织和结构的适当穿透力；第二，在被穿透的组织之间存在密度和厚度的差异，以便在穿透后 X 线的剩余量有差异；第三，穿透后余下的 X 线是不可见的，通过 X 线胶片感光产生一幅具有黑白对比的 X 线片。

人体对于成像来说是一个复杂的对象，它不仅由不同厚度的物质而且由 X 线吸收程度有差异的含有不同元素的不同物质构成。如果组织中每单位体积元素的总量不同则密度不同，因此人体内部组织密度可分为三类：①高密度组织，如骨骼和钙化；②中等密度，如韧带、肌肉、神经、实质脏器、结缔组织和体液；③低密度组织，如脂肪组织，呼吸道内、消化道内、鼻窦内和乳突窦内的空气。

X 线吸收和厚度的关系显而易见，任何较厚的物质比任何较薄的相同物质吸收的 X 线量多，如 10 cm 的水比 3 cm 的水吸收更多的 X 线。对于密度（每单位体积质量）有差异的物质来说，在其他一致的情况下，5 cm 的水比 5 cm 的蒸汽吸收的 X 线量多，因为每立方厘米蒸汽重量小于水。构成物质的原子序数可影响它的 X 线吸收特性。总的来说，物质的原子序数越小，所吸收的 X 线量就越小，例如铝的原子序数是 13，铅则为 82，因此一片铝要比一片较薄的具有同样面积和重量的铅所吸收的 X 线量要少。这就是铅为何用来封装 X 线球管和作为 X 线室的墙壁防护以及制作保护性手套和衣服的原因。

疾病可以改变人体内的组织密度。例如，肺结核可在低密度肺组织内产生中等密度的纤维化病变和高密度的钙化病灶。胸片能够显示纤维病变、钙化和肺组织之间的这种差别。因此具有不同组织密度的病变能够产生相应的病理学 X 线影像。

由此可见，组织结构和器官内部密度和厚度的差别是产生影像对比和形成影像的基础。

3. X 线系统组成

用于医学 X 线摄影的 X 线是使用电力产生的。图 1-1 是描述一个 X 线系统的主要组成部分的方块图。一个 X 线系统的目的是将电能转变为 X 线能，并应用于疾病检查。

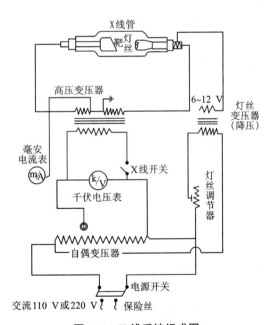

图 1-1　X 线系统组成图

（1）X 线发生器：X 线发生器可把电能转变为产生 X 线束所需要的高压电能，可把 120 伏、208 伏和 220 伏的交流电转变为更加适合产生 X 线的波形，它也可为 X 线管和 X 线系统的其他部分提供其他形式的电能。

（2）X线球管：图1-2是描述一个X线球管的结构图。X线球管可把发生器提供的电能转变为X射线束，这可通过在X线球管的阴极和阳极之间施加高电压实现。无论何时，电子在充满负电荷的阴极产生并向阳极加速运行，最终撞击在充满正电荷的阳极的目标区域而产生X射线。应用于产生X线的大多数能量在靶上转变为热能，仅有不到1%的能量转变为X线。

（3）控制台：控制台是操作者能够控制X射线束产生的 两个位置之一，无 论是简单还是复杂，控制台的目的是允许操作者预先选择X线曝光的参数设置，启动曝光程序。

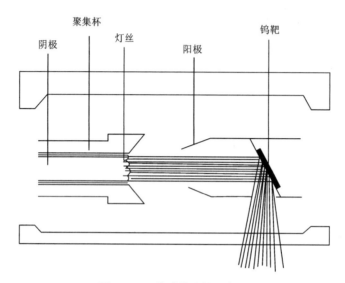

图1-2　X线球管结构示意图

4.X线检查技术

正如前述，人体组织中存在着密度差异，这是产生X线影像对比的基础，即自然对比。至于缺少自然对比的组织和器官，为了在这些结构之间产生对比，常有意把较高或较低的对比剂引入到这些结构，称为人工对比。因此，自然对比和人工对比两者都是X线检查的基础。

（1）常规检查（包括X线透视和X线摄片）。

1）X线透视：X线穿过人体到达荧光屏，产生动态的X线影像，即为透视。通常用于人体天然对比较好的部位，如胸部，可实时观察肺、心血管系统的活动。此外，将透视与对比剂联合使用，可追踪观察对比剂通过身体的情况，如胃肠道钡餐、钡灌肠，以及血管造影。X线透视拥有操作简单、费用低和即时可获得结果等优点。但是，X线透视也有影像对比度和清晰度差的弱点，很难观察那些缺乏密度和厚度差别的器官以及诸如头颅、脊柱、盆腔等密度高和厚度较大的部位，缺乏客观记录也是一大缺点。

2）X线摄片：X线摄片广泛应用于临床以帮助医生诊断疾病和制订治疗方案，具有对比度和清晰度好的特点，易于显示具有高密度和厚度较大的病灶或者密度和厚度差别不足以产生良好对比度的部位。影像对比度是用于描述一张X线片中两个区域密度差别的术语，即密度差大，则对比度高，反之则低。具有高影像对比度的图像是指在对X线吸收大的区域表现为很白，而X线吸收小的区域则表现为很黑。在许多情况下，较高的影像对比度可提高区别一张X线片中不同结构的能力。X线片可留下客观记录以供评阅和随时比较以观察病理变化和治疗后疗效，且患者接受X线量少。但是，它不能像X线透视那样动态观察器官功能，检查的范围受胶片大小限制。因此，为了得到更多有关病变的信息，X线摄片应包括正位片、侧位片。

（2）X线体层摄影：体层摄影可获得所选择的层面上的结构影像，而所选择层面外的其他结构则在投影过程中模糊掉。X线体层摄影常用于显示普通X线片所不能显示的病变，如具有许多重叠结构的病变，或者位置较深的病变。这样就能了解病变内是否有破坏、空洞或钙化,病灶边缘是否锐利,以及病变的确切位置和范围。目前,随着CT、MRI的出现,X线体层摄影在临床上的应用已很少。

(3)造影检查:在常规X线片中,绝大多数软组织不能清晰地显示。为了观察空腔器官内部或组成循环系统的大血管,必须在体内引入对比剂。

高密度对比剂是比周围组织更能有效地吸收X线的物体。为了观察胃肠道和内分泌管道,患者常需要吞下一种像钡化合物类的对比剂混合物。如果医生想检查循环系统中的大血管或其他组成部分,常把对比剂注入患者的血液内。造影检查扩展了X线检查的应用范围。

对比剂与一般治疗药物不同,其使用方法特殊,如剂量大、浓度高、速度快等。实际上,对比剂给药等于将大量的药物直接引入人体内的某一部位,所以操作者应技术熟练,熟悉各种对比剂的性能、用途和禁忌证等。造影检查前必须采取以下措施以预防或应对不良反应的发生:①按产品说明书要求决定是否做过敏试验;②严格控制禁忌证,对有变态(过敏)史者、甲亢患者、心脏功能不全及无尿症患者都禁用对比剂;③准备好各种不良反应及并发症的急救药品。

5.放射防护

X线对医学界来说是一个惊人的意外。可让医生观察患者身体内部结构而无须通过手术。比起打开患者的伤口直接观察,使用X线观察骨折更容易和安全。但是,X线也有害,在应用X线的早期,许多医生让患者和他们自己长时间暴露在X光线下,最终医生和患者开始发生放射性皮肤病,医学界才了解到在应用的过程中一定在某些方面出现了错误。

问题在于X线是一种电离辐射,当正常光线撞击一个原子时,它不能使原子发生任何意义上的变化。但是当X线撞击一个原子时,它能够使电子脱离原子而产生一个离子,一个带电的原子。自由电子然后与其他原子相撞而产生更多的离子。

一个离子的电荷可导致细胞内发生非自然的化学反应。电荷可破坏DNA链,带有一股断开的DNA的细胞或者死亡,或者DNA发生突变。如果许多细胞坏死,则身体会发生疾病。如果DNA突变,一个细胞可能变成癌性的,则癌症也会形成。如果突变发生在精细胞或卵细胞内,则可导致出生缺陷。由于所有这些风险,今天医生对于X线的使用显得很小心。

我们在使用X线时要遵循下列原则:①时间防护,指的是尽可能减少在X线场内的时间,尽量缩短照射时间;②距离防护,指X线机工作时,应尽可能使工作人员远离X线源;③屏蔽防护,指的是在X线源和人员间放置一种能吸收X线的物质,如铅玻璃、混凝土。

即使具有以上这些危险,X线扫描仍然是一个比手术检查安全的选择。X线机是医学中一个无可估价的工具,在科学研究领域中的价值重大,X线确确实实是最有用的发明之一。

第二节 X线诊断的新进展

近几年,图像获得和交流系统(PACS)得到了快速发展,是随着放射信息系统(RIS)而出现的。PACS是以高速计算机设备以及海量存储介质为基础,以高速传输网络联接各种影像设备和终端,管理并提供、传输、显示原始的数字化图像和相关信息,具有查找医学图像及相关信息快速、准确、图像质量无失真、影像资料可共享等特点。X线影像的数字化对于PACS是非常重要的;高质量的数字化X线医学影像对于PACS数据源是必不可少的。数字化的X线影像的优点是把数据采集和图像显示分开,数据采集器可被调整至满意的程度以接受X线光子,准确记录信息和更有效地抑制散射线,而同时分开显示影像可以利用较好的影像对比增强度来诊断病变。更为重要的是,分开采集影像数据和分开显示影像以后,就有可能进行包括影像增强在内的影像处理工作和智能化的电脑协助诊断。

有三种使X线影像数字化的方式,即计算机化X线摄影(CR),数字化X线摄影(DR)和影像数字化采集(VDA)。CR和DR二者都可把模拟影像信息转变为数字化影像信息。影像数字化采集可把X线探测器产生的影像信号直接进行A/D转换,从而获得单框或一系列的影像。这里我们对CR和DR进行详细介绍。

1．CR

（1）CR 的基本结构和原理：目前 CR 系统影像处理操作的组成图见图 1-3。应用到影像数据流的全部操作可大概命名为"影像增强"。这种数据通路之内的影像处理功能的作用应该是在空间分辨力、清晰度、对比度、动态范围和信噪比方面改善 CR 影像的视觉质量。在主要通路中的处理就是把信息最大化地传输给观察者。

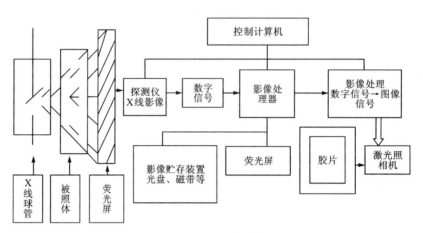

图 1-3　CR 系统组成图

当前 CR 是以光刺激介质磷光体，即众所周知的储存磷光体的使用作为其基础的。它们是数字化 X 线摄影最成功的商用探测器。所用的磷光体是粉末状钡氟卤化物中最常见的，而且放在感光胶片的底层形成成像板或荧光屏。X 线吸收机理与普通磷光体荧光屏是一样的，区别在于有用的光学信号并不来自对入射辐射的即时反应所散发的光线，而是来自于由捕获的电荷所组成的潜在的影像受到光刺激且从亚稳态释放出来时所散发的光线。这样可触发所谓的光刺激发光（PSL）的过程，从而导致在量上与原始 X 线照射成比例的较短波长的光线（蓝光）的发射。在 CR 系统中，一个含有储存磷光体的成像板（IP）放在一个光密处进行曝光，然后用激光扫描光栅读出释放 PSL。蓝色 PSL 光使用一种光线向导仪收集，采用光电倍增器管（PMT）探测。PMT 信号数字化以点对点为基础形成影像。CR 得到广泛的认可源于它的大动态范围、数字化特性、容易携带以及它的独特性而非它的内在影像质量。CR 系统在近 20 年应用中得到了改善而能够被应用。它们是当代技术和工程的奇迹，但是它不能超越其固有的影像质量弱点。

（2）CR 的影像特点：

1）高灵敏度：即采集极弱的信号时不致被噪声所掩盖。

2）高分辨力：影像分辨力可理解为区别二个最小微粒的能力。CR 的像素可达 2000×2000，足以观察其他检查技术所不能发现的细节。

3）高线性度：所谓线性是指在整个光谱范围内得到的信号是否与真实影像的光强度成线性比例，即得到的影像是否与真实图像很好吻合。IP 所发出的荧光量依赖于一次所激发的 X 线量。在 1∶10 范围内具有较好的线性度，非线性度低于 1%。

4）数字化输出和储存：CR 系统能够直接产生且可长期储存在目前各种储存介质中的数字化影像，也可以直接输入到影像储存和转换系统以及远程医疗系统、英特网系统。

5）强大的后处理功能：数字化 CR 影像具有许多后处理功能，例如测量、局部放大，对比度转换、影像增强、减影等。

（3）CR 的临床应用：CR 可以根据 X 线吸收率的差异再处理影像资料，比传统 X 线平片更好地显示解剖结构。

1）头部和骨关节系统：CR 可以进一步测量骨盐的含量。对于关节来说，由于数字化影像特点，CR 经过再处理可以显示关节软骨及其周围软组织。

2）CR 在胸部平片中的应用：胸部平片是最常用的 X 线检查，总体上 CR 胸片优于传统的胸部 X 线平片，特别是在显示纵隔和膈肌等重叠结构时。在显示肺部结节病灶和气管、大血管等病灶和气管、大血管等纵隔结构时，CR 也优于传统的 X 线平片。但是，对于间质性病变和腺泡性病变的显示，CR 则不如传统 X 线平片。

3）CR 在胃肠道和泌尿系统中的应用：CR 的密度分辨力明显高于传统 X 线平片，在显示肠道积气、结石等病变也优于传统的 X 线平片。在双对比造影检查中，CR 对于胃小弯、微小病变和黏膜皱壁等结构的显示优于传统 X 线造影检查。CR 可以压缩泌尿系的高密度影像并使用调谐和空间频率处理功能来增加密度层次和软组织影像的锐度，以及大大改善软组织的分辨力，特别是肾体层摄影时。此外，CR 可提高显示结石和微小钙化的能力。

2. DR

（1）DR 的基本结构和工作原理：DR 由电子暗盒、扫描控制器、系统控制器和影像监视器等组成。它可通过电子暗盒把 X 线转变为数字化影像。其原理是影像增强管把作为信息载体的 X 线转变为可见光，然后光电管把可见光转变为视频信号，视频信号再经模/数转换转变为数字化矩阵影像。DR 与 CR 技术均是将 X 线影像信息转换为数字影像信息的系统，并且可根据临床的需要来进行后期处理。两者均是当今医学影像诊断中较为有效的手段，具有各自的特点，但两者相比 DR 系统整体效果更优于 CR。DR 比 CR 具有更高的图像质量、分辨力、响应速度，通过采用 DR 技术进行相关影像的采集，有助于减少成像时间、减少工作人员的任务量、及时有效的获取到较高质量的图像，便于进一步提高对患者摄片的诊断率。

（2）DR 的优点：

1）DR 具有较宽的曝光容忍度以及较广的动态范围，摄片时可允许技术上出现一定的差错。

2）所呈图像的质量高，层次丰富，其具有 3.6 LP/mm 的空间分辨力。

3）DR 也可以像 CR 一样具有各种强大的后处理功能，并且具有远程会诊的潜力。

4）无 X 线胶片，在计算机对图像进行传输、存储时能够节省冲片和胶片的费用，方便快捷减少不必要的开支。

（3）DR 的应用：数字化 X 线摄影是指把数字化影像处理技术应用到投照 X 线摄影。由于 DSA 的广泛应用，在下一节对 DSA 进行重点介绍时简要叙述它在临床上的应用。

第三节 数字减影血管成像（DSA）

数字减影血管成像（DSA）是 20 世纪 80 年代兴起的一门新的医学成像技术。正如命名所指，是特指把应用对比剂前后获得的两幅影像相减的技术，旨在研究血管和产生图像质量较普通血管造影大大提高数字减影血管造影（图 1-4）。

1. DSA 的主要组成

DSA 包括 X 线球管、影像增强器、电视透视、高分辨摄像机、模/数转换器、计算机和影像储存系统。

2. DSA 的基本原理

（1）视频图像的获取：在电脑的控制下，传输到 X 线发生器的定时信号触发 X 线的产生并穿过患者为影像增强器接收。位于影像增强器和摄影机之间的一个光圈控制到达摄影机的光线量。摄像机从影像增强器接受光学图像并把它转变为以模拟形式输送到影像处理器进行处理的电子视频信号。影像处理器可使图像数字化，储存在存储器，并使它能以数字化形式与在不同的时间或能量水平获得的另一幅影像进行减影，包括 X 线球管和发生器、影像增强器、电视摄像机等在内的成像系统的基本组成与那些用于普通透视中的相似，但在质量上较高。显示在视频监视器上的不同灰阶影像称为视频图像。

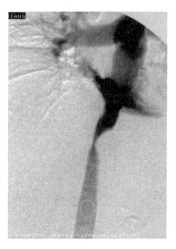

布-加氏综合征,下腔静脉近端明显狭窄清晰显示,而骨骼和软组织未显示。

图 1-4　DSA 图像

(2)对数增幅:对数增幅或振幅是指视频信号是怎样在实际减影步骤之前被处理的。对于对数增幅,从视频摄影机读出的信号在减影之前通过电路传输,其输出量与输入的对数成比例。这种情况下 DSA 信号差等于:

$$DIFF_{LOG} = (\mu/\rho)_I \, \rho_I d.$$

$(\mu/\rho)_I$ 是指碘的质量衰减系数,而 $\rho_I d$ 是碘的浓度与血管直径的乘积或投射浓度。通过一个特殊电路系统的视频增幅器处理后,可压缩和调节视频信号强度的显示范围,然后将视频信号强度的对数函数变化转变为线性函数变化,扩大低视频信号强度区和缩小高视频信号强度区的显示,从而二者都可同时显示于视频影像上。

(3)模拟/数字转换:是经过对数增幅处理后的视频影像仍属于由不同灰阶度组成的模拟像;在计算机处理前必须数字化。我们假定,由 X 线系统、影像增强器和电视摄影仪获取模拟视频影像,模拟信号传递到影像处理器,后者可提供一些前处理工作以调整视频信号的幅度和水平以满足数/模转换器的输入要求。视频信号的一系列不同的电压值经模拟/数字转换器处理后,既可转换成不同的二元值,输入计算机并经处理后,则可转变为一组不同的象素值,这样视频影像就可转变为数字化影像。

3. DSA 影像的产生

数字减影血管成像(DSA)是一个使用计算机技术强化 X 线影像质量的方法。这涉及到把未使用对比剂的 X 线图像与使用对比剂的 X 线图像进行相减,减影可显示血管而没有周围结构的干扰。减影所处理的主要物理学变量包括时间、能量和深度。

(1)时间减影:目前为此,数字 X 线摄影系统使用的最常用运算方法是时间减影。它指的是某一时间获取的图像与随后某一时间获取的图像相减所依赖的许多计算机协助的技术。在介入操作期间,对比剂引入血管,减影图像将只包含充满对比剂的血管影像。

(2)能量减影:能量减影交替使用两种不同的 X 线束从而产生一幅由于光电相互作用中的差异所指的减影图像。

(3)杂交减影:一些 DSA 系统具有把时间减影和能量减影结合起来的能力。如果患者能够制动,则杂交减影技术理论上可获得高质量的图像。

4. DSA 成像模式

(1)经静脉 DSA(IVDSA):IVDSA 是指导管插入静脉以注射对比剂的任一 DSA 模式。例如把导管头端或套管针置于外周静脉(外周法)或上腔静脉或右心房(中心法)注射对比剂的技术称为非选择性 IVDSA，即再循环法；把导管头端置于目标静脉或邻近目标静脉的位置或心腔内注射对比剂称为选择性 IVDSA。

非选择性 IVDSA，不论是外周法还是中心法，都属于经静脉注入对比剂显示动脉的再循环法。进入静脉的对比剂经由肺循环流入体循环，然后使动脉显示。目前，非选择性 IVDSA 主要用于主动脉及其大分支疾患的诊断，如主动脉炎、主动脉狭窄、颈动脉体瘤等的诊断，目前临床上用的较少，常在动脉插管有困难或不适合作 IADSA 时采用。

选择性 IVDSA 混合的血容量较非选择性 IVDSA 小，对比剂稀释少，因此常用于上下腔静脉、股髂静脉、肾静脉疾病，累及右房、肺动脉和静脉的先天性心血管畸形等疾病的诊断和治疗，如先天性上下腔静脉畸形、腔静脉狭窄和 Budd-Chiari 综合征等。

(2)经动脉 DSA(IADSA)：DSA 显示血管的能力与血管内对比剂的浓度密切相关。在 IADSA 中，对比剂直接注入靶动脉或邻近靶动脉的区域，因而较少被稀释，靶动脉内的对比剂浓度仍然高于使用大剂量、较高浓度注射的 IVDSA，因此 IADSA 可较清楚显示细小血管。

IADSA 也可分为选择性和非选择性两种。非选择性 IADSA 是指导管头端置于靶动脉的主动脉近端注射对比剂的技术；而选择性 IADSA 是指进一步把导管头端置于靶动脉的主要分支以注射对比剂的技术。IADSA 可克服 IVDSA 的许多缺点。它可增加感兴趣区的对比剂浓度以提高空间分辨率到绝大多数细小的动脉都显示满意的程度。可以使用较低的对比剂浓度，而且检查速度快于常规血管造影技术。

5. DSA 特殊成像技术及临床应用

DSA 的优势在于高分辨力、对比剂用量少、实时显示和入路监视等。DSA 在诊断和治疗血管性疾病的过程中得到广泛的认可。介入放射学是一门新兴的介于传统内科学和传统外科学之间的学科，具有诊疗一体化、可视化的鲜明学科特点，是与内科、外科并列的三大医学学科之一。总体上它可分为血管介入和非血管介入两种。绝大部分涉及使用有关血管介入技术，因此 DSA 在介入放射治疗中起着不可替代的重要作用。其特殊的成像技术有以下几点：

(1)透视路径图技术与造影转化路径图技术：透视路径图技术是在透视条件下一气完成，可以随时取消路径图，成像方便。造影转化路径图技术可以从一个序列中选取一幅较满意的图作为参考，靶血管区的病灶有初步了解，其功能在某些方面优于透视路径图技术。该技术能引导微导丝、微导管进入病变血管，评价脑动脉瘤填塞是否致密，亦能清楚地显示分支血管的轨迹，特别是对于走行纤曲、重叠、成角的血管的显示。

(2)旋转 DSA 技术与 3D-DSA 技术：旋转 DSA 技术是利用血管造影 C 臂旋转来达到检查要求的新技术，它可以多方位显示兴趣区的造影血管解剖。3D-DSA 技术是近几年在旋转 DSA 技术上发展起来的一项新技术，是旋转血管造影技术、DSA 技术及计算机三维图处理技术相结合的产物。该技术主要用于脑血管瘤的诊断和治疗，判断脑动脉狭窄，对胸、腹盆部、骨肿瘤的供血动脉可清晰显示，并指导进一步治疗。

(3)步进 DSA 技术：步进 DSA 技术采用快速脉冲曝光采集，实时减影成像。该技术提供了一个观察全程血管结构的新方法，解决了以前血流速度与摄影速度不一致，而出现血管显示不佳或不能显示的问题。该技术的特点是对比剂用量少，一次序列曝光显示全程下肢血管影像，尤其适用于不宜多用对比剂的受检者。目前应用于临床的步进 DSA 有单向的，即从头侧至足侧；亦有双向的，既能从头侧向足侧，也可以从足侧向头侧观察受检者。该技术适用于双下肢血管性病变的诊疗。

(4)C 臂 CT 技术：C 臂 CT 技术是应用在 DSA 系统中进行的旋转血管造影采集的图像进行血管造影形成的计算机断层成像。其原理和 CT 三维重建技术相似，但是 C 臂 CT 技术数据采集数量不同于普通 CT 三维重建采集。C 臂 CT 旋转采集 500F 原始数据，普通三维重建旋转采集 150F 原始数据，因此其获得图像质量也不同于三维重建影像。正在进行介入手术的患者，通过 C 臂 CT 技术，可以直接在血管造影检查室内观察出血的程度，这样就避免了将患者运送至其他设备上进行检查。高分辨 C 臂 CT 技术可以清晰显示置入的支架，判断支架释放后的伸展情况及贴壁情况。类 CT 技术能够不使用对比剂即可实现高质量的检查，可以扩展腹部操作的范围(包括穿刺和引流)并提供诊断和介入方面的帮助。C 臂 CT 技术在肿瘤应用方面也具潜在价值,它能显示密度较大部位的肿瘤、因此可用作导引活检和术中治疗肿瘤的评估及指导肿瘤的栓塞等。

(5)3D 路径图:应用 3D 的血管重建技术将容积数据与实时透视匹配,代替传统二维路图功能;优点在于当医生更换感兴趣区时不必重复注射对比剂制做路图。3D -Roadmap-与 C 臂旋转、床面升降及移动、FOV 改变等相关联。

(6)虚拟支架植入术:是应用在 DSA 系统中进行的旋转血管造影采集的图像进行计算机后处理血管三维立体成像。在三维后处理工作站中对重建出来的狭窄血管或者载瘤血管进行血管分析,根据测量数据及支架厂家提供的数据进行虚拟支架放置,供医生选择。

(肖恩华,张洁,禹成,郭建伟,谭长连)

Chapter 1

X-ray imaging

X-ray imaging includes general radiography, digital radiography (DR) and digital substraction angiography (DSA). They will be described in detail in the following three sections

Section 1 General X-ray imaging

1. The principles and instruments of radiography

(1) X Rays production

X-rays are electromagnetic waves whose wavelengths range from 0.0006 to 50 nm. They are produced when rapidly moving electrons strike a solid tungsten target and their kinetic energy is converted into radiation. If the material is a metal with a high atomic number, and the electrons have sufficient energy (speed), X-rays are produced. Therefore, the device for producing X-rays mainly includes X-rays tube, transformer and operating table.

The most efficient means of generating X-rays is an X-ray tube. The simplest form of an X-ray tube uses a stationary anode housed in a sealed glass envelop from which air has been evacuated. Two important parts of the tube are the cathode and the anode. In an X-ray tube, a "cloud" of electrons is produced at the tungsten filament wire and repelled by the negative charge of the cathode. The electrons stream is shaped by the focusing cup and it is attracted at high speed to the positively charged metal target area of the anode. Interact with the atoms. The voltage difference between the cathode and anode is extremely high, so the electrons fly through the tube with a great deal of force. When a speeding electron collides with a tungsten atom, it knocks loose an electron in one of the atom's lower orbitals. An electron in a higher orbital immediately falls to the lower energy level, releasing its extra energy in the form of a photon. It's a big drop, so the photon has a high energy level — it is an X-ray photon. In other words, as the electrons interact with the atoms of the tungsten target, the electrons give up most of their energy in the form of heat. In medical radiolography, only about 1% of their energy is emitted as X-radiation.

(2) Properties of X Rays

X rays have many properties in common with light. However, the unique properties of X rays are what make them invaluable in diagnostic imaging. Some of these are:

1) Penetrating effect: X rays are able to penetrate materials that absorb or reflect visible light.

2) Fluorescent effect: When X-rays are absorbed, they cause certain substances to fluoresce, that is, to emit radiation of lower energy (for example, visible and ultraviolet radiation).

3) Sensitization effect: Like light, X-rays can produce an image on photosensitive film, such as photographic film or X-ray film, which can then be made visible by development.

4) Ionization effect: Because of their high energy content, X rays can produce ions, that is, remove electrons from atoms to form positively charged ions and negative electrons. When formed and collected in a controlled manner, these ions may be used for measuring and controlling radiographic exposures.

When ions are formed in living tissue, there is a chance that they can produce biologic changes. When deliberately brought about by the use of high radiation doses, these biologic changes are used to treat tumors in radiation therapy. The substantially lower doses used in diagnostic imaging carry with them only a remote possibility of producing injury to humans. However, it is not a zero risk. Caution and care are the key approaches in the use of x-radiation.

These properties of X rays are applied in medical and industrial radiography, radiation therapy, and research.

2. The principles of radiography

Why X rays can make the structures inside human body visible on fluorescent screen or film are attributed to this two reasons: 1) The properties of X rays, namely penetrating effect, fluorescent effect and sensitization effect; 2) There are differences in density and thickness between human tissues. When X rays penetrate different tissues and instructures with X-rays absorption in varying degree inside human body, there exists difference in the amount of X-ray photons that can reach the fluorescent screen or films, therefore differences in X-ray absorption produce the shades of gray that contain the information in a radiography or fluoroscopy.

Therefore, there are three basic conditions in producing a radiography. The first, X rays must have certain penetrating power that can penetrate tissues and structures inside body; The second, there are difference in density and thickness between penetrated tissues so that the remains of X-ray photons are different after penetration; The third, the remaining X ray after penetration is invisible and produces a radiography with black-white contrast through sensitization such as X-ray film.

The human body is a complex subject for imaging, composed of not only different thickness but also different materials containing different elements that absorb X rays in varying degrees. The density is different if the amount of elements per unit volumn in tissues is different. Therefore the density of tissues inside human body can be divided into three: 1) High density tissues, such as bones and calcification; 2) Moderate density tissues, such as cartilages, muscles, nerves, parenchymal organs, connective tissues and body fluid; 3) Low density tissues, such as fatty tissues, and air inside respiratory tract, gastro-intestinal tract, paranasal sinus and mastoid sinus.

The relationship betweenX-ray absorption and thickness is intuitively obvious—a thick piece of any material absorbs more X-radiation than a thin piece of the same material. For example, 10 cm of water will absorb more X rays than 3 cm of water. For materials that differ in density (mass per unit volume), for example, g/cm^3, higher density materials absorb more X-radiation than those of lower density, other things are equal. For example, 5 cm of water will absorb more X rays than 3 cm of steam because steam weighs less per cubic centimeter than water. The atomic number of the material of which the object is composed affects its X-ray absorption characteristics. In general, the lower the atomic number of a material, the less it absorbs X-radiation. For example the atomic number of aluminum is 13; Lead is 82. Therefore, a sheet of aluminum absorbs a smaller amount of X rays than does a thinner sheet of lead of the same area and weight. This is why lead is used in the tube housing and as a lining for the walls of X-ray rooms, as well as in protective gloves and aprons.

Diseases can change the tissues density in human body. For example, pulmonary tuberculosis can produce moderate density fibrous lesions and high density calcifying lesions inside lower lung tissue. Thoracic film can show this difference among fibrous lesion, calcifying lesion and lung. Therefore pathological changes with different tissue density can produce corresponding pathological X-ray images.

Thus it can be seen that the difference in density and thickness inside tissue structures and organs is the basic for producing image contrast and formation.

3. The X-ray system

X rays used inmedical radiography are electronically produced. Figure 1-1 is a block diagram that depicts the major components of an x-ray system. The purpose of an X-ray system is to convert electrical energy into X-ray energy as specified by the user, and to direct the X rays toward the patient.

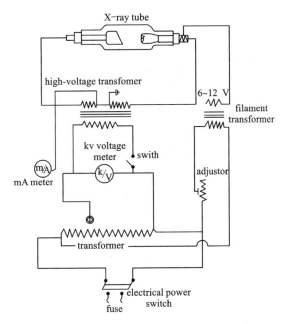

Figure 1-1 A block diagram that depicts the major components of an x-ray system

The X-ray generator converts the electrical power into high voltage power, which the X-ray tube requires to produce the X-ray beam. The generator converts the alternating current (AC)electrical power of 120, 208 and 220 volts into a waveform more suitable for the production of X rays. It also provides other forms of electrical power for the X-ray tube and other components of the X-ray system.

The X-ray tubes convert the electrical energy provided by the generator into an X-ray beam. This is accomplished by imposing a high voltage between the negative cathode and the positive anode of the tube. Whenever electrons are produced at the negatively charged cathode and accelerated toward the anode, they strike the positively charged target area of the anode, and produce X rays (Figure 1-2). Most of the energy used in the production of x rays is converted to heat in the target. Less than 1% is typically converted into x-radiation.

The control panel is one of the two places where the X-ray machine operator can control the x-ray beam. Whether rudimentary or complex, the purpose of the control panel is to allow the operator to select predetermined settings of X-ray exposure and to initiate the exposure.

4. X-rays examination techniques

As described before, there exists density difference in human tissues, which is the basis for producingX-ray images contrast, namely natural contrast. As for tissues or organs lack of natural contrast, higher or lower contrast media are deliberately introduced into these structures in order to produce contrast between these structures, it calls artificial contrast. Therefore natural and artificial contrast are both basis of X-ray examination.

(1)Conventional examinations

It includes fluoroscopy and radiography.

1)Fluoroscopy

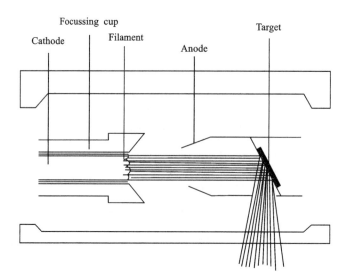

Figure 1-2   X-ray tube

In fluoroscopy, the X-rays pass through the body onto a fluorescent screen, creating a moving X-ray image. Fluoroscopy is most suitable for the position in human body with good natural contrast, such as thoracic fluoroscopy, which allows us to peer the dynamic function of inside lung and cardiovascular system timely, without any surgery at all. Contrast media are often used in conjunction with a fluoroscope. Doctors may use fluoroscopy to trace the passage of contrast media through the body, such as gastrointestinal barium, barium enema, and angiography. In addition, it possesses other advantages such as simple operation, low expense and immediately getting results. But fluoroscopy has poor images contrast and clearness, and it is difficult to observe organs lack of density and thickness differences and parts with high density and more thickness, such as head, spinal column, pelvis and so on. Lack of objective record is another disadvantage.

2) Radiography

Radiography is applied broadly in clinics to help physician diagnose diseases and make therapeutic strategies. It has good contrast and clearness and is not difficult to visualize lesions with high density and more thickness. Radiographic contrast is the term used to describe the density differences between two areas in a radiography. When this density difference is large, the radiographic contrast is high. When the density difference is small, the radiographic contrast is low. An image with high radiographic contrast is one in which regions on the film corresponding to areas of high X-ray absorption in the patient appear very white, while regions corresponding to areas of low X-ray absorption are very dark. In many cases, higher radiographic contrast improves the ability to differentiate structures in a radiography. The X-ray film can leave objective record to review and compare at any time to understand pathological changes and therapeutic effect after treatment. But it cannot observe the organ function dynamically as fluoroscopy, and the examined area is limited by the film size. In general, entopic and lateral films must be considered to get more information about lesions.

(2) X-ray tomography

Tomography can acquire image of structures on a selected slice and other structures outside the selected slice are blurred during projection. Tomography is usually used to visualize those lesions that cannot be visualized by radiography, or has many overlapping structures, or locates deeply. Thus we can know whether there are destruction, cavity or calcification inside lesions, or the lesion edge is sharp, and the exact position and range of lesion. At present, X-rays tomography has been seldom used in clinics with the advent of CT and MRI.

（3）Contrast examination

In a normal X-ray picture, most soft tissue doesn't shows up clearly. To observe the inside of the cavity organs, or to examine the blood vessels that make up the circulatory system, doctors must introduce contrast media into the body.

Contrast media are liquids that absorb X-rays more effectively than the surrounding tissue. To observe the gastrointestinal tract and endocrine ducts, a patient will swallow a contrast media mixture, typically a barium compound. If the doctors want to examine blood vessels or other elements in the circulatory system, they will inject contrast media into the patient's bloodstream. Contrast examination obviously enlarges the scope of X-rays examination.

Contrast media is different from general therapeutic medicaments with special betaken methods, such as big dosage, high concentration, high injected speed and so on. Actually, contrast media administration means to introduce a large amount of medicine into a certain position of the patient, therefore, the operator must be familiar with operating techniques and the quality, application purpose, and contraindications of various contrast media. We must take the following measures before contrast examination: 1）Decide whether to do allergy test according to the product specification; 2）Strictly controlling the contraindications of contrast media. Contrast media is prohibited for patients with hypersusceptibility history, hyperthyroidism, cardiac insufficiency and anuria; 3）The preparation of all kinds of emergency medicines is necessary for dealing with by-production reactions and complications.

5. Radiation protection

X-rays are a wonderful addition to the world of medicine, they let doctors peer inside a patient without any surgery at all. It's much easier and safer to look at a broken bone using X-rays than it is to open a patient up. But X-rays can also be harmful. In the early days of X-ray science, a lot of doctors would expose patients and themselves to the beams for long periods of time. Eventually, doctors and patients started developing radiation sickness, and the medical community knew something was wrong.

The problem is that X-rays are a form of ionizing radiation. When normal light hits an atom, it can't change the atom in any significant way. But when an X-ray hits an atom, it can knock electrons off the atom to create an ion, an electrically-charged atom. Free electrons then collide with other atoms to create more ions.

An ion's electrical charge can lead to unnatural chemical reactions inside cells. Among other things, the charge can break DNA chains. A cell with a broken strand of DNA will either die or the DNA will develop a mutation. If a lot of cells die, the body can develop various diseases. If the DNA mutates, a cell may become cancerous, and this cancer may spread. If the mutation is in a sperm or an egg cell, it may lead to birth defects. Because of all these risks, doctors use X-rays sparingly today.

We must comply with the following protection principles in order to avoid X-rays harmful to our health: （1）Time protection means all relative people reduce the time staying at X-rays room, the time exposing to X-rays as more as possible ; （2）Distance protection means the operators must be away from the X-rays resources as far as possible; （3）Shield protection means an object with X-rays absorption is placed between the X-rays resources and the operators, such as Lead glass and concrete.

Even with these risks, X-ray scanning is still a safer option than surgery. X-ray machines are an invaluable tool in medicine, as well as an asset in security and scientific research. They are truly one of the most useful inventions of all time.

Section 2　New advances in diagnostic radiology

In recent years, PACS (Picture Archving and Communication Systems) have undergone a rapid development.

PACS is merging with RIS (Radiology Information System). The digitalization of X-ray imaging is very important for PACS; high-quality digital X-ray medical images are indispensable for PACS data source. The advantage of digital X-ray image is by separating detecting and display, detector can be optimized to receive photon, record information accurately and suppress scattering more effectively, while separated display can work more better with best contrast enhancement to diagnose pathological changes. Most important issue is that, after separating detecting and display, it will be possible to perform image processing including enhancement and intelligent computer-aided diagnose.

There are three ways to digitalize x-ray imaging, that's computed radiography (CR), digital radiography (DR) and video digital acquisition. Both CR and DR convert analog imaging information to digital image. Video digital acquisition performs A/D convert directly upon video signal produced by x-ray detector, and acquires images by single frames or by series.

1. Computed radiography (CR)

(1) Basic structures and principles of CR

A simplified diagram of the image processing operations in current CR systems is depicted in Figure 1-3. The ensemble of operations applied to the stream of image data could be roughly entitled 'image enhancement'. The role of image processing functions within this data path is to improve the visual quality of the CR image in terms of spatial resolution, sharpness, contrast resolution, dynamic range, SNR. The processing efforts in the main path have to do with maximizing the information transfer to the viewer.

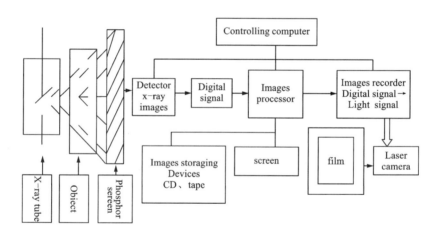

Figure 1-3 A diagram of the image processing operations in CR systems

Present day computed radiography (CR) is based on the use of photostimulable phosphors, which are also known as storage phosphors. They are commercially the most successful detectors for digital radiography. The phosphors used are most often in the barium fluorohalide family in powder form and deposited onto a substrate to form an imaging plate or screen. X-ray absorption mechanisms are identical to those of conventional phosphor screens used with film. They differ in that the useful optical signal is not derived from the light emitted in prompt response to the incident radiation, but rather from subsequent emission when the latent image, consisting of trapped charge, is optically stimulated and released from metastable traps. This triggers a process called photostimulated luminescence (PSL) resulting in the emission of shorter wavelength (blue) light in an amount proportional to the original X-ray irradiation. In CR, an imaging plate (IP) containing the storage phosphor is positioned in a light-tight enclosure, exposed to the x-ray image and then read out by raster scanning with a laser to release the PSL. The blue PSL light is collected with a light guide and detected with a photomultiplier tube (PMT). The PMT signal is digitized to form the image on a point-by-point basis . The broad acceptance of CR has been due to its large dynamic range, digital nature, easy portability and uniqueness rather than its intrinsic image quality. CR systems have improved in the almost 20 years that they have been available. They are now technological and engineering marvels, but have been unable to transcend their inherent image quality weaknesses.

(2)Images characteristics of CR

1)High sensitivity: Namely images cannot be covered by noise when acquiring very low signal.

2)High resolution: Images resolution can be described as the defined size as soon as possible or ability to differentiate two particles. The pixel of CR can be more than 2000 × 2000 enough to observe the details not described by other techniques.

3)High linearity: So called linearity is whether signals getting within the whole spectrum range are linear proportionate to the light intensity of real images, namely whether acquired images fit real images very well. The amount of fluorescence emitted by IP depends on the amount of stimulated X rays one time. It has good linearity within 1: 10, non-linearity is lower than 1%.

4)Digitalized export and storage: CR system can directly produce digitalized images that can be stored in all kinds of the present storage media for long time, and directly imported into the images storing and transferring system and distant medicine system, as well as internet system.

5)Powerful post-processing function in CR system: Digitalized CR images have many post-processing function, such as measurement, local magnification, contrast transformation, images intensification, substraction and so on. It is easier to visualize histological structures and lesions and has improved the accurate rate of diagnosis.

(3)Clinical application of complete CR systems

CR can reprocess imaging data according to the difference in the X-rays absorption rate, and display the anatomic structures more advantageous than traditional X-rays plate film.

1)Head and osteoarticular system: CR can further quantify the amount of bone salt. As for joints, CR can display the changes of articular cartilage and surrounding soft tissues by reprocessing because of its digitalized images.

2)The application of CR system in thoracic plate films: Thoracic plate film is a x-rays examination in the most common use, CR thoracic films are generally superior to traditional thoracic films, especially displaying the overlapping part of mediastinum and diaphragmatic muscle. CR is also superior to traditional x-rays film in diaplaying of nodular lesions in lungs and mediastinal structures such as trachea, blood vessels. But CR system is not as good as traditional plate films in displaying interstitial disease and alveolar disease.

3)Gastrointestinal system and urinary system: The density resolution of CR images is clearly higher than that of traditional x-rays films and superior to traditional x-rays films in displaying intestinal air, stone and so on; In dual-contrast examination, CR is also superior to traditional x-rays contrast examination in visualizing the lesser curvature of stomach, tiny lesions, mucous membrane folders and so on; CR can compress the high-density images of urinary structures and use tuning and space frequency processing function to improve density layers and sharpness of soft tissues images and the resolution of soft tissues greatly, especially kidney tomography; Improving the ability to display stone and tiny calcification .

2. Digital radiography(DR)

(1)The basic structures and principles of DR

DR is comprised of electric dark box, scanning controller, system controller and image monitor and so on, it can transfer X rays into digitalized images by electric dark box. It principles is that image intensified tube transfers X rays as information carrier into visualized light, and photoelectric tube transfers the visualized light into vedio signal, then vedio signal can be transferred into digital matrix images by A/D . Both DR and CR technologies are systems that convert X-ray image information into digital image information, and can be post processed according to clinical needs. Both of them are effective methods in medical imaging diagnosis and have their own characteristics, but the overall effect of DR system is better than CR. DR has higher image quality, resolution, and response speed than CR. By adopting DR technology to collect related images, it helps to reduce imaging time, reduce the workload of staff, and obtain high-quality images in a timely and effective manner. It is convenient to further improve the diagnosis rate of patients taking pictures.

(2)The advantages of DR

1)DR permits very broad exposure latitude and has wide dynamic range, allows technical error happened in the process of taking a film. It can also get a very good image in some position where the exposing parameters is difficult to control.

2)The image presented is of high quality and rich in layers, with a spatial resolution of 3.6 LP/mm.

3)DR can also perform all kinds of images postprocessing as CR, and has the potential of remote consultation.

4)Without X-ray film, it can save the cost of developing film and film when the computer transmits and stores the image. It is convenient and quick to reduce unnecessary expenses.

(3)The application of DR

Digital radiography refers to the application of digital image processing techniques to projection radiography. These applications are briefly reviewed below with the treatment concentrating on digital subtraction angiography (DSA) because of its relatively widespread application.

Section 3   Digital substraction angiography(DSA)

DSA is a new medical imaging technique springing up in 1980's. As the name implies, refers specifically to techniques which subtract two images that are obtained before and after contrast media is administered to the patient for the purposes of studying blood vessels (angiography) and produces digital substraction angiography (DSA) of which the quality is improved greatly than conventional angiography (Figure 1-4).

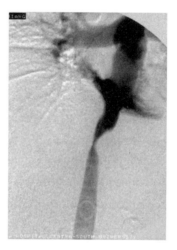

Budd-Chiari Syndrom, A stenosis at the approximate
side of the inferior vena cava was visualized clearly, but
soft tissues and bone were not visualized.

Figure 1.4   DSA image

1. The main components of DSA

DSA system includes X-rays generator and tube, image intensifier, TV fluoroscopy, high-resolution video camera, A/D conversion, computer and image storage.

2. The basic principles of DSA

(1) Obtaining video image

The image acquisition process begins when timing signals, delivered to the X-ray generator under computer control, initiates the production of X-rays which are transmitted through the patient and received by the image intensifier. An aperture, placed between the image intensifier and the video camera, controls the amount of light delivered to the camera. A video camera receives the light image from the image intensifier and converts it into an electronic video signal which is delivered to the image processor in analog form. The image processor digitizes the image, stores it in memory, and makes it available in digital form for subtraction with another image set acquired at a different time or at a different energy. The basic components of the imaging system including the X-ray tube and X-ray generator, the image intensifier, and the television camera are similar to but must be of higher quality than, those used in conventional fluoroscopy. Different grey scale images displaying in vedio monitor are called vedio images.

(2) Logarithmic amplitude

The term amplitude refers to how the video signal is processed prior to the actual substraction step. For logarithmic amplitude, the signal read from the video camera is passed prior to substraction through electric circuitry, the output of which is proportional to the logarithm of input. The DSA difference signal in this case is:

$$DIFF_{LOG} = (\mu/\rho)_I \rho_I d.$$

$(\mu/\rho)_I$ is the mass attenuation coefficient of iodine, and $\rho_I d$ is the product of iodine concentration and vessel diameter, or projected concentration. The video frequency signal with different intensity can be compressed and its display range can be adjusted after processed by a video frequency amplifier through a special circuitry, and then the logarithmic function change of the video signal intensity can be converted into the linear function change, namely the area of low video frequency intensity is enlarged and the area of high video frequency intensity is compressed, thereby both area s of low and high video frequency can be displayed clearly on video images at the same time.

(3) Analog-to-digital conversion

The video image after logarithmic amplitude process is still an analog image comprised of different grey scale. It must be digitalized before computer processing. We will assume that an analog video image has been acquired by the x-ray system, image intensifier, and television camera. The analog signal is delivered to the image processor that provides some preprocessing to adjust the amplitude and level of the video signal to satisfy the input specifications of the digital-to-analog converter. A series of different voltage values of video signal can be converted into different duality value after processed by A/D converter, then it can be converted into a group of different pixel values after imported into computer and processed. Thus video image can be transferred into digital image.

3. Formation of DSA image

Digital subtraction angiography (DSA) is a procedure, using computer technology to enhance the image quality of X-rays. This involves subtracting the radiographic image obtained without a contrast agent from an image taken with a contrast agent. Subtraction allows for visualization of blood vessels without interference from surrounding structures. The main physics variations processed by subtraction include time, energy and depth.

(1) Temporal subtraction

By far the most common algorithm using digital radiographic systems is temporal subtraction. It refers to a number of computer-assisted techniques whereby an image obtained at one time is subtracted from an image obtained at a later time. If, during intervening period, contrast material was introduced into the vasculature, the subtracted image will contain only the vessels filled with the contrast material.

(2) Energy subtraction

Energy subtraction uses two differentX-ray beams alternately to provide a subtraction image resulting from differences in photoelectric interaction.

(3) Hybrid subtraction

Some DSA systems are capable of combining temporal and energy subtraction techniques into what is called hybrid subtraction. If patient motion can be controlled, hybrid subtraction can theoretically produce the high-quality DSA images.

4. DSA imaging modes

(1) Intravenous DSA(IVDSA)

IVDSA refers to any DSA mode that inserting a catheter into vein to inject contrast media. For example, The technique that places the head of catheter or cannula needle in peripheral vein (peripheral method) or superior vena cava or right atrium(central method) to inject contrast media is named non-selection IVDSA, namely recirculation method; the technique that places the head of catheter in targeted vein or the position near targeted vein or heart cavity to inject contrast media is called selected IVDSA .

Non-selected IVDSA, whether peripheral or central method, belongs to recirculation method that displays arteries by intravenously injecting contrast media. Contrast media that enters into vein must flow from lung circulation to body circulation and then artery can be visualized . At present, non-selected IVDSA is mainly used in the diagnosis of aortic disease and its main branches's disease, such as aortitis, aortic stenosis, carotid body aneurysm and so on. it is seldom used in clinics and only used when it is difficult to insert a catheter into an artery or it is not suitable for intraarterial DSA(IADSA).

The mixed blood volume of selective IVDSA is smaller than that of non-selective IVDSA, and the contrast medium is less diluted. Therefore, it is often used for diseases such as the superior and inferior vena cava, femoral iliac vein, renal vein disease, and congenital cardiovascular malformations involving the right atrium, pulmonary artery and vein. Diagnosis and treatment, such as congenital vena cava malformations, vena cava stenosis and Budd-Chiari syndrome.

(2) Intraarterial DSA (IADSA)

The DSA ability to display blood vessels is closely related with the concentration of contrast media inside blood vessels. In IADSA, the contrast media is injected directly into targeted artery or area near targeted artery and thereby less diluted, the concentration of contrast media inside targeted artery is still higher than IVDSA with large dose and injection at high concentration. Therefore IADSA can display clearly tiny blood vessels.

IADSA can be divided into non-selected or selected groups. The non-selected IADSA refers to technique that places the head of catheter in the aortic approximate part of targeted artery to inject contrast media; The selected IADSA refers to technique that puts the head of catheter further into the main branches of targeted artery to inject contrast media. The intraarterial injection can obviate many of the disadvantages of the intravenous studies. It will increase the contrast concentration in the region-of-interest improving the spatial resolution to the point that all, but the most minute arterial changes can be appreciated. A lower concentration of contrast material can be used and the examination can be performed more rapidly than conventional film screen angiogram.

5. The clinical application and special imaging technology of DSA

The advantages of DSA are high resolution, low contrast agent consumption, real-time display and access monitoring. DSA is widely recognized in the process of diagnosing and treating vascular diseases. Interventional radiology is an emerging discipline between traditional internal medicine and traditional surgery. It has the distinctive characteristics of integrated diagnosis and treatment and visualization. It is one of the three major medical disciplines alongside internal medicine and surgery. In general, it can be divided into vascular intervention and non-vascular intervention. Most of them involve the use of related vascular interventional techniques, so DSA plays an irreplaceable role in interventional radiotherapy. Its special imaging technology has the following points:

(1)Perspective road map technology and radiography conversion road map technology

The perspective path diagram technology is completed under fluoroscopy conditions. The path diagram can be cancelled at any time, which is convenient for imaging. Contrast conversion path map technology can select a more satisfactory map from a sequence as a reference. The lesions in the target vessel area have a preliminary understanding, and its function is better than the perspective path map technology in some aspects. This technology can guide the micro-guide wire and micro-catheter into the diseased blood vessel, evaluate whether the cerebral aneurysm is densely packed, and can clearly show the trajectory of branch blood vessels, especially for the display of curved, overlapping, and angle

(2)Rotating DSA technology and 3D-DSA technology

Rotating DSA technology is a new technology that uses the rotation of the angiographic C-arm to meet the inspection requirements. It can display the shadow vessel anatomy of the area of interest in multiple directions. 3D-DSA technology is a new technology developed in rotating DSA technology in recent years. It is a combination of rotating angiography technology, DSA technology and computer three-dimensional image processing technology. This technology is mainly used for the diagnosis and treatment of cerebral hemangioma, to determine cerebral artery stenosis, to clearly display the blood supply arteries of chest, abdomen, pelvis, and bone tumors and to guide further treatment.

(3)Stepping DSA technology

Stepping DSA technology uses fast pulse exposure acquisition, real-time subtraction. This technology provides a new method of observing the whole vascular structure, and solves the problem that the blood flow speed is inconsistent with the photography speed, and the blood vessels are displayed poorly or cannot be displayed. The feature of this technology is that the amount of contrast agent is small, and a sequence of exposure shows the entire blood vessel image of the lower extremities, which is especially suitable for subjects who are not suitable to use more contrast agents. The stepping DSA currently used in clinical practice has one-way, that is, from the head side to the foot side; there are also two-way, which can observe the subject from the head side to the foot side or from the foot side to the head side. This technology is suitable for the diagnosis and treatment of vascular diseases of the lower extremities.

(4)C-arm CT technology

C-arm CT technology is a computer tomography that uses images collected by rotating angiography in the DSA system to form angiography. The principle is similar to that of CT 3D reconstruction technology, but the number of C-arm CT technology data collection is different from that of ordinary CT 3D reconstruction collection. C-arm CT rotates to collect 500F raw data, and ordinary 3D reconstruction rotates to collect 150F raw data, so the image quality obtained is also different from that of 3D reconstruction. Patients undergoing interventional surgery can directly observe the degree of bleeding in the angiography examination room through the C-arm CT technology, thus avoiding transporting the patient to other equipment for examination. High-resolution C-arm CT technology can clearly display the inserted stent, and judge the extension and adhesion of the stent after release. CT-like technology can achieve high-quality examinations without the use of contrast agents, can expand the scope of abdominal operations (including puncture and drainage) and provide assistance in diagnosis and intervention. C-arm CT technology is also of potential value in tumor applications. It can display tumors with a higher density, so it can be used for guided biopsy and intraoperative evaluation of tumor treatment and guide tumor embolization.

(5) 3D path map

Application of 3D vascular reconstruction technology to match volume data with real-time fluoroscopy, instead of the traditional two-dimensional path function; the advantage is that when the doctor changes the area of interest, there is no need to repeatedly inject contrast agent to make the road map. 3D-Roadmap-is associated with C-arm rotation, bed surface elevation and movement, FOV changes, etc.

(6) Virtual stent implantation

It uses the images collected by rotating angiography in the DSA system to perform computer post-processing for three-dimensional three-dimensional imaging of blood vessels. Perform vascular analysis on the reconstructed stenosis or tumor-bearing blood vessel in the three-dimensional post-processing workstation, and perform virtual stent placement based on the measurement data and the data provided by the stent manufacturer for doctors to choose.

(Xiao Enhua, Guo Jianwei, Zhang Jie, Yu Cheng, Tan Changlian)

第二章

电子计算机 X 线断层摄影术(CT)

电子计算机 X 线断层摄影术(CT)作为一种无创性放射学方法，开创了人体任何部位断层成像之先河，而且邻近结构不会叠加，尤为重要的是它所获得的对比分辨率首次使放射学方法可以分辨高密度颅骨内的脑组织。通过 1972 年、1994 年、2019 年典型的 CT 扫描参数比较，我们不难发现 CT 技术在前 20 年内从未停止其进步的步伐，如表 2-1 所示，其中扫描时间的缩短及空间分辨率的提高最引人注目。目前，低剂量 CT 扫描方案也逐渐应用于临床，可显著降低患者的辐射剂量。接下来要介绍的螺旋 CT 如同其他成像形式一样，开始从层层间成像向容积成像技术转变，该技术的优点是在三维空间中具有更好地各向同性的空间分辨率，从而能更精确地从三维空间中描绘扫描的解剖结构。

历史上有三位科学家对 CT 的发展贡献卓越：Radon，Hounsfield 和 Cormack。Radon 于 1917 年就首次明确地叙述投影的重建功能；Hounsfield 于 1972 年首先完成实验性 CT 机的装配和测试；Cormack 的最大贡献是得出 CT 的数学计算方法。Hounsfield 和 Cormack 在 1979 年共享诺贝尔医学奖。

表 2-1　前 20 年 CT 技术不断进步

扫描参数	1972 年经典值	1994 年经典值	2019 年经典值
矩阵大小	80×80	1024×1024	1024×1024
空间分辨率	3Lp(线对)/cm	15 Lp(线对)/cm	32 Lp(线对)/cm
对比分辨率	5 mm/5 Hu/50 mGy	3 mm/3 Hu/30 mGy	2 mm/3 Hu/12.3 mGy
扫描时间	5 min	<1 s	66 ms
每次扫描的数据大小	50KB	2 MB	47 MB
X 线功率	2 kW	40 kW	2 * 120 kW

注：mGy=毫格雷，格雷是指 SI 单位的辐射量。Hu=Hounsfield 单位，CT 密度值。空气(零衰减)CT 值= -1000 HU，水的 CT 值=0 HU。

第一节　基本概念

CT 与传统 X 线片比较，CT 图像是真正的 X 线断层图像，能使人体部位任何层面的组织密度分布图像化。当然 CT 仍采用 X 线作为投射源，获得因通过选定层面从不同方位被吸收衰减后的 X 线值，该值通过模拟/数字(A/D)转换器处理后输入电脑并获得选定层面组织衰减系数的数字矩阵，然后将该数字矩阵的数据通过数字/模拟(D/A)转换器转变为黑白灰阶，从而可以在荧屏上清楚显示。CT 图像具有图像清晰、分辨率高、且没有非选择层面组织干扰的优点。

1. 体素和像素

实际上，CT 图像是一定厚度人体组织的断层图像。断层图像按矩阵排列分成若干个很小的基本单位，通常任一小单位内的物质密度由一个CT值表达,这些小单位就叫体素。CT图像也是由许多按矩阵排列的小单位组成,这些小单位即像素。体素是三维概念,像素是二维概念。图2-1示,在图像中像素可以代表体素,像素越小,图像分辨率越高。

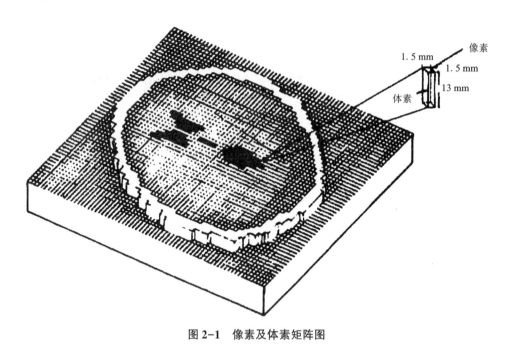

图2-1　像素及体素矩阵图

2. 矩阵

矩阵是数学概念,代表横行和垂直的数字排列,将所扫描层面分割成许多立方体,即体素。如果图像面积恒定,体素体积越小,图像矩阵越大,其清晰度越高。

3. 空间分辨率

空间分辨率是影像中能够分辨的最小细节,也称为高对比分辨率,是物体与均质环境的X线衰减系数差别的相对值大于10%时CT图像分辨该物质的能力。即保证分辨一定密度差别的先决条件下,清楚显示组织几何形状的能力,它代表能分辨最小物体的直径。

CT图像的空间分辨率取决于许多因素,其中最主要的影响因素如下:

(1)焦点的大小,即电子撞击阳极面积。

(2)探测器元件的大小,探测器元件的大小和焦点的大小决定电子束的宽度。

(3)患者前方和后方的准直器,决定层厚。

(4)重建中心(或卷积过滤)可调整为高频(决定边缘)或低频(为了减少噪声和假影)。

(5)可以通过以下途径提高分辨率:①增加探测器数量;②缩小体素(或像素)的体积,但要以增加噪声为代价;③采用减少平滑化的重建中心,也要以增加噪音为代价。

现代标准CT机的分辨率在扫描层面内可达到亚毫米级,在轴线上也可达到小于1 mm的级别。

4. 密度分辨率

密度分辨率能显示最小密度差别,也可称为对比分辨率,即在低对比度的情况下使组织间的细微密度差别显示出来的能力,CT图像的密度分辨率高于常规X线片10~20倍。

5. 时间分辨率

时间分辨率指成像设备单位时间内采集影像的帧数,是设备的性能参数,与每帧影像的采集和重建时间、显示方式及连续成像的时间与能量有关,对CT成像来说,就是机体活动的最短时间间距,指在相邻2

次观测的最小时间间隔。

6. CT 值

X 线通过穿透人体组织后，可计算出每一单位体积的 X 线衰减系数，即 μ 值，μ 值可转变为 CT 值，代表同一单位的组织密度。

物质的 CT 值等于该物质的吸收系数（μ_m）减去水的吸收系数（μ_w）后除以水的吸收系数并乘上 1000，其单位为 Hu（Hounsfield）。物质 CT 值计算公式：CT 值 = $(\mu_m - \mu_w)/\mu_w \times 1000$。人体组织的 CT 值界限为 2000 个分度，骨骼的 CT 值最高（+1000 Hu），空气的 CT 值最低（-1000 Hu）。

7. 窗宽和窗位

窗宽代表 CT 值的范围，在荧屏上包括 16 个灰阶。人体组织的 CT 值范围为 2000 Hu（-1000~1000 Hu），如果用 2000 个不同的灰阶代表 2000 个 CT 值，人眼无法区分如此细微的差别（通常只能区分 16 个灰阶差别）。假如用 16 灰阶反映 2000 Hu，能区分的 CT 值差别为 125 Hu（2000/16），也就是说很难分辨 CT 值差别小于 125 Hu 的组织。对荧屏上的图像运用不同的窗宽是为了提高组织结构细节的显示，分辨 CT 值差别很小的组织。例如当窗宽为 100 Hu 时，能分辨的 CT 值差别为 6.25 Hu（100/16），CT 值差别大于 6.25 Hu 的两种组织均可被区分出来。

窗位是窗宽的中心位置，为了详细地观察某一组织结构，该组织结构的 CT 值被视为窗中心。例如脑的 CT 值为 35Hu，因此窗位定位 35 Hu，窗宽通常为 100 Hu，荧屏上 16 灰阶代表的 CT 值范围为-15~85 Hu，CT 值小于-15 Hu 的组织结构的灰阶与 CT 值为-15 Hu 的组织结构无差别，CT 值大于 85 Hu 的组织结构的灰阶与 CT 值为 85 Hu 的组织结构也无差别，只有 CT 值在-15~85 Hu 之间的组织结构的 CT 值差别可用 16 灰阶表现出来。

在荧屏上，增加窗宽可以提高图像的阶层，但减低了组织对比度，图像的细节显示较差。假如窗宽调至最低，图像中没有阶层，只有黑白两种图像。提高窗位，图像渐黑，减低窗位，图像渐白。因此实际上窗宽和窗位技术对显示病变很重要。

8. 假影

根据其来源可以将 CT 系统的图像假影分为以下几种。

（1）物理相关因素：

1）量子噪声：X 线光子的强度难免存在空间上和时间上的统计变化，其中较活跃成分在投射数据中表现为信号依赖性的噪声，减少噪声需通过增加 X 线强度、采集时间和患者接受 X 线的剂量。量子噪声的信号依赖性导致重建图像中典型的辐射状假影。

2）由患者产生的 X 线散射：在扇形束射线系统中，可以通过充分准直作用后减少散射效应；但在环形探测器系统中，必须采用精确的散射模型来矫正此类效应。

3）线束硬化：为了达到所有诊断目的，单纯的经验矫正通常可以补偿此类效应，特殊情况下，当某一层骨骼组织较多，残留的线束硬化效应就显示出来了，较典型的如头颅扫描时两侧岩骨之间的暗带。

4）非线性部分容积效应：当成像层面含有高对比度的组织结构时，辐射衰减呈指数关系而并非线性关系，检测的数据与重建的数学模式不一致，尽管已经设计了一些矫正方法，但由于花费增高和检测时间延长以及操作复杂而未能被广泛应用。减少非线性部分容积效应最简单且最有效的方法就是缩小层厚。

（2）患者相关因素：

1）患者或某个器官的运动：典型的运动假影为条纹状或斑纹状，其强度受运动器官的对比度影响。尽管很容易辨认图像中的运动假影通常与某一运动有关，但多个运动假影混合在一起就很难解释该假影与哪些运动有关了。如前所述，减少运动假影的最有效的方法就是加快数据采集速度。

2）金属异物：因为金属（如假牙）的衰减系数很大，探测器和数据采集系统的动态变化范围尚不足以精确适应投射数据的采集，更有甚者，在某些情况下非线性部分容积效应常加重投射数据中的不协调性，因此，图像上出现来自金属物体的条纹状假影。

（3）系统相关因素：

1）探测器灵敏度的校准不充分。

2）探测器灵敏度的时间、温度和辐射记录相关性漂移。

3）重建算法不适当。

4）扫描移动不同步。

5）X线球管电压波动。

所有以上误差均因受扫描系统采用几何结构的影响而以不同类型在重建图像中显示出来，如在扇形束系统中，探测器相关的误差通常显示为环形假影，而在静止的环形探测器系统，常为条纹状假影。

9. 部分容积效应

如果在同一扫描层面内含有两种以上不同密度物质，则测得的CT值代表它们的平均值而不能如实反映其中任何一种物质的CT值，这种现象即为部分容积效应。

由于X线束宽度有限，每一测量值只代表X线束平均强度，该平均值通过对数转换获得X线束有效衰减值，通常低于实际衰减值。垂直X线束的衰减梯度越大，有效衰减值越低于实际衰减值，从而导致边缘的条纹切线影。

小于层厚的病变虽然可以在CT图像中显示，但由于部分容积效应，测得的CT值并不能真正反映该病变组织的CT值。如果病变组织密度比周围组织密度高而且其厚度小于层厚，则所测得的CT值比其本来CT值小。相反如果病变组织密度比周围组织密度低而且其厚度小于层厚，则所测得的CT值比其本来CT值大。因此，临床诊断中对小病变CT值进行评价时要考虑部分容积效应。

第二节　CT成像原理

1. CT成像（图2-2）

（1）X线扫描数据的采集和转化：X线通过人体后因被吸收而衰减，衰减程度与层面中病变的组织、器官和密度（原子序数）有关，密度越大，X线衰减系数越大。CT探测器将已衰减的X线转变为电信号，然后这些电信号转变为相应的数字信号并输入计算机内。

（2）扫描数据的处理和图像重建：计算机能调整和处理输入的原始数据以重建图像。

（3）图像的储存和显示：重建图像矩阵中的数据可转化为不同灰阶的光斑以形成可以在荧屏和胶片上显示的图像，也可通过打印机以数据的形式打印出来或用磁带、光盘、软盘永久保存。

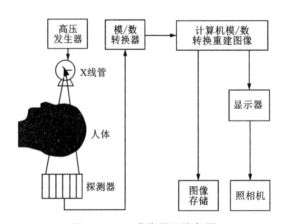

图2-2　CT成像原理线条图

2. CT 扫描基本装置

CT 扫描装置主要由 X 线管、探测器、准直器、模拟/数字(A/D)转换器、检查床、高压发生器、计算机系统、图像显示存储输出系统组成。

(1)X 线管:在过去的 20 年内,传统的非电子束 CT 机性能的显著提高依赖于使用的 X 线球管工艺的重大进步。如今,金属靶(钨、铼、钼)镶饰在厚石墨块上以提高散热能力,靶的直径达到 20 cm,旋转速度达到 10 000 rpm,通常靶的运作温度达到 1 200℃,焦点温度可超过 2 500℃,球管的最大散热可达 10 kW。然而受 X 线球管影响,CT 扫描机的最大限制是最大容许承受的 X 线功率。更进一步的发展应是靶的冷却系统(如液体旋转冷却)、轴承系统的进步和电子束的产生。

(2)探测器:CT 机有两类探测器,均通常由 1 000 个探测元件线性排列或由更多的探测元件排成环形的几何图形。商用螺旋 CT 机探测器已发展至宽体 320 排,320 排相邻的探测元件以同时进行 16 cm 范围扫描。闪烁类探测器大多数采用闪烁体物质,如碘化铯、钨酸镉以及用稀土氧化物制成的陶瓷闪烁体。CT 探测器闪烁体特别关键的参数是余辉。因为 CT 数据采集不能像核技术那样使用脉冲计数,而是采用整合探测器电流,所以余辉导致在组织/气体或组织/骨骼界面出现测量误差。数据采集的方案最起码要能补偿探测器余辉相关的首序效应。与稀有气体电离探测器相比,闪烁类探测器的几何效率(活性与无活性区的比率)通常较低,但常超过其量子效率的代偿。扇形束系统中,为了减少散射的 X 线,在闪烁体元件前通常使用准直器。气体探测器使用室墙能达到与准直器相同的目的,而由于 X 线球管的靶与探测器元件一起移动,气体探测器的这种自准直效应在环形探测器系统中不适应。

(3)准直器:准直器分别位于患者前方与 X 线球管出口之间及患者后方与探测器入口之间,用来限制到达感兴趣区解剖部位的已滤过的 X 线束。准直器孔径决定层厚,通常其范围为 1~10 mm。

(4)模拟/数字(A/D)转换器。

(5)检查床:检查床的主要功能是将受检者移至扫描孔内,在对扫描部位的扫描过程中,传统 CT 机的检查床步序水平移动,而螺旋 CT 检查床是均匀水平移动。

(6)高压发生器:为 X 线管提供高电压。

(7)计算机系统:CT 计算机系统有两大类,①主计算机;②阵列计算机。主计算机是整个 CT 机的控制系统,控制 X 线管、探测器、准直器、检查床的运动和 X 射线产生、数据的产生收集以及各个部件的信息交流。阵列计算机主要完成图像的重建。

(8)图像显示、存储、输出系统。

第三节 CT 扫描机的发展

20 世纪 80 年代螺旋 CT 未发明之前,CT 的发展通常以"代"称呼。螺旋 CT 问世以后,已不再称呼几代 CT,取而代之的是单排螺旋 CT、多排螺旋 CT、能谱 CT、双源 CT 等。

1. 第一代 CT

第一代 CT 扫描机追溯至 Hounsfield 开发的电磁干扰扫描机。该类 CT 机采用单一笔形束 X 线和单个探测器,两者同步平移和旋转。对检查对象进行平移扫描,平移结束后旋转 1°角,再准备行另一方向扫描。采集重建图像所需的投射数据一般需要数分钟。第一代 CT 扫描机特点:射线利用率低、单一笔形束、单个探测器、平移-旋转-平移、扫描时间为数分钟。

2. 第二代 CT 机

第二代 CT 机设计为小角度扇形束 X 线和一组探测器。由于采用扇形束通过患者增加了数据采集通道,从而减少旋转次数,所以扫描时间相应缩短,约 20 秒。为了覆盖整个扫描对象,第二代 CT 机仍然使用了平移和旋转。第二代 CT 扫描机特点:单一小角度扇形束、探测器组、旋转-平移-旋转、扫描时间为 20 秒;第二代 CT 扫描机的优点:时间缩短,矩阵提高(探测器孔径变小);第二代 CT 扫描机的缺点:探测器直线排列，射线束到探测器中间和两边不对称，需要射线校准避免假影。

3.第三代 CT 机

第三代 CT 机的扇形束角度加宽，扇形束可以覆盖整个扫描对象，每束投射路径由相匹配的探测器决定，探测器可以是小且窄的闪烁探测器板，也可以是气体电离室。由于扫描对象完全位于扇形束中，无需平移，因此 X 线球管和探测器组只需围绕固定轴中心作单一旋转运动。旋转 360° 可获得全部扫描数据，扫描时间缩短至 1~3 秒。该类 CT 机构造的主要缺点是探测器漂移效应的累积，从而在重建图像中出现假影。为了利用连续扫描间的停顿时间(dead time)几乎所有第三代 CT 机都采用了脉冲 X 线源。图 2-3 示第三代 CT 机的结构。第三代 CT 扫描机特点：单一宽角度扇形束、探测器组、X 线源-探测器配对的旋转运动(无平移)、扫描时间 1~3 秒；第三代 CT 扫描机的优点：时间缩短到 2~9 秒，不用做射线校准(射线到探测器的距离相等)；第三代 CT 扫描机的缺点：容易出现环形假影。

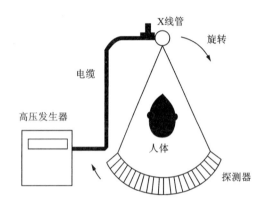

图 2-3　第三代 CT 成像的结构示意图

4.第四代 CT 机

探测器固定环形排列是第四代 CT 最显著的特点，X 线源旋转但探测器组固定不动。宽角度扇形束 X 线覆盖整个扫描对象，600 个或更多的固定的探测器排列成环形。第四代 CT 机通常很昂贵，是因为使用了大量的闪烁探测器和 PMTs。第四代 CT 机的扫描速度大大提高，当运动器官成像时，可以与心电图等生理信号做同步旋转运动。第四代 CT 扫描机特点：单一宽角度扇形束、探测器环形排列、X 线源旋转运动(无平移)；第四代 CT 扫描机的优点：球管扇形夹角到 50°~90°，避免同心环假影；第四代 CT 扫描机的缺点：一个角度内只有部分探测器工作，成本增加。

5.第五代 CT

第五代 CT 即超高速 CT，也称电子束 CT(EBCT)，主要由电子枪、聚焦线圈、偏转线圈、多排探测器组群、高速移动的检查床及控制系统组成(图 2-4)。穿过人体的电子束能量衰减后可被探测器检测，然后通过模拟/数字(A/D)转化和数字/模拟(D/A)转化形成与传统 CT 一样的图像。与传统 CT 不同的是电子束 CT 无需球管和探测器移动。迄今为止，电子束 CT 是断层成像速度最快的 CT 机之一，最快可达每层的扫描时间仅为 0.05 秒。第五代 CT 扫描机特点：它可以完成许多传统 CT 机不能完成的工作，如评价搭桥手术的开通情况；检查心内疾病和先天性心脏病；定量测量左右心室壁肿块、心室容积、收缩和舒张功能(如心输出量、射血分数)、冠状动脉钙沉积的检测；第五代 CT 扫描机的优点：时间分辨率高，有效减少运动假影，可进行形态学研究；第五代 CT 扫描机的缺点：机架笨重，架构复杂，维修困难，价格昂贵。

6.螺旋 CT

任意方位的图像重建(包括重叠重建)使三维图像显示得到很大的进步，而且螺旋 CT 能快速覆盖更大体积的扫描对象，使得呼吸控制技术能更好地应用以提高对呼吸运动敏感的体内脏器的成像质量。螺旋

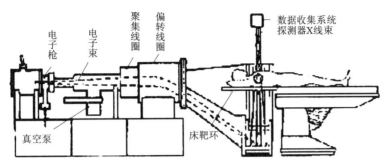

图 2-4　电子束 CT 成像示意图

CT 大大地改善了肺结节的成像, 提高了三维表面成像质量, 而且第一次在使用对比剂的情况下获得前所未有的血管成像质量(图 2-5)。目前螺旋 CT 图像的限制仍是 X 线球管可承受功率, 如单层扫描的有效功率是 40 kW, 30 秒或更长时间螺旋扫描的功率必须减低以避免球管超负荷。由于相关的量子噪声增加, 软组织成像通常必须采用平滑卷积核心重建。另一方面由于骨骼组织对比度高, 可采用薄层扫描获得足够的空间分辨率以用于矫形外科检查。选择合适的移床方式, 采用旋转 180°重建图像而非常规的 360°, 可以减少因移床而产生的图像模糊化。依赖螺旋 CT 特殊的成像方式, 目前扫描机每旋转 360°进床深度是层厚的 1 至 2 倍(图 2-5 示), 单层扫描除外。螺旋 CT 的 X 线球管可承受功率就像计算机的处理器性能一样, 必须在预期的时间内从技术上进一步提高。对未来技术发展产生另一重大影响的是多层面探测器应用和扩展平面探测器为立体角探测器, 以便更好地利用 X 线球管可承受功率并能在规定时间内覆盖更大的体积, 因此这些探测器被认为是螺旋 CT 未来发展最重要的方向, 依赖于生产工艺的进步, 这些探测器可能使得扫描机轴线方向的空间分辨率进一步提高。

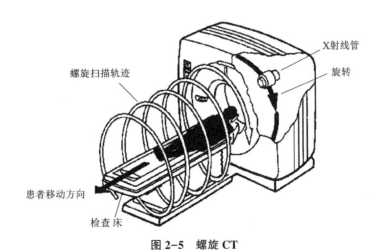

图 2-5　螺旋 CT

第四节　CT 检查方法和临床应用

1.非增强扫描或注射对比剂前扫描

非增强扫描或注射对比剂前扫描是指对比剂还未注入血管期间所进行的扫描, 一般采用横断位, 有时采用冠状位, 层厚为 1~10 mm。扫描时患者保持体位不动, 螺旋 CT 进行螺旋容积扫描后重建 1 mm 左右薄层并用其进行多平面重建(MPR)及曲面重建(CPR), 行腹部扫描时要口服阴性(如水)对比剂。

2. 注射对比剂后扫描

注射对比剂后扫描是指对比剂注入血管后进行的扫描，其目的是提高病变组织与正常组织的密度差别，以更好地显示非增强扫描图像中不能显示或显示较差的病变，并且可以根据病变是否增强或增强类型做出定性诊断。

3. 造影 CT 检查

造影 CT 检查是指使用造影检查后对器官或组织进行 CT 扫描，可以更好地显示组织结构和发现病变，如脊髓造影 CT 检查、膀胱造影 CT 检查等，现应用较少。

4. 特殊 CT 扫描

（1）薄层扫描：其目的是观察某些病变细节，避免部分容积效应，例如观察肺部小球形病变时，应采用薄层 CT 扫描。

（2）重叠 CT 扫描：检查床移动距离小于层厚，如层厚为 10 mm，移床 8 mm，扫描层面部分重叠，可以避免部分容积效应的出现和微小病变的漏诊，其缺点是过多的重叠会引起 X 线照射量增加。

（3）靶 CT 扫描：也称目标 CT 扫描或放大 CT 扫描，通过采用小视野（FOV）和薄层（1~5 mm）针对感兴趣区做局部 CT 扫描，可以明显提高空间分辨率，临床多用于小器官和小病变的 CT 扫描，如肺小结节、垂体和肾上腺。

（4）高分辨率 CT（HRCT）：采用薄层、更锐利或最锐利重建方法（或骨算法重建）以及特殊滤过过程以获得组织细微结构的图像，这种技术称为高分辨 CT。高分辨率 CT 主要用于肺部弥漫性病变和结节性病变，骨算法重建主要用于颞骨 CT 扫描以显示内耳、中耳听骨链等微细结构。

（5）延迟 CT 扫描（DCT）：延迟 CT 扫描是指注入对比剂后等待数分钟或数小时重复扫描，例如为了对肝海绵状血管瘤作定性诊断要延迟数分钟或半小时扫描，对于小肝细胞癌要延迟 4~8 小时扫描，因为含碘对比剂大部分通过肾脏排泄，但有 10% 通过肝脏排泄，正常肝实质细胞具有吸收和排泄有机碘的功能，其 CT 值在注入对比剂后 4~6 小时可增加 1~10 Hu，而肝癌细胞无此功能。

（6）动态扫描：它是指注入对比剂后运用 CT 机软件进行快速连续扫描，然后一帧帧处理和显示图像的一种方法。动态扫描分为两种：摇篮床进出式大范围连续动态扫描和单器官连续动态扫描，除了发现病变外，可以更好地评价病变的性质。

（7）三维 CT（3DCT）：三维 CT 是指在相应的工作站软件的支持下利用来自螺旋 CT 的容积数据构造三维图像，这些三维图像可以实时旋转以便从不同角度观察病变，或者利用减影功能有选择性地去掉一些遮盖病变的血管和骨骼组织，以便更好地观察或模拟手术过程。这些方法包括表面遮蔽重建技术和容积重建技术，大多数用于大范围 CTA 检查或是外伤后骨的 VR 重组等。

（8）CT 血管造影（CTA）：也称螺旋 CT 血管造影，注入对比剂后，当对比剂在血循环和目标血管内达到最高峰时对其进行螺旋 CT 容积扫描，最后通过计算机将这些容积数据重建为目标血管的数字立体图像。这些成像方法包括表面遮蔽重建技术（SSD）和最大密度投影技术（MIP），前者可获得彩色图像。该技术多用于人体主要器官血管结构的显示。CTA 开创了螺旋 CT 在临床上应用的新领域，其优点有：①无需插管；②可从任何角度观察血管；③结合 MRI 可了解血管解剖以观察血管腔内的改变；④图像处理操作简捷，且能显示血管的细小分支（如左侧冠状动脉的对角支）。

（9）CT 仿真内镜检查（CTVE）：CT 仿真内镜检查是螺旋 CT 容积扫描和计算机仿真技术相结合的结果，通过对 CT 容积扫描的图像数据进行后处理重建，类似纤维内镜效果的腔器官内表面立体图像。

（10）CT 灌注：CT 灌注扩展了 CT 用途的新方向，是多层面断层成像技术的发展结合计算功能提高和高压注射器同步功能进步的结果。图像处理速度的提高除了提供详细的解剖图像外，使进一步研究组织的功能改变成为可能。采集过程包括团注含碘对比剂前和注入中立刻对选定的感兴趣区进行快速重复的扫描，因此灌注 CT 代表快速扫描技术与先进的计算机图像处理技术相结合的一种技术，可以反映组织富含血管度和灌注情况，以获得一些关于血流量的信息，所以它属于功能成像范畴。它的基本原理是在对比剂首过期对选定层面进行快速动态扫描获得一系列动态图像,通过分析首过期与每一像素相应的体素的密度变化,获得能反映血流灌注情况的参数以得到新的数字矩阵,该数字矩阵可以通过 D/A 转换转变为以相应的灰阶或颜色显示出来,获得灌注图像。因此碘基对比剂团注速度和时间分辨率是灌注 CT 面临的两个技术问题。灌注 CT 首先用于脑梗塞的诊断,然后应用于肝、肾、肿瘤的血流灌注分析。电子束 CT 灌注用于心脏灌注情况的评估以协助缺血性心脏病的早期诊断。

(11)双能 CT:双能 CT 通过两种不同能量的光子束穿透进行成像,利用不同物质能量吸收曲线的差异,能够准确地推算出该物体的成分构成。一般采用 140 kV 和 80 kV 两种不同的能级获取图像,临床上可用于显示尿酸盐结晶、结石成分定性分析、肌骨成像(显示肌腱、软骨和韧带)、肿瘤特征分析等。

(12)低剂量 CT 扫描:所谓低剂量 CT 是相对常规辐射的扫描方案,以采取降低管电压、管电流等方式来降低总的辐射剂量来实现的。最被人所熟悉的是肺部低剂量 CT 筛查。低剂量 CT 结合迭代重建技术可在减少放射剂量的同时保持影像质量。

(13)CT 透视:CT 透视是运用螺旋 CT 快速连续扫描实现实时显示被检组织的体层成像,图像显示率达 6 幅/秒,扫描速度达 2~8 层/秒,主要用于穿刺活检及介入治疗,显著提高了穿刺定位的准确性和效率。

(肖恩华,康振,梅习龙,罗志凌,谭长连)

Chapter 2

Computerized tomography

Computed tomography (CT) was the first non-invasive radiological method allowing the generation of tomographic images of every part of the human body without superimposition of adjacent structures. Even more importantly, a contrast resolution could be achieved that for the first time in radiology permitted the differentiation of soft tissue inside the highly attenuating skull. The technological improvements in the first and the latest 20 years of CT can best be characterized by a comparison of typical scan parameters from 1972, 1994, and 2019, as shown in Table 2.1. The greatest progress has been made in reducing scan times and in improving spatial resolution. At present, the low-dose CT scanning protocol is gradually applied in clinical practice, which can significantly reduce the radiation dose of patients. The following introduction of spiral CT, like other imaging modalities, has started to move from a slice-by-slice to a volume imaging method, with more isotropic spatial resolution in all three dimensions, allowing better three-dimensional representation of anatomical structures.

Table 2. 1 Technological Improvements in the First 20 Years of Computed Tomography

Scanner parameters	Typical Values, 1972	Typical Values, 1994	Typical Values, 2019
Matrix size	80×80	1024×1024	1024×1024
Spatial resolution	3 line pairs/cm	15 line pairs/cm	32line pairs/cm
Contrast resolution	5 mm/5 HU/50 mGy	3 mm/3 HU/30 mGy	2 mm/3 HU/12. 3 mGy
Scan time	5 min	<1 sec	66ms
Data size per scan	50 kByte	2 MByte	47 MByte
X-ray power	2 kW	40 kW	2×120 kW

Definitions: mGy = milligrays, where a gray is the SI unit for radiation dose. HU = Hounsfield units; the contrast scale used in CT is defined by zero attenuation (air) = −1000 HU and attenuation coefficient of water = 0 HU.

Historically, three contributors are most important: Radon, Hounsfield and Cormack. Reconstruction of a function from its projections was first formulated by Radon in 1917. The first experimental X-ray CT scanner was fabricated and tested by Hounsfield in 1972. An important contribution to the mathematics of X-ray CT was made by Cormack. Hounsfield and Cormack shared the 1979 Nobel Prize for medicine.

Section 1　Basic concepts

Compared with traditional X-ray films, CT images, which visualize tissue density distribution at a selected slice in the human body, are real tomographic images. It still uses X rays as projection sources and receives the value of the attenuated X-ray after human tissue absorption in different orientations at a selected slice. This value is imported into the computer by A/D transformer to get digital matrix about tissue attenuated coefficients of a selected slice, and these data from the digital matrix can be visualized on screen by different white-black degrees through D/A transformer. CT images possess characteristics of clearness, high resolution and no interference from the non-selective slice.

1. Voxel and pixel

CT images are tomography of a position inthe human body with a certain thickness. The imaging tomography can be divided into several small basic units according to matrix arrangement. The matter density within every small unit can be generally expressed by CT value, and these small units are named voxel. A CT image also composes of many small units according to matrix arrangement, these basic units are named pixels. The voxel is a 3-D concept, and the pixel is a 2-D concept. Pixel is the representation of voxel when imaging (see Figure 2-1). The smaller the pixel, the higher the image resolution.

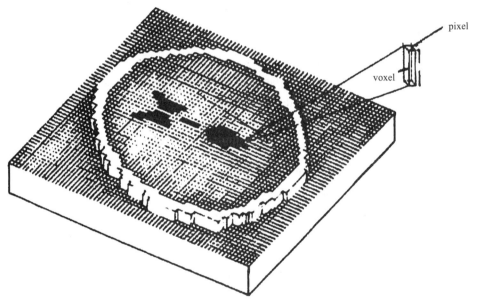

Figure 2-1 Pixel and voxel

2. Matrix

Matrix is a mathematical concept which represents ahorizontal and vertical digital array and divides the scanned slice into numerous cubes, namely pixel. If the image area is constant, the smaller the size of the pixel and the larger the matrix of CT images, the higher the definition of images.

3. Spatial resolution

The smallest detail that can be resolved in the image, also known as high contrast resolution, which is the ability of CT image to distinguish the material when the relative value of X-ray attenuation coefficient difference between the object and homogeneous environment is greater than 10%. Which is the capability of visualizing the geometrical shape of tissue under the prerequisite of ensuring a certain density difference. It's often expressed by the diameter of the smallest objects that can be differentiated.

The spatial resolution of a CT image depends on several factors, the main influencing are as follows:

(1)Size of the focal spot, which is the area on which the electrons hit the anode.

(2)Size of the detector elements: The size of the detector elements and the size of the focal spot determine the beam width.

(3)Collimators anterior and posterior to the patient, which determine the slice thickness.

(4)Reconstruction kernel (or convolution filter), which can be tuned to high frequencies (determining edges), or low frequencies (reduce noise and other artifacts).

(5)Better resolution can be obtained by:

1)Increasing the number of detectors.

2)Using a smaller pixel (or voxel) size, at the expense of more noise.

3)Using a reconstruction kernel with less smoothing, at the expense of more noise.

A typical modern CT machine has sub-mm in-plane resolution, and up to <1 mm axial resolution.

4. Density resolution

The minimum density difference that can be displayed. It's also named contrast resolution which is the capability of visualizing the small density difference between tissues in the case of low contrast. The CT density resolution is 10~20 times higher than that of conventional X rays.

5. Tempotal resolution

It originally refers to the number of frames of images collected by the imaging equipment in unit time. It is a performance parameter of the equipment and is related to the acquisition and reconstruction time of each frame of image, the display mode and the time and ability of continuous imaging. Specifically in CT imaging, it is the shortest time interval of body activity. It refers to the minimum time interval between two adjacent observations.

6. CT value

X-rays attenuated coefficients per unit volume, namely μ value, can be calculated afterX rays penetrated through the human body. The μ value can be converted into CT value to express tissue density as a unified unit.

The CT value of a matter is equal to the difference that the absorption coefficient of this matter (μm) minus the absorption coefficient of water (μw), and divided by μw, and multiplied by 1000. Its unit is named Hu (Hounsfield). Here is the formula calculating CT value of a matter: CT value = (μm−μw)/ μw×1000.

TheCT value limit of human tissues is 2000 Hu, the upper is the bone CT value (1000Hu), the lower is the air CT value (−1000 Hu).

7. Window width and window level

Window width represents the range of CT values, including 16 grey scales on screen. The range of CT values in human tissues is 2000 Hu (−1000~+1000). If 2000 different grey scales are used to represent 2000 Hu, the human eye cannot differentiate such a small difference (generally only 16 grey scales). If 16 grey scales are used to reflect 2000 Hu, the CT value difference that can be distinguished is 125 Hu (2000/16), namely, it is difficult to distinguish tissues with CT value difference less than 125 Hu. Different window width should be applied to observe images on the screen to improve visualization of detailed tissue structures and differentiate two tissues in which the CT value difference is small. For example, the distinguishable CT value is 6.25Hu (100/16) if the window width is 100, namely, it can differentiate two tissues if the CT value difference is larger than 6.25Hu.

Window level is also namedas a window center, the CT value of a matter can be viewed as a center to observe its tissue structures in detail. For example, the brain CT value is 35Hu, thus 35Hu can be chosen as the window level, whereas 100 Hu is often used as window width, the range of the CT value of 16 grey scales on screen is −15 ~85 Hu. The greyscale of tissues of which CT value is lower than −15 Hu is the same as −15 Hu, and the greyscale of tissues of which CT value is larger than 85Hu is the same as 85Hu, only tissues whose CT value range from −15 to 85 Hu can be visualized clearly in 16 grey scales.

On screen, increasing window width can increase image grey scales, but reduce tissue contrast and the ability of detail visualization poorly. If the window width is adjusted to the lowest, there are no grey scales inside the images and only black-white images. If the window level is increased, the images displayed on screen become dark, whereas if the window level is lowered, the images become white. Therefore, the window technique is very important to visualize lesions.

8. Artifacts

Image imperfections or artifacts observed in CT systems can be classified according to their origin:

(1) Physics-related causes

1) Quantum noise: Physically unavoidable spatial and temporal statistical variation of the X-ray beam intensity exist, and the more active ones will show up as signal-dependent noise in the projection data. A reduction of the noise level requires an increase in x-ray intensity or data acquisition time, along with an increase in patient dose. The signal dependency of the quantum noise leads to typical radial noise structures in the reconstructed images.

2) X-ray scattering by the patient: In fan-beam systems it is possible to use detectors that are sufficiently collimating to reduce the effect of scattering adequately. In detector ring based systems, however, mathematical scatter models have to be used to correct this effect.

3) Beam hardening: Simple empirical corrections are usually sufficient to compensate for this effect for all diagnostic purposes. In particular situations such as when the amount of bone in a particular slice is very large, residual beam hardening effects (e.g., the dark bands typically seen between the petrosal bones in head scans) may show up.

4) Nonlinear partial volume effects: As a consequence of the exponential, rather than nonlinear attenuation of radiation when high-contrast structures are immersed only partially in the imaged slice, the measured data become inconsistent with the mathematical model used for reconstruction. Although correction methods have been devised, they have not been widely accepted owing to the associated increase in expense, measurement time, and complexity. The simplest and most effective way to reduce nonlinear partial volume effects is to reduce the slice thickness.

(2) Patient-related effects

1) Movement of the patient or organs: Typical motion artifacts are striated or spotted. Their intensity is affected by the contrast of the moving organs. Although in the images these artifacts can usually be easily identified as motion-related, the combination of several artifacts can make it considerably more difficult to interpret the images. The most effective way to reduce motion artifacts, of course, is to speed up the data acquisition time accordingly.

2) Metallic foreign objects: Due to the strong attenuation of metal (for example, in dental -fillings), the dynamic range of the detector and data acquisition system is often not large enough to accurately accommodate the measurement of the projection data. To make things worse, in such a situation nonlinear partial volume effects usually amplify inconsistencies in the projection data. As a consequence, the images show streaking artifacts originating from the metallic objects.

(3) System-related causes

1) Insufficient calibration of detector sensitivity.

2) Time−, temperature−, or irradiation-history-dependent drift in detector sensitivity.

3) Inadequacies of the reconstruction algorithm.

4) Desynchrony of scanning and move.

5) Fluctuations of X-ray tube voltage.

All of the above errors will show up in the reconstructed images with different typical patterns that vary further with the scanning geometry employed. For example, detector-related problems in fan-beam systems usually manifest themselves as ring-shaped artifacts, whereas in systems based on stationary ring detectors they will have the character of streaks or stripes.

9. Partial volume effect

If there are two or more objects of different density within the same scanned slice, the measured CT value represents their average and does not accurately reflect the CT value of any object, this phenomenon is named partial volume effect.

Due to a finite beam aperture, every measurement represents an intensity that is averaged over the beam aperture. This average intensity is log-converted to give an effective beam attenuation. This value is always an underestimate of the actual attenuation. The larger the attenuation gradients perpendicular to the beam, the larger the underestimate, and this results in streaks tangent to edges.

Although lesions smaller than slice thickness can be displayed in CT images, the measured CT value cannot reflect the CT value of the lesions due to the partial volume effect. If the density of a lesion is higher than that of surrounding tissues and its thickness is less than slice thickness, the measured CT value of the lesion is less than itself, whereas if its density is lower than surrounding tissues and its thickness is less than slice thickness, the measured CT value is larger than itself. Therefore, the partial volume effect should be considered in the evaluation of small lesions in clinical diagnosis.

Section 2　The principles of CT imaging

1. CT imaging(Figure 2-2)

(1)Collection and transformation of x-ray scanning data

X rays will be absorbed to attenuate when passing through the human body, the degree of attenuation is related with tissues, organs and density (atomic ordinal number) of pathologicalchanges in a selected slice, the larger the density, the larger x-ray attenuation coefficient.

CT detectors convert attenuated X-ray signals into electrical signals, then these electrical signals can be converted into corresponding data signals to be imported into computers.

(2)Procession of scanned data and images reconstruction

The computers can adjust and process the imported original data to reconstruct images.

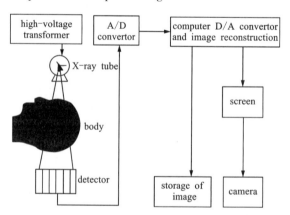

Figure 2-2　The principles of CT

(3)The display and storage of images

The data in reconstructed images matrix can be converted into different grey-scale light spots to form images, which can be displayed on the screen, as well as the films. It also can be printedin data by printer or recorded into tapes, compact disc and floppy disk for permanent storage.

2. Basic structures of CT scanner

CT scanner is mainly composed of X-ray tubes, detectors, collimators, A/D convertor, examining couch, high-voltages transformer, computer system and instruments for displaying, storing and exporting images.

(1)X-ray tubes

The dramatic increase in the performance of conventional-i. e. , nonelectron-beam based-CT scanners over the past 20 years has required significant improvements in the technology of the x-ray tubes used. Today, typically, a metal (tungsten-rhenium molybdenum) target is brazed to a thick graphite block for improved heat dissipation. Target diameters of up to 20 cm are used with rotational speeds of up to 10, 000 rpm. Typically the target is operated at a temperature of 1200℃ and the area around the focal spot reaches over 2500℃. The maximum heat dissipation of these tubes can reach up to 10 kW. Still, the major limitation in the use of CT scanners imposed by the x-ray tube is the maximum permissible sustained x-ray power. A further increase will require major developments in target cooling (e. g. , liquid cooled-rotating targets), bearing systems, and generation of the electron beam.

(2)Detector systems

There are two types of detector systems employed with CT. Both types of systems are usually arranged in linear arrays with up to about 1, 000 detector elements or as rings with even more elements in the case of systems with a geometry. Commercial spiral CT detector has been developed to 320 rows of wide body. 320 rows of adjacent detection elements can scan the 16 cm range at the same time. For scintillation based detectors the most commonly used scintillator materials have been cesium iodide (CsI) and cadmium tungstate, as well as ceramic scintillators employing rare-earth oxides and oxysul_des. A particularly critical parameter for CT detector scintillators is their afterglow behavior. Since CT data acquisition systems do not use pulse counting as in most nuclear applications, but rather integrate the detector current, the afterglow leads to measurement errors near tissue/air and tissue/bone interfaces. Data correction schemes have been developed to at least compensate for first-order effects related to the detector afterglow. Compared to the rare-gas ionization detector, the scintillation detector usually has a lower geometric efficiency (ratio of active versus ineffective frontal area), which is, however, generally more than compensated for by the latter's higher quantum efficiency. In fan beam systems a collimator is usually employed in front of the scintillator elements to reduce the effects of scattered x-rays. In gas detector arrays the chamber walls effectively serve the same purpose by acting as a collimator aligned with the position of the x-ray focal spot. This self-collimating effect of gas detectors, on the other hand, excludes their application in ring detector based systems, since the focal spot of the x-ray tube moves relative to the detector elements.

(3)Collimator

Collimator locates between the outlet of x-ray tubes and the input of the detectors receiving x rays. Pre-and post-patient collimators restrict the filtered X-ray beam to the anatomy of interest. The width of collimator aperture, which can adjusted with the scope of 1~10 mm, decides the slice thickness.

(4)A/D convertor

(5)Examination couch

The main function of the examination table is to move the examinee into the scanning hole. During the scanning process of the part to be scanned, the couch of conventional CT scanner moves horizontally by steps, and the couch of spiral CT moves horizontally by uniform motion.

(6)High-voltage transformer

It mainly provides high voltage for theX-ray tubes.

（7）Computer system

There are two main computer systems in CT: 1）Main computer; 2）Array computer. The main computer is responsible for running control of the whole system, including the movements of X-ray tubes, detectors, collimator and couch; X-rays production; the production and collection of data; information exchange between parts. The array computer is responsible for the reconstruction of images.

（8）The instruments for images displaying, storing and exporting

Section 3　Development of CT scanners

Before the invention of spiral CT in the late 1980s, the development of CT was usually called "generation". After the advent of spiral CT, it is no longer called several generations of CT, but replaced by single row spiral, multi row spiral, energy spectrum, dual source and so on.

1. The first generation

The first generation of X-ray CT naturally entailed the first EMI scanner developed by Hounsfield. This scanner used a single pencil beam and a single detector, which translated and rotated synchronously. There was translational motion across the object being scanned, and at the end of each translational motion an incremental 1° rotation followed in preparation for the upcoming scanning. The collection of a set of projection data needed for tomographic image reconstruction of a slice usually took several minutes. Features of the first generation of CT scanner: Low ray utilization rate; Single pencil beam; Single detector; Translation-rotation-translation; Several minutes acquisition time.

2. The second generation

The design of the second generation CT incorporated a small-angle fan-beam X-ray and an array of multiple detectors. Since the diverging fan beams passing through the patient increased data collection channels, the number of angular rotations required could be reduced. Therefore the scan time in this second generation scanner was shortened substantially, the normal scan time was approximately 20 sec. The second-generation scanner still entailed translational motion as well as rotational motion in order to cover the object fully.

（1）Features of the second generation CT scanner: Single small-angle fan beam; Detector array; Translation （smaller）-rotation （fewer）-translation; 20 sec acquisition time.

（2）Advantages: Shorter time, higher matrix （smaller detector aperture）.

（3）Disadvantages: The detector is arranged in a straight line, and the ray beam to the middle and both sides of the detector is asymmetric, so ray calibration is required to avoid artifacts.

3. The third generation

In the third generation the fan-beam angle was widened, thereby allowing the fan to cover the entire object to be scanned. Each projection path is defined by a matching detector, which can be either a small and narrow Scintillation detector slab or a segment of a gas ionization chamber. Because the entire object is covered or encompassed, no translational movement is required. Therefore both the X-ray tube and the detector array need only Simple rotational motion around a fixed axial center. The entire 360° is usually scanned for whole data collection. The scan time can be as short as 1 to 3 sec. The major drawback of this configuration is that the effects of the drift of the detectors are cumulative, so artifacts appear in the reconstruction image. Almost all third-generation scanners use pulsed X-ray sources in order to take advantage of significant dead time between successive views. Figure 2-3 illustrates the configuration of the third-generation CT scanner. （1）Features of the third generation CT scanner: Single wide-angle fan beam; Detector array; Rotation of source-detector pair only （no translation）；1-3 sec acquisition time

　（2）Advantages：The time is shortened to 2 ~ 9 seconds, and there is no need for ray calibration（the distance between the ray and the detector is equal）.（3）Disadvantages：Prone to ring artifacts.

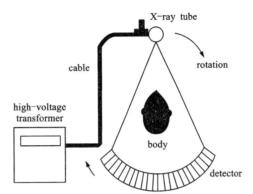

Figure 2-3　The third generation of CT

4. The fourth generation

　The construction of a stationary circular ring detector array is probably the ideal choice for a rotating X-ray source. A striking analogy is the circular ring PET scanners of various types developed during the 1970s. This stationary ring is the most distinct feature of the fourth-generation X-ray CT. The X-ray source rotates, but the detector array does not. A wide-angle fan-beam X-ray encompasses the entire patient, and 600 or more stationary detectors form a circular ring array. With this kind of configuration, detector drift is not cumulative and therefore can be corrected. The advantages of this system are similar to those of the third-generation systems, but the main drawback of the third-generation systems, the drift effects, have been eliminated since detector drifts no longer accumulate over successive views. The fourth-generation systems are generally more expensive due to the large number of scintillation detectors and PMTs are employed. The speed of fourth-generation scanners allows for the synchronized rotational motion with physiological signals such as that obtained from electrocardiograph（ECG）when the imaging of moving organs is required.（1）Features of the fourth generation CT scanner：Single wide-angle fan beam；Ring detector array；Rotation of source only（no translation）.（2）Advantages：The fan-shaped angle of the ball tube is 50 ~ 90 ° to avoid concentric ring artifacts.（3）Disadvantages：Cost increases since only parts of detector work in each angle.

5. The fifth generation

　The fifth generation CT scanner is also named ultrafast CT or electron beam CT（EBCT）. It's mainly composed of electronic gun, focusing coils, deflecting coils, groups of multi-rows detectors, high-speed moving couch and control system（shown in Figure 2-4）. It applies electron beam to passing through human body and can be detected by detectors after energy attenuation, and then forms a image as same as the conventional CT image by A/D convertion and D/A convertion. It has no tubes and detectors movement different from conventional CT. Electron beam（ultrafast）computerized tomography is to date one of the fastest modalities to provide sectional images. The fastest scanning speed is 0. 05 second per slice, so it can finish many tasks that conventional CT cannot finish.（1）Features of the fifth generation CT scanner：It's particularly useful to evaluate bypass graft patency, intra-and congenital cardiac lesions, and quantify right and left ventricular muscle mass, chamber volumes, and systolic and diastolic function（such as cardiac output and ejection fraction）, and detect the calcium deposition in coronary arteries.（2）Advantages：High temporal resolution, effective reduction of motion artifacts.

（3）Disadvantages：Heavy frame，complex structure，difficult maintenance and exorbitant price.

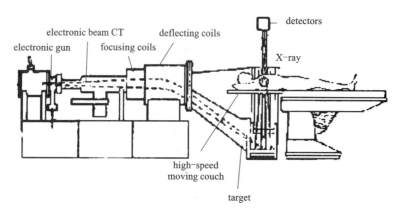

Figure 2-4　The electron beam CT

6. The spiral CT

The reconstruction of images with arbitrary position and spacing, including overlapping reconstruction improved three-dimensional displays. Further, the improvement in rapidly covering larger volumes in spiral CT allows a better and more comfortable use of breath-holding techniques for improved imaging of internal organs that are susceptible to respiratory motion. Thus spiral CT, in particular, has improved the assessment of pulmonary nodules, has significantly increased the quality of three-dimensional surface-rendering type image representations, and with the use of contrast agents for the first time has allowed the display of vascular structures with previously unachievable quality. The main limitation in spiral CT image quality today still is due to the available sustained power from theX-ray tube. While 40 kW are available typically for single scans, the power has to be reduced for spiral scans of 30 seconds and more to avoid overloading of the tube. As a result of the associated increase in quantum noise, soft tissue images frequently have to be reconstructed with smoothing convolution kernels. On the other hand, because of the high contrast of bone structures, the full spatial resolution can be made available for orthopedic examinations employing thin slice width settings. Blurring of the images in the direction of the patient's movement through the gantry can be minimized by appropriate choices for the table motion, and by reconstructing images for every 180℃ of scanner rotation rather than using the customary 360° scan coverage. Depending on the specific imaging situation, table feed values of one to two times the slice thickness per 360° of scanner rotation are being used today (see Figure 2-5). Single-slice scanning will then be the exception. Required technical improvements will have to come in the available sustained x-ray power, as well as in the advances in computation time expected through increased processor performance. Another important impact of future technological developments will come from the use of multislice detectors or planar detector arrays extending over a larger solid angle, thus allowing better use of the available x-ray power and covering larger volumes within a given time. Such detectors are considered a most important future development. Depending on the technology employed, these detectors possibly will also allow improvement of the spatial resolution in the scanner axis direction.

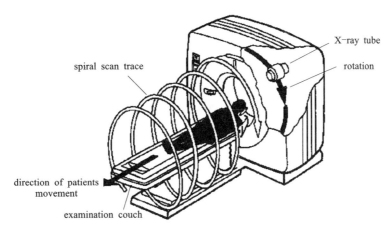

spiral scan trace

X-ray tube

rotation

direction of patients
movement

examination couch

Figure 2-5 Scan of spiral CT

Section 4 CT examination methods and clinical applications

1. Non-contrast scan or pre-contrast scan

It refers to the scan during which contrast media is not injected intothe blood vessel. In general, transverse scanning is often considered, and sometimes coronal scanning. The slice thickness is 1~10 mm. When scanning, the patient remained in a fixed position. After spiral CT volume scanning, a thin layer of about 1 mm was reconstructed and used for multiplanar reconstruction (MPR) and curved surface reconstruction (CPR). Negative contrast agent (such as water) should be taken orally during abdominal scan.

2. Post-contrast scan

It refers to the scan during which contrast media is injected into the blood vessel. The purpose is to improve the density difference between lesions and normal tissues to display lesions not displayed or poorly displayed on non-contrast scanning images. It can make a qualitative diagnosis of lesions according to whether the lesions are enhanced or the type of enhancement.

3. CT contrast examination

Contrast examination represents a method that scans an organ or a structure after contrast examination, which can better visualize structures and find lesions, such as myelography CT, cystography CT et al. However, this method is scarcely used in clinical practice now. .

4. Special scans

（1）Thin-slice scan

Its purpose is to observe the details of some lesions and avoid partial volume effect, for example, a thin-slice scan should be considered when observing small spherical lesions in the lung.

（2）Overlapping scan

The distance the examination table moves is less than slice thickness, for example, if the slice thickness is 10 mm, and the distance the examination table moves is 8 mm, it can make scanning slices overlap partially to avoid partial volume effect or missed diagnosis. The disadvantage is that too much overlap can lead to an increase in X-ray exposure.

(3) CT-targeted scanning

It's also named target CT scanning or magnifying CT scanning, which can perform local CT scanning of the region of interest by using small FOV (field of view) and thin slice(1~5 mm). It can improve spatial resolution greatly and mainly used in scanning of small organs or lesions, such as pulmonary nodules, pituitary and adrenal gland.

(4) High-resolution CT (HRCT)

If applying thin-slice with sharper or sharpest reconstruction method (or bone arithmetic reconstruction) and special filtrating process to obtain images of microstructure of tissues, this technique is called high-resolution CT (HRCT). HRCT is mainly used in pulmonary diffuse lesions and nodular lesions, bone arithmetic reconstruction mainly used in temporal bone CT scanning to visualize the micro-structures of inner ears and the middle ear auditory ossicular chain.

(5) Delayed CT (DCT)

DCT represents repeated scans with delays of minutes or hours after contrast media injection. For example, to make a qualitative diagnosis of hepatic cavernous hemangioma, it is necessary to delay the scanning for several minutes or half an hour, and for small hepatocellular carcinoma, it should be delayed for 4-8 hours. Because iodine contrast media is mainly excreted through the kidney, but 10% through the liver. Normal liver cells have the function of iodine absorption and excretion, and their CT value can increase by 1~10 Hu after 4~6 hours after contrast media injection, while liver cancer cells do not possess such this function.

(6) Dynamic CT scan

It means a method to use machine software to perform continuous rapid scanning after contrast media injection, then process and display images one by one after scanning. The dynamic scan can be classified into two types. In addition to finding the lesions, cradle in and out large-scale continuous dynamic scanning and single organ continuous dynamic scanning can better evaluate the nature of the lesions.

(7) Three dimensional CT (3DCT)

This method means to utilize volume data from spiral CT to construct 3D images under the support of workstation software, these 3D images can be rotated in real-time to observe lesions from different angles; or use subtraction function to selectively remove some blood vessels and bones covering lesions to further observe and imitate operation procedure. The common methods include shaded surface display (SSD) and volume-rendering technique. Most of them are used for large-scale CTA examination or VR reconstruction after trauma.

(8) CT angiography (CTA)

Also called spiral CT angiography (SCTA), a technique which performs spiral CT volume scanning when the concentration of contrast media within blood circulation and target vessels arrives at the peak after contrast media injection, and finally reconstruct these volume data into digitalized cubic images through a computer. These imaging methods include SSD and maximum intensity projection (MIP), the former can obtain color images. This kind of technique is mostly used in visualizing vasculatures in the main organs of the body. CTA opened up a new field of clinical application of spiral CT, which has the following advantages: 1) Do not need catheterization; 2) Observation of vessels from any angle; 3) Dissecting blood vessels to observe luminal changes combining with MR images; 4) The operation of image processing is simple, and it can show the small branches of blood vessels (such as the diagonal branch of the left coronary artery).

(9) CT virtual endoscopy (CTVE)

CTVE is a resultof a combination of spiral CT volume scanning and computer simulation technology. It can perform post-processing of images data from CT volume scanning to reconstruct surface cubic images of lumen organs similar to fibre endoscopy.

（10）CT perfusion

CT perfusion expands the new direction of CT application. It is the result of the development and deployment of multi-slice computed tomography (MSCT) technology combined with increased computing power and synchronized high-pressure injectors. In addition to more detailed anatomic imaging, improved speed and processing make it possible to study the functional changes of tissues. The acquisition procedure includes rapid, repetitive scanning of a defined region of interest before and immediately after the injection of a bolus of iodine contrast agent. Therefore, perfusion CT represents a technology combining rapid scanning technology with advanced computer image processing technology. It can reflect the vascularity and blood perfusion of tissues to obtain information about blood flow, so it belongs to the scope of functional imaging. Its basic principle is to perform rapid dynamic scanning of a selected slice during the first pass of contrast agent and obtain sequential dynamic images, then analyzes the density change of each voxel corresponding to every pixel during the first pass of contrast agent and gets parameters reflecting blood perfusion to obtain new digital matrix, which can be transformed through D/A converting into corresponding greyscales or colors to get perfusion imaging. So the injecting speed of a bolus of iodine contrast agent and high temporal resolution are two technical questions of CT perfusion imaging. Perfusion CT was first used in the diagnosis of cerebral infarction and then the blood perfusion of the liver and kidneys, neoplasms. Electron beam CT perfusion imaging can be used in evaluating cardiac perfusion to help the early diagnosis of ischemic heart diseases.

（11）Dual-energy CT

Dual-energy CT imaging can accurately calculate the composition of the object through two different energy photon beams and the difference of energy absorption curve of different substances. Two different energy levels of 140KV and 80KV are generally used to obtain the image. Clinically, it can be used to display urate crystals, qualitative analysis of stone components, musculoskeletal imaging (showing tendons, cartilage and ligaments), and tumor characteristics analysis, etc.

（12）Low dose CT scan

The so-called low-dose CT is achieved by reducing tube voltage and tube current to reduce the total radiation dose compared with the conventional scanning scheme. It is best known for low-dose CT screening of the lungs. Low-dose CT combined with iterative reconstruction can reduce radiation dosewhile maintaining image quality.

（13）CT fluoroscopy

CT fluoroscopy is the application of spiral CT rapid continuous scanning to realize real-time display of the body tomography of the examined tissues, with the image display rate up to 6 images per second and the scanning speed up to 2-8 slices per second. It is mainly used for puncture biopsy and interventional therapy, significantly improving the accuracy and efficiency of puncture positioning.

（Xiao Enhua, Kang Zhen, Mei Xilong, Luo Zhiling, Tan Changlian）

第三章

磁共振成像

核磁共振（NMR）或称磁共振成像（MRI）是一项新的无创性检查技术，主要应用于描绘人体的内部结构，并可获得人体内部结构的高质量图像，它完全没有电离辐射，目前看来对人体无任何明显的危害。MRI 基于核磁共振、波谱技术的原理，从而获取分子结构微弱的化学和物理信息。该技术之所以称为磁共振成像而非核磁共振成像，是因为 20 世纪 70 年代后期"核"这个词汇的负面涵义。MRI 初期作为一种体层成像技术，获取人体薄层 NMR 信号图像。目前 MRI 已从体层成像技术发展为三维成像技术。

简单地回顾 MRI 的发展史有助于我们学习 MRI。1946 年 Bloch F 和 Purcell E 分别发现磁共振现象，1952 年两人因此获诺贝尔奖。1950 至 1970 年期间，NMR 用于分子结构的化学和物理分析。1971 年 Damadian R 发现正常组织和肿瘤的核磁弛豫时间有差别，因此激励了科学家研究将磁共振用于疾病的检测。1973 年 Hounsfield 发明基于 X 线的计算机辅助体层（CT），医院愿意花巨资购买医疗影像设备，从而刺激了 MRI 的发展。同年，Lauterbur P 采用类似于 CT 的背投技术完成小试管内样本的磁共振成像。1975 年 Ernst R 将相位、频率编码和傅利叶转换这些现代 MRI 技术的基础应用于磁共振成像。1977 年 Damadian R 推出了全身 MRI，同年 Mansfield P 发明了平面回波成像（EPI）技术，在随后数年内该技术的成像速度达到电视速度（30 毫秒/帧），1980 年 Edelstein 与同事采用 Ernst 的技术获得人体的图像，一帧图像约需时 5 分钟，到 1986 年成像时间降至 5 秒左右，而且对图像质量的影响不大。同年，发展中的 NMR 波谱在约 1 cm 大小的样本上能获得 10μm 的空间分辨率。1987 年平面回波成像能在单个心动周期内获取实时电影成像。同年，Dumoulin C 完善了磁共振血管成像（MRA），MRA 不需对比剂而获得流动血流的图像。1991 年 Ernst R 因将脉冲傅利叶转换运用于 NMR 和 MRI 方面的成就而获得诺贝尔化学奖。1993 年功能 MRI（fMRI）得到发展，该技术可将人脑各部位的功能信息图像化，平面回波成像出现的头 6 年内多数临床医生认为其主要用途在心脏的实时成像，fMRI 的发展使 EPI 有了新的用途，如脑的思维、运动控制区的描绘。1994 年，纽约洲立大学、斯托尼布鲁克和普林斯顿大学的研究人员作了极化 12q 硒气成像用于呼吸系统的研究，很显然，MRI 仍是一支年轻而生气勃勃的学科。

第一节　磁共振成像系统的基本组成

所有 MRI 成像仪均由巨大磁体，其内的梯度线圈、适当大小的 RF（射频）发射和接收线圈及辅助设备组成，可产生和分析 MRI 信号并最后获得图像。一般来说，MRI 成像仪由主磁体、梯度系统、射频系统、线圈、计算机系统及其他辅助设施组成。

1. 主磁体

主磁体产生静磁物场，MRI 对磁场的强度、稳定性和均匀性有严格的要求。目前用于成像的磁场强度为 0.5 至 11.7 特斯拉（T），该磁场强度对人体健康无害，且能获得良好质量的图像。磁场均匀性是要求在较大的空间内磁场强度相差范围为 $10^{-4} \sim 10^{-6}$（百万分之几，ppm）。磁场稳定性是指磁场不同时期的变化率，短期稳定性要求在几个 ppm/h 以内，长期稳定性在 10 ppm/h 以内。非常均匀和稳定的强磁场对高质量的图像至关重要。

磁体有三种：永久磁体、超导磁体即阻抗磁体和超导磁体。

阻抗磁体由许多线圈组成，电流通过线圈产生磁场，关闭电源则磁场消失。这种磁体的制造成本低于超导磁体，但开机时因线圈存在电阻故电流消耗明显，0.3T 的阻抗磁体开机时电流消耗巨大。

永久磁体意如其名，磁场永远存在且强度不变，维持磁场不需成本。其主要缺点为磁体非常重，0.4T 的磁体重达数吨，难以制造强度较大的磁体，较小的永久磁体则限制了磁场强度。

超导磁体是目前最常用的，超导磁体有点类似于阻抗磁体，与阻抗磁体比较其主要的差别在于线圈浸泡于零下 268.8° 的液氦内，如果你在 MRI 机器里面，你的唯一感觉就是冷，不过别担心，磁体被真空很好地隔离。线圈在如此低温的情况下，耗电量减少，开机成本显著下降。超导磁体的制造成本仍很高，但很容易达到 0.5T 至 3.0T 的高场强，从而获得更高质量的图像。

2. 梯度系统

MRI 系统内另一种磁体称为梯度磁体。MRI 机内有三组梯度线圈，各负责 z、x、y 方向。梯度线圈在主磁场内用于产生精确的场强变化，与主磁场比较梯度磁场的强度很小，180 至 270 高斯即 18 至 27 毫特斯拉（特斯拉的千分之几），梯度磁场的变化可作图像层面的定位以及相位、频率编码。

3. 射频系统

射频系统是用于发射射频脉冲的一组装置。质子吸收能量后被激发、产生并获取 MR 信号。射频系统包括发射和接收两部分，由发射器、放大器、发射线圈、接收线圈和低噪信号放大器等组成。射频线圈是 MRI 系统的"天线"，它发射射频信号给患者并接收返回的信号。射频线圈也可仅为接收信号之用，而由体线圈作为发射器，或发射和接收均由体线圈完成（发射接收器）。在成像仪中带有内置发射线圈的射频（RF）发射器，使用高灵敏度的 RF 接收器来接受和放大 MR 信号。或者也可以使用在发射和接收模式之间切换的单个 RF 线圈。

4. 计算机图像处理系统

计算机图像处理系统的作用是将 MRI 扫描所获得的资料进行处理并形成图像。为了完成资料采集、图像处理和显示，必须配置大功率计算机和高分辨模数转换器。模数转移器将探测器传入的模拟信号转换为数字信号以形成体层图像资料，数模转换器再以不同灰阶或颜色的形式显示图像。各种用于控制扫描仪和梯度的计算机（控制计算机），用于创建 MR 图像（阵列处理器），以及用于协调所有过程（与操作员控制台和图像档案相连的主计算机）。

5. 附加成像线圈

附加成像线圈包括接收线圈或者发射/接受线圈。

6. 其他外围设备

其他外围设备，例如检查床控制，心电（ECG）设备和专门的 MRI 序列的呼吸触发监测，磁体的冷却系统，操作员控制副台（例如用于图像处理），用于打印胶片的设备，或 PACS（图片存档和通信系统）。

第二节　磁共振成像的原理

某些原子具有磁偶极运动，源于原子的电荷和角运动即自旋。氢质子就是具有磁偶极运动的原子核，具有广泛的生物学关联。磁共振成像的基础就是控制磁偶极运动，从而产生信号而获取人体的图像。当一个质子放置在一个强大恒定的外加磁场中，质子的偶极运动将平行于外加磁场，自旋的质子其偶极运动维持圆圈运动称之为进动，质子本身的自旋轴与外加磁场方向轴成角旋转，这种现象最简单的比喻就是具有自旋轴的陀螺绕地球引力缓慢旋转（图 3-1）。由于质子的偶极运动在任一特定时间都具有其方向和强度，即具有一定的向量，向量由两部分组成：与进动轴一致的纵向成份和垂直于外加磁场方向的横向成份，质子按一定的进动频率旋转。进动频率称为拉莫（Larmor）频率，与外加磁场的强度有关，可由简单公式 $W = rT$ 表示，其中 W 代表进动频率，T 代表磁场强度，r 代表每种原子的特定常数（旋磁率）。

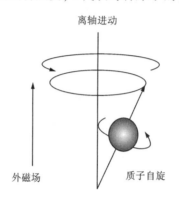

图 3-1　在磁场中的质子进动

事实上，在外加磁场中顺应磁场方向的偶极运动质子处于低能态，逆外加磁场方向的则处于高能态（图 3-2）。高、低能态质子的相应分配决定于样本的温度和外加磁场的强度，这些所谓"上旋"（低能态）与"下旋（高能态）质子的数量差异产生了净磁化。体温状态下质子的净磁化强度很小，低能态质子仅略多于高能态质子（百万分之几）。为方便起见用矢量描述质子的净磁化。

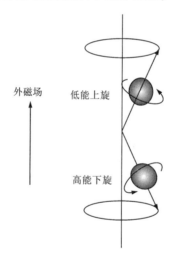

图 3-2　磁场中质子自旋方向

机体或组织置入强磁场中，数秒内就产生净磁距。采用一个垂直于外磁场且为拉莫频率的电磁脉冲将打破质子的平衡状态，自旋频率在射频频率范围内的质子产生所谓共振，射频脉冲的能量将传递给磁场中的进动质子，这些质子获能后有两个结果：一是为随着这些质子偶极运动的方向相应改变，低能态质子跃迁为高能态，于是纵向净磁矩减小（由于上旋与下旋质子数量的差别减小）；二是为射频脉冲使所有质子产生同相进动，从而产生横向净磁矩并以拉莫频率旋转。因此，使用射频的结果是净磁矩的纵向分量减小而横向分量增加。当给予的射频能量足够大时，纵向分量又开始增加，但其方向将与外磁场相反，此时横向分量又相应减小。

关闭射频脉冲后，质子从射频脉冲获得的能量被释放，从而恢复原来的平衡状态。能量释放称为弛豫，探测其释放的能量是产生 MR 成像信号的基础。净磁矩的纵向分量和横向分量弛豫速度不同，纵向分量恢复至原先的平衡状态的过程表现为指数曲线，可用时间常数 T1 来表示。横向分量衰减至原先的平衡状态同样呈指数曲线，而用时间常数 T2 来表示。两种弛豫过程反映了进动质子与其局部环境之间互相作用的两种不同类型，T1 弛豫是能量释放过程，质子从高能态恢复至低能态，能量从质子转移给周围的分子称之为晶格，T1 弛豫称为自旋—晶格弛豫。反之，T2 弛豫是质子自旋相干性的丧失，相干性是由于质子之间、质子与其他具磁性运动的核子之间的相互作用改变了局部磁场的均匀性，即均匀磁场的固有稳定性，因为涉及其他核子的互相作用，T2 弛豫称之为自旋—自旋弛豫。由于生物组织和体液的组成和结构的不同，T1 和 T2 弛豫时间差别相当明显。

MRI 信号强度主要取决于三个参数：①组织内质子的密度（质子密度越大信号越强）；②T1 弛豫时间；③T2 弛豫时间。组织间的视觉对比取决于组织间这些参数的差别，体内大多数软组织间的对比明显。通过改变核子的电磁能从而控制 MR 信号，改变三个参数对图像信号的影响程度：质子密度、T1 和 T2，可选用许多 MR 成像技术（权重）以观察组织某些特性。

敏感的接收器采集机体组织的信号，计算机系统分析处理并将获得的可视图像显示在屏幕上。获得图像后，可选择性地重点显示某组织或人体某部分。图像重建技术可将常规的灰阶图像转换为彩色图像、表面三维模拟图像或组织、器官及人体某部位图像。几种典型 MRI 图像（头、颈、肾脏）见图 3-3。

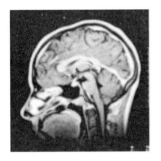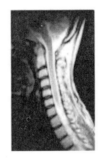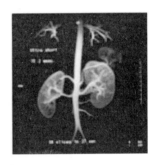

图 3-3 头、颈、肾脏的 MRI 图像

第三节 射频脉冲序列

1. 自旋回波序列

自旋回波脉冲序列是最常用的脉冲序列。通过调节脉冲序列的变量可获得 T1 加权、质子即自旋密度和 T2 加权像，双回波和多回波系列可同时获得质子密度和 T2 加权像。

自旋回波序列两个重要的变量是重复时间（TR）和回波时间（TE），所有自旋回波序列包括先发射一个选层的 90°射频脉冲，继而再发射一个或多个 180°重聚射频脉冲（图 3-4）。

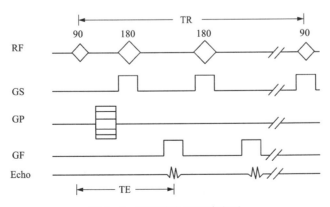

图 3-4 双回波自旋回波序列

2. 反转回复序列

反转回复序列可获得重 T1 加权像。此外，STIR(短 TI 反转回复)序列可用于脂肪抑制，该序列采用很短的反转时间以抑制脂肪信号，而水和软组织信号不受影响。反转回复序列的基本组成为先发射 180° 射频脉冲将磁化翻转，继之 90° 射频脉冲将剩余的纵向磁化转为 X~Y 轴即横向磁化，从而使射频线圈能检测信号，成像时通常再给一个类似于自旋回波 180° 射频脉冲使信号重聚，第一个 180° 射频脉冲与 90° 射频脉冲之间的时间称为反转时间(TI)。5T 的 MRI 机 TI 为 140ms 左右时，脂肪信号被抑制，而水的质子信号保留，这是因为脂肪的 TI 显著小于水的 TI。

3. 梯度回波序列

梯度回波序列(图 3-5)与自旋回波和反转回复序列比较种类更多。其基本序列的变化可在序列末加去相或聚相梯度、改变 TR 和 TE 及脉冲翻转角。自旋回波序列的脉冲翻转角一般接近 90°，而梯度回波序列的脉冲翻转角可在 10°~80° 之间选择。梯度回波的基本序列 FLASH 如图 3-5 所示。采用较大的翻转角而获取准 T1 图像，较小的翻转角获取准 T2 图像。

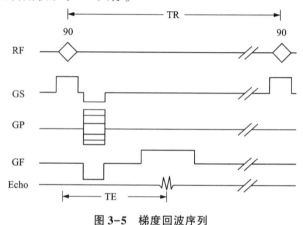

图 3-5　梯度回波序列

其他的梯度回波序列例如 GRASS 和 FISP，其组织对比特征不如 FLASH 直观。FLASH 和 SPGR 序列比较 GRASS 和 FISP 序列，前两者对脑和脊髓的灰白质对比优于后两者，采集时间略长时尤为如此。短 TR 时间的 GRASS 和 FISP 序列的 SNR(倍躁比)优于 FLASH 序列，故适合呼吸门控技术时使用。

4. 平面回波脉冲序列

平面回波成像是与梯度回波相关的快速梯度回波成像，在单个 TR 采集时间内获取整套 64 或 128 个回波信号。平面回波序列可以采用整套梯度回波，也可采用一个自旋回波加梯度回波链如图 3-6 所示。平面回波成像可短于 1/10 秒，因而可用于心脏成像和其他快速成像，如弥散成像和灌注成像。

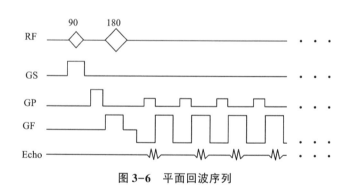

图 3-6　平面回波序列

第四节 磁共振波谱学

活体生物组织的磁共振波谱学(MRS)首先由两组科学家报道:Moon 和 Richards 1973 年使用^{31}P-MRS 检查鼠的腿肌运动。由此开始 MRS 检查几乎遍及所有器官,包括脑、心脏、肝、肾、前列腺和肢体。MRS 有助于检查代谢性疾患、肿瘤、一些炎症性和缺血性疾病。人类活体的 MRS 主要运用于脑,MRS 时常先于除活检外的其他诊断手段,包括原发性脑肿瘤、炎症,如 AIDS、脱髓鞘疾病、多发性硬化、癫痫和脑血管意外。

MRS 敏感的原子核,例如氢(^{1}H),碳(^{13}C),氟(^{19}F)和磷(^{31}P)等,氢质子波谱最有价值的优点在于同样的硬件不仅能进行波谱成像,而且能进行磁共振成像,此外,氢谱比磷谱敏感 7 倍。

可以通过^{1}H MRS 方法进行研究的代谢物,包括但不限于 N-乙酰天门冬氨酸(NAA)、胆碱(Cho)、肌酸(Cr)、乳酸、谷氨酸(Glu)、谷氨酰胺(Gln)和脂质。

MRS 的临床应用包括对肿瘤生化变化的连续评估,分析代谢紊乱,感染和疾病以及评估肿瘤复发与放射损伤的治疗方法。早期的应用专门用于脑部疾病,但是现在还进行了乳腺、肝脏和前列腺的 MRS 波谱结果与 MR 影像的相关性

在作出最终诊断之前,始终作为参考的^{31}P-MRS 磷谱中的主要代谢物信号是磷酸化形式的单峰肌酸(Cr),即磷酸肌酸(PCr)。PCr 中的高能磷酸盐键充当快速可用的能量储备,当能量增加支出时,准备补充催化的能量来自三磷酸腺苷(ATP)。ATP 包含三个非等价的磷酸基团(α-、β-和 γ-)的共振频率不同,在^{31}P-MRS 波谱中产生三个单独的信号。作为磷酸盐,ATP 中的核与附近的其他自旋相互作用,即经历所谓的同核 J 耦合,ATP 信号的线分裂可以观察到 α-和 γ-ATP 形成双峰,β-ATP 形成三重峰。在^{31}P-MRS 波谱中可见的另一个重要的代谢产物是无机磷酸盐(Pi),它也可以作为能量代谢化学反应的底物或产物。其他可检测的^{31}P 代谢产物包括细胞膜前体,即磷酸单酯(PME)和细胞膜降解产物,即磷酸二酯(PDE)。体内 PME 信号中主要贡献者是磷酸胆碱(PC)和磷酸乙醇胺(PE),而主要的 PDE 是甘油磷酸胆碱(GPC)和甘油-磷酸乙醇胺(GPE)

波谱改变见于多种酶缺乏、线粒体异常、营养不良、炎性肌病和甲状腺疾病,肌病包括磷酸果糖素缺乏、淀粉酵素缺乏、Duchenne 肌营养不良、Becker 肌营养不良、皮肌炎;多肌炎包括全肌炎、甲状腺功能减低症(甲低)和充血性心衰。

磁共振波谱学检查可使用多种脉冲序列,最简单的序列包括一个 90°的 RF 脉冲,不使用梯度场,每个 RF 脉冲后立即由 RF 线圈采集信号。许多成像序列也可用于波谱检查(比如自旋回波序列),成像序列与波谱序列的重要差别是后者的 RF 线圈在采集信号时不使用读出梯度场,而使用频率信息(由读出或频率梯度场提供)以提供空间或位置信息,频率信息用于确定不同的化合物,这是因为不同的化合物其周围的电子云对波谱成像的共振原子屏蔽程度不同,而屏蔽程度则取决于特定的化合物以及共振原子在化合物内的特定位置,电子屏蔽导致原子共振频率有细微的差异,因此 MRS 能确定不同的化合物。

MRS 利用不同的化学物质当磁场刺激时其震动频率不同(像音叉)而成像。MRS 检测信号既类似于 MRI 而获取脑或人体其他组织图像(图 3-7 示前列腺癌的波谱成像),也类似于功能 MRI(fMRI)让我们看到脑组织"工作",而 MRS 获取的信息则告诉我们有什么化学物质存在于脑内?量有多少?一种 MRS 类型^{31}P-MRS 可检测脑内的脂类化学物质,有两种脂类化学物质:磷酸单脂(PME's)告诉我们脑内脂质的形成;磷酸二脂(PDE's)告诉我们脑内脂质的降解。

MRS 已经用于显示精神分裂症和双相精神障碍(狂躁、抑郁)患者脑内脂质化学的异常。MRS 有望能研究上述和其他一些疾病患者的脑部改变,使这些患者得到更快更准确的诊断,甚至探索新的治疗方法。

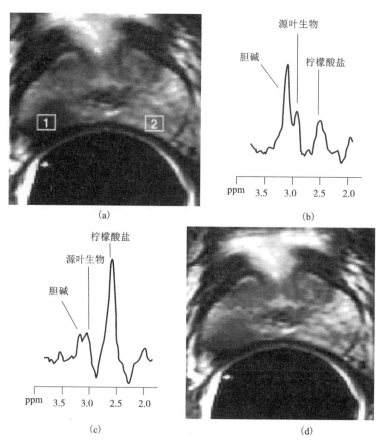

(a)经前列腺中部的 T2 加权横向 MR 图像显示肿瘤病灶：①的信号强度降低，正常左侧周围区域；②的信号强度降低。(b)从影像异常区域获得的磁共振波谱显示胆碱升高，柠檬酸盐减少，这种模式与确定的癌症一致。(c)从正常左外周区获得的 MR 波谱显示柠檬酸盐占优势的正常波谱模式，胆碱无异常升高；(d)三维磁共振波谱成像显示肿瘤区域呈红色覆盖。

图 3-7　MR 波谱和 3D-MR 波谱成像

第五节　功能 MRI

　　功能 MRI(fMRI)是一项近年来发展起来的技术，用以获得中枢神经系统的功能信息。fMRI 基于流向局部血管的血流增加伴随着大脑特定区域的神经元激活，导致脱氧血红蛋白局部相对减少，因为血流增加而没有相应耗氧量、氧气提取量增加。由于脱氧血红蛋白是顺磁性物质，它会改变 $T2^*$ 加权 MRI 图像信号。因此，这种内源性对比增强剂用作功能磁共振成像的信号。fMRI 旨在识别大脑对特定外部刺激做出反应的区域信号变化。通常采集功能图像使用 $T2^*$ 加权技术，用于诱导神经元反应的经典任务是视觉(例如观察变化的模式)或感觉运动(例如一系列定义的手指运动)激活，各种各样的存在用于神经元激活和在功能性 MRI 图像上观察到的变化。fMRI 可探测脑组织激活部分的血流量细微增加，且有助于神经外科术前计划、癫痫评价以及脑"地形图"描绘。

　　fMRI 不同于 MRI，后者仅显示解剖结构，前者还能显示脑组织活动信息。fMRI 通过探测神经活动对局部血流量、血流速度和血氧饱和度的间接作用，从而获得激活脑组织图像。fMRI 开始于 1990 年代，当时 MRI 设备配置了快速记录处置装备，再与计算机相连，能快速获得二维图像，记录时间短至 40 毫秒，分辨率 1 mm×1 mm。由于 fMRI 的图像采集和处理时间与 MRI 相近，放射学界容易接受。

　　最常用的 fMRI 方法是获取脑不同部位的氧耗图像。激发某部位的脑组织，该部位的氧需求增加，血流量因此增大。结果导致供应该部位的血管内氧含血红蛋白量增加而脱氧血红蛋白量相对减少。脱氧血红蛋白属顺磁性物质，致使该部位脑组织 $T2^*$ 缩短、信号降低。血流量增加时脱氧血红蛋白相对减少导致信号增强，称为血氧水平依赖成像即 BOLD。为获取这种血流改变的图像其成像技术复杂，1.5T 的磁共振成像机可检测到 1%~5% 信号增强的变化。

组织血流量的变化与脑组织活动有直接关系，刺激与非刺激状态下图像的差别已经阐明了这一点。另一种成像方法是动态磁敏增强即 DSC，可获取对比剂流经脑组织血管的动态图像。

fMRI 技术应用于病理状态的患者，其图像变化恒定，故该技术也常用于研究正常脑功能成像，而且 fMRI 还有另一重要的优势，其功能图像与解剖图像对应，使其功能定位具有解剖基础。同样，fMRI 技术易于确定多部位脑激活区，不像其他成像技术需要复杂的模拟定位。fMRI 较其他技术如 PET 的另一优势是 BOLD 技术在扫描前不需注入或摄取任何对比剂等物质。但是，fMRI 在采集图像时要求人体维持静止以保证图像清晰。

功能性 MRI 基于以下假设：刺激会增加被它激活的特定大脑区域的需氧量。为了满足更高需求，激活区的毛细血管血流量和血容量增加通过局部血管舒张。此外，假设多余的氧气被供应到激活区域，因为血液增加一段时间后，流量超过了代谢需要。比例较高与氧结合的血红蛋白分子（氧合血红蛋白）延长了 $T2^*$ 周围水的时间，可观察到 $T2^*$ 加权图像信号增加。这种对比机制被称为血氧依赖（BOLD）对比（图 3-8）。BOLD 对比度随 MR 成像仪的磁场强度增加而增加，与 MR 扫描相关的噪声使其有些难以通过听觉刺激来测量大脑的激活。而且，标准的刺激技术只有有限的时间分辨率用于生理变化的配准。因此，与事件相关的范例仅有短时间的激活变得越来越常用。BOLD 成像的空间分辨率有限，因为血液中增加的氧饱和度可能比实际已激活的区域大。最后，$T2^*$ 受许多混杂因素影响是微观层面上可能难以分离的因素。这就是为什么观察到的信号变化幅度不能提供定量测量刺激引起的生理变化。尽管许多研究活动都集中在功能性 MR 成像上，大多数影像中心在常规临床应用中仅起很小的作用。临床上，BOLD 成像用于计划神经外科手术干预。

尽管有局限性，但功能性 BOLD 成像可实现完全无创的和无辐射评估大脑活动的细微变化，空间分辨率为 1~2 mm 或更高，时间分辨率为 100 毫秒的范围。

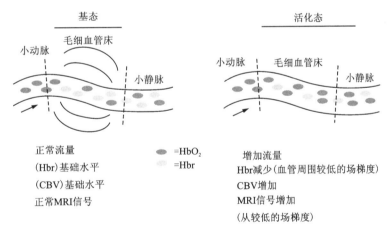

图 3-8 功能磁共振血氧依赖（fMRI BOLD）

第六节 MRI 假影

MRI 图像中与实际解剖结构不相符的虚假影像称为 MRI 假影，表现为图像变形、缺失、模糊等。常见的 MRI 假影有以下三种。

（1）图像处理假影：包括有化学位移假影、截断假影、部分容积效应和卷褶假影等。

（2）运动假影：运动假影表现在图像的相位编码方向有明亮躁音或重复的高信号，是由于成像序列采集过程中成像器官运动所致。可源于动脉博动、吞咽动作、呼吸运动、肠蠕动和身体移动。根据运动假影的原因可采用不同的技术使之减少。

(3)磁化率假影及金属假影：磁化率是物质的基本特征之一，为某物质进入外磁场后磁化强度与外磁场强度的比值。在 MRI 成像时，两种磁化率差别较大的组织界面上将出现假影，即磁化率假影，常出现在脑脊液与颅骨间、空气与组织之间等。体内或体外的金属物质可以导致局部磁化率发生显著变化，出现严重的磁化假影，也称为金属假影。

第七节　MRI 的优点与缺点

1. MRI 的优点

MRI 与传统的诊断设备，如 X 线和 CT 比较有许多突出的优点，如 X 线及 CT 检查电离幅射对人体有害，MRI 则无电离幅射而采用射频波。X 线及 CT 显示骨骼良好但显示软组织不佳，MRI 采用多参数成像，可得出详尽的解剖学图谱，软组织对比度明显高于 CT；另外，传统 X 线技术常使被投照物体的影像变形，因为被投照物体为三维物体，而 X 线片为二维影像，MRI 能多方位断层成像，使医学界能从三维空间上观察人体成为现实。人体能量代谢研究，可直接观察细胞活动的生化蓝图，磁共振波谱 MRS 的研究可以观察组织器官的能量代谢情况；此外不使用造影剂可以观察心脏和血管结构，无骨假影干扰，后颅窝病变清晰可辨。

2. MRI 的缺点

MRI 成像速度慢，不适合于运动性器官和危重患者的检查；对钙化灶和骨皮质病灶不够敏感；此外，对一些肥胖患者的成像效果欠佳，对一些体内有金属移植物的患者存在危险性。图像易受多种假影影响。

第八节　MRI 的安全性

MRI 的安全性是很重要的问题，尽管 MRI 没有电离幅射，可用于产生信号的射频能量非常强大，对人体器官有潜在危害，但已经证实目前医用 MRI 没有明显的危害。四种可能的不良反应需考虑：静磁场、改变磁场的电流、对敏感组织的热效应和噪音。

第九节　MRI 增强

MRI 普通检查时某些组织的对比度不够，为了使这些组织有足够的对比度，在检查时使用对比剂。对比剂可增强人体器官和血管的成像效果。MRI 最常用的对比剂为钆。钆注入血管后，异常组织如肿瘤或瘢痕容易吸收钆，造成这些异常组织的信号增高。人体对钆的耐受性优于其他对比剂如 X 线检查常用的碘。

（肖恩华，卞读军，李华兵，韦小芳，刘宁远，谭长连）

Chapter 3

Magnetic resonance imaging

Nuclear magnetic resonance(NMR) or magnetic resonance imaging(MRI) is a new noninvasive technique used primarily in medical settings to map the internal structures of the body and produce high quality images of the inside of the human body which completely avoids the use of ionizing radiation and appears to be unassociated with any significant hazards. MRI is based on the principles of nuclear magnetic resonance (NMR), a spectroscopic technique used by scientists to obtain microscopic chemical and physical information about molecules. The technique was called magnetic resonance imaging rather than nuclear magnetic resonance imaging (NMRI) because of the negative connotations associated with the word nuclear in the late 1970's. MRI started out as a tomographic imaging technique, that is it produced an image of the NMR signal in a thin slice through the human body. MRI has advanced beyond a tomographic imaging technique to a volume imaging technique.

Before beginning a study of the science of MRI, it will be helpful to reflect on the brief history of MRI. Felix Bloch and Edward Purcell, both of whom were awarded the Nobel Prize in 1952, discovered the magnetic resonance phenomenon independently in 1946. In the period between 1950 and 1970, NMR was developed and used for chemical and physical molecular analysis. In 1971 RaymondDamadian showed that the nuclear magnetic relaxation times of tissues and tumors differed, thus motivating scientists to consider magnetic resonance for the detection of disease. In 1973 the x-ray-based computerized tomography (CT) was introduced by Hounsfield. This date is important to the MRI timeline because it showed hospitals were willing to spend large amounts of money for medical imaging hardware. Magnetic resonance imaging was first demonstrated on small test tube samples that same year by Paul Lauterbur. He used a back projection technique similar to that used in CT. In 1975 Richard Ernst proposed magnetic resonance imaging using phase and frequency encoding, and the Fourier Transform. This technique is the basis of current MRI techniques. A few years later, in 1977, Raymond Damadian demonstrated MRI of the whole body. In this same year, Peter Mansfield developed the echo-planar imaging (EPI) technique. This technique will be developed in later years to produce images at video rates (30 ms/image). Edelstein and coworkers demonstrated imaging of the body using Ernst's technique in 1980. A single image could be acquired in approximately five minutes by this technique. By 1986, the imaging time was reduced to about five seconds, without sacrificing too much image quality. The same year people were developing the NMR microscope, which allowed approximately 10μm resolution on approximately one cm samples. In 1987 echo-planar imaging was used to perform real-time movie imaging of a single cardiac cycle. In this same year Charles Dumoulin was perfecting magnetic resonance angiography (MRA), which allowed imaging of flowing blood without the use of contrast agents. In 1991, Richard Ernst was rewarded for his achievements in pulsed Fourier Transform NMR and MRI with the Nobel Prize in Chemistry. In 1993 functional MRI (fMRI) was developed. This technique allows the mapping of the function of the various regions of the human brain. Six years earlier many clinicians thought echo-planar imaging's primary applications was to be in real-time cardiac imaging. The development of fMRI opened up a new application for EPI in mapping the regions of the brain responsible for thought and motor control. In 1994, researchers at the State University of New York at Stony Brook and Princeton University demonstrated the imaging of hyperpolarized ^{129}Xe gas for respiration studies. MRI is clearly a young, but growing science.

Section 1   Basic components of an MR imaging system

All MRI scanners have the same basic components: A large magnet, within which are situated gradient coils and an appropriately sized RF (radio frequence) tranmitter and receiver coils. Ancillary equipment is required to generate and analyze the MRI signals from which the final image is construted. In general, a MRI scanner is composed of magnetic system, gradient system, radiofrequency (RF) system, computerized images processing work station and other peripheral devices

1. Magnetic system

Magnet system is comprised of main magnet, gradient system, radiofrequency (RF) transmitter and receiver, additional coils, various computers for controlling the scanner and the gradients, and other peripheral devices.

Mainmagnet can produce a quiet magnetic field. MRI has strict demands on strength, stability and homogeneity of magnetic field. Magnetic field strengths used for imaging currently range from 0.1 tesla (T) to 2.0 T, which are harmless to human health and produce good quality images. Magnetic field homogeneity requires that a high homogeneous magnetic field can be produced within a large space and needs to be $10^{-4} \sim 10^{-6}$ (several parts per million, ppm). Magnetic field stability is variable rate of magnetic field per time, short-term stability required to be within several ppm/h, long-term within 10ppm/h. A very uniform, or homogeneous, magnetic field of incredible strength and stability is critical for high-quality imaging.

Magnet includes permanent magnet, conventional magnet, namely resistive magnets and superconducting magnet.

(1) Resistive magnets consist of many windings or coils of wire wrapped around a cylinder or bore through which an electric current is passed. This causes a magnetic field to be generated. If the electricity is turned off, the magnetic field dies out. These magnets are lower in cost to construct than a superconducting magnet (see below), but require huge amounts of electricity (up to 50 kilowatts) to operate because of the natural resistance in the wire. To operate this type of magnet above about the 0.3-tesla level would be prohibitively expensive.

(2) A permanent magnet is just that — permanent. Its magnetic field is always there and always on full strength, so it costs nothing to maintain the field. The major drawback is that these magnets are extremely heavy: They weigh many, many tons at the 0.4-tesla level. A stronger field would require a magnet so heavy it would be difficult to construct. Permanent magnets are getting smaller, but are still limited to low field strengths.

(3) Superconducting magnets are by far the most commonly used. A superconductive magnet is somewhat similar to a resistive magnet — coils or windings of wire through which a current of electricity is passed create the magnetic field. The important difference is that the wire is continually bathed in liquid helium at 268.8 degrees below zero. If you're in an MRI machine, the only thing you feel is cold, but don't worry, the magnet is well insulated by the vacuum. This almost unimaginable cold causes the resistance in the wire to drop to zero, reducing the electrical requirement for the system dramatically and making it much more economical to operate. Superconductive systems are still very expensive, but they can easily generate 0.5-tesla to 2.0-tesla fields, allowing for much higher-quality imaging.

2. Gradient system

Another type of magnet found in every MRI system is called a gradient magnet. There are three gradientcoils inside the MRI machine, one for each direction. Gradient coils are used to produce deliberate variations in the main magnetic field (Bo). These magnets are very, very low strength compared to the main magnetic field; they may range in strength from 180 gauss to 270 gauss, or 18 to 27 millitesla (thousandths of a tesla). The variation in the magnetic field permits localization of image slices as well as phase encoding and frequency encoding.

3. RF system

RF system is a unit devicethat is used to emit RF pulse, resonate protons after proton energy absorption, produce and receive MR signal. In fact, RF system is composed of transmitting part and receiving part, which includes transmitter, amplifier, transmitting coils, receiving coils, low noise signal amplifier and so on. RF coils are the "antenna" of the MRI system that broadcasts the RF signal to the patient and/or receives the return signal. RF coils can be receive-only, in which case the body coil is used as a transmitter; or transmit and receive (transceiver). A radiofrequency (RF) transmitter with a transmit coil built into the scanner. A highly sensitive RF receiver to pick up and amplify the MR signal. Alternatively, imagers may use a single RF coil switched between the transmit and receive modes.

4. The computer images processing system

This system is mainly used to process data from MRI scanner and get reconstructed images. It must equip with large-load computer and high-resolution A/D transformation in order to complete data collection, images procession and display. Imitated signals transferred by the detector are transformed into digital signals to produce slice images data through A/D transformation, and display images in different grey scales or colors again through D/A transformation. Various computers for controlling the scanner and the gradients (control computer), for creation of the MR images (array processor), and for coordinating all processes (main or host computer, to which are connected the operator's console and image archives)

5. Additional coils, either receive coils or transmit/receive coils.

6. Other peripheral devices

such as a control for the patient table, electrocardiography (ECG) equipment and respiration monitors to trigger specialized MR sequences, a cooling system for the magnet, a second operator's console (e. g. for image processing), a device for film exposure, or a PACS (picture archiving and communications system).

Section 2　Principles of MR imaging

Certain atoms have an inherent magnetic dipole moment that arises from their electrical charge and their angular momentum, or spin. The proton is one such atomic nucleus with a magnetic dipole moment that also has wide biological relevance. MR imaging is founded on the manipulation of magnetic dipole moments in such a way that signals generated from these interactions that can be translated into visual images of the body. When a proton is subjected to a strong, steady, externally-applied magnetic field, a force will act on the magnetic moment in such a way that the dipole moment of the proton aligns itself in parallel with the external field. Because of its spin, however, the dipole moment performs a maintained circular movement known as a precession in which its own spin axis rotates at an angle around another axis that is parallel with the external field. The simplest analogy to this phenomenon is that of a spinning toy top which spins on its own axis while is slowly revolves around the earth's gravitational pull (Figure 3-1). Because the dipole moment of the proton has both a direction and a magnitude at any given time, the most useful description of the moment is made using vectors. The vector is thus comprised of two components, the longitudinal component aligned with the axis of precession and the transverse component aligned perpendicular to the external field and rotating at the frequency of precession. This frequency of precession is known as the Larmor frequency and is related to the strength of the applied external field by a simple equation (W = rT) , in which w is the precessional frequency, T is the magnet field strength and r is a constant (gyromagnetic ratio) unique for each atom.

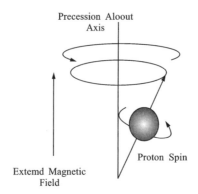

Figure 3-1　Proton Precession in a Magnetic Field

In practice, the longitudinal component of the dipole moment for protons exposed to an external field can either be aligned with (lower energy state) or against (higher energy state) the direction of the external field (Figure 3-2). The relative distribution of protons in one or the other of these energy states depends on both the temperature of the sample as well as the strength of the external field, but the difference in these so-called "spin-up" (lower energy) versus "spin-down" (higher energy) alignments creates a net magnetization. The net magnetization of protons at body temperature is very weak, with only a very small excess (i. e. , a few parts per million) of protons being in the lower energy spin level. Conveniently, the net magnetization of the protons can also be described using a vector.

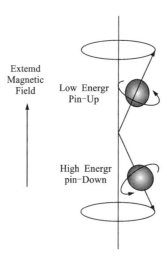

Figure 3-2　Proton Spin Orientation in a Magnetic Field

When a body or tissue is placed in a strong magnetic field, the net magnetization vector is established in a matter of seconds. This equilibrium of spin states can be displaced by the introduction of a pulse of electromagnetic waves applied perpendicular to the external field and at the Larmor frequency. For protons, this frequency lies within the radiofrequency (RF) range. Through a process known as resonance, energy in an RF pulse will be transferred to the precessing protons in the field. This energy input will cause two effects on the protons. Firstly, protons in the low spin-energy level will be bumped into the high spin-energy level with a corresponding shift in the orientation of their dipole moments. As such, the magnitude of the longitudinal component of the net magnetization vector decreases (due to the reduction in difference in the relative numbers of spin-up and spin-down protons). Secondly, the RF pulse serves to force all of the protons into coherent precession, resulting in the formation of a transverse component of the net magnetization vector that now rotates at the Larmor frequency. Thus, as RF energy is applied, the longitudinal component of the net magnetization vector decreases and the transverse component increases. Given enough energy, the magnitude of the longitudinal component can begin to increase again, but its direction will be antiparallel to that of the applied field. Corresponding decreases in the transverse component will accompany this increase (in the antiparallel direction) of the longitudinal component.

After the RF pulse is turned off, the protons release or re-radiate the energy they acquired from the pulse so that they return to their initial state of equilibrium. This energy release is known as relaxation and detection of this process forms the basis of the MR imaging signal. The relaxation of the longitudinal and transverse components of the net magnetization vector do not even occur at the same rate. The recovery of the longitudinal component back to its equilibrium value can be described using an exponential function with a time constant denoted T1. The decay of the transverse component back to its equilibrium value can also be described using an exponential function, but with a time constant denoted T2. Not surprisingly, the two relaxation processes reflect two different types of interactions between the precessing protons and their local environment. T1 relaxation is representative of the energy loss associated with high energy spins returning to their low energy state and giving the energy back to neighboring molecules which collectively make up what is known as the lattice. Accordingly, T1 relaxation is commonly referred to as spin-lattice relaxation. By contrast, T2 relaxation is representative of the loss of proton spin phase coherence associated with the protons interacting with other protons, other nuclei with magnetic moments that alter the local magnetic field homogeneity, or inherent instability in the homogeneity of the magnetic field. Because of these interactions with other nuclei, T2 relaxation is also known as spin-spin relaxation. Because of the differences in the composition and structure of tissues and biological fluids, the T1 and T2 relaxation times vary considerably within the body.

The strength of the MRI signal depends primarily on three parameters: 1. Density of protons in a tissue (the greater the density of protons, the larger will be the signal); 2. The T1 relaxation time; and 3. The T2 relaxation time. The visual contrast between tissues is dependent upon how these parameters differ between tissues. For most soft tissues in the body, the proton density is very homogeneous and therefore does not contribute in a major way to signal differences seen in an image. However, T1 and T2 can be dramatically different for different soft tissues, and these parameters become responsible for the major contrast between soft tissues. Fortunately, it is possible to manipulate the MR signal by changing the way in which the nuclei are initially subjected to electromagnetic energy. This manipulation can change the dependence of the observed signal on the three parameters: proton density, T1 and T2. As such, a number of different MR imaging techniques ("weightings") are available from which to choose that accentuate some properties and not others.

The signals from the body's tissues are detected by a sensitive receiver, and are analyzed by a computerized system to create a visual representation for display on a computer screen. Once the image is created, data can be selectively visualized so as to optimize the examination of the desired tissue or body compartment. Image reconstruction algorithms can be used to present the normally grayscale images as color-coded pictures, as surface-rendered three-dimensional models, or as tissue-, organ-or compartment-specific isolation views. Several typical MR images of the head, neck and kidneys are shown in Figure 3-3.

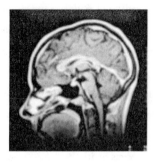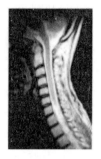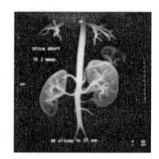

Figure 3-3   Typical MR images of the head (left), neck (middle) and kidneys (right)

Section 3   Radio frequency pulse sequences

1. Spin echo sequence

The spin echo pulse sequence is the most commonly used pulse sequence. The pulse sequence timing can be adjusted to give T1-weighted, Proton or spin density, and T2-weighted images. Dual echo and multiecho sequences can be used to obtain both proton density and T2-weighted images simultaneously.

The two variables of interest in spin echo sequences is the repetition time (TR) and the echo time (TE). All spin echo sequences include a slice selective 90 degree pulse followed by one or more 180 degree refocusing pulses as shown in Figure 3-4.

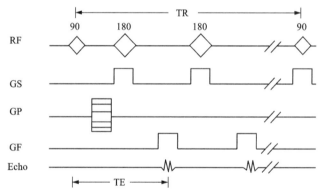

Figure 3-4   Double echo spin echo sequence

2. Inversion recovery sequence

Inversion recovery pulse sequences are used to give heavy T1-weighting. In addition, the STIR (short TI inversion recovery) sequence can be used for fat suppression, where a relatively short inversion time is used to null the fat signal while maintaining water and soft tissue signal. The basic part of an inversion recovery sequence is a 180 degree RF pulse that inverts the magnetization followed by a 90 degree RF pulse that brings the residual longitudinal magnetization into the x-y or transverse plane where it can be detected by an RF coil. In imaging, the signal is usually refocused with a 180 degree pulse as in a spin echo sequence. The time between the initial 180 degree pulse and the 90 degree pulse is the inversion time (TI). A diagram of the sequence is shown below.

With a TI of about 140 ms on a 1.5 T MRI machine, the fat signal is nulled while the water proton signal is still present. This occurs because the T1 of fat is significantly smaller than the T1 of water.

3. Gradient echo sequences

The gradient echo sequences show a wide range of variations compared to the spin echo and inversion recovery sequences. Not only is the basic sequence varied by adding dephasing or rephasing gradients at the end of the sequence, but there is a significant extra variable to specify in addition to things like the TR and TE. This variable is the flip or tip angle of the spins. The flip angle is usually at or close to 90 degrees for a spin echo sequence but commonly varies over a range of about 10 to 80 degrees with gradient echo sequences. For the basic gradient echo sequence FLASH (Figure 3-5), illustrated below, the larger tip angles give more T1 weighting to the image and the smaller tip angle give more T2 or actually T2 * weighting to the images.

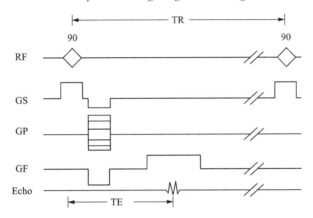

Figure 3-5   Gradient echo sequences

Images from other gradient echo sequences such as GRASS and FISP have less intuitive tissue contrast characteristics than FLASH. The FLASH and SPGR sequences show better tissue contrast between white matter and grey matter in the brain and spinal cord than GRASS or FISP and are preferred when the time of acquisition does not have to be very short. GRASS and FISP maintain better SNR than FLASH at short TR times and are therefore preferred with breath-holding techniques, for example.

4. Echoplanar pulse sequences

Echoplanar imaging is a gradient echo technique related to fast gradient echo imaging. The entire set of 64 or 128 phase steps is acquired during one acquisition TR. Echoplanar sequences may use entirely gradient echoes or may combine a spin echo with the train of gradient echoes as illustrated in the diagram below (Figure 3-6). Echoplanar images may be acquired in less that 1/10th of a second and therefore may be useful in cardiac imaging and other rapidly changing processes, such as diffusion weighted imaging and perfusion weighted imaging.

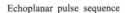
Echoplanar pulse sequence

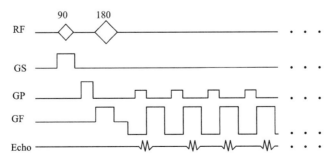

Figure 3-6   Echoplanar pulse sequence

Section 4　MR Spectroscopy

Magnetic resonance spectroscopy (MRS) of intact biological tissues was first reported by two groups: Moon and Richards using [31]P−MRS to examine intact red blood cells in 1973, and Hoult et al. using [31]P−MRS to examine excised leg muscle from the rat in 1974. Since then MRS has been applied to almost every organ of the body including brain, heart, liver, kidney, prostate, and extremities. MRS is useful for looking at disorders of metabolism, tumors and certain inflammatory and ischemic diseases. Most of the work with in vivo MRS in humans has been in the brain. Abnormalities have been seen, sometimes with earlier detection than for any other diagnostic procedure short of biopsy, in primary brain tumors, infections such as AIDS, demyelinating disorders such as multiple sclerosis, epilepsy, and stroke.

MRS-sensitive nuclei such as hydrogen (^{1}H), carbon (^{13}C), fluorine (^{19}F) or phosphorus (^{31}P). ^{1}H MRS, however, has the most valuable advantage that the same hardware for magnetic resonance imaging (MRI) as well as for MRS can be used. Moreover, its sensitivity is by a factor of 7 higher than that of phosphorus. The metabolites that can be investigated via ^{1}H MRS methods include but are not limited to N-acetylaspartate (NAA), choline (Cho), creatine (Cr), lactate, glutamate (Glu), glutamine (Gln) and lipids.

The dominant metabolite signal in the ^{31}P-MR spectrum is singlet of the phosphorylated form of creatine (Cr), i. e. phosphocreatine (PCr). The high energy phosphate bond in PCr serves as a rapidly available energy reserve, ready to replenish energy catalyzed from adenosine-triphosphate (ATP) during increased energy expenditure. ATP contains three non-equivalent phosphate groups ($\alpha-$, $\beta-$, and$\gamma-$) that differ in their resonance frequencies, which yield three individual signals in the ^{31}P-MR spectra. As the phosphate nuclei in ATP interact with other nearby spins, i. e. undergo so-called homonuclear J-coupling, line splitting of the ATP signals can be observed, which forms doublets forα-and γ-ATP, and atriplet for b-ATP. Another important metabolite visible in the ^{31}PMRS spectrum is inorganic phosphate (Pi), which also serves as a substrate or product in chemical reactions of energy metabolism. Other detectable ^{31}P metabolites include cell membrane precursors, i. e. phosphomonoesters (PMEs) and cell membrane degradation products, i. e. phosphodiesters (PDEs). The major contributors to the PME signal in vivo are phosphocholine (PC) and phosphoethanolamine (PE), while the main PDEs are glycerolphosphocholine (GPC) and glycerol-phosphoethanolamine (GPE).

Uses of MRS include serial evaluation of biochemical changes in tumors, analyzing metabolic disorders, infections and diseases, as well as evaluation of therapeutic oncology treatments for tumor recurrence versus radiation damage. Early applications were dedicated to brain disorders, but now breast, liver, and prostate MRS are also performed. Correlation of spectroscopy results and MR images are always advised before making a final diagnosis.

Spectroscopic changes are documented in a variety of enzyme deficiencies, mitochondrial abnormalities, dystrophies, inflammatory myopathies, and thyroid disease. In muscle these diseases include phosphofructokinase deficiency, amyloglucosidase deficiency, Duchenne muscular dystrophy, Becker muscular dystrophy, dermatomyositis, polymyositis, inclusion body myositis, hypothyroidism, and congestive heart failure.

Magnetic resonance spectroscopy (MRS) is performed with a variety of pulse sequences. The simplest sequence consists of a 90 degree RF pulse without any gradients with reception of the signal by the RF coil immediately after the single RF pulse. Many sequences used for imaging can be used for spectroscopy also (such as the spin echo sequence). The important difference between an imaging sequence and a spectroscopy sequence is that for spectroscopy, a read out gradient is not used during the time the RF coil is receiving the signal from the person or object being examined. Instead of using the frequency information (provided by the read out or frequency gradient) to provide spatial or positional information, the frequency information is used to identify different chemical compounds. This is possible because the electron cloud surrounding different chemical compounds shields the resonant atoms of spectroscopic interest to varying degrees depending on the specific compound and the specific position in the compound. This electron shielding causes the observed resonance frequency of the atoms to slightly different and therefore identifiable with MRS.

MRS uses the fact that different chemicals vibrate at different frequencies (like a tuning fork) when stimulated by a magnet (Figure 3-7). The machine used to detect these signals is similar to an MRI (magnetic resonance imager) that produces pictures of the brain or other body tissues (The prostate cancer is demonstrated in Figure 7d with 3D MR spectroscopic imaging), and to functional MRI (fMRI) that allows us to see the brain 'working'. With MRS however a signature is produced which is used to tell

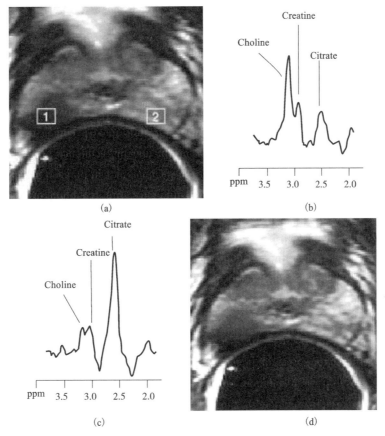

(a) T2-weighted transverse MR image through the middle prostate gland shows decreased signal intensity in a tumor focus (1) and middle signal intensity in normal left peripheral zone (2). (b) MR spectrum obtained from area of imaging abnormality (1 in a) demonstrates elevated choline and reduced citrate, a pattern consistent with definite cancer. (c) MR spectrum obtained from a normal left peripheral zone (2 in a) demonstrates a normal spectral pattern with citrate dominant and no abnormal elevation in choline. (d) 3D MR spectroscopic imaging shows the tumor area is overlaid in red.

Figure 3-7   MR Spectroscopic and 3D MR Spectroscopic Imaging

what chemicals are present in the brain, and in what amounts. A special type of MRS, $^{31}P-MRS$, can be used to investigatelipid chemicals in the brain. There are two types of chemicals: 1. Phosphomonoesters (PME's). These tell us about how lipids are formed in the brain. 2. Phosphodiesters (PDE's). These tell us about how lipids are broken down in the brain.

MRS has been used to show that lipid chemistry is abnormal in the brain of people suffering from schizophrenia and bipolar affective disorder (manic-depression). It is hoped that MRS can be used to study what is happening in the brain of sufferers of these and other conditions, allowing quicker and more accurate diagnosis, as well as finding new ways to treat these conditions.

Section 5 Functional MRI

Functional MRI (fMRI) is a technique that has recently been introduced to obtain functional information from the central nervous system. fMRI is based on the increase in blood flow to the local vasculature that accompanies neural activity in the specific areas of the brain, resulting in a local reduction of deoxyhemoglobin because the increase in blood flow occurs without an increase in oxygen extraction. As deoxyhemoglobin is a paramagnetic agent, it alters the $T2^*$-weighted MRI image signal. Thus, this endogenous contrast enhancing agent serves as the signal for fMRI. FMRI of the brain aims at identifying cerebral areas that respond to a well-defined external stimulus by a change in signal. Functional images are typically acquired using $T2^*$-weighted techniques. Classical tasks used to induce neuronal responses are visual (such as looking at changing patterns) or sensorimotor (such as a sequence of defined finger movements) activation. A wide variety of protocols exist for neuronal activation and the interpretation of the changes observed on functional MR images.

The fMRI detects subtle increases in blood flow associated with activation of parts of the brain. The fMRI may be useful for preoperative neurosurgical planning, epilepsy evaluation, and "mapping" of the brain.

The fMRI technique differs from MRI in that it localizes brain activity rather than only structures. It produces images of activated brain regions by detecting the indirect effects of neural activity on local blood volume, flow, and oxygen saturation. FMRI was developed in the early 1990s, when MRI equipment was fitted with devices that sped up the recording process. The equipment is then connected to a computer which rapidly produces two-dimensional images. The recording time can be as little as 40 milliseconds, and the resolution 1x1 mm. Because the image acquisition and processing times are similar to those for structural MRI, this allow for fMRI to be readily used into existing radiological practice.

The most common fMRI method yields images of oxygen consumption of different parts of the brain. Activation of an area of the brain causes an increase in blood flow to that area that is greater than that needed to keep up with the oxygen demands of the tissues. This results in a net increase in intravascular oxyhemogobin and a decrease in deoxyhemoglobin. Deoxyhemoglobin is paramagnetic, resulting in shorting of the $T2^*$ of the brain and decrease in signal. Less deoxyhemoglobin as a result of increase in blood flow results in an overall increase in signal. It is called blood oxygen level dependent imaging (BOLD). Sophisticated image processing techniques are used to obtain images of these flow changes. The increase in signal detected ranges from 1%~5% on a 1.5T MR system.

These changes in tissues blood volume have been directly correlated with evoked brain activity. These conclusions have been made by the differences in results obtained during both stimulated and nonstimulated states. Another method is dynamic susceptibility contrast (DSC), which produces images of a contrast agent flowing through the blood vessels of the brain.

The fMRI technique is mostly used in research on normal brain functioning because it has yet to be proved that consistent results could be obtained in patients with pathological conditions. However, a major research advantage to fMRI is that there is a natural correspondence to MRI structural images. This provides an anatomic basis to the functional localizations. It can also easily identify multiple regions of activation without the modeling or registration complications of other imaging techniques. Another advantage of fMRI over other technology, such as PET, is that the BOLD method does not require injection or ingestion of any substances prior to the scan. It does, however, require the subject to remain still during the procedure in order to prevent the images from being blurred.

Functional MRI is based on the assumption that a stimulus increases the oxygen demand of a specific brain region that is activated by it. To meet the higher demand, capillary blood flow and the blood volume in the activated region are increased by local vasodilatation. Moreover, it is assumed that excess oxygen is supplied to the activated area because the increased blood flow exceeds the metabolic needs after some time. The higher proportion of hemoglobin molecules bound with oxygen (oxyhemoglobin) prolongs the T2* time of the surrounding water, which is observed as a signal increase on T2*-weighted images. This contrast mechanism is known as blood oxygen level-dependent (BOLD) contrast (Figure 3-8). The BOLD contrast increases with the magnetic field strength of the MR scanner. The noise that is associated with MR scanning makes it somewhat difficult to measure cerebral activation by auditory stimuli. Moreover, the standard techniques of stimulation have only a limited temporal resolution for the registration of physiologic changes. Therefore, event-related paradigms with only short periods of activation are becoming more popular. The spatial resolution of BOLD imaging is limited because the area with an increased oxygen saturation of the blood may be much larger than the region that has actually been activated. Finally, T2$*$ is affected by many confounding factors at the microscopic level that may be difficult to isolate. This is why the magnitude of the observed signal change does not provide a quantitative measure of the physiologic changes induced by stimulation. While much research activity is focused on functional MR imaging, it has only a very small role in routine clinical applications at most radiologic centers. Clinically, BOLD imaging is used to plan neurosurgical interventions. Despite its limitations, functional BOLD imaging enables fully noninvasive and radiation-free evaluation of subtle changes in cerebral activity with a spatial resolution of 1~2 mm or better and a temporal resolution in the range of 100 msec.

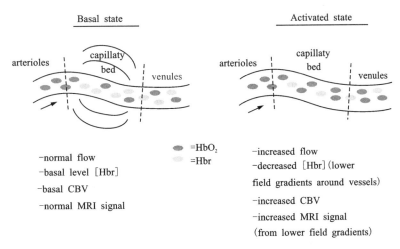

Figure 3-8   fMRI BOLD

Section 6   MRI artifacts

False images existing in MRI that do not match the actual anatomical structure are called artifacts. MRI artifacts usually appear as image distortion, deletion, blur, etc. There are several common MRI artifacts.

1. Imagingprocessing artifacts

The imaging processing artifacts includes chemical shift artifacts, truncation artifact, partial volume effect and "wrap-around" artifacts.

2. Motionartifacts

Motion artifacts appear as bright noise or repeating densities oriented in the phase direction, occurring as the results of motion during acquisition of a sequence. These artifacts may be seen from arterial pulsations, swallowing, breathing, peristalsis, and physical movement of a patient. Motion artifacts can be reduced by various techniques depending on their cause.

3. Magneticsusceptibility artifact and metal artifacts

Magnetic susceptibility is one of the basic characteristics of substance. It is the ratio of the magnetization intensity of a substance to the external magnetic field intensity after entering the external magnetic field. During MR imaging, artifacts appear on the interface of two tissues with large differences in magnetic susceptibility, that is, magnetic susceptibility artifacts, which often appear between the cerebrospinal fluid and the skull, the air and the tissue. Metallic substances inside or outside the body can cause significant changes in partial magnetic susceptibility, resulting in severe magnetization artifacts, also known as metal artifacts.

Section 7   Advantages and disadvantages of MRI

1. Advantages of MRI

MRI offers some major advantages over traditional diagnostic tools such as the X-ray and computed tomography (CT)scanning. MRI is a unique imaging method because, unlike X-rays, it does not rely on ionizing radiation; instead it uses radiofrequency waves. The ionizing radiation used in X-rays and CT is proven to be dangerous. X-rays and CT are usually reserved for bone imaging since soft tissue does not show up very well in the images produced, whereas MRI uses multi-parameter imaging to get a detailed anatomical atlas and is exceptional at showing the contrast in soft tissue. Additionally, objects often appear distorted when imaged using traditional X-ray techniques. This is because the object being imaged by an X-ray is three-dimensional, but the film is only two-dimensional. MRI can perform multi-directional tomographic imaging, making it a reality for the medical community to observe the human body in three-dimensional space. Human energy metabolism research can directly observe the biochemical blueprint of cell activity. Magnetic resonance spectroscopy(MRS)research can provide insight into the energy metabolism of tissues and organs. In addition, MRI can observe the structure of the heart and blood vessels without the use of contrast agents, without bone artifacts, posterior fossa lesions are clearly distinguishable.

2. Disadvantages of MRI

A disadvantage to MRI is that it doesn't image bone tissue or calcium deposits very well when compared to other techniques. Certain sequence done with MR can also be uncomfortable and require more time when compared to other techniques, not suitable for examination of motor organs and critically patients. Additionally, it is unavailable to certain patient populations such those who are obese. Also it is dangerous for other patient populations, such as those with certain metallic implants, to undergo an MRI examination. Picture quality is easily affected by various artifacts.

Section 8   MRI safety

The safety of MRI is an important consideration. Although it does not use any ionizing radiation, the radiofrequency energy that is used to produce a signal from the patient is still fairly intense and has the potential to damage internal organs. Yet provided the machine is used sensibly, no basic hazard has been identified. Four possible adverse effects were considered, including the static magnetic field; induced currents due to changing magnetic fields; heating effects on vulnerable tissues; and acoustic noise

Section 9   MRI enhancement

MRI can be enhanced in order to achieve enough contrast in tissues that do not normally exhibit enough contrast for effective viewing during the examination by using contrasts agents.

Contrast agents enhance images of organs or blood vessels. The most popular contrast agent used in MRI is an element called gadolinium. When gadolinium is injected into the bloodstream, it is readily absorbed in abnormal tissues such as tumors or scar, causing them to appear brighter in an MRI scan. Gadolinium is generally better tolerated than other contrast agents, such the Iodide commonly used in X-ray exams.

(Xiao Enhua, Bian Dujun, Li Huabing, Wei Xiaofang, Liu Ningyuan, Tan Changlian)

第二篇

骨骼系统

骨骼系统由骨和关节组成，构成躯体的支架。骨骼系统的运动功能有赖于骨间的连结、关节及韧带才能完成。

骨质含有钙，在 X 线片上呈高密度，与周围软组织形成良好对比。骨皮质和骨松质结构不同，亦使两者在 X 线片上具有良好的对比并得以显示细节。骨骼的 X 线照片能显示骨骼系统各种疾病的大体病理改变，如先天异常、炎症、代谢异常、外伤和肿瘤等。因此，骨骼系统是医院放射科最常见的 X 线检查部位之一。

在临床实践中，有些骨关节疾病的放射学特征非常典型，易于作出诊断；有些则不典型，难以作出肯定诊断。另一方面，有些疾病，如骨感染和肿瘤等，其放射学征象出现比临床症状和体征晚，只有在临床表现出现一段时间后，放射学征像才变得较明显。CT 和 MRI 能显示骨髓和骨关节周围软组织的异常表现，因此更易于早期诊断骨骼系统疾病。总之，骨骼系统的放射诊断是最依赖于放射射线、临床和实验室检查有机结合的一门诊断学科。

Part 2

Skeletal system

The skeletal system, which forms the supporting system of the body, consists of bones and joints. The mobility of the skeletal system depends much more on the connections between the individual bones, the joints and the ligaments.

Bone substance, because of its calcium content, which is high density and differs apparently from the surrounding soft tissue, and its constitutional difference between the cortex bone and the sponge bone, is full of contrast and detail on a film. Bone radiography may provide clues to the presence of various pathologic categories of skeletal diseases, such as congenital, inflammatory, metabolic, traumatic and neoplastic diseases. So the skeletal system is one of the most common X-ray examinations you will encounter in a radiology department in a hospital.

In clinical practice, the roentgen diagnosis of bone and joint diseases may be apparent, but there are instances, however, those roentgen findings are atypical and present diagnostic problems. And again, the radiographic findings may lag behind the clinical symptoms and signs, as in case of infection and tumors; it requires a period of time before radiographic changes are apparent. Computed tomography and magnetic resonance imagine can show the abnormal changes in bone marrow and the soft tissue around the bones and joints, so the diseases can be demonstrated easier and earlier by them. In no other medical field than in skeletal radiology is the diagnosis so dependent on the intelligent integration of information from roentgenologic, clinical and laboratory sources.

第四章

骨骼

第一节　检查方法

1. X 线检查

除用于金属异物定位、骨折复位和固定外，透视一般不用于骨关节疾病的检查与诊断。

X 线平片优于透视，是骨关节的常用放射学检查方法。常规摄片应注意以下几点：

（1）可能的情况下，被检查的任何解剖部位至少应包括正位、侧位两个摄影位置。如果 X 线表现与临床诊断不符，应加摄其他位置。如果忘记这一原则，很可能造成诸如无移位的骨折等较严重的漏诊。

（2）长骨照片应包括邻近的一个关节；颈椎、胸椎或腰椎照片，应包括齿状突、第 1 肋骨、腰骶角等解剖学标志，以便对脊椎计数定位。

（3）照片中应尽可能包括骨关节周围的软组织。

（4）当一侧肢体照片的诊断可疑时，就加摄对侧骨或关节照片，以供比较；这一点在儿童患者及疾病的早期阶段尤其重要。

目前，随着 CT 的普及，体层摄影已很少用于骨关节检查；MRI 亦越来越多地代替关节造影。关节软骨与关节囊均为软组织密度，X 线平片不能显示；关节造影是在关节腔内注入阳性或阴性造影剂，以显示关节结构，多用于膝关节，以评价半月板与韧带是否撕裂。

2. CT 检查

CT 对于许多骨关节疾病，特别是头颅、脊椎及骨盆疾病的检查与诊断具有重要作用。目前，CT 已是大多数脊椎疾病的首选影像检查方法。CT 的主要优点是具有良好的密度分辨力与影像对比度，可以提供骨及相邻软组织结构的断层图像。

近几年，螺旋 CT 已经普及，其相对于传统 CT 具有两大优点：降低辐射剂量，缩短检查时间。在低辐射剂量范围内获得层面重叠图像有利于进一步行多方位图像及三维图像重建。

（1）CT 平扫：CT 检查时常将躯体或两侧肢体同时扫描以便处于对称位置，有利观察。骨骼系统一般行横轴面扫描，在矢状面或冠状面定位像上定位后，常规采用螺旋扫描，电压 120 kV，电流 80~100 mAs，重建层厚和层间距为 2~3 mm 或更薄，均采用标准算法。所有骨骼系统图像都要用骨窗（窗位 300~400 Hu，窗宽 1000~1500 Hu）及软组织窗（窗位 40~50 Hu，窗宽 200~400 Hu）分别观察骨及软组织，通常要进行三维图像重建，以利于显示病变全貌。

（2）增强 CT 扫描：对于软组织病变及向软组织扩展的骨病变，静脉注射碘对比剂的增强 CT 扫描有利于不增强病变、坏死组织与强化病变的鉴别。与平扫相比，增强扫描能更精确地确定病变的范围与性质。

3.MRI 检查

目前，MRI 亦成为骨和软组织检查的重要手段。MRI 可以很好地显示骨髓、关节软骨、骨与关节周围软组织的形态和信号及其中的实质性、囊性与出血病变。一般认为，骨与软组织的 MRI 检查是在 X 线平片或 CT 检查的基础上进行的。但是，MRI 已是某些脊椎与关节疾病，特别是半月板、韧带、骨肿瘤或肿瘤样疾病的首选检查方法。

（1）MRI 平扫：骨与软组织的 MRI 检查亦分 MRI 平扫与增强扫描。可分别选择体部或表面线圈以增强图像的信噪比和对比度。对于四肢检查，横轴面像是基础扫描层面，因为在所有扫描层面中，横轴面像最易显示细微的皮质断裂、小的软组织肿块及其与神经血管的关系。冠状面与矢状面像可提供有益的补充信息。但是，对于脊椎检查，矢状面像有利于显示较长的范围，以便发现临床难以定位的病变。当在首次扫描层面发现可疑区域时，应加扫横轴面、冠状面或其他层面图像以更详细评价病变。自旋回波或快速自旋回波 T1 及 T2 加权像是骨 MRI 检查的主要序列，脂肪抑制序列亦很常用。更短时间的脉冲序列、心脏及周围门控技术、运动假影抑制技术使 MRI 对骨骼疾病的检查适应性更好。

（2）MRI 增强扫描：某些骨与软组织疾病需行钆增强 MRI 检查。MRI 增强扫描的应用不但可提高某些疾病诊断的敏感性，亦可判断病变的血供情况并且更精确地确定病变的范围与特性。

4.其他检查

除上述三种常规检查方式以外，还有一些检查手段也可应用于骨骼系统，如单光子发射计算机断层成像术（SPECT）和正电子发射断层成像术（PET）用于恶性骨肿瘤，超声用于骨密度测定等。

第二节 正常表现

人类的 206 块骨骼是由致密、坚硬并略有弹性的结缔组织构成。骨骼由骨膜包裹，外层为致密骨，其内包裹松质骨，松质骨内充满血管和神经。根据形态不同，人类骨骼分为四种类型，长骨或管状骨、短骨、扁骨及不规则骨。长骨干的骨髓腔内含有黄骨髓，其两关节骨端内则充有红骨髓。扁骨、短骨、椎体、颅骨板障、胸骨及肋骨骨髓腔内亦含有红骨髓，血细胞由活动性红骨髓产生。骨细胞产生骨组织，后者呈同心圆层状环绕哈氏管组成复杂的哈氏系统。哈氏系统内相互交错的管道含有血管、淋巴管和神经纤维。

1.管状骨

四肢骨分为长骨与短骨两类。长骨又称管状骨，可再分为长管状骨和短管状骨。长管状骨包括上肢骨与下肢骨，短管状骨包括手之掌指骨与足之跖趾骨。短骨是指腕骨与跗骨，类似正方体，其外为薄层骨皮质，内为松质骨。籽骨是位于肌腱和关节囊外的小骨，髌骨是最大的籽骨。

（1）小儿长骨：小儿长骨（图 4-1）明显不同于成人长骨，它由骨干、骨骺和干骺端组成，并有典型的 X 线特征。

骨骺是一块软骨，其中会出现 X 线照片时可显示的二次骨化中心。骨骺未骨化软骨的量随骨化中心的增大而变小。二次骨化中心的出现时间、增大及其与骨干融合的时间代表着长骨的生长与成熟状态。有许多放射学测量方法根据骨化中心的出现时间、大小及特点来评价骨龄。但骨龄只是个体骨成熟水平的简单评侧，骨龄的估计尚要根据其他特点，如种族、性别、地区、身高、体重及营养状态等因素进行校正。

干骺端是骨干紧邻骨骺的末端部分。这是一个软骨生成松质骨的移行区。干骺端血供丰富、代谢活跃。因此，干骺端是一个对许多疾病易感的特别重要的部分。

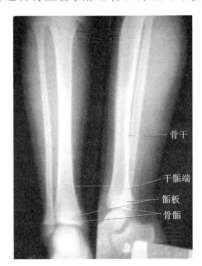

长骨的关节端称为骨骺。邻近骨骺的骨性部份称为干骺端。骨骺与干骺端之间被骺板分开。远离关节端的骨质部分称为骨干。

图 4-1 正常儿童胫骨、腓骨的分区

X 线平片上,干骺端是紧邻骨骺软骨的增宽部分,其中有致密网格结构,称为骨小梁。干骺端的末端终止于横行的钙化软骨盘或临时钙化带。在二次骨化中心与临时钙化带之间有一未钙化的软骨形成的透明线,即骺线或骺板,青春期后该线消失。

骨干是由致密骨壁,即骨皮质环绕而形成的管状结构,其中的圆柱状低密度腔,称为骨髓腔。骨皮质富含钙,投影呈不透明的高密度影。骨皮质在骨干中部最厚,往干骺端逐渐变薄,在骺板融合前与骺板相续。穿过骨皮质的营养动脉显示呈管状低密度。

X 线平片上,小儿长骨骨化部分投影呈不透明的含钙高密度影,未骨化部分投影呈类似周围软组织的水样密度影。骨干的两端为骺软骨,其中有二次骨化中心生成,骨化中心周围环绕一层类似临时钙化带的钙化软骨。嵌于骨骺骨化中心与骨干之间的条状低密度影为骺线。

(2)成人长骨:成人长骨(图 4-2)不同于小儿长骨,只有骨干和两侧骨端组成。骨干中部骨皮质最厚,向两端逐渐变薄并与骨端的软骨下骨性关节面相续。长骨两端膨大以形成关节,并有骨性结节突出以供肌肉或韧带附着。长骨骨皮质外被覆坚韧的袖套状结缔组织,称为骨外膜。骨外膜呈软组织密度,通常在 X 线平片上不显影。

2. 脊椎与骨盆

(1)脊椎的影像解剖:正常脊椎由 33 个椎骨构成,从上到下依次为 7 个颈椎、12 个胸椎,5 个腰椎,5 个骶椎和 4 个尾椎。成人时,骶椎和尾椎分别融合形成骶骨和尾骨,其他脊椎终生保持相互独立且能两两间相互活动。

胎儿和新生儿时期,脊柱有一个原发的后突曲度。生后,胸椎和骶尾椎仍保持后突状态,但继发前突相继出现。首先,约于生后 6 个月,婴儿学坐时出现颈部前突。然后,约于 1 岁半,幼儿能站立时完成腰椎前突。原发和继发曲度相互移行自然,但腰骶联合部曲度改变突然,并形成腰骶角。脊椎曲度可因脊椎疾病或椎旁肌肉痉挛而变化。

除了第 1、第 2 颈椎、骶骨和尾椎,每个脊椎均由前方略呈圆柱状的椎体及后方的椎弓环(椎管)组成,椎管前壁为椎体的后面,侧壁为椎弓根,后壁为 2 块椎板,椎板骨皮质比椎体骨皮质厚而致密。椎板在后部汇合形成棘突。两侧的椎弓根与椎板联合处发出横突及上关节突、下关节突。横突与棘突像一个强大的支柱,其中有许多肌肉和筋膜附着。

两个脊椎之间为椎间盘(图 4-3),椎间盘由两部分组成,中心部分称为髓核,周围是纤维环。髓核含有胶冻状物质并随年龄增大而逐渐纤维化。纤维环含有纤维软骨与致密的胶原纤维,外层环状纤维呈板层状并与上下相邻的椎体终板连续。

胚胎发育时,第 1 颈椎即环椎的椎体与该椎分离并与第 2 颈椎相连构成齿状突,致第 1 颈椎(图 4-4)呈卵圆形的环状,该环状前后部分甚薄,侧方的上下面张开形成小关节面,称为侧块,环的前部及后部中央有分界明确的小结节以代替前方的椎体与后方的棘突。环椎前弓的后面光滑,称为齿状突窝,其表面与齿状突相关节。环椎侧块的下面宽阔、呈圆形,扁平或轻微凹陷,其表面向内倾斜并与枢椎相关节。

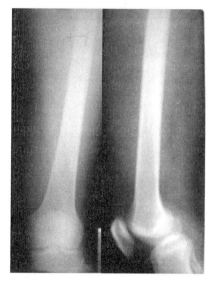

成人长骨,如股骨,由骨干和两个骨端构成,骨端常膨大以组成关节。

图 4-2 正常成人股骨

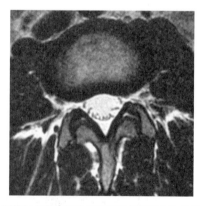

腰椎间盘中央部分的髓核呈高信号并被呈低信号的纤维环环绕。

图 4-3 正常成人腰椎间盘轴面

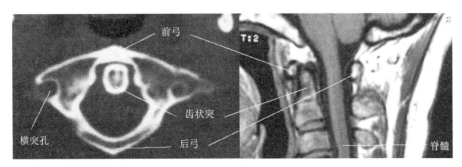

图 4-4 正常成人环椎及枢椎的轴面 CT 像和磁共振矢状面

第 2 颈椎即枢椎（图 4-4）是因为其作为环椎旋转的枢轴而得名，其突出的特征是胚胎发育时形成了一向上突出的齿状突。枢椎的上关节面宽阔、稍微上凸并稍向外下倾斜，并与环椎侧块的下关节面相关节，含有横突孔的枢椎横突只有单一的前结节。颈椎棘突较长，每一颈椎两侧横突各有一横突孔供椎动脉通过。

第 3 颈椎（C_3）至第 7 颈椎（C_7）椎体的侧后缘两椎体间相互形成较小的滑膜关节，称为"构椎关节"或"Luschka 关节"，该关节与神经、血管关系密切。

胸椎体从上致下逐渐增大并与 12 对肋骨相关节。腰椎较颈椎及胸椎大，腰椎体高度较矮、横径大于前后径。

骨性骨盆由 2 块髋骨和骶骨、尾骨组成。髋骨又由髂骨、坐骨和耻骨三块骨骼组成，在成年人，该三块骨骼在髋臼处融合呈单一的髋骨。

（2）正常 X 线表现：颈椎照片应包括正侧位及第 1、2 颈椎的特殊位置，为了观察椎间孔常常要加摄斜位片。胸椎、腰椎通常应摄正侧位片，如要显示腰椎椎弓峡部则要加摄斜位片。

脊椎（图 4-5）投影呈含钙的高密度不透明影，椎间盘呈透明的软组织密度。脊椎前后位片上，椎体显示清晰，除第 5 腰椎外，上一脊椎的棘突均投影于下一脊椎椎体中部。每一椎体两边有横突呈直角伸出。椎弓根呈卵圆形或环状与椎体重叠。椎弓根的上下方有上、下关节突及小关节间隙。一般情况下，上、下关节之相邻脊椎等大或逐渐增大。颈椎之椎弓根呈卵圆形，腰椎与胸椎椎弓根则呈环状。成人椎弓根之内侧面均膨凸，但在儿童，可有变异或呈凹陷状。两侧椎弓根之间的距离称为椎弓根间距，又叫椎管横径。椎管横径在颈与腰膨大及脊髓圆椎处最大，而在胸椎中段最小。椎弓根形态及椎弓根间距的变化均具有较大诊断价值。前后位像上我们还应注意脊椎的排列顺序，正常棘突应位于中线呈垂直排列。

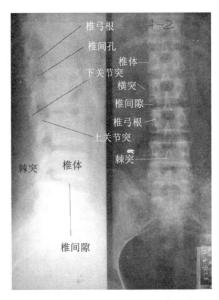

图 4-5 正常成人腰椎的侧位与前后位像

侧位片上，椎体呈致密的方形骨块，其间为半透明的椎间盘，被称为椎间隙。椎体后方为椎弓根及其间的椎间孔，再后方为棘突，椎间孔的方向随脊椎平面不同而异。颈椎间孔方向斜行，胸椎间孔走行趋向冠状方向，腰椎呈正冠状位走行。

侧位观椎体与椎间盘的外形及内部结构均能清晰显示，但椎弓等后部结构相互重叠。椎体前缘或后缘的连线、椎小关节的连线在侧位片上都应呈一条连续、自然的曲线。

第二节 基本病变

尽管骨骼疾病病理变化与X线征象各种各样，但其中有不同疾病共存的X线征象，称为基本病变。在一种疾病中，这些基本病变可以单独存在或混合存在。

1. 骨质疏松

骨质疏松(图4-6)通常是由骨代谢异常所致，其特点是骨量减少，但骨的质正常，即矿物质含量在正常范围。骨质疏松患者成骨活动减弱或蛋白质缺乏、血清钙、磷、碱性磷酸酶在正常范围内。骨质疏松可伴发于各种疾病，并可分为广泛性、区域性与局限性。

广泛性骨质疏松包括年龄相关骨质疏松(如老年性骨质疏松、绝经后骨质疏松)、内分泌疾病致骨质疏松(如巨人症、甲状旁腺功能亢进症、甲状腺功能亢进症、皮质醇功能亢进症)或与妊娠和酒精中毒有关。广泛性骨质疏松主要累及中轴骨及四肢长骨近侧部，脊椎骨不但有骨量的减少、尚有形态的变化。广泛性骨质疏松骨密度弥漫降低，但在X线平片上有时与骨质软化很难鉴别。

区域性骨质疏松可发生于废用、反射性交感神经萎缩、髋关节一过性骨质疏松及区域性迁移性骨质疏松，主要累及四肢骨。该类骨质疏松较重者由于骨内膜与骨外膜下及骨皮质内的骨吸收会引起骨皮质变薄、松质骨变化，主要发生于骨端关节面下及干骺端。

局限性骨质疏松常常伴发于局限性骨病，如骨肿瘤、骨感染。

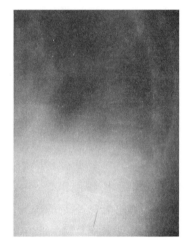

胸椎侧位片示脊椎弥漫性密度减低，并有椎体压缩与凹透镜样改变。

图4-6 老年妇女绝经后脊椎骨质疏松

骨质疏松只有在较严重时才有X线方面的改变，包括骨透亮度变化，骨小梁变化及外形变化，椎体的改变包括压缩致楔形椎、鱼脊椎、许莫氏结节、其他急性及不全骨折与椎体内骨小梁栅栏样变。不同类型骨质疏松具有相同的X线表现，其主要特点是广泛骨密度减低伴有长骨骨皮质变薄。

在长骨，骨质疏松的骨吸收可能在骨内膜、皮质内哈氏管或骨外膜最明显，但这些变化需要放大摄影及计量X线摄影才能显示。骨皮质变薄、但结构正常，骨小梁稀疏、数量减少，剩余的骨小梁较粗大并位于应力方向，这在骨质疏松与骨质软化的鉴别诊断中具有较大意义。

2. 骨质软化

骨质软化与骨质疏松不同，骨质软化(图4-7)是一组由于皮质骨或松质骨之骨样组织矿化异常或延迟而引起的疾病，维生素D缺乏病(佝偻病)主要与骨质软化有关。

正常人骨样组织的形成与矿化呈动态平衡，当骨样组织生成过多或矿化不足均可引起骨质软化。胃肠道血钙吸收不足或磷排泄过多均可引起血钙过低或骨质软化。骨质软化的常见原因为维生素D缺乏，在婴幼儿形成维生素D缺乏病，在成人则引起骨质软化症。骨质软化常有血生化异常，包括低血钙、低血磷与碱性磷酸酶增高。

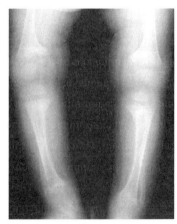

**图4-7 2岁患儿维生素D缺乏病
胫骨、腓骨骨质软化图像**

骨质软化的特征性X线改变有骨密度减低，骨皮质较厚但边缘模糊，与周围软组织分界欠清，骨小梁边缘模糊，形成所谓"磨玻璃样"改变，这是由于多余的骨样组织覆盖于骨小梁表面及哈氏管内壁所致。由于有多余的骨样组织形成，骨质变软，承重骨骼如脊椎、骨盆容易变形或骨折。Looser 带或 Milkman 假骨折线是骨质软化另一重要 X 线特征。这是一些与骨皮质垂直的带状低密度区，1~2 mm 宽，常两侧对称发生于肩胛骨的腋缘、股骨颈、耻骨与坐骨肢及肋骨。这代表骨质软化时不全骨折的不良愈合现象。

3. 骨质破坏

骨皮质或骨松质被破坏并被病理组织代替称为骨质破坏，其可单发、多发、局限性或弥漫性。

X 线片上，骨质破坏显示为密度减低的无骨结构骨质溶骨区(图 4-8)。根据 X 线表现，骨质破坏分为三类：一类是呈地图样分布的大块骨质破坏，此类在 X 线平片上容易显示；另一类是虫蚀样骨质破坏，提示病变进展较快，如急性骨髓炎；还有一类是浸润型骨质破坏，破坏区弥漫扩展，如恶性骨肿瘤。一般认为，破坏较慢的病变较破坏较快的病变边缘更光滑、锐利。

4. 骨质增生硬化

骨质增生硬化(图 4-9)是指 X 线片显示骨质异常增多、密度增高，如象牙质样改变。骨质增生硬化可见于许多疾病，如肾性骨营养不良、骨关节病、镰状细胞贫血、Paget 病、骨转移瘤、骨髓纤维化、骨创伤及慢性骨髓炎。

慢性骨感染或骨低毒感染时，骨对疾病的反应与急性骨髓炎不同，不是骨质溶解，而是新骨形成，在 X 线片上表现为骨密度增高、骨骼增大、骨皮质增厚、骨小梁增粗，骨小梁及骨髓腔均消失。

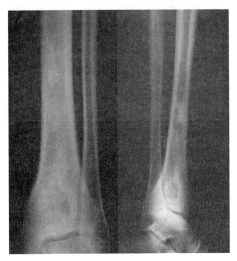

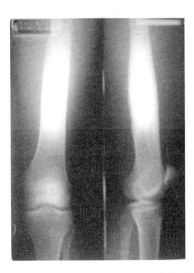

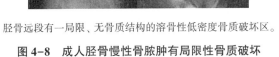

胫骨远段有一局限、无骨质结构的溶骨性低密度骨质破坏区。

X 线照片示股骨干密度增高，外形增粗，髓腔消失，如象牙质样。

图 4-8　成人胫骨慢性骨脓肿有局限性骨质破坏

图 4-9　成人股骨干慢性骨髓炎致骨质硬化

5. 骨膜反应

骨膜反应(图 4-10)又称骨膜增生。骨膜系覆盖于骨表面的膜状结缔组织，骨借骨膜与周围的软组织相连。除非患病，正常骨膜不能在 X 线片上显影。骨膜反应表现为形状不同的高密度投影，可以是分层状、花边状或爆花状。但在疾病早期，骨膜反应多表现为与骨皮质稍分离的线状密度增高影，其中间隔有裂隙状低密度区，随病变进展，该低密度裂隙会被不定形的新骨填充而与骨皮质融合。单纯根据骨膜反应的形态难以作出正确诊断，应综合其他 X 线表现及临床资料。

许多疾病可引起骨膜反应，常见的有葡萄球菌骨感染、骨梅毒、伤寒骨感染、应力骨折、骨白血病、原发和继发的恶性骨肿瘤及增生性骨关节病。

6. 骨质坏死与死骨

局部骨组织血液供应中断、骨细胞代谢完全停止称为骨坏死。骨坏死是指部分或完全与周围正常骨组织分离的坏死骨组织(图 4-11)。

骨坏死的组织学特征是骨细胞及细胞核的丧失,骨基质中的细胞陷窝呈空虚状态。在破骨细胞清除前,骨基质形态正常,这一过程需要较长时间。因此,骨坏死在数周或更长的时间内 X 线表现会显示正常。

骨坏死的主要 X 线表现是骨密度增高,这有两个原因,一是新骨沉积于原有骨小梁上或骨髓腔内,形成绝对密度增高;二是与充满炎性肉芽组织和脓液的死骨腔对比,死骨呈相对高密度。不同的疾病或疾病的不同阶段死骨形态各异。恶性骨肿瘤的残留骨可能为死骨或活骨。

骨坏死常见于慢性化脓性骨髓炎、骨缺血坏死及骨创伤后,偶尔见于骨结核。

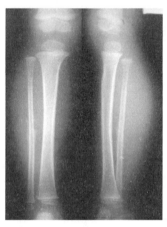

腓骨干皮质稍外侧的线状、花边状密度增高影即腓骨急性化脓性骨髓炎的骨膜反应,其与骨皮质间有一较窄的透明间隙。

图 4-10 儿童腓骨急性化脓性骨髓炎的骨膜反应

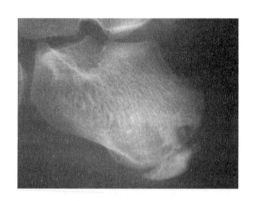

图 4-11 儿童跟骨结核病灶中有砂粒样死骨

7. 骨折线

骨折线是指贯穿骨骼、使骨的连续性中断的条状低密度影(图 4-12)。骨折线是骨折的特征性 X 线征象。由于骨小梁的嵌插,压缩性骨折之骨折线会变模糊并形成条状高密度影。评价骨创伤时应注意如下 2 点:①具有骨创伤病史并有可疑骨折体征但首次 X 线检查阴性者,特别是腕、脊椎和肋骨等部位创伤,应行 CT 或(和)MRI 进一步明确诊断;②当不能肯定骨折时,特别是可能会与骨折线混淆的骺线尚存的婴儿或儿童,应加照对侧的 X 线摄片,以供比较。

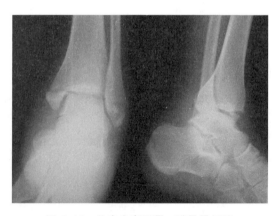

图 4-12 儿童患者胫骨、腓骨骨折线

8.软组织变化

一张好的骨骼 X 线片，应尽量包括周围软组织。软组织肿胀或炎性水肿表现为密度稍增高的肿块，软组织内脂肪线模糊或消失。软组织内钙化多是由于陈旧损伤或结缔组织疾病所致。软组织内积气可能是由于含气感染或与外界相通的损伤所致。

9.骨病变基质

某些肿瘤及其他疾病均具有骨病变基质，基质可能是软骨性、骨性或混合性的。一个具有明确壁性结构的透明区域可能是含有液体或血液的囊肿，如其内伴有斑点样或爆玉米花样钙化可能是软骨组织，如其中有粗糙的骨小梁或不规则骨质硬化则可能是纤维组织。

为了能作出正确诊断，骨骼系统阅片时应注意如下几点：

(1)病变部位：是骨骺、干骺端、骨干，还是大关节的持重面。

(2)侵犯骨骼：某些疾病好发于某些骨骼，病变系单发还是多发。

(3)病变类型：是溶骨性、成骨性还是混合性。

(4)病变边缘：病变边缘分界清晰还是模糊。

(5)周围骨反应：骨膜反应是条状、分层还是针样。

(6)骨组织：是软骨性、骨性还是纤维性。

(7)软组织是否有变化。

(8)患者的年龄与性别。

(9)疾病的发作形式：属急性、慢性还是进行性的。

(10)有无外伤史。

第四节　常见疾病诊断

普通 X 线检查在骨与关节损伤的诊断中具有重要作用。这不但能确定是否有骨折存在，在 X 线透视下尚能帮助骨折与脱位的复位。

1.骨折

(1)长骨骨折：

1)临床及病理表现：骨皮质及骨小梁的连续性中断，骨骼中出现裂缝称为骨折。长骨骨折多见于四肢骨，其形态随外伤的部位及施力的方向不同而不同，骨折可发生于长骨的任何部位，包括骨骺。

2)影像学表现：骨折线是长骨骨折的特征性 X 线征象。新鲜骨折在 X 线片上显示为骨折端或骨折碎片间的透明线，其边缘不规则而锐利。注意不要将骺线误诊断骨折线。有些骨折线在某一方向的照片上难以显示，但另一方向的照片可能显示清晰(图4-13)。对于压缩性骨折，不能显示透明骨折线，而显示为高密度线。

放射学通常对骨折进行如下分类：①根据骨折线的方向和形态，骨折可分为纵型、斜型、Y 型及螺旋型，粉碎性骨折是指骨折片大于 2 块的骨折；②根据骨折线的延伸情况，骨折可分为完全性骨折和不完全性骨折，前者是指骨折线累及长骨横径

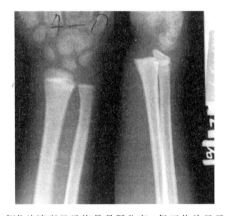

侧位片清晰显示桡骨骨骺分离，但正位片显示不清。

图4-13　儿童患者桡骨远端骨骺分离

全长，后者只有部分骨皮质断裂或产生皱折，多发生于儿童，被称为青枝骨折；③病理性骨折，是指在原先有病的骨骼，如骨髓炎、骨肿瘤及其他骨骼疾病的基础上发生的骨折。

当骨折被确诊时,我们应注意观察骨折远端与近端之间的位置关系。相对于骨折近端,骨折远端是否有前后、内外侧移位,骨折碎片是否有重叠、压缩、分离或旋转;骨折两端是否有成角,因为骨折是否成角是决定治疗方案的重要方面。

骨折的愈合:

无并发症的骨折在损伤2~3天后开始愈合,愈合是骨折处血肿机化和肉芽组织生长的过程。开始,在骨折片间有纤维性骨痂形成,这种骨痂多在伤后5~10天形成,又叫临时性骨痂。软骨性骨痂及纤维性骨痂的形成均较缓慢,且这种骨痂在X线片上不显影,因此,骨折线仍可见,但变得较模糊。随着骨折愈合进一步发展,在骨折两断端间及骨膜下有骨性骨痂形成并逐渐演变成骨性愈合。此时骨折线消失。

骨折愈合速度变异较大,患者的年龄、营养状态、骨折部位与类型及骨折后是否得到恰当治疗均与骨折愈合有关。无并发症骨折的平均愈合时间常为8~10周。新骨塑形是骨折愈合的最后阶段并常需要数月。这样,全部骨痂完成骨化过程,正常骨结构得以恢复。

骨折愈合的诊断:正确评价骨折愈合必需有赖于临床与X线的综合应用。

骨折愈合的X线表现:骨折愈合的最早征象是骨膜骨痂的出现,即紧邻骨皮质环绕骨折处的模糊阴影并随骨化的进展密度逐渐增高。骨内骨痂位于骨折片之间并使骨折线变模糊。随着骨内骨痂的增多,骨折线变得更加模糊,骨折线内逐渐有不透明骨化影出现,最后,骨折线消失,骨髓腔重新形成。

骨折愈合的常见并发症有以下两种:

延迟愈合:骨折处新骨形成过程受损,但形成新骨的能力仍然存在,会产生延迟愈合。假如创造合适的条件,骨折仍能愈合,但要经历较长时间。如果未能提供合适条件并进行不恰当治疗将会导致骨折不愈合。X线片上,延迟愈合者骨痂出现延迟且量少,骨折线较长期存在,但在骨折两断端间没有骨质硬化。

骨折不愈合:在一定的时间内不发生骨折愈合,新骨形成能力消失称为骨折不愈合。X线片上,骨折线始终存在,骨折片分离,骨折断端变圆钝并硬化,常没有骨痂或只有微量骨痂出现且骨痂不跨过骨折线,可有假关节形成,即骨折两端硬化,近折端呈膨突状、远折端近侧表面凹陷形成关节样改变。骨髓腔在骨折两端处封闭。

常见骨折类型有以下几种:

柯雷骨折:柯雷骨折是最常见骨折的一种,多见于老年。骨折线位于桡骨腕关节面2.5 cm以内。移位的柯雷骨折,骨折线几乎均呈横贯性,远折端向背侧及桡侧移位,断端向掌侧成角,并常伴有尺骨茎突骨折及桡尺远侧关节分离。

肱骨髁上骨折:这是常见于儿童的肱骨下段最常见损伤。骨折线与骺线距离不等。可以通过干骺端、肱骨髁或通过骺线,通过骺线者称为骨骺分离。骨折线的形状可以是T形或Y形。远侧骨折端可能向后、向前并向内或向外移位。远折端向后移位更常见,称为伸展型骨折。骨折端向前移位少见,称为屈曲型骨折。

股骨颈骨折:股骨颈骨折最常见于老年人,特别是伴有骨质疏松者。根据解剖学部位,骨折可分为头下型、经颈型、基底型及粗隆间型等。经颈型与粗隆间型较其他型常见。头下型、经颈型及基底型骨折均位于关节囊内,由于该三型股骨头血液供应受到影响,容易并发缺血坏死。当股骨头发生缺血坏死时,其密度增高,关节面变形并关节面下小囊形成。

(2)脊椎骨折

1)临床及病理表现:脊椎骨折的发生概率仅次于长骨骨折。尽管全脊椎均可能受到损伤,但一般情况下,最常发生于脊柱的屈曲部位,如下胸段与上腰段脊椎。

2)影像学表现:

①X线表现:由于压缩的关系,骨折的椎体呈楔形变(图4-14)。由于骨小梁嵌插,椎体压缩骨折不能见到透明的骨折线,反而被高密度线代替。椎间隙多正常或轻微变窄,这与脊椎结核完全不同。

②CT表现:对于骨折的诊断,CT可以作为平片的补充手段,尤其是脊椎及大多数骨盆骨折。对于脊椎暴裂骨折(图4-15),CT比X线平片能提供更有价值的信息,因为CT容易显示碎骨片的数目,碎骨片突入椎管的程度及其与脊髓的关系。对于大多数骨盆骨折,CT能很好地确认髋臼碎骨片的状况,提供较X

线平片更多的信息，而不是简单地证实 X 线平片的信息而进行诊断。

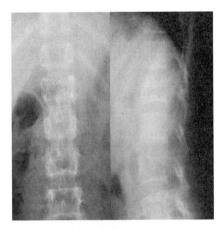

图 4-14　L_1 椎体压缩骨折

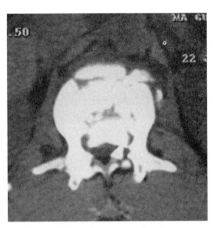

图 4-15　CT 轴面像示 L_1 椎体暴裂骨折

③MRI 表现：尽管 MRI 在显示骨折线方面不如 CT，但 MRI 很容易显示骨折断端邻近的血肿、软组织水肿、出血及其他软组织损伤。偶尔，MRI 能显示 X 线平片不易诊断的长骨隐匿性骨折和轻微的椎体压缩骨折(图 4-16)。骨挫伤有骨小梁断裂，骨髓水肿与出血，但 CT 与 X 线平片表现正常。MRI T1 WI 表现为在高信号的骨髓像中有低信号病变，T2 WI 病变呈高信号，在抑脂像中表现尤其明显。尽管 MRI 对如脑和脊髓等软组织与骨髓的损伤十分敏感，但尚不能代替详细的临床检查与骨骼的常规 X 线检查。

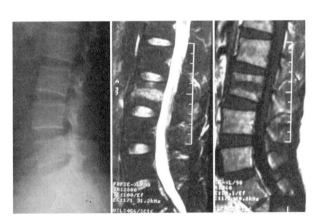

T1 WI 与 T2 WI 示 L_3 椎体隐匿性压缩骨折。

图 4-16　椎体压缩性骨折的 X 线片及磁共振影像片

2. 椎间盘突出

(1)临床及病理表现：椎间盘突出多发生于 20 至 40 岁的青壮年，男性多见。下腰段最常受累及，颈椎次之。典型的侧后方腰椎间盘突出压迫椎管侧隐窝或椎间孔内的神经根，引起疼痛、感觉异常、麻木、肌无力及被压迫神经根区域的反射减弱。颈与胸段椎间盘突出不但可引起神经根性异常，尚可压迫脊髓引起脊髓病，导致神经束表现，如压迫平面的双侧肢体乏力、麻木和痉挛。要准确定位其被压迫的神经或脊髓平面往往非常困难。

椎间盘的中央部分为胶冻状的髓核，周围部分为纤维环，有弹性。椎间盘的上、下方在儿童为透明软骨板，成人为终板。纤维环的后方及外后方最薄弱，容易产生裂缝，当髓核物质疝入裂缝时即形成椎间盘突出。当椎间盘物质突出超过椎体边缘压迫附近结构即产生临床症状和体征。

(2)影像学表现：

1)X 线表现：当患者以神经根病或脊髓病为主诉并怀疑与椎间盘突出有关时，X 线平片是基本检查手段，这有利于病变正确定位及作为 CT、MRI 检查的前期准备。除罕见的游离髓核碎片钙化外，脊椎平片不能确诊椎间盘突出。椎间隙变窄、椎体边缘骨质增生、骨赘形成、小突关节间隙变窄或增宽、关节面骨质增生与骨赘形成及椎间盘内"真空征"都提示有椎间盘退变，但不管有无症状及有无椎间盘突出，椎间盘退变患者都可见到这些表现。过去，X 线平片主要是作为初筛方法显示脊椎是否有临床表现类似椎间盘突出的炎症或肿瘤存在。但 X 线平片对骨结构早期变化的诊断很不敏感。放射性核素骨扫描、CT 及 MRI 均优于 X 线平片。

2）CT 表现：CT 是腰椎间盘突出的首选检查方法，但是，要评价颈与胸段椎间盘突出应首选 MRI。CT 可显示椎间盘退行性变的三种类型：膨出、突出和脱出。40 岁以上的成年人椎间盘膨出很常见。椎间盘膨出是指椎间盘在所有方向都超过相邻椎体的边缘。典型的椎间盘膨出呈对称性，中线部最明显。但是，偶而一边的膨突会大于另一边的膨突。下腰部的椎间盘膨出常不引起神经根压迫，但椎管较小者，弥漫性椎间盘膨出可能压迫硬脊膜囊前缘。严重的椎管狭窄患者，尚可压迫脊髓或神经根。椎间盘突出是指椎间盘组织局限性突出超出椎体的边缘。此种突出可发生于椎间盘的任意点位，甚至可向上或下突入相邻椎体内形成骨内突出，或称"许莫氏"结节。椎间盘突出的 CT 诊断标准如下：①椎间盘密度的组织局限性、角样或息肉样突入椎管，突出的椎间盘组织密度（CT 值 60~100 Hu）明显高于硬膜外脂肪（CT 值-50-0HU）或充满液体的硬膜囊（CT 值 20~50 Hu）；②突出物局部硬膜外脂肪组织移位；③硬脊膜囊前外侧边缘局部变形；④突出物压迫使神经根汇合部或下降部或出口部移位（图 4-17）。

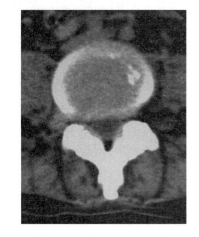

椎间盘突出伸入右侧椎间孔内。

图 4-17 CT 轴面像示椎间盘组织局部突出

椎间盘脱出是指突出的椎间盘组织突破后纵韧带与椎间盘本体分离。椎间盘碎片位于椎管内硬膜外间隙的疏松脂肪组织内并与椎间盘分离向上或向下移位。移位的碎片最终压迫同一椎间盘上部或下部平面的神经根。椎间盘脱出也称游离碎片性突出。当突出物位于椎间盘平面，CT 难以鉴别单纯性突出与游离碎片性突出；偶尔，游离碎片性突出在碎片与原椎间盘之间有脂肪裂隙显示。当椎间盘以上或以下平面硬膜外间隙出现与椎间盘密度一致的软组织块时，游离碎片性突出即可确立。

3）MRI 表现：到目前为止，MRI 是诊断所有节段脊椎椎间盘突出的最佳方法。矢状面 T1WI 不但能显示椎间盘组织向后突入椎管内，还能评价椎间孔的大小、轮廓及是否有狭窄。突出的椎间盘组织常表现为与同一平面的椎间盘组织呈相同信号，而与相邻的硬膜外间隙脂肪组织的高信号及硬膜囊内蛛网膜下隙的低信号形成明显对比。矢状面 T2WI 示椎间盘突出呈肿块状超过低信号的椎体后部边缘。突出物常与同一平面椎间盘呈相同信号，而与低信号的硬膜及高信号的蛛网膜下腺有明显分界。尽管仔细辨认矢状面图像上突出物对椎间孔内神经周围脂肪组织的压迫可能提示最外侧性突出的可能，但横轴面更易于显示最外侧性椎间盘突出对椎间孔内神经周围脂肪组织及出口段神经根的压迫。联合矢状面和横轴面 T1WI，很容易显示向上或向下移位的游离碎片性椎间盘突出（图 4-18）。表现为与椎间盘组织呈相同信号的块状物，

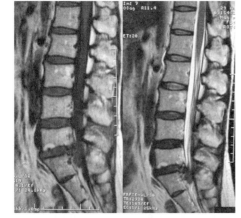

图 4-18 磁共振矢状面 T1WI 及 T2WI 示 L_5-S_1 椎间盘突出游离碎片向下移位

使硬膜外间隙的脂肪组织移位或消失，容易与呈低信号的蛛网膜下隙鉴别。在 T2WI 上，移位的髓核碎片信号不一致，常呈高信号，这可能为水化作用所致。此时，碎片与许多肿瘤一样与高信号的蛛网膜下隙难以区分。碎片虽与椎间盘分离但未移位，MRI 及其他任何影像学方法都难以诊断。

3.骨髓炎

（1）临床及病理表现：病原微生物可通过邻近感染的软组织、关节或通过伤口或开放性骨折直接进入骨内。血源性感染的骨髓炎是最常见的感染方式，实际上是一种由血液输送的骨病，常见于婴儿和儿童，新生儿亦可累及。金黄色葡萄球菌是最常见的病原菌，病变几乎均始发于干骺端，开始形成小脓肿，随着脓腔内压力增高，脓肿逐渐增大，并穿破骨皮质进入骨膜下间隙，脓肿顺骨膜下扩散则累及骨干。如果感染没有控制，骨骼全长即被累及，导致广泛的骨膜反应。在生长期，感染很少越过骺板，但易于突破邻近干骺端的骨质，当干骺端位于关节囊内时，即会引起化脓性关节炎。被破坏的骨质，特别是骨皮质难以被吸收，即留下较大块的死骨，死骨会逐渐与活骨分离。死骨表现为特征性的高密度，其周围有死腔。如没有适当的治疗，化脓性骨髓炎很容易慢性化。在慢性期，骨质破坏过程减慢并有明显的修复反应。慢性化脓性骨髓炎可能有很长的病程，并有持续排脓的窦道及死骨排出。

（2）影像学表现：

1）X线表现：在早期，尽管临床表现明显，急性化脓性骨髓炎的X线表现仍很轻微并容易被漏诊。仔细观察，此期可发现骨骼邻近的软组织水肿。起病头3天，软组织内有轻微变化。由于充血和骨内水肿，病变局部深部软组织肿胀。继之，肌肉肿胀、软组织之间的间隙模糊或消失。稍后表现为软组织内急性脓肿形成，这是由于感染导致骨皮质破坏所致。骨骼变化要在起病2周后才变得明显，首先在长骨的干骺端出现斑片状骨质破坏区，随后，小的斑片状骨质破坏区融合形成边界欠清的大的骨质破坏。接着，骨皮质破坏，骨干周围有明显的花边样骨膜反应，骨皮质坏死即形成死骨。急性化脓性骨髓炎的显著X线特点（图4-19）是广泛骨质破坏、明显的骨膜反应、修复反应轻微。与急性化脓性骨髓炎不同，慢性化脓性骨髓炎有明显的骨质增生、骨密度明显增高、骨皮质增厚、骨轮廓不规则，其中可点缀低密度骨质破坏，死骨腔中可能会有大块死骨。慢性化脓性骨髓炎愈合后，骨质破坏及死骨消失，但患病的骨骼会增粗。

2）CT表现：CT能发现X线平片难以显示的软组织与骨髓内炎症和脓肿，小骨质破坏区及小死骨片。

3）MRI表现：MRI具有良好的软组织分辨力，容易显示软组织形态与含水量的早期变化。脓肿在T1WI表现为低信号，T2WI及STIR表现为明显的高信号。增强扫描有更利于显示软组织异常，提高病变的显示力并更易准确显示脓肿的范围，这有利于骨髓炎与蜂窝织炎及软组织脓肿的鉴别。MRI能清晰地分辨骨髓坏死与骨髓水肿。

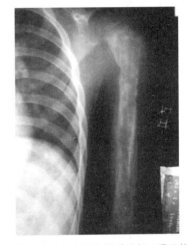

X线照片示有广泛的骨质破坏，明显的骨膜反应与不明显的反应性骨质增生。

图4-19 左肱骨急性化脓性骨髓炎

4.结核

（1）临床及病理表现：骨与关节结核几乎总是继发于身体其他部位的结核，特别是肺结核。骨结核好发于青少年，如同其他血源性感染的疾病一样，骨结核的原发病灶亦位于干骺端。长骨结核较脊椎及关节结核少见。

（2）影像学表现：

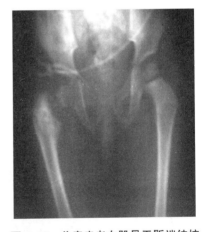

图4-20 儿童患者右股骨干骺端结核

1）X线表现：长骨结核的典型部位在干骺端及骨骺（图4-20）。青年患者，骨结核象化脓性骨髓炎一样，病变可从干骺端累及骺板。成年人，可累及骨干。不象化脓性骨髓炎，尽管偶而可见到砂粒样死骨，骨结核较少有骨膜反应、骨质硬化或死骨形成。薄层骨膜反应往往与窦道形成有关。根据感染结核菌的毒力不同,骨结核 X 线可表现为类似慢性骨脓肿或良性骨肿瘤的局灶性病变,亦可表现类似尤文肉瘤、淋巴瘤或白血病骨病等弥漫浸润性病变。随病变进展,骨结核有破坏骨骺累及关节的趋势,亦可突破骨皮质、骨膜侵及周围软组织并形成窦道。

当结核发生于手足等短管状骨,并呈溶骨性病变时,病变可使所在整个骨干膨大呈梭形,称为"骨气臌"。这与慢性生长的诸如内生软骨瘤、良性骨肿瘤类似。

脊柱是骨结核的最常见部位,好发于儿童及青少年,无性别差异。脊柱结核的好发节段依次为:腰椎、胸腰段及颈椎,尾椎发病最少见。脊椎结核的首发部位多为椎体,椎弓很少累及。原发感染病灶可能位于椎体中央、边缘或前方骨膜下,但在日常所见到的常为此三者的混合型。脊椎结核在 X 线表现为慢性、进行性、局限性骨质破坏,受累椎体由于压缩骨折而塌陷呈楔形变。相邻椎体连续受累及很常见,并可沿着前侧方的脊椎韧带累及远离病变部位之椎体。椎旁软组织形成冷脓肿很常见,脓肿内可能见到钙化灶。

脊椎结核(图 4-21)的基本 X 线征象有:①单个或多个椎体骨质破坏,常常形成楔形变;②两个相邻受累脊椎之椎间隙变窄或消失,这一点是脊椎结核与椎体压缩骨折、脊椎转移瘤的主要不同点及鉴别诊断的要点;③冷脓肿形成,椎旁软组织增宽、边缘模糊,并向两侧膨出呈梭形肿胀;根据受累的是腰椎、胸椎或颈椎等位置不同,软组织肿胀可能是腰大肌、椎旁软组织或咽后间隙;④骨质破坏使脊柱形成局限性后突畸形或侧弯畸形。

2)CT 表现:CT 对于显示脊椎病变在软组织的累及范围极小的砂粒样死骨或砂粒体优于 X 线平片(图4-22)。CT 对感染性脊椎炎更重要的作用是对诊断不明确患者在 CT 引导下引流或活检。

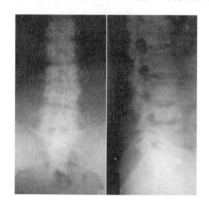

图 4-21　X 线平片示脊椎结核

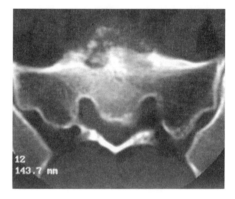

图 4-22　CT 影像显示骶骨结核的砂粒体

3)MRI 表现:像 CT 一样,MRI 对于长骨结核病变的定位、累及范围及骨质破坏的分类能提供较 X 线平片更多的信息。MRI 对脊椎结核具有重要的诊断意义。矢状面 T1WI 及 T2WI 能够显示普通 X 线平片不能显示的椎体病变。更重要的是,MRI 能确定软组织脓肿的范围、病变对椎管的侵犯及其对脊髓的影响情况(图4-23),这能给外科手术提供非常有价值的信息。增强扫描能更好地显示冷脓肿的壁。

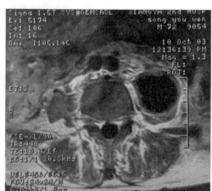
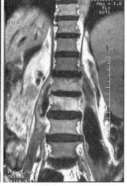

图 4-23　增强 MRI 影像显示双侧腰大肌冷脓肿

5. 骨肿瘤

骨肿瘤为 X 线诊断提出了一个十分重要而复杂的问题。临床医生、病理科医生和放射科医生之间常常为某一肿瘤的良性、恶性诊断而存在分歧，但其最后诊断结果又决定着患者的治疗方法及预后情况。几乎所有骨疾病研究者都同意：要作出正确的骨肿瘤诊断，临床、放射学及病理学应相互结合，必要时还应考虑生化及血液学检查的结果。

放射学检查在骨肿瘤的诊断中有重要的地位。如未阅读 X 线片，病理科医生不应作出骨肿瘤的肯定诊断。详细的临床资料，如症状的类型及病程，以前是否有创伤、放射治疗及病理性骨折对于作出正确的病理诊断亦是十分重要的。

骨肿瘤的放射学诊断应包括：①骨骼病变是否是肿瘤；②是良性肿瘤还是恶性肿瘤，是原发性肿瘤还是转移性肿瘤；③肿瘤可能是何种组织学类型；④肿瘤相邻骨骼及软组织侵犯范围的评价。

骨肿瘤分为良性骨肿瘤、恶性骨肿瘤和转移性骨肿瘤。患者的年龄、发病部位、病变数目及临床症状、体征和实验室检查在骨肿瘤的诊断中均具有重要作用。X 线诊断可能鉴别大多数骨肿瘤的良性、恶性。良性骨肿瘤生长较慢，常常表现为边界清晰的膨胀性骨质破坏，病变与正常骨组织的分界锐利而清晰。膨胀的骨皮质完整，没有软组织肿块，没有骨膜反应，没有远处转移。恶性骨肿瘤的表现则相反。在观察骨肿瘤的 X 线表现时应注意以下几点：

(1)发病骨的类型(长骨还是扁骨)及病变的位置，病变是位于骨骺、骺板还是干骺端或骨干，病变是位于骨髓腔、骨皮质还是骨皮质旁，不同的骨肿瘤具有不同的好发部位，如骨巨细胞瘤好发于长骨骨端，骨肉瘤则多发于长骨干骺端，骨髓瘤好发于扁骨。

(2)病变是单发还是多发：原发性骨肿瘤常单发，骨髓瘤及转移性骨肿瘤常多发。

(3)病变受累的长度及范围。

(4)骨质变化：是大块骨质破坏还是虫蚀样骨质吸收，是浸润性骨质破坏还是囊样骨质破坏，是否有骨质增生，是否是混合型。

(5)肿瘤组织的密度，特别注意是否有钙化存在及其 X 线表现特征：均质、斑点状还是棉絮状。

(6)骨内病变相邻骨质边缘的变化：是锐利还是模糊，病变边缘密度是增高还是降低，反应边的宽窄。

(7)病变相邻骨皮质的变化：是骨髓腔面受累还是骨外膜面受累，是浸润性破坏还是压迫性吸收。

(8)骨膜反应：是否有骨膜反应存在，是层状还是洋葱皮样，是均质的还是日光放射状，是否有Codman 三角。

(9)病变邻近软组织是否有变化，应特别注意肌间隙，软组织内是否有肿瘤组织。

除少数特殊情况外，CT 对骨肿瘤的诊断亦有限。肿瘤的近皮质钙化或骨化在 X 线平片上可类似骨化性肌炎。CT 扫描能显示骨化性肌炎之钙化在骨骼周围，而未附着于骨上，颇具特征。CT 能显示较浅表骨肉瘤同样具有浸润性生长的特点，中央呈钙化的高密度，边界不清，皮质受累，而不像骨软骨瘤一样骨骼的皮质、骨髓与肿瘤相连续。CT 对于显示骨样骨瘤的瘤巢敏感性与特异性亦较高，表现为中央斑点状的高密度区，周围有透明带环绕，其外周邻近骨质有不同程度的骨质增生硬化区。常规 X 线照片的高度空间分辨力能更精确地显示肿瘤基质中的钙化或骨化类型。CT 虽然能侦测到微量的钙化或骨化，但这并不能比X 线平片提供更有意义的鉴别诊断信息。

MRI 对于骨骼肌肉肿瘤的分期具有较大作用。其多方位成像、软组织对比度的特性使其能精确地评价肿瘤的范围、皮质受侵、邻近软组织肿瘤形成及关节受累的程度。

为了保证适当地切除肿瘤而尽可能地多保留肢体，鉴别恶性骨肿瘤与瘤周水肿是非常必要的，尽管这可能很困难，但要较广泛地切除肿瘤，常要包括病变周围数厘米范围组织，这是保肢手术的基础。过度地估计真正肿瘤的范围，可能导致保肢手术变为截肢手术。应用不同梯度回波的动态增强 MRI 可以相当可靠地鉴别肿瘤与瘤周水肿。水肿呈特征性均匀强化，其信号高于或等于邻近肿瘤的信号。动态增强对于计划活检者亦能提供有用的信息，坏死区域应避免活检，高血供区比低灌注区活检更有效。使用或不使用对比剂的脂肪抑制序列可显示肿瘤的假包膜。T2WI 加饱和技术的脂肪抑制序列可以消除化学位移假影，更好地显示肿瘤对骨皮质的侵犯与骨膜反应。TE 时间大于 10 的梯度回波序列容积采集法可以更好地显示骨基质中的矿化物。当临床诊断欠清，通过对骨内与骨外病变信号强度的比较可帮助鉴别肿瘤与感染。

良性、恶性骨肿瘤的鉴别诊断可参考表 3-1。

表 3-1 良性、恶性骨肿瘤的鉴别诊断

鉴别诊断	良性	恶性
生长状况	生长缓慢。无邻近组织受侵或只有推压移位	生长迅速。邻近组织或器官受侵
转移	无	有
局部骨变化	膨胀性骨质破坏，边界清晰、锐利，骨皮质变薄、膨胀但连续	浸润型骨质破坏，分界不清、边缘不规则。邻近骨皮质被破坏。可有肿瘤骨形成
骨膜反应	无或病理性骨折后有，不被肿瘤破坏	各种各样，常易被肿瘤破坏
邻近软组织变化	无或边界清晰的肿块	浸润性软组织肿块，边界不清

（1）骨巨细胞瘤（破骨细胞瘤）：

1）临床及病理表现：骨巨细胞瘤是一个由骨内结缔组织及多核巨细胞组成的呈进行性增生的肿瘤，巨细胞形态类似破骨细胞并散布于充满梭形细胞的基质中，故该肿瘤又称为破骨细胞瘤。骨巨细胞瘤有良性、恶性及过渡性之分。

骨巨细胞瘤好发于 20~40 岁，偶而可发生于骺板尚未闭合的 20 岁前的青少年。病变大部分位于长骨骨端，尤多见于骨骼已成熟的膝关节、桡骨远端、脊椎及髋骨。尽管肿瘤可能起源于干骺端，当被确诊时，长骨骨骺部多已被广泛累及。临床所见的干骺端发病者多为儿童及青少年。骨巨细胞瘤的常见和首发症状为进行性加重的疼痛，伴有局部肿胀、触痛。许多患者有运动受限，常见于膝关节。病理骨折不常见，但可能是首发症状。

2）影像学表现：

①X 线表现：许多放射学医生认为骨巨细胞瘤（图 4-24）具有特征性的 X 线表现。它是一个位于长骨骨端的偏心性、溶骨性病变，病变可位于或紧邻干骺端区域并可扩展至软骨关节面下方。肿瘤可呈皂泡样改变、其中有少许骨

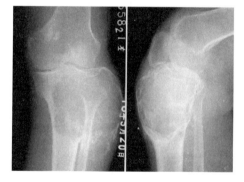

图 4-24 胫骨近端巨细胞瘤

嵴，此种骨嵴实际来自于膨胀、变薄的骨皮质的影像重叠。骨皮质表面被破坏、肿瘤累及邻近软组织强烈提示骨巨细胞瘤生长活跃或恶变。累及扁骨的巨细胞瘤多呈溶骨性改变，椎体内的巨细胞瘤可引起压缩性骨折。

②CT 表现：CT 扫描除可显示受累骨骼与 X 线平片一样的征象外，还可显示许多 X 线平片及血管造影难以显示的病变细节，如肿瘤的大小、位置、肿瘤与肌肉及筋膜的关系，肿瘤边缘的细节及肿瘤与神经、血管及邻近骨结构的关系。CT 可能显示实质性软组织肿瘤内有囊变区或液-液平面。注射对比剂后，囊变区以外的实质性肿瘤会强化。

③MRI 表现：MRI T1 加权像示肿瘤呈低或中等信号强度，T2 加权像呈高信号。偶而病变内会出现不同信号的液平面及囊变区。增强后 T1 加权抑脂像示实质性肿瘤强化，囊变区无变化。

（2）骨囊肿（单纯性或单房性骨囊肿）：

1）临床及病理表现：骨囊肿并不是一个真正的骨肿瘤，而是一个原因不明的常见肿瘤样病变。骨囊肿好发于青少年，尤以 20 岁以前多见。大宗病例显示病变好发于肱骨，尤以肱骨上段靠近骺板处常见。次常见部位是股骨上段。骨囊肿常因不明显的外伤引起骨折，或因其他疾病行 X 线检查时被偶然发现。但部分

患者在被诊断前可能有轻微疼痛或运动受限。

骨囊肿的大体病理特征为弧立性的囊腔内充满清亮的血清样液体。囊的内表面常常衬有不同厚度的、灰白、红棕或偶而呈黄色光滑的膜。囊内的膜由含血管的疏松结缔组织构成，其中散在分布破骨巨细胞、新形成的不成熟骨或骨样小梁，后者常与囊壁表面平行。骨皮质常变薄呈透明的蛋壳样膜状物，很容易用刀切破。

2）影像学表现：

①X线表现：骨囊肿的X线表现特征为干骺端边界清晰的透明样病变，常位于骨的中心，局部骨皮质膨胀并变薄。囊肿偏骺侧边界清晰，远侧边缘欠清，其径线小于骨骺侧。随长骨增长，囊肿可远离骺板而进入骨干内。病变外骨皮质常常甚簿，但不会完全消失。骨囊肿偶而可被梁样结构横贯并形成多囊样表现，这是由于囊壁的骨嵴所致，而非真正的骨隔。

骨囊肿最重要的并发症是病理性骨折。此时，变簿的骨皮质塌陷，形成所谓碎片陷落征。骨折后，小的骨囊肿因有骨痂形成而消失，大的骨囊肿可变小。除合并骨折外，骨囊肿常没有骨膜反应。

②CT表现：骨囊肿CT表现为边界清晰的，单发水样密度囊状病变。增强后扫描无强化。其他CT表现类似X线平片上的表现。

③MRI表现：磁共振（MRI）T1WI示病变为薄壁、边界清晰的低信号囊样病变，T2WI呈与水类似的高信号。骨检查前有骨折，囊内可见多种信号强度，并可见到液平面。

（3）骨肉瘤：

1）临床及病理表现：骨肉瘤是最常见的原发性恶性骨肿瘤，常见于青壮年，80%发生于30岁以前。男性是女性患者的2倍。骨肉瘤常起源于长骨的干骺端，尤以股骨远端，胫骨和肱骨近端多见。

2）影像学表现：

①X线表现：骨肉瘤（图4-25）可引起多种X线表现。随肿瘤的类型不同，骨肉瘤可表现为无结构的致密肿块（成骨型），也可表现为程度不同的骨质破坏（溶骨型）或两者的混合型。当肿瘤中具有丰富的肿瘤骨及肿瘤骨基质时，X线表现为高密度。当其中肿瘤骨稀少，则多会形成溶骨性骨质破坏。骨肉瘤的骨膜反应常见而不规则，形成所谓高密度的"日光放射状"骨膜反应，一般认为这一征象较具诊断特异性，但也有例外情况。骨肉瘤的两端可见到Codman三角（骨膜三角或骨膜袖）。这是由于骨膜反应形成的新骨被快速生长的肿瘤组织侵蚀破坏所致。受累骨骼邻近的软组织可见肿块并可能见到新形成的肿瘤骨。肿瘤可以突破骺板侵犯邻近的关节。

②CT和MRI表现：一般认为MRI在确定肿瘤的骨内及骨外浸润范围较X线平片及CT优越。因此，当骨肉瘤只在骨髓腔内浸润，骨小梁不被破坏时，MRI是显示肿瘤的最敏感方法（图4-26）。MRI T1WI示典型的骨肉瘤呈不均匀低信号，T2WI呈不均匀高信号。MRI对显示肿瘤是否侵及周围肌肉、血管、神经亦优于X线平片和CT。但MRI显示肿瘤骨或钙化的能力不及X线平片和CT。

（4）转移性骨肿瘤：

1）临床及病理表现：身体他处的恶性肿瘤可以通过血流或淋巴循环转移到骨骼。常见的原发肿瘤为乳腺、甲状腺、肺、肾或前列腺，胃肠道转移致骨骼者较少见。骨转移瘤可发于老年红骨髓丰富的骨骼。脊椎、骨盆、肋骨、颅骨系常见部位，病变常为多发性。

2）影像学表现：

①X线表现：有时X线平片只表现为骨质疏松而没有其他异常改变。骨转移瘤可以为溶骨型、成骨型或混合型，溶骨型最常见。

溶骨型转移瘤：表现为不规则的斑片状透光区。骨皮质从内受侵而无膨胀改变。病变边界不清，周围无硬化反应。当转移瘤累及脊椎时，病变常为多发性和跳跃性的，椎体与椎弓根无选择性破坏。椎体压缩骨折呈楔形变，但椎间隙完整。这点有助于转移瘤与脊椎结核鉴别。病理性骨折可能是骨转移瘤的首发征象。

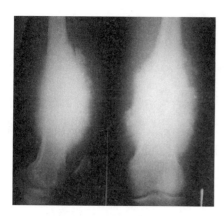

图 4-25　左股骨骨肉瘤

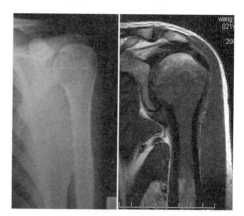

图 4-26　MRI 示左肱骨早期骨肉瘤，但
X 线照片显示正常

成骨型转移瘤：少见且常提示原发肿瘤生长速度较慢。成骨性转移瘤多见于前列腺癌、肺癌、乳腺癌，甲状腺癌偶可产生成骨性转移。受累骨骼常为脊椎、骨盆或肋骨，表现为局部骨结构丧失的骨密度增高区。

②CT 表现：放射性核素骨扫描阳性患者进一步行 CT 检查有助于了解病变的细节。CT 对于了解转移瘤的累及范围亦非常有用。偶尔，只有 CT 才能显示偶见于转移性骨肿瘤的软骨与骨样组织钙化。CT 是评价骨盆与骶骨病变的有效方法，尤其是评价软组织的累及范围。

③MRI 表现：MRI 已广泛用于脊椎转移癌的诊断。T1WI 示脊椎转移性病变呈低信号，类似于急性（30天以内）良性压缩性骨折，但表现没有压缩性骨折明显。T2WI 转移瘤可表现为等、高或混杂信号，在 T2 加权抑脂像上则呈高信号。同 CT 一样，MRI 很容易显示转移癌对软组织的侵犯及其累及范围。

（陈柱，吴海军，罗涛，肖恩华，谭利华）

Chapter 4

Skeleton

Section 1 Method of examination

1. X-ray examination

Fluoroscopy should play no part in the examination of bones or joints, apart from the localization of metallic foreign bodies, reduction and fixation of fractures.

Radiography, which is superior to fluoroscopy, should play the leading role in the examination of bones or joints. There are certain elementary rules in routine radiography of bones and joints, which require emphasis.

(1) At least two views of the anatomic part under examination should always be taken at right angles to each other if possible. Additional views are necessary sometimes if the radiological diagnosis do not accord with the clinical manifestations. Failure to comply with this rule could result in serious risk of missing, for example, a fissure or fracture without displacement.

(2) For study of a long bone, a near-by joint should be included, and for study of any segment of cervical, thoracic or lumbar vertebrae, some signs, such as odontoid process of axis, first ribs, or sacrovertebral angle, should be included in one film so as to make localization of vertebrae easy.

(3) The surrounding soft tissue of the bones and joints should be included in the film as much as possible.

(4) The bone or joint on the other side should be examined whenever possible in addition to the one in question, for comparison. These are very useful, particularly in children and the forepart of the disease.

Nowadays, tomography has seldom been used in the study of the bones or joints since the prevalence of the computed tomography and the magnetic resonance imaging has also taken the place of pneumoarthrogrphy in the study of the joint more and more, which is a procedure to show the articular cartilage and the articular capsule, which are of soft tissue density and are invisible to X-ray, by injection of positive or negative contrast agents into the joint, and often used to evaluate the knee joint for meniscal and ligament tear.

2. CT examination

Computed tomography is now recognized as an important technique for the study of a wide range of diseases of the bones and joints, especially of the skull, spine and pelvis. CT has now become the primary imaging procedure for most spinal diseases. The major advantages of CT for osteal studies are that it has excellent contrast resolution and can provide accurate tomographic sections of the osseous structure and related soft tissues in any plane.

Recently helical (spiral) CT has been introduced and popularized and has two main advantages over conventional CT: Reduced radiation dose and decreased time for the examination. The ability to obtain overlapping images with decreased radiation exposure allows one to obtain this section for multiplanar or three-dimensional reconstruction.

(1) Plain CT

We often examine truck or both of the limbs simultaneously to maintain a constant symmetrical position. For scanning the bone in axial planes, helical scanning is performed routinely after locating on the sagittal or coronal scout image. Standard algorithms are used for all scanning. Generally, the tube voltage is 120kV, tube current is 80~100 mAs, and the layer thickness and layer space for reconstruction is 2~3 mm or thinner. All images should be reviewed at window and center settings appropriate for visualization of both bone (center = 300 to 400 HU, window = 1000 to 1500 HU) and soft tissues (center = 40 to 50 HU, window = 200 to 400 HU). Three-dimensional imaging reconstruction is usually performed to show the full picture of the lesion.

(2) Enhanced CT

In the soft tissue lesions or soft tissue extensions from bone, intravenous injection of iodinated contrast medium concomitantly with CT results in clear differentiation of the non-enhanced lesions and necrosis from the enhancing lesions. Compared with plain CT without intravenous contrast, this technique more accurately defines the scope and properties of the lesions.

3. MRI examination

In current practice, MR imaging has also become the important method of choice for the evaluation of bones and soft tissues. Magnetic resonance imaging can present the most contrast for the bone marrow, the articular cartilage, the soft tissues around the bones or joints and the solid, cystic, and hemorrhagic processes in them. In general, the need for MR imaging is based on the interpretation of the radiograph or CT. But MRI is the first choice for the evaluation of some of spinal and articular diseases, especially for meniscal and ligament tear, osteal tumors or tulmorlike diseases.

(1) Plain MRI

There are plain and enhanced MR imagefor the evaluation of bones and soft tissues as well. Body coils or surface coils may be selected to increase the signal-noise ratio and contrast of the images. Axial imaging must always be performed for the assessment of extremities because among all available imaging planes, it most reliably shows subtle cortical disruption, small soft tissue masses, and their relationship to neurovascular structures. This should be complemented with coronal or sagittal imaging. But, in the sagittal plane, MR can be employed for global survey of a long segment of the spine for the detection of lesions that may be difficult to localize clinically. Suspicious areas on the survey examination can be more completely evaluated in the axial, coronal, or other planes. Spin echo or fast spin echo sequences with T1 and T2 weighting have been the mainstay for the MRI of bones and soft tissues. Fat-suppressed sequences are also common sequences. Shorter pulsing sequences, cardiac and peripheral gating, and motion artifact suppression methods enhance the capabilities of MR imaging for the diagnosis of bone disease.

(2) Enhanced MRI

The use of gadolinium-enhanced MR imaging for the boneand soft tissue lesions has been evaluated. The goal of the application has not only been to enhance specificity of diagnosis, but also to monitor the blood supply of the lesions and more accurately to define the scope and properties of the lesions.

4. Other examination techniques

In addition to the three conventional examinations mentioned above, some other examinations are also available in the skeletal system. For example, Single Photon Emission Computed Tomography (SPECT) and Positron Emission Computed Tomography (PET) are used in malignant bone tumors, and ultrasound is used in bone density measurement.

Section 2　Normal appearance

The dense, hard and slightly elastic connective tissue comprises the 206 bones of the human skeleton. It is composed of compact osseous tissue surrounding spongy cancellous tissue permeated by many blood vessels and nerves and enclosed in membranous periosteum. There are four kinds of the bones by shape, the long or tubular, the short, the flat and the irregular. Long bones contain yellow marrow in longitudinal cavities and red marrow in their articular ends. Red marrow also fills the cavities of the flat and the short bones, the bodies of the vertebrae, the cranial diploe, the sternum, and the ribs. Blood cells are produced in active red marrow. Osteocytes form bone tissue in concentric rings around an intricate Haversian system of interconnecting canals that accommodates blood vessels, lymphatic vessels, and nerve fibers.

1. Tubular bones

There are two kinds of bones in the extremities: The long bones and the short bones. The long bones are also known as the tubular bones, which are divided into long tubular bones that include arm and leg bones, and short tubular bones, which are in the hands and feet. The short bones of the wrist and the ankle, whose dimensions are approximately equal, consist of a layer of cortical substance enclosing spongy substance. Sesamoid bones are small bones situated in the tendon and articular capsules. The patella is the largest sesamoid bone.

(1) Growing tubular bone

A growing tubular bone (Figure 4-1), which consists of a shaft or diaphysis, epiphysis and metaphysis, has distinct roentgenologic features which are quite different from that of an adult bone.

The epiphysis is a mass of chondral bone, in which the secondary ossification center develops and is readily visible on radiography. The epiphysis consists of varying amount of ossified and non-ossified cartilage. The proportion is depending on the size of the ossified center. The first appearance of the secondary ossification center, its enlargement and the fusion with the shaft represent the progressive stage in the growth and maturation of the tubular bones. Numerous roentgen methods have been proposed for assessing the skeletal age according to the time of appearance, the size, the differentiation of the ossification centers and the time of fusion. Skeletal age is only one measure of the maturation level of an individual and of course, the skeletal age estimation must be correlated with other findings such as races, sex, district, height, weight and nutritional state, etc.

The metaphysis is the terminal segment of the shaft immediately adjacent to the epiphyseal cartilage. It is a transitional deep zone in which the spongy bone contains cartilaginous cores. The metaphysis is richly supplied with blood, highly vascular and active in metabolic process. As a result, the metaphysis is special vulnerable to many diseases processes and is of the greatest importance. On the film it

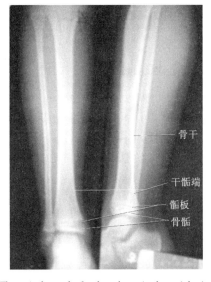

骨干
干骺端
骺板
骨骺

The articular end of a long bone is the epiphysis. The zone of bone adjacent to the epiphysis is the metaphysis. The epiphysis and metaphysis are separated by a physis. The zone of bone away from the articular end is the diaphysis.

Figure 4-1　Zones of child long bone

appears to be a widened portion just next to the epiphyseal cartilage, and consists of a tightly meshed network of fine linear shadows known as trabeculations. At the end of the shaft it terminates in a transverse disk of calcified cartilage, the provisional zone of calcification or designated as epiphyseal plate which anchors the epiphysis and the diaphysis. In between the secondary ossification center and the provisional zone of calcification there is a transparent line formed by the noncalcified cartilage named the epiphyseal line. It disappears after puberty.

The shaft (diaphysis) is a tube like structure with a surrounding compact wall, the cortex, which encloses a cylindrical space of decreased density, the medullary cavity. The cortex is the calcified portion and casts opaque shadow. It isthickest in the middle and tapers off toward the metaphysis and continues with the epiphyseal plate before fusion. The nutrient artery canal appears as a defect of decreased in the cortex.

On the film of a growing bone, the calcified portions cast opaque shadow of calcium density, the uncalcified portions of a growing bone cast shadow of water density similar to that of surrounding soft tissues. The shaft or the diaphysis is capped at each end by a mass of cartilage, the epiphysis, in which the secondary ossification center develops. This epiphyseal ossification center is surrounded by a thin layer of calcified cartilage corresponding to the disk-shaped transverse provisional zone of calcification at the end of the metaphysis. The strip of uncalcified cartilatge interposed between the epiphyseal ossification center and the end of the shaft represents the epiphyseal line of water density.

(2) Adult tubular bone

Adult tubular bones (Figure 4-2) differ from the growing bones. Each long bone is composed of a shaft and two extremities. The shaft is usually strong and the cortex is thick in mid-portion and become thinner toward the extremities and in continuation with the subchondral articular surface. The extremities of the long bones are usually expanded in afford articulation. Bony protuberances are present for muscular or ligament attachment. Externally the cortex is covered by sleeve of tough connective tissue, the periosteum. It is a soft tissue structure density and casts no visible shadow in the films.

2. Spine and pelvis

(1) Roentgen anatomic consideration

The normal spine consists of 33 vertebrae, grouped according to their situation as follows: 7 cervical, 12 dorsal, 5 lumbar, 5 sacral and 4 coccygeal. The sacral and coccygeal groups fuse in the adult to form two bones, the sacrum and coccyx, while the other groups remain separate throughout life and can move between each other.

In the foetus and newborn infant the vertebral column has a continuous primary curvature which is convex backwards. Throughout

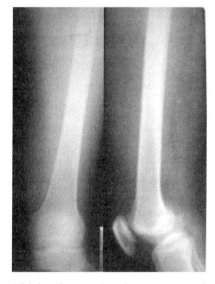

Adult long bone, such as femur, is composed of a shaft and two extremities, which are usually expanded in affording articulation.

Figure 4-2   Normal adult femur

postnatal life the thoracic, sacral and coccygeal parts of the column retain this form, but secondary curves which are convex forwards appear, first in the cervical region when the child learns to sit up at about 6 months, and later in the lumbar region when standing is accomplished at about 18 months. The primary and secondary curvatures smoothly go into one another except at the lumbosacral junction where the change in direction is abrupt (lumbosacral angle). Thesecurvatures may be altered by disease of the vertebrae or by spasm of the vertebral muscles.

With the exception of the 1st and 2nd cervical vertebrae, the sacrum and the coccyx, each vertebra is composed of an anterior portion, the approximately cylindrical body and a posterior ring (spinal canal) that is formed anteriorly by the posterior surface of the corresponding vertebral body, laterally by pedicles and posteriorly by two laminae, which are covered with a layer of compact bone that is much thickened and stronger than the thin cortex of the vertebral body. The laminae converge posteriorly to unite in a single spinous process. On both sides a transverse process and superior and inferior articular processes arise from the junction of pedicle and lamina. The transverse and spinous processes are strong struts which give attachment to many of the vertebral muscles and their associated fascial layers.

In between the vertebrae, there are intervertebral disks (Figure 4-3); each disk contains two parts, the central nucleus pulposus and the peripheral annulus fibrosus. The nucleus contains gelatinous material that becomes more fibrotic with age. The annulus contains fibrocartilage and dense fibrous tissue with laminar fibers joining the adjacent vertebral end-plates.

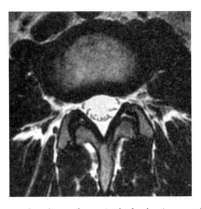

The central nucleus pulposus in the lumbar intervertebral disk, which is hyperintense, is surrounded by hypointense peripheral annulus fibrosus.

Figure 4-3　Axial T2WI of a normal lumbar intervertebral disk of an adult man

Since embryologically the body of the first cervical vertebra has been contributed to the second cervical vertebra as the odontoid process, the general configuration of the first cervical vertebra (Figure 4-4) is that of an oval ring. Anteriorly and posteriorly the ring is quite thin, flaring at its lateral extremities into large facets. At the midpoint in the ring, both anteriorly and posteriorly, are small but well-defined tubercles in stead of body or spinous process. Along the dorsal aspect of the anterior ring of the atlas, the bone is smooth; this area is called "fovea dentis."

It is this surface which articulates with the dens, or the odontoid process. The inferior facets are also broad, round, and flat or slightly convex. Their plane is directed caudalward, medially articulating with the axis.

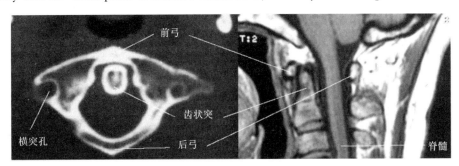

Figure 4-4　Axial CT image & sagittal T₁WI of normal atlas and axis in adult man.

The second cervical vertebra (Figure 4-4) is named the "axis" because it serves as a pivot upon which the atlas can rotate. Its most outstanding characteristic is also a result of its embryological development in the form of the superiorly projecting dens or odontoid process. The superior articular facets are broad and match those of the atlas, being round, slightly convex, and directed cranially and laterally. Here the transverse processes forming the vertebra foramen end in a single anterior tubercle.

The cervical vertebra has a long spinous process; each cervical vertebra has two vertebral foramina one on each side for the passage of the vertebral arteries. Small synovial joints are present, covertebral joint or "joint of Luschka", from C_3-C_7, situated between the poster lateral margin of the lower five cervical vertebral bodies and that are in close relationship to nerves and vessels.

The bodies of thoracic spines progressively increase in size caudally and carry 12 rib pairs. The lumbar vertebrae are larger than the thoracic or cervical vertebrae. The transverse diameter is larger than anteroposterior in the lumbar vertebral body with small height.

The bony pelvis is composed of two hip bones, the sacrum and the coccyx, which are described above. Each hip bone is composed originally of three distinct bones, the ilium, the ischium and the pubis. In the adult these three bones are fused together at the acetabulum.

（2）Normal roentgen appearance

A cervical spine radiography series should include anteroposterior and lateral viewsand a special view for the 1st and 2nd vertebrae, occasionally oblique views are necessary for the inspection of the intervertebral foramina. Anteroposterior and lateral views are required in general for study of thoracic or lumbar spine. Oblique views are necessary for special study of the pars interarticularis of lumbar spine.

The vertebrae (Figure 4-5) cast opaque shadows of calcium density in contrast with interposed radiolucent intervertebral disk spaces that are of soft tissue density. In the antero-posterior view of a vertebra we see clearly the body, with the shadow of a spinous process projected through the middle of it. This spinous process belongs to the vertebra immediately above, except in the case of the fifth lumbar vertebra. On each side of the body the transverse processes stick out at right angles. The pedicles in this view appear as oval or circular rings. Above and below the pedicle are the superior and inferior articular processes and the transparent articular space between them. Generally speaking, a vertebra is always as big as or bigger than the one immediately above it. In the cervical region the pedicles are oval, and in the lumbar and dorsa region they are circular. In adults the medial surface of the pedicle is always convex, but in children there are

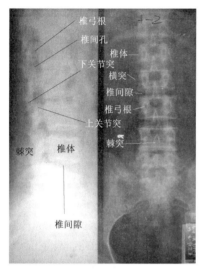

Figure 4-5　Normal adult lumbar vertebrae in the lateral and antero-posterior views.

considerable variations and it may be concave. The distance between the pedicles of the same vertebra is called interpedicular distance, which represents the transverse diameter of the spinal canal. This distance is greatest at the cauda equina and at the cervical and lumbar enlargements. It is least in the mid-thoracic region. Alterations in the shape of the pedicles or in the interpedicular distance may have great diagnostic significance. In antero-posterior view, one should always note the alignment of the spinal column and the correct vertical alignment of the centers of the spinous processes.

In the lateral view we see the bodies of the vertebrae as dense rectangular masses and the disks as transparent spaces between double bodies; behind bodies the pedicles separating the intervertebral foramina, and behind these again the spinous processes. The direction of the intervertebral foramina varies in different parts of the column. In the cervical region the foramina run obliquely, in the dorsal region more laterally, and in the lumbar region they run in a true lateral plane.

In the lateral view, the configuration and their internal structures of the bodies of vertebrae and the intervertebral disk spaces can be showed clearly, but the posterior elements of the neural arches are superimposed. One should note the alignment of the anterior and posterior borders of the vertebral bodies, the alignment of the articular surfaces. All these should form a smooth, gentle curve.

Section 3　Basic pathological changes

There are various pathologic processes and roentgenologic signs in skeletal diseases, but we can find some radiological features that are the fundamental building blocks for roentgenologic diagnosis. It may occur alone or in combination.

1. Osteoporosis

Osteoporosis（Figure 4-6）is given risen to by a common metabolic disorder of bone, which is characterized by qualitatively normal, that is the normal mineralization of the bone, but quantitatively deficient bone. There is lack of osteoblastic activity or from protein deficiency. The serum calcium and phosphorus, alkaline phosphate are normal usually. It can be divided into generalized, regional, and localized types and accompanies a variety of disease processes.

Generalized osteoporosis may be age-related (senile and postmenopausal osteoporosis) or may accompany endocrine disorders (acromegaly, hyperparathyroidism, hyperthyroidism, Cushings disease), pregnancy or alcoholism. Involvement of the axial skeleton and proximal portions of the long bones of the appendicular skeleton predominates. In the spine not only osteopenia but also changes in vertebral contour occur. Usually a uniform decrease in radiodensity is noted. Differentiating generalized osteoporosis from osteomalacia radiographically may be extremely difficult.

Regional osteoporosis occurs in osteoporosis of disuse or immobilization, reflex sympathetic dystrophy, transient osteoporosis of the hip and regional migratory osteoporosis. Changes predominate in the appendicular skeleton. A more aggressive type of bone resorption in these conditions can lead to cortical bone changes at endosteal, intracortical and subperiosteal bone envelopes and to spongy bone changes at subchondral and metaphyseal locations.

Localized osteoporosis is commonly associated with focal skeletal lesions, such as neoplasm and infection.

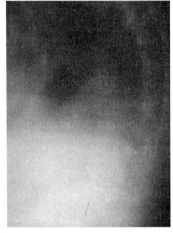

A uniform decrease in radiodensity of the spine with compressed or concave-lens-like bodies is noted on the lateral view of the dorsal spine.

Figure 4-6 Postmenopausal osteoporosis of the spine in an old woman

The radiographic changes of osteoporosis often are discovered when well advanced andinclude changes in radiolucency, trabecular pattern, and shape or vertebral bodies in the spine (wedge-shaped vertebrae, compressed vertebrae, fish vertebrae), Schmorls nodes, acute and insufficiency fractures and bone bars (reinforcement lines). It has the same roentgenologic appearance in all conditions producing it. It is characterized by generalized decrease of bone density with thinning of cortex of the long bones.

In the tubular bones, bone resorption may be distinguished in three sites (endosteal envelope, intracortical [haversian] envelope and periosteal envelope). These changes are best detected with magnification radiography and quantitated with radiography. It is worthwhile to note that the thinning of the cortex maintains normal content and appear dense, in contrast with that of decalcification. The trabeculations appear loosely arranged and coarse, decrease in number; those remaining are in line of stress.

2. Osteomalacia

Just in contrast to the former, osteomalacia (Figure 4-7) is a group of disorders resulting from inadequate or delayed mineralization of osteoid in mature cortical and spongy bone, which in some ways is closely related to rickets (an interruption in orderly development and mineralization of the growth plate).

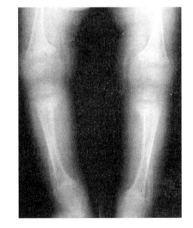

Figure 4-7 Osteomalacia of rickets of the tibia and fibula in a child aged 2.

Normally there is a balance between osteoid formation and mineraliztion and osteomalacia may be considered as a result of either excessive osteoid formation or insufficient mineral. Insufficient absorption of calcium from the gastrointestinal tract or excessive secretion of phosphates ultimately results in calcium deficiency and osteomalacia. A frequent cause of osteomalacia is vitamin D deficiency, ricket in early life while osteomalacia in adult. Blood chemical changes usually present; Low serum calcium and phosphorus, elevated alkaline phosphotase level.

The radiographic changes are characterized by general marked decrease of bone density, thick cortex, the normal outline of the bone is blurred, being indistinguishable from the surrounding soft tissue, giving a so called "ground glass" appearance without trabecular details, forabnormal quantities of osteoid coats the surfaces of trabeculae and lining the haversian canals in the cortex (osteoid seams). Because of excessive osteoid formation, the bones are softened, fracture and deformity may occur in weight bearing region, such as vertebrae, pelvis. Loosers zones or Milkmans pseudofractures are other important features. These are band like of decrease of density at right angle to the cortex, usually bilateral and symmetrical, about 1~2 mm in width and occurs at the axillary region of the scapula, femoral neck, pubic and ischial rami and ribs. It represents a healing reaction to infraction in osteomalacia bone.

3. Destruction of bone

Bone substance, both the cortex and the spongy bone are destroyed and replaced by pathological tissue. It may be localized or diffused, single or multiple.

Roentgenologically, it shows osteolytic bone areas of decreased density and loss of bone structures (Figure 4-8). There are three patterns according to the radiographic manifestation. One is geographic distribution, which consists of large areas of bone being destroyed and is easily detectable. Another is a moth-eaten appearance in which there are many small holes suggestive of a more aggressive lesion as in acute osteomyelitis. Still other is permeative pattern that gives a melting appearance as in cases of malignant bone tumors. As a rule, a slow growing process gives sharper margin than that of a rapid growing process.

4. Hyperostosis osteosclerosis

Osteosclerosis (Figure 4-9) is abnormal hardening or increased density of bone on radiographs, such as occurs with eburnation. Osteosclerosis may accompany a great variety of disorders, including renal osteodystrophy, osteoarthritis, sickle cell anaemia, Pagets disease, skeletal metastasis, myelofibrosis, trauma of bone, and chronic osteomyelitis.

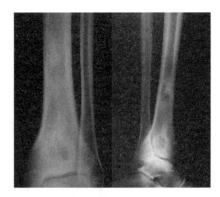

There is a local osteolytic bone area of decreased density and loss of bone structures in the caudal tibia.

Figure 4-8   Local destruction of Brodie's abscess of the tibia in an adult man

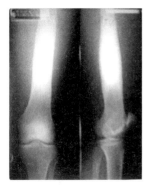

There is increased density of the femur shaft on radiographs, such as occurs with eburnation. The shaft appears to be thickened and loss of medullary cavity.

Figure 4-9   Osteosclerosis of chronic osteomyelitis of the femur shaft in an adult man

In chronic infection or infection caused by low virulence organisms, the bone reaction differs, instead of osteolysis, there is marked new bone production characterized roentgenologically by increase of bone density. The bone appears to be thickened and loss of trabeculations and its medullary cavity.

5. Periosteal reaction

Periosteal reaction(Figure 4-10) is also known as periosteal proliferation. The normal periosteum, which casts no shadow on the film unless it is diseased, is a connective-tissue membrane covering the surface of the bone and connecting it with the surrounding soft tissues. Periosteal reaction casts shadow of increase of density and occurs in various forms. It may be laminated, lace-like or sunburst appearance. But, in the forepart of a disease, the X-ray appearances of the periosteal reaction may be those of a linear opacity curving slightly away from the cortex of the bone and separated from it by a narrow, clear space which fills in later, resulting in a uniformly dense, structureless area of new bone formation, continuous with the underlying cortex. It is not easy to form a correct diagnosis upon a disease only through the shapes of the preriosteal reaction. Other radiographic signs and clinic materials should take into account when a diagnosis is made.

Periosteal reaction occurs in a great many conditions. Among the more important are staphylococcal infection, syphilis, typhoid, trauma, 'stress' fractures, lekemia, malignant tumors both primary and secondary, and hypertrophic oseoarthropathy.

6. Osteonecrosis and sequestrum

Osteonecrosis occurs when metabolism of bone cells cease forever from local ischemia of bone. Sequestrum (Figure 4-11)is a fragment of dead bone that is partially or entirely detached from the surrounding or adjacent healthy bone.

Osteonecrosis is characterized histologically by the loss of nuclei and disappearance of the bone cells, so that the cell-spaces in the bone matrix appear empty. The bone matrix itself remains unchanged in appearance until removed by osteoclasts. This will last for some time. So X-ray changes of the dead bone may remain normal for a few weeks or even longer.

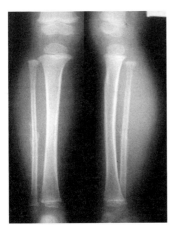

A linear and lace-like opacity curving slightly away from the cortex of the fibula shaft and separated from it by a narrow, clear space is the periosteal reaction of the acute osteomyelitis.

Figure 4-10 Periosteal reaction of acute osteomyelitis of the fibula in a child

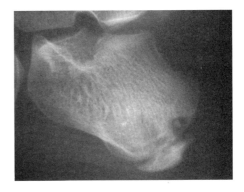

Figure 4-11 Sand-like sequestrum (↑) of teberculosis of the calcaneus in a child.

The chief characteristic that is responsible for the radiographic definition of dead bone is its apparent increase in density, which is due either to (1)an increased amount of additional bone deposited on existing bone trabeculae or medullary cavity or (2)contrast with surrounding necrotic bone cavity, which contains inflammatory porosis, granulation tissue and/or pus. The shape of sequestra varies in different diseases or in different periods of the illness. The remnant bones in malignant bone tumors may be dead bone or living bone.

Osteonecrosis is usually seen in chronic osteomyelitis, ischemic necrosis and traumaof bones, occasionally in tuberculosis of bones.

7. Fracture line

It is a pathognomonic sign of a fracture, represent by a line of decreased density across the bone with interruption of bone continuity(Figure 4-12). The fracture line may be obscured by impaction resulting a line of increased density with interrupted bone trabeculations. Some principles should be kept in mind in evaluating skeletal trauma: (1)patient with history of trauma and suggestive signs of fracture but negative X-ray finding for the initial examination. CT or MRI should be performed for more accurate diagnosis, especially in those fractures occurring in the wrist, vertebrae and ribs. (2)comparison of the sound side should be made, whenever you are uncertain about a fracture, particularly in babies or children, whose epiphyseal lines could be confused for a fracture.

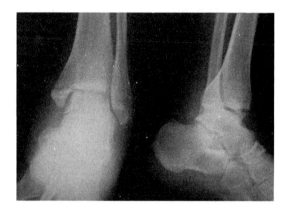

Figure 4-12　Fractures lines (↑)of the tibia and fibula in a child.

8. Soft tissue changes

A good X-ray film of bones, the surrounding soft tissue should be included as much as possible. The presence of soft tissue swelling may be indicative of a mass of increase density or of inflammatory edema, by loss of the definition or displacement of the fat lines in the soft tissue. Calcifications may result from old trauma or indicative of connective tissue disorder. Gas in the soft tissue may indicate gas infection or trauma that is open to air.

9. Bone matrix

It is produced by certain tumor or some other pathologic processes. It may be cartilageous, osteoid, fibrous tissue, or mixed. A large area of lucent with distinct wall may be a cyst containing blood or fluid. It may appear as fine stippled calcifications or popcorn-like calcification representing a chondroid matrix or it may be replaced by fibrous tissue giving an appearance with coarse trabeculation mixed with irregular bony sclerosis.

A logic approach to skeletal radiology is essential in making a correct diagnosis. The following factors should be kept in mind.

(1)Site of the lesion: epiphysis, metaphysis or diaphysis, weight bearing surface of a large joint.

(2)Bone involved: Some diseases have a predilection for certain bones, single or multiple.

(3)Behavior of the lesion: osteolytic, osteobalastic or mixed.

(4)Margin of the lesion: sharply defined or poorly defined.

(5)Bone reaction: Periosteal reaction, solid, laminated, spiculated bony sclerosis.

(6)Matrix production: Chondroid, osteoid or fibrous formation.

(7)Soft tissue changes.

(8)Age, sex of the patient.

(9)Onset of the disease, acute, chronic, progressive etc.

（10）History of trauma.

Section 4　Diagnosis of common diseases

Routine X-ray examination plays an important note in the diagnosis of traumatic lesions of bone and joints. It determines not only the presence or absence of fracture but also help in the reduction of a fracture or dislocation under television-fluoroscopic guidance.

1. Fracture

（1）Fracture of long bone

1）Clinical and pathological manifestations: Fracture is defined as a break across the bone with discontinuity of the cortex and interruption of the bony trabeculations. It commonly occurs in the extremities. Fracture may occur in any portion of the bone including separation of epiphysis, depending on the site of injures and direction of force exerted.

2）Imaging manifestations

Fracture line is a definite radiologic feature of a fracture. A fresh fracture appears radiologically as a translucent line between the fractured fragments and often shows an irregular and sharp margin. One should not mistake an epiphyseal line for a fracture line. Sometime, the fracture line may hardly be identified onone film but clearly seen on the other angular view (Figure 4-13). In case of impaction of the fracture fragments this translucent line may not be seen but a dense line instead.

Fracture ordinarily be classified radiologically: ①According to the direction and shape of the fracture line. It may be oblique, spiral, longitudinal or y-shaped. A comminuted fracture denotes a fracture with more than two fragments. ②According to the extend of the fracture, It may be a complete fracture, involving the entire width of the bone or it may be incomplete in which only on part of the cortex is buckled, or broken, it is called greenstick fracture and this condition usually occurs in children. ③Pathologic fracture: Fracture occurs in a diseased bone, such as in osteomyelitis, tumors and some other bone diseases.

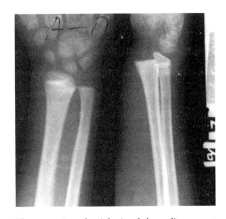

The separation of epiphysis of the radius cannot be identified on the anteroposterior view film and clearly seen on the lateral view.

Figure 4-13　Separation of epiphysis at lower end of radius in a child

Once a fracture is identified, one must pay attention to the position of the distal fragment in relation to the proximal fragment. The distal fragment may be displaced either anteroposteriorly or lateromedially. The fragments may be overlapped, impacted, separated or rotated. There may be angulation between the fragments. These features are of primary importance when treatment is considered.

Healing of a fracture:

Healing takes place usually 2 or 3 days after injury in a case of an uncomplicated fracture. Healing process is accomplished through the organization of a hematoma and in growth of granulation tissue at the site of fracture. A fibrous callus is formed initially in between the fragments. This newly formed mass also called temporary callus and usually takes place between the 5th to 10th day after injury. Deposition of further callus in the form of cartilaginous and fibrous mass takes place slowly. Since this type of callus casts no shadow on X-ray film, so the fracture line remains visible but burred on the film. New bones are laid down as the progress of union proceeds. The new bone when effectively formed is deposited between the ends of the bone and in the subperiosteal space and finally becomes a firm bone union. At this time, the fracture line disappears.

The speed of union is variable and related to age of the patient, site and type of fracture, status of nutrition and available proper treatment. Average time for union of a fracture, in uncomplicated case, usually takes about 8 −10 weeks. Remolding of the new bone is the final stage and may involve a period of several months. The whole callus now ossified and normal bone structure is restored.

Diagnosis of union of fracture: A satisfactory union of the bone must be assessed by both clinical and radiological findings.

Radiological evidence of union: The earliest evidence of union is the presence of periosteal callus, a hazy shadow around the site of fracture and becomes denser with progressive calcification, adjacent to the cortex. The endosteal callus is formed between the fracture fragments and the fracture line becomes hazy. With the formation of more endosteal callus the fracture becomes hazier. The space between the fragments is found to be occupied by an opaque shadow, finally the fracture line disappears and the medullary cavity is reformed.

The common defects in bone union are:

Delayed union: The power of developing new bone at the site of fracture has been impaired but the capacity for the growth of new bone still exists. If the condition is properly managed, the union will take place but after a longer time. Failure to recognize this condition and improperly treated will lead to nonunion. Radiologically, there is minimal or delayed callus formation. Fracture line remains visible for a longer time than expected but there is no sclerotic change atthe bone ends.

Non-union: Union can't take place at the expected time. The osteogenic capacity to lay down new bone has already disappeared. Radiologically the fracture lime remains visible through out the course with separated fragments. The bone ends becomes rounded and dense sclerosis develops. There is usually absence of callus or only minimal periosteal callus is seen but without tendency to bridge over the gap. False joint (pseudoarthrosis) may be produced. The proximal end of the fragment becomes convex while the distal end assumes a concave surface with sclerosis of both ends. The medullary cavity is closed at the ends.

The common fracture typesare as follows:

Colles' fracture: This is one of the most common bone injury and is commonly seen in elderly person. The fracture line is within 2.5 cm from the articular end of the radius. In displaced Colle's fracture, the fracture lime passes almost transversely and the distal fragment is displaced dorsally and radially, and the end of fracture forms an palmar angle, and is often associated with fracture of the styloid prosess of the ulna and separation of the radioulnar joint.

Supracondylar fracture of the humerus: It is the most common injury at the lower end of the humerus and commonly seen in children. The fracture line may pass at a variable distance from the epiphyseal line. It may pass through the metaphysis or through the condyles or pass through the epiphyseal line (epiphyseal separation). The shape of fracture may be T or Y-shaped. The distal fragment may be displaced posteriorly or anteriorly with associated medical or lateral displacement. Posterior displacement is much more common, known as extension type of fracture. Anterior displacement of distal fragment is uncommon, known as flexion type of fracture.

Fracture of the neck of the femur: This injury is common in elderly patient especially liable to occur in those cases with osteoporosis. Fracture may be classified according to the anatomic site, such as subcapital, transcervicle, basal, intertrochanteric etc. Subcapital, transcervicle and basal fractures are all intracapusular in position, because the interference of blood supply and are prone to develop avascular necrosis. The transcervicle and intertrochanteric types are more common than the rest. When there is avascular necrosis, the femoral head becomes increase in density, deformed and with cystic degeneration.

(2) Fracture of spine

1) Clinical and pathological manifestations: Fracture of spine occurs next to the fracture of long bones. Although any part of the vertebral column may subject to injury, but in general, it occurs most in the flexible portion of the vertebral column, such as lower thoracic and upper lumbar region.

2) Imaging manifestations

① X-ray findings: The affected vertebral body becomes wedge shaped due to compression(Figure 4-14). The translucent fracture lime may be hardly visible and often replaced by a dense line as a result of impaction of the fragments. The intervertebral disk space may be narrowed slightly but usually well preserved. This feature is quite different from that of tuberculosis of spine.

② CT findings: Computed tomography may be a supplement to plain radiography, especially for vertebral and major pelvic fractures. Computed tomography gives a more accurate evaluation of vertebral burst fractures (Fig. 4-15)than plain radiography, since it readily demonstrates the number of fragments present, as well as the degree of their retropulsion into the spinal canal and their relationship to the spinal cord.

Use of computed tomography has long been advocated in the identification of acetabular fragments in major pelvic fractures. Computed tomography thus provides additional information in the evaluation of major pelvic fractures rather than simply confirming plain radiographic findings.

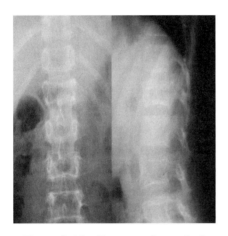

Figure 4-14　Compressed vertebral fracture(L1).

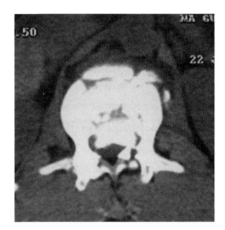

Figure 4-15　Vertebral burst fracture of the L_1 body on the CT axial image

③ MRI findings: MRI readily demonstrates the hematoma between and around the ends of the fractured bones and the edema, breeding or other injuries of the proximal soft-tissue, although it has proven less useful in detecting the fracture line than CT. Occasionally, MRI can identify the occult bone fractures of the long bones and the subtle compression fracture of the vertebral bodies that don't easily appear on films (Figure 4-16). Bone bruise, which has broken trabeculae and edema or bleeding in the marrow and can not be displayed by CT and plain film, demonstrate decreased signal contrasted with high signal of the bone marrow on T1-weighted images and markedly increased signal on T2-weighted, especially on short tau inversion recovery (STIR) images. Though high sensitive to the changes in the medullary and soft-tissue trauma, such as the brain and spine, MRI should not be used as a substitute for a careful clinical examination and standard radiologic studies.

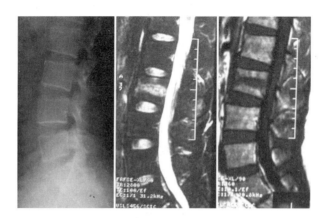

**Figure 4-16　Occult compressed fracture of the L₃ vertebral
bodies on X-ray film & T1 weighted and T2 weighted MR images**

2. Intervertebral disk herniation

(1) Clinical and pathological manifestations: The intervertebral disk herniation occurs most commonly in the 2nd to 4th decade of life, and preferentially for the men. The low lumbar intervertebral disks are affected most frequently, and the cervical in the next place. Posterolateral lumbar disk herniations typically compress the adjacent nerve root in the Lateral recess of the spinal canal or in the intervertebral foramen, with resultant pain, paresthesias, numbness, muscle weakness, and diminished reflexes in a radicular distribution characteristic of the nerve root being compressed (radiculopathy). Cervical and thoracic disk herniations may cause not only radiculopathy but also myelopathy due to compression of the spinal cord, resulting in long tract findings with bilateral weakness, numbness, and spasticity below the level of compression. Clinical localization of the specific level of nerve or cord compression is often very difficult.

The intervertebral disks consist of a central gellike nucleus pulposus that is surrounded by a peripheral elastic annulus fibrosus. Superiorly and inferiorly, a disk is marginated by hyaline cartilaginous plates in the children or end-plate in the adult. Intervertebral disk herniation occurs when nuclear material herniates into the fissure that usually occurs posteriorly or posterolaterally where the annulus is narrowest. Thus, protrusion of disk material beyond the margin of the disk compresses things hereabout and gives rise to signs and symptoms.

(2) Imaging manifestations

1) X-ray findings: In the evaluation of patients presenting with signs and symptoms (radiculopathy or myelopathy) suggesting a herniated disk, radiologic imaging is essential for accurate localization and spinal canal preliminary to CT or MR imaging. With the rare exception of a calcified free fragment herniation, a conclusive diagnosis of herniated inter-vertebral disk cannot be made on plain film examination of the spine. Narrowing of the disk space, eburnation and spurring at the margins of the vertebral bodies, narrowing or widening of the apophyseal joint spaces with eburnation and spurring of the opposing articular processes, and the "vacuum disk" sign are all indications of disk degeneration, and any or all of these findings may be recognized in both symptomatic and asymptomatic individuals with or without disk herniation. In the past, the main value of plain films was as a screening device to demonstrate the presence of vertebral lesions, such as metastatic malignancy or inflammation, that might clinically simulate herniated disk. However, plain films are relatively insensitive for detection of early structural change in bone; radionuclide bone scanning, computed tomography (CT), or magnetic resonance (MR) imaging better fulfill this purpose.

2) CT findings: CT has been the most widely accepted initial examination for the diagnosis of a lumbar

herniated disk, however, in the cervical or thoracic region, MRI has been recommended for the first choice to access the disks.

The intervertebral disk degeneration shows three kinds on the CT image: diffuse bulging, herniation and free fragment herniation.

Diffuse bulging of the intervertebral disks is a common finding in individuals older than 40. A bulging disk extends diffusely outward in all directions beyond the margins of the adjacent vertebral bodies. Disk bulging is typically symmetrical and maximal in the midline, but the degree of protrusion occasionally is greater on one side than the other. Bulging of a lower lumbar intervertebral disk does not usually cause nerve root compression, but in a relatively small spinal canal, a diffusely bulging disk may impinge on the anterior margin of the thecal sac; in severe spinal stenosis, such impingement often affects the underlying spinal cord or nerve roots.

Herniation of an intervertebral disk represents a focal protrusion of disk material beyond the margin of the disk. Such focal protrusions may occur at any point around the disk margin or even superiorly or inferiorly into the adjacent vertebral bodies (intraosseous herniation, Schmorl's node).

The criteria for the diagnosis of disk herniation by CT include the following: ① Focal (angular or polypoid) extension of disk density into the spinal canal. The herniating mass of disk material is significantly more dense (60 to 100 HU) than either the extradural fat (− 50 to 0 HU) or the fluid-filled thecal sac (20 to 50 HU). ② Displacement of extradural fat at the site of herniation by the protruding mass. ③ Focal deformity of the anterolateral margin of the thecal sac by the impinging mass. ④ Displacement of the emerging/descending/exiting nerve root by the impinging mass (Figure 4-17).

Free fragment herniation is a term indicating separation of the focal herniation from the remainder of the disk, with penetration of the separated fragment through the fibers of the posterior longitudinal ligament. The fragment lies free in the loose fatty areolar tissue of the extradural space of the spinal canal and can migrate superiorly or inferiorly away from the disk space. A migrated free fragment disk herniation may thus compress a nerve root above or below the level from which it originated.

When the focal herniation is at the disk level, it is usually not possible to differentiate a simple herniated disk from a free fragment herniation by CT; only rarely can a cleavage fatty plane be demonstrated between the protruding mass and the remainder of the disk margin. When the extradural impinging mass that is as dense as the intervertebral disc is visualized above or below the disk level, the diagnosis of a migrated free fragment is evident.

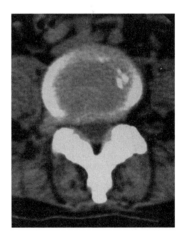

Figure 4-17　Axial CT section shows a focal polypoid herniation from intervertebral disk extends into right lateral intervertebral foramen(↑).

3)MRI findings: By far, MRI has been the best way to diagnose the intervertebral disk herniation in all spines.

The T1-weighted sagittal study is useful not only in demonstrating posterior disk protrusion into the spinal canal but also in evaluating the size, contour, and patency of the intervertebral foramina. On T1-weighted sagittal images, a herniated disk frequently appears isointense with the adjacent disk of origin, in distinct contrast to the adjacent hyperintense extradural fat and the hypointense sub-arachnoid space

On T2-weighted sagittal images, disk herniation usually appears as a focal polypoid mass protruding posteriorly beyond the hypointense posterior vertebral margin. The herniation frequently appears relatively isointense with the disk of origin and can be sharply delineated from the hypointense dura and hyperintense subarachnoid space

On axial images, far lateral disk herniation impinging on the perineural fat and exiting nerve root at the foraminal level can be readily identified. The diagnosis of far lateral disk herniation can be suggested on parasagittal images by careful recognition of impingement by the protruding mass on the perineural fat within the affected foramen.

A free fragment disk herniation (Figure 4-18) that has migrated superiorly or inferiorly from the disk level can be readily identified on T1-weighted spin-echo images, both sagittal and axial. The disk fragment typically appears as a polypoid mass, isointense with intervertebral disc tissue, which can be distinctly differentiated from the hypointense subarachnoid space. It displaces or obliterates the hyperintense epidural fat. On T2-weighted images, the signal intensity of the migrated disk fragment is variable. It frequently is predominantly hyperintense, perhaps related to increased hydration, merging almost imperceptibly with the hyperintense subarachnoid space in a manner similar to many neoplasms. Free fragment herniation without migration cannot be distinguished on MR imaging or by any other diagnostic imaging method from simple disk herniation without separation of the herniated portion from the disk of origin.

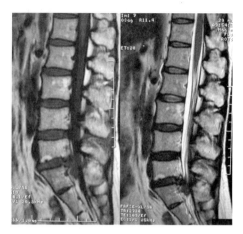

Figure 4-18　A free fragment disk herniation migrated inferiorly from the L_5-S_1 disk level on sagittal T_1WI and T_2WI.

3. Osteomelitis

(1) Clinical and pathological manifestations: Pathogenic organisms enter the bone by direct extension from neighbouring infected soft tissue, infected joint, or through penetrating wound or compound fractures. Hemotogenous infection, being the most common types, is a blood born disease of bones and is frequently a disease of infants and children. Newborn babies may also be affected. Staphylococcus aureus is the most common infecting organism. The initial lesion is almost always located in the metaphysis. It starts with a small abscess and the abscess enlarges as the tension within the abscess increases. The infected material breaks through the cortex to reach the subperiosteal space, thus elevating the periosteaum and infection spread along the shaft of the long bone. If the infection is not checked, the whole bone is involved. As a rule, there is extensive formation of periosteal new bone. The infection rarely spread across the epiphyseal plate during the growth period but does tend to break through the bone near the metaphysis. When the metaphysis is intracapasular in position, pyogenic arthritis will occur. The destroyed bone, especially the cortex may not be absorbed, leaving a large piece of dead bone and is pradually detached from the living bone. This is the sequastrum and is characterized by its abnormal high density and is situated in a pus cavity. This disease has a great tendency to become chronic, if it is not properly treated. In the chronic stage, the destructive process slows down and replaced by marked reparative change. Chronic osteomyelitis may give a long drown out course with persistent discharging sinuses and expelling of sequastua.

(2) Imaging manifestations

1) X-ray findings: In the early stage, radiological changes may be minimal and escape from detection even there are marked symptoms and signs clinically. By careful observation, at this stage, one may discover some changes in the adjacent soft tissue due to inflammatory edema. Subtle changes in the soft tissues may appear within the first 3 days. Focal deep soft-tissue swelling is related to the vascular changes and edema occurring within the bone. Subsequently, muscle swelling and obliteration of soft-tissue planes occur. Actual abscess formation in the soft tissues is a later phenomenon that relates to violation of the cortex by the infection. Bone changes become evident two weeks later after the onset of the disease. Discrete and mottled areas of bone destruction first appear in

the metaphysis of long bone. These small lytic areas become coalesce to form a larger area of destruction with ill-defined margin. The cortex is destroyed subsequently within a short time. There is marked periosteal reaction giving a lace-like appearance along the shaft. Dead cortical bone may be separated to form sequeastrum. The outstanding features of acute osteomyelitis (Figure 4-19) are manifested by extensive bone destruction with marked periosteal reaction but little reparative changes. In the chronic stage, there is marked bone proliferation, and there is a striking different radilogic appearance from that to acute stage. The affected bone shows marked increase of density, thickened and irregular in contour pocked of decreased densities may be noted indicating the residual bone destruction. Large piece of sequastrum often presents in a bone cavity.

In healed case, bone destruction and sequastrum disappear, leaving only some thickening of the affected bone.

2)CT findings: CT can identify the inflammation and abscess in the soft-tissues or in the marrow, little destruction of the bones and small sequestua not suspected from conventional radiographs.

3) MRI findings: MRI provides superior tissue contrast and readily demonstrates early alterations in soft-tissue morphology and water content. Abscesses demonstrate decreased signal on T1-weighted images and markedly increased signal on T2-weighted and short tau inversion recovery (STIR) images. Gadolinium chelate enhancement has been utilized in

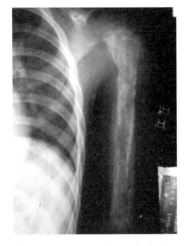

There are extensive bone destruction with marked periosteal reaction but little reparative changes on the X-ray film.

Figure 4-19　Acute pyogenic osteomyelitis of the left humerus

characterizing these soft-tissue abnormalities and has been reported to increase lesion conspicuity and improve delineation of abscesses and differentiation of osteomyelitis from cellulitis and soft-tissue abscess. MRI clearly depicts medullary destruction as well as surrounding reactive marrow edema.

4. Tuberculosis

(1)Clinical and pathological manifestations: Tuberculosis of bones and joints are almost always secondary to tuberculosis elsewhere in the body, especially pulmonary tuberculosis. It affects most commonly among the young subjects, teenagers. Just as the other hematogenous infection of the bone, the initial focus usually starts in the metaphysis. Tuberculosis of long bones is less frequent than tuberculosis of spine or joints.

(2)Imaging manifestations

1) X-ray findings: The classic location of the long bone infection (Figure 4-20) is in the metaphysis or epiphysis. In the youngest patients, extension from the metaphysis through the physis occurs, similar to pyogenic infections. In adults, the diaphysis may be infected. Unlike pyogenic osteomyelitis, there is

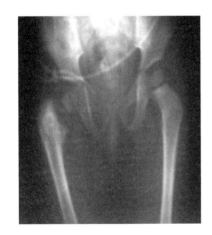

Figure 4-20　Tuberculosis of the right femur metaphysis in a child.

less likely to be periosteal reaction, bone sclerosis, or formation of a sequestrum, although, occasionally, small, sand like sequestrum may be noted. Spiculated periosteal reaction is often associated with chronic sinus formation. Depending on the virulence of the tuberculous infection, the radiographic appearance may be focal, mimicking a Brodie's abscess or benign bone tumor. It may have an aggressive permeative pattern, identical to a round cell tumor（Ewing's sarcoma, lymphoma, leukemia）. As this disease progresses, it has a tendency to break through the epiphysis to involve the joint. It may break through the cortex, periosteum and invade the surrounding soft tissue forming a fistula.

When a lytic lesion occurs in the short tubular bones of the hands or feet, it often produces fusiform enlargement of the entire diaphysis, termed spina ventosa tuberculosa. The appearance is identical to a slow-growing benign bone tumor such as an enchondroma.

The spine has been the most frequent site of skeletal tuberculosis and most prevalent in children and young adults. There is no difference between two sexes. Common occurrence in such order: lumbar, thoraco-lumbar region and cervical spine. Coccyx is the least affected. Initial focus usually lies in the vertebral body while the neural arches are seldom involved. The initial focus of infection may be central, marginal or subperiosteal（anterior）, but in fact in our daily practice, it often appears as a mixture of the three. Radiologically, it appears as slow but progressing localized area of bone destrution, the affected vertebra becomes collapsed due to compression, giving a wedge shaped appearance. Involvement of the contiguous vertebral body is frequent and extension to distant vertebral bodies may occur along the aterolateral ligament of the spine. Cold abscess formation is common in the adjacent paravertebral soft tissue. Calcium deposition may be present within the abscess.

Cardinal radiological features of the tuberculosis of the spine（Figure 4-21）include: ①Destruction of the vertebral body or bodies and usually gives a wedge shaped appearance; ②Narrowing or total obliteration of the disc space between the two affected vertebrae, This feature is different and distinguish from those of fracture of spine or metastatic tumor of spine; ③Cold abscess formation, the paravertebral soft tissue shadow is blurred, widened and bulges to a fusiform swelling. The soft tissue swelling may be in the psoas muscle, in the paraspinal soft tissue or in the retropharyngeal space, depending on the location of the vertebra affected, lumbar, thoracic or cervicle respectively; ④The destructive process causes a local Kyphosis or scoliosis of the spine.

2）CT findings: CT identifies the soft tissue extension from the vertebra and small, sand like sequestra or the rice bodies（Figure 4-22）better than conventional radiographs. Its most important place in the evaluation of infectious spondylitis is for CT-guided aspiration or biopsy in undiagnosed cases.

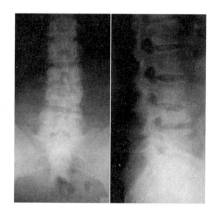

Figure 4-21　Tuberculosis of the lumbar
vertebra on the X-ray film.

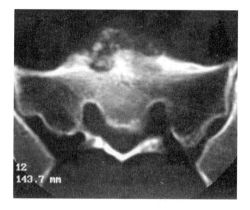

Figure 4-22　Rice bodies of the tuberculosis
of the sacrum on CT image(↑).

3）MRI findings: Like CT, MRI is an outstanding tool in the evaluation of spinal TB（Figure 4-23）. Both sagittal T1WI and T2WI reveal involvement of vertebral bodies not suspected from conventional radiographs. More importantly, the ability to define the soft tissue abscesses and extension into the spinal canal and the effect on the spinal cord by axial sequences is helpful to the surgeon if he or she plans to drain the abscess. The use of gadolinium can depict the wall of the abscess better.

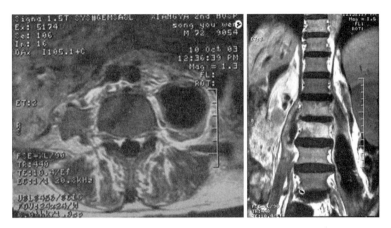

Figure 4-23　Cold abscesses in the double psoas muscles on enhanced MR images

5. Bone tumor

Bone tumors present a most interesting and complicated problem in X-ray diagnosis. This subject is often confused by disagreement and argument as to benignity or malignity of the tumor between the clinician, pathologists and radiologists. Often the final diagnosis determines the treatment and prognosis of patients. All those dedicated to the study of skeletal disorders agree that a combined clinical, radiologic, and pathologic study, supplemented whenever necessary by biochemical and hematologic investigations, is essential in order to arrive at the precise diagnosis of an osseous tumor.

Radiology is of great importance in the diagnosis of bone tumors. Radiographs should always be available to the pathologist, who should never make a definite diagnosis without knowing the radiologic features. It is also of fundamental importance to provide the pathologist with detailed clinical information (such as duration and type of sympotoms, previous trauma or irradiation, pathologic fracture).

Radiologically, the diagnosis of the bone tumors should includes: (1) Whether the bone lesion is tumor; (2) Whether the tumor is benign, or malignant, primary or metastatic? (3) Which kind of the tumor is according to the histologic types? (4) An assessment of the circumstances of the bone and soft tissue are affected.

Bone tumors are classified into benign, malignant and metastatic. Patient's age, site of the tumor, number of the lesion, (single or multiple) together with clinical symptoms and signs and laboratory findings should always be considered in making a diagnosis. Radiologically, the differentiation between benign and malignant lesion may be possible. A benign tumor usually shows a lesion with well defined and usually expanded border or margin. The demarcation between the normal and affected bone is sharp and clear cut. The expanded thin bone cortex remains intact and shows no invasion of the surrounding soft tissue. There is usually no periosteal reaction. No evidence of distant metastasis. Benign tumors often run a slow course. A malignant tumor behaves just opposite. The following points should be ascertained from a radiographic examination of a bone tumor:

(1) The type of bone affected (tubular or flat) and the site of the lesion with reference to the epiphysis, growth plate, metaphysis, or diaphysis, and with reference to its medullary, cortical, or juxtacortical location: The different bone tumors show their preferential location, such as giant cell tumors located at the end of long bones, osteosarcomas ususlly aroused in the metaphysis of long bones and myelomas often from flat bones.

(2) Whether the lesion is monostotic or polyostotic: The primary bone tumors often are monostotic and the myelomas and metastases are polyostotic.

(3) An estimate of how much of the total length and circumference of the bone is affected

(4) The nature of any bone changes present: destructive or radiolucent of moth-eaten, permeative or geographic type, proliferative, or mixed

(5) The density of tumor tissue, with particular regard to the presence of calcification and its roentgenographic characteristics: Solid, punctate, smokey)

(6) The character of the margins of the lesion in the bone: sharp, ill-defined, thick, thin, increased or decreased density

(7) The nature of any cortical bone changes: The involvement of medullay or periosteal surfaces, cortical invasion, pressure atrophy

(8) The character of periosteal reaction: The presence or absence, laminated or "onion peel," solid, sunburst, or Codman's triangle

(9) The presence or absence of adjoining soft-tissue changes with particular mention of fascial planes, tumor tissue, etc.

The role of computed tomography (CT) is also quite limited with the occasional exception. A juxtacortical calcified or ossified lesion may simulate the appearance of myositis ossificans. CT scan should demonstrate the peripheral pattern of ossification and lack of attachment to the underlying bone that is characteristic of myositis ossificans. The aggressive nature of a surface osteosarcoma will be well-demonstrated on CT, with the dense central pattern of mineralization, ill-defined margins, and cortical attachment without the cortical and medullary continuity necessary for the diagnosis of osteochondroma. CT is also both sensitive and specific in identifying the nidus of an osteoid osteoma with a punctate, radiodense circumferential radiolucent zone, and varying degrees of circumferential sclerosis in the adjacent bone. The superior resolution of routine radiography allows more accurate characterization of the type of mineralization within tumor matrix. Although detection of minute amounts of calcification or ossification is possible due to the tomographic technique of CT, this really adds little of significance to the radiographic differential diagnosis. In addition, gradient echo MR sequences can fulfill the same function while obtaining additional information.

MRI is the imaging modality of choice in staging of musculoskeletal lesions. Its multiplanar capability and soft tissue contrast allows accurate determination of the intraosseous extent of tumor, cortical disruption, adjacent soft tissue mass, or articular extent.

Differentiation ofmalignant tumor margin from adjacent, reactive edema is difficult but necessary to ensure that optimum resection is performed in limb sparing surgery. As several centimeters of surrounding disease-free tissue must be included during a wide resection, which is essential to the success of a limb salvage procedure, overestimation of true tumor extent may necessitate amputation instead. Dynamic contrast enhanced MRI using various gradient echo sequences has been shown to provide fairly reliable means of differentiating reactive edema from tumor. Edema characteristically demonstrates homogenous enhancement with an intensity greater than or equal to that of the adjacent tumor. Dynamic contrast studies also provide useful information for planning a subsequent biopsy by demonstrating the necrotic areas to be avoided, and the well-vascularized foci, which provide a higher yield of diagnostic tissue than less well perfused areas. In addition, use of a fat suppressed sequence with or without contrast will allow demonstration of a pseudocapsule. The use of fat saturation techniques with T2-weighted imaging, as well as with contrast sequences, will eliminate chemical shift artifact, allowing better visualization of cortical involvement and periosteal reaction. Gradient echo sequences with TE greater than 10, particularly volume acquired sequences will accentuate and aid in detection of mineralization within tumor matrix. The comparison of relative signal intensity within the intraosseous and extraosseous portion of a lesion aids in the differentiation of tumor versus infection when the clinical diagnosis is ambiguous.

The table 3-1 should be kept in mind to differentiate the benign bone tumors from the malignant.

Table 3-1 Differentiation of Benign Bone Tumors from the Malignant

	Benign	Malignant
Development	Slowly. No adjoining tissue extension or only displacement by pressuring	Rapidly. Adjoining tissue or organs extensions common
Metastasis	No	Yes
Local bone changes	Expanding lesion with well-defined and sharp endosteal margin. Cortex thinned and expanded with continuity	Permeating destructive pattern with ill-defined margin and wide zone of transition. Adjacent cortex frequently destroyed. Probable tumor bone formation.
Reactive periosteal bone	Absence or presence after pathological fracture without destruction	Variousness frquently with destruction.
Adjoining soft-tissue changes	Absence or mass with well-defined margin	Permeating soft tissue mass with ill-defined margin

(1) Giant cell tumor(osteoclastoma):

1) Clinical and pathological manifestations: Giant cell tumor is a local aggressive neoplasm composed of connective tissue and multinucleated giant cells that resemble osteoclasts scattered in a matrix of spindle stromal cells, so it is also called osteoclastoma. The tumor of this kind may be benign, malignant and transitional.

The age incidence of these tumors is most from 20-40. Rarely, does it develop before 20 years of age when the epiphyseal plate is still ununited. The sites affected most frequently are the long tubular bones, bones about the knee, the lower end of the radius, spine, and innominate bone in a skeletally mature patient. The epiphyses of the tubular bones will have been involved extensively by the time of diagnosis, although the tumour may originate in the metaphysis. Metaphyseal location is especially noted in children and adolescents. The most frequent, and generally first symptom was pain of increasing intensity, associated with local swelling and tenderness of the affected area. Limitation of motion of the adjacent joint, most frequently the knee, was present in many patients. A pathologic fracture was infrequent and was, occasionally, the first symptom.

2) Imaging manifestations

① X-ray findings: Most radiologists agree that the giant cell tumor (Figure 4-24) has a fairly characteristic radiologic feature. It is usually an accentrally situated osteolytic lesion in the end of a long bone and in or adjacent to the metaphyseal region. It may expend to the subchondral bone and abuts on the joint surface. It often gives a soap-bubbling appearance with scanty trabeculatic. A delicate trabecular pattern results from subsequent cortical thinning and expansion. Violation of the cortical surface and spread into contiguous soft tissues is striking evidence of the aggressiveness or the malignancy of some giant cell tumors. Tumors involving the flat bones may also be osteolytic; vertebral collapse may occur if the spine is affected.

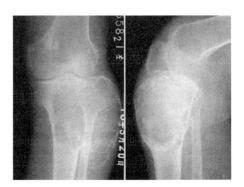

Figure 4-24 Giant cell tumor of the proximal tibia.

② CT findings: CT scanning not only can demonstrate the same signs of the affected bone by giant-cell tumor as the radiography but also may provides information not previously available by plain film and angiography regarding precise size of the tumor mass, its location and relationship to muscle bundles and fascial planes, definition of the margins of the tumor and the relation to neural, vascular, and adjoining bony structures. There may appear cysts or fluid-fluid levels in the solid soft mass on the CT images. After contrast media administration, the tumor can enhance except cysts.

③ MR findings: With MR imaging, T1-weighted image of the tumor often demonstrates the low or mediate signal intensity and T2-wighted image the high signal intensity. Occasionally, intraosseous fluid levels and multiple cysts in the lesion with different signal intensity may be seen. Fat-suppressed T1-weighted MR image after gadolinium administration demonstrates enhancement of the mass, but the cyst in the tumor remains unchangeable.

(2) Bone cyst (Simple or Unicameral bone cyst)

1) Clinical and pathological manifestations: Bone cyst, tumor-like lesion, is a common non-neoplastic process of uncertain pathogenesis. There was a great preponderance of young children, with the highest frequency in the first two decades of life. The majority of large series indicate a predilection for the humerus, particularly the upper metaphysis, close to the growth cartilage. The next most common site was the upper end of the femur. Bone cysts are generally discovered because of a fracture due to an insignificant trauma or incidentally after a roentgenologic examination for other reasons. However, some patients may experience mild pain or limitations of motion at variable times prior to the diagnosis.

The gross appearanceof the bone cyst is characterized by a unicameral cavity filled with a clear serosanguineous fluid. The inner surface of the cyst is lined by a usually smooth membrane of variable thickness, grayish white, reddish brown, or occasionally yellow in color. The cyst membrane consists of loose vascular connective tissue, showing scattered osteoclast giant cells and newly formed immature bone or osteoid trabeculae, usually oriented paralled to the surface of the cyst wall. The cortex is often reduced to a thin translucent membrane resembling an eggshell that can be cut relatively easily with the knife.

2) Imaging manifestations:

①X-ray findings: The roentgenographic features are characterized by a well-outlined, radiolucent metaphyseal lesion, usually located centrally, expanding and thinning the cortex. The cyst has its broader base and greatest diameter near the epiphyseal plate and its conic end in the shaft. The edge of the cyst is rather sharp at the plate, but the margin near the marrow distal end may be indistinct. As the long bone growths, the cyst moves away from the epiphyseal plate and is found in the shaft at variable distances. The bone cortex is usually extremely thin but never completely destroyed. The cyst is occasionally traversed by bone trabeculae giving a multilocular appearance, which is due to prominent bone ridges of the cortical wall and not to true bone septum.

The most important complication is a pathologic fracture whereby the thinned cortex is crushed, giving rise to the so-called fallen fragment sign. A small cyst can disappear spontaneously through osteocartilaginous callus formation after the fracture, and a large cyst may get smaller as well after this. Periosteal reaction is generally absent in bone cysts, except at sites of infraction.

②CT findings: CT scan shows a focal unilocular area of water-like attenuation with the well-marginated wall in the affected bone. After contrast material administration, the attenuation in the cyst remains unenhanced. The rest of the CT signs are the same as the plain film shows.

③MRI findings: T1-weighted MR image shows the cyst with the low signal intensity and the well-defined, thin-wall and T2-weighted MR image with homogeneous high signal intensity like water. Intraosseous fluid levels and various signal intensity may be seen if there is fracture before the examination.

(3) Osteosarcoma

1) Clinical and pathological manifestations: It is the most common type of primary malignant bone tumor and is a disease of young adults. About 80% of the tumor appears before the age of 30. Males are twice as common as

females. Osteosarcomas usually arises in the metaphysis of long bone, more frequently at the distal end of the femur, the proximal end of the tibia or the humerus.

2) Imaging manifestations

①X-ray findings: Radiologically, osteosarcoma (Figure 4-25) produces all varieties of bone changes. It may be very dense and structureless (osteoblastic type) or varies but little from the normal or almost total destruction of the bone (osteolytic type) or present as an admixture. These depend on the composition of various type of tumor cells. Tumors with abundant tumorous bone or tumor ostoid matrix, may reveal a dense tumor bone radiologically. A tumor in which tumor bone formation is sparse appears largely osteolytic. The periosteum is frequently involved and is highly irregular; giving a so called "sunburst" appearance-dense radiating bony speculations, and often considered to be diagnostic. Of course, exceptions do exist. Codman's triangle (reactive triangle or periosteal cuff) near the edge of the mass may be seen. This phenomenon is considered to be due to direct erosion of the already formed periosteal new bone by fast growing tumor. Occasionally a Codman's triangle may be seen with a benign lesion such as a healing fracture, subperiosteal haemorrhage, osteomyelitis or aneurysmal bone cyst. Soft tissue mass immediately adjacent to the affected bone maybe detected radiologically due to soft tissue invasion and tumor bone formation may occur in the soft tissue mass. Tumor may break through the epiphyseal plate to invade the nearby joint.

②CT and MRI findings: MR imaging appears to be superior to the plain film and CT scanning in defining the intraosseous and extraosseous extent of the tumor. Therefore, MRI is thought to be able to show the osteosarcoma (Figure 4-26) earliest when the tumor only infiltrates in the marrow and the trabeculae are not destroyed and to reveal it better whether soft tissues such as muscles, vessels or nerves around the mass are infiltrated by it. But MRI is inferior to the plain film and CT in confirming tumor bone or calcification in the osteosarcoma.

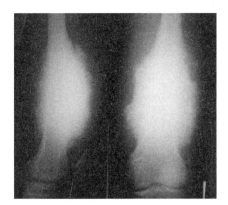

Figure 4-25   Osteosarcoma of the left femur.

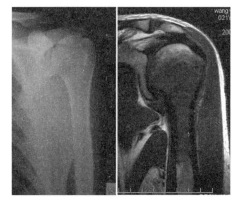

Figure 4-26   Early osteosarcoma of the left humerus on MR image appears normal on the X-ray film (left).

On T1-weighted spin-echo MR images the tumour is typically of heterogeneously low signal intensity, whereas on T2-weighted spin-echo MR images it is usually of inhomogenously high signal intensity.

(4) Metastatic bone tumor

1) Clinical and pathological manifestations: Carcinoma elsewhere in the body may show distant metastasis to bone through blood stream or lymphatics. It is common from the breast, thyroid, lung, kidney or prostate but rarely from the gastrointestinal tract. Metastasis occurs often in elderly person and in the bones rich of red marrow. The verbebrae, pelvis, ribs and skull are often the sites of metastasis. Lesions are usually multiple.

2) Imaging manifestations

①X-ray findings: Occasionally the involved bones may show no apparent change at all except for some generalized osteoporosis on the film. The lesions may be osteolytic, osteoblastic or mixed. Osteolytic lesions are more common.

Osteolytic metastasis: They shows irregular radiolucent patches of bone destruction. The cortex is invaded from inside and often shows little expansion. They are poorly circumscribed with no condensation of bone surrounding the lesion. When the vertebral column is involved. The lesions are frequently multiple and jumping. Both the body and the pedicle may be destroyed. The verbebral body become compressed and assumes a wedge shape but the intervertebral disc space remains intact. This point helps distinguish metastases from tuberculosis of spine. Pathologic fracture may be the first evidence of bone metastasis.

Osteoblatic metastasis: Less common type and usually represent a slow growing tumor. It is usual with prostatic carcinoma. Carcinoma of the lung, breast, thyroid occasionally produce osteoblastic metastasis. The involved bone, usually the spine, pelvis or ribs, shows increase of bone density on the film with loss of normal bone architecture.

② CT findings: On CT scans, further delineation of the nature of a scintigraphically positive bone scan may be possible. CT is an excellent tool in determining the extent of metastatic lesions. Occasionally, matrix calcification in mineralized cartilage or osteoid will be appreciated only on CT. Rarely are these patterns of mineralization found in metastatic lesions. Computed tomography is the method of choice for studying pelvic or sacral lesions, particularly to evaluate the extent of soft tissue involvement.

③ MRI findings: MR imaging has been used most extensively in the evaluation of spinal metastasis. On T1-weighted images, vertebral lesions are low signal intensities are similar but less pronounced in acute (less than 30 days old) benign compression fractures. On T2-wighted image, metastatic lesions show similar, increased or heterogeneous signal intensity, and usually hyperintense on fat-suppressed T2WI. Like CT, MRI readily demonstrates the extent of soft tissue involved by metastasis.

(Chen Zhu, Wu Haijun, Luo Tao, Xiao Enhua, Tan Lihua)

第五章

关节

第一节　检查方法

人体关节分为三种类型：纤维关节(不动关节)、软骨关节(微动关节)、滑膜关节。滑膜关节是可动关节，如四肢关节，这种关节包括三个部分：骨端、关节软骨、关节囊。透明软骨覆盖在骨端表面，可起到保护关节面的作用，但破坏后不能再生。评价关节疾病有多种影像检查方法，其中 X 线平片是最基本的、最常用的方法，计算机体层、磁共振成像、数字减影血管造影的应用也越来越广泛。关节影像学检查的目的是发现关节病变、明确病变程度和范围、选择适当的治疗方法、评估治疗效果和发现并发症，建立关节疾病的病因学诊断还必须结合临床表现和实验室指标。

1. X 线检查

(1)X 线平片：透视已很少应用。X 线平片是日常工作中评价关节疾病的首选，是其他影像检查的基础。骨质因内含钙质呈高密度而有别于周围软组织，X 线平片影像对比良好，这是 X 线平片的优点。关节囊、韧带、关节软骨因缺乏自然对比，X 线平片不能显示，这是 X 线平片的劣势。关节 X 线平片的基本要求同骨骼摄影。

(2)数字减影血管造影：数字减影血管造影用于诊断肿瘤和血管性疾病，是侵入性检查，关节疾病不常应用。

(3)关节造影：关节造影是通过向关节腔注射阴性或阳性造影剂以显示关节内结构的方法，也属侵入性检查。在 CT 和 MRI 广泛用于诊断关节疾病以前，关节造影较常用，但现已逐渐被 CT 和 MRI 取代。

2. CT 检查

CT 是诊断关节疾病的重要工具，是一种快速、准确、非侵入性检查方法。CT 的重要特性，如横断位成像、良好的分辨率、能够测量衰减值，使 CT 在关节疾病诊断方面较 X 线平片具有明显的优势。所以 CT 广泛用于显示位于解剖复杂部位的病变和 X 线平片难以发现的病变。CT 扫描方法包括平扫、增强扫描、CT 关节造影。平扫不使用造影剂；增强扫描静脉内注射碘剂，它具有两个目的，一是提高病变和正常组织的密度差以发现病变，另一目的是显示病变的强化特征以便正确诊断；CT 关节造影是指关节造影之后的扫描。轴位扫描和重建最常用。扫描参数同骨骼，所有图像分别用设定的适合于观察骨骼和软组织的窗宽和窗位观察。

3. MRI 检查

MRI 显示正常的关节结构，如关节骨端、骨性关节面、关节软骨、关节囊、肌腱、韧带、脂肪组织和关节周围的软组织；它也能发现病变组织，如肿块、水肿、关节积液、出血、创伤和退变组织，能够发现病变的早期改变，所以 MRI 在关节疾病诊断方面起着重要和独特的作用。利用表面线圈能够提高信噪比。MRI 是多参数成像方法，常用自旋回波或快速自旋回波的 T1 加权、T2 加权和脂肪抑制序列。MRI 是多平面成像方法，根据诊断需要可选择横断位、冠状位、矢状位和斜位扫描。静脉内注射钆喷替酸二葡甲胺盐(Gd-DTPA)的增强 MRI 能够增加诊断的准确性，了解病变的血供特点。

第二节　正常表现

1. 关节骨端和关节软骨

关节骨端的骨皮质构成骨性关节面，因其富含钙质，在 X 线平片(图 5-1~R)和 CT 图像上显示为光滑、规则的高密度线状影，在 MRI 各种序列图像上呈薄的低信号影；骨端的髓质富含脂肪，T1WI 和 T2WI 序列上均表现为高信号；覆盖在骨性关节面表面的 X 线关节软骨平片和 CT 不能显示，T1WI 和 T2WI 序列上均表现为弧形中等信号；在脂肪抑制序列则表现为高信号；骨骺为一软骨团块，包含数量不同的钙化成分和非钙化软骨，二者的比例取决于钙化中心的大小，非钙化部分的影像表现同关节软骨。

2. 关节囊、韧带及关节盘

关节囊、韧带以及一些关节内存在的关节盘是维持关节稳定性和完整性的主要结构，由纤维组织构成，X 线平片不显影，CT 表现为软组织密度影，MRI 各种序列上呈低信号。

3. 关节间隙

关节间隙在 X 线平片(图 5-2~R)和 CT 上表现为关节相对的骨端之间的低密度间隙，它包括真正的解剖腔隙、关节软骨和少量滑液，儿童因骺软骨未完全骨化，在 X 线平片及 CT 上关节间隙较成人宽。MRI 能区分真正的解剖腔隙、关节软骨和少量滑液，滑液在 T1WI 序列呈低信号，在 T2WI 序列呈高信号。

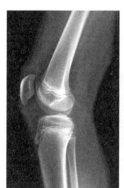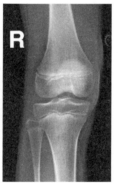　　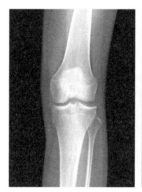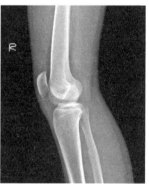

图 5-1　正常小儿关节 X 线平片　　　　　　　　图 5-2　正常成人关节 X 线平片

第三节　基本病变

关节疾病具有一些共同的影像表现，通过分析这些表现可得到大量的诊断信息。这些影像表现包括关节破坏、关节间隙改变、关节肿胀、关节强直和关节脱位。当患有关节疾病时它们可单独或同时出现。

1. 关节破坏

关节破坏是指关节软骨和软骨下骨性关节面被病理组织侵犯和取代。当关节软骨受累时关节间隙变窄；当骨性关节面和关节面下骨质受累时，在 X 线平片和 CT 表现(图 5-3)为低密度区，内部失去骨质结构，磁共振成像时，松质骨的破坏表现为正常骨髓的高信号被病理组织的低信号或混杂信号代替，密质骨的破坏表现为正常骨皮质的低信号被病理组织的高信号或混杂信号代替，关节破坏是诊断关节疾病的重要证据，最初累及的部位因病因不同而异，如化脓性关节炎的关节破坏先累及持重区，而结核性关节炎的关节破坏先累及非持重区。CT 发现隐匿的或微小的骨质破坏较 X 线平片敏感，MRI 又优于 CT。

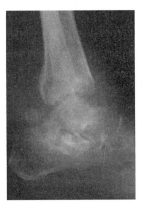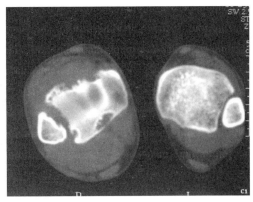

图 5-3　关节破坏 X 线平片和 CT 影像

2.关节间隙改变

大量关节积液可导致关节间隙增宽。关节间隙狭窄提示关节软骨破坏，根据破坏的部位、分布和方式，可对关节疾病作出相当准确的影像学诊断。关节间隙狭窄可见于下列情形：化脓性关节炎、结核性关节炎、关节退行性变、类风湿关节炎等。除非和健侧的正常关节对比，否则关节间隙的轻微改变难以发现。

3.关节肿胀

关节肿胀可因关节炎症、创伤和出血等引起，滑膜充血、关节周围软组织和关节囊肿胀、关节内积液和出血是关节肿胀的病理基础。关节肿胀时，关节的优质平片可显示关节周围软组织密度增加，脂肪间隙模糊或移位。CT 和 MRI 显示此征象远较 X 线平片敏感。肿胀的关节周围软组织和关节囊在 CT 上表现为轮廓增大、密度减低、软组织内脂肪线移位(图 5-4)。关节积液在 CT 上显示为水样密度影，合并出血或积脓时密度升高，急性血肿的衰减值(CT 值)大约波动于 60~80 Hu。MRI 不仅能够显示增厚的关节囊，还能显示出各种病变的异常信号：关节肿胀在 T1WI 序列呈低信号，在 T2WI 序列呈高信号，增强扫描无强化；关节积液在 T1WI 序列呈低信号，在 T2WI 序列呈高信号，增强扫描无强化；急性血肿在 T1WI 和 T2WI 序列均呈低信号，亚急性血肿在 T1WI 和 T2WI 序列均呈高信号，慢性血肿在 T1WI 序列呈低信号，在 T2WI 序列呈高信号，有时血性关节积液会出现液平面，上部为血清，下部为血液的细胞成分，两者具有不同的 CT 和 MRI 表现。脓肿在 CT 上表现为低密度区，增强 CT 有环状强化；MRI 图像上，脓肿在 T1WI 序列呈低信号，在 T2WI 序列呈高信号，静脉内注射钆喷替酸二葡甲胺盐(Gd-DTPA)后增强扫描呈环状强化。脓肿的强化环代表周围的炎性细胞浸润带，中心的无强化区代表坏死组织。

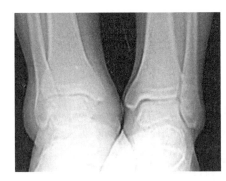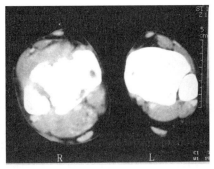

图 5-4　关节肿胀 X 线平片和 CT 影像

4.关节强直

关节强直是关节破坏的后果，分为骨性强直和纤维性强直。骨性强直是指关节间隙完全消失，且有骨小梁通过，多见于化脓性关节炎，平片易发现。纤维性强直指关节间隙有纤维组织穿过，常见于结核性关节炎，单凭 X 线平片不能确诊，诊断必须结合临床。

5.关节脱位

关节相对应骨端的位置改变称为关节脱位，意味着关节连续性的丧失，可分为完全性和非完全性脱位，后者又称半脱位。任何能引起关节破坏的疾病都可造成关节脱位。通常根据 X 线平片可诊断关节脱位，但有时须将患侧关节和健侧关节对比，否则一些隐匿性脱位难以发现。CT 比 X 线平片更容易发现解剖复杂部位的关节脱位，MRI 不仅能发现脱位，而且能发现脱位的合并症，如关节内出血、韧带损伤、肌腱撕裂。

第四节　常见疾病诊断

关节疾病虽种类繁多，其分类却并无统一标准。根据病因学分类，可将其分为：感染性、退行性、免疫性、外伤性、先天性、代谢性及肿瘤性五种类型，以下将介绍几种常见的关节疾病。

1.化脓性关节炎

(1)临床及病理表现：化脓性关节炎是由于关节感染后炎症反应所引起的急性的关节病变。常见致病菌有：金黄色葡萄球菌、α 或 β 溶血链球菌、淋球菌和肺炎球菌。病菌可经血行感染、由邻近感染灶蔓延、关节外伤后直接植入感染。该病可发生于各年龄阶段，多见于儿童。受累关节主要为承重大关节，如髋关节、膝关节。单关节发病多见，多关节发病者只占该病的 20% 左右。急性化脓性关节炎起病急骤，伴发热、寒战等全身症状，典型的局部表现为受累关节红、肿、热、痛。实验室检查：白细胞增多，关节渗液或外周血细菌培养阳性，红细胞沉降率和 C-反应蛋白增高。病理学改变：滑膜充血、水肿，渗出和增厚；关节内渗出液可逐渐增多，这些渗液中含有大量的白细胞、纤维素和蛋白溶解酶，其中蛋白溶解酶可起到迅速破坏关节软骨的作用。随着液体积聚和滑膜增生，关节囊肿胀增大，周围软组织明显水肿，骨质破坏亦随之而至。晚期可出现骨性强直。

(2)影像学表现：

1)X 线表现：X 线出现异常与其病理改变是同步的。疾病早期，临床症状和体征可明显，而影像学改变甚微，但仍可能在最初几天发现某些改变，例如关节周围软组织密度增高，筋膜层及关节囊脂肪垫移位，易见于膝关节、踝关节。由于液体积聚，关节间隙可增宽。随后，关节间隙因关节软骨破坏而变窄，以关节持重部出现早，发病 2 周后可见明显骨质改变，骨质破坏的部位亦以关节持重部为常见，该病变特点可区别于结核性关节炎。偶见死骨，关节内和周围软组织充气征罕见。因关节囊破坏可继发病理性脱位和半脱位，感染后数周可见关节周围钙化。晚期，关节软骨严重破坏，出现骨性强直。有效抗生素治疗对控制疾病的发展有积极作用。

2)CT 表现：CT 检查有如下优点：①疾病早期，对显示软组织改变较敏感；②较之普通 X 线检查，能更早发现关节渗出；③明确显示骨质和软骨受累的范围；④更易发现轻微的骨质破坏、死骨及解剖复杂部位的病变；⑤充气征的发现是诊断化脓性关节炎的可靠依据；⑥合并有腐败菌感染的关节炎时，CT 可观察到关节内碎骨片。

3)MRI 表现：MRI 是诊断化脓性关节炎最敏感的检查方法。较之 CT 更易显示软组织改变，关节囊、关节软骨及韧带的病变，能明确炎症侵犯周围软组织的范围，MRI 可用于早期诊断，但其特异性不高。软组织和骨髓肿胀在 T1WI 呈低信号，脂肪抑制和 T2WI 呈高信号，MRI 增强后无强化。骨质破坏则在 T1WI 上呈低信号病灶，T2WI 和脂肪抑制后呈高信号，增强后有明显强化，且病灶内信号强度不均匀，边界不清楚。MRI 还能显示脓肿和死骨：脓肿在 T1WI 上呈低信号，T2WI 上呈高信号，增强后有边缘强化；死骨在 T1WI 和 T2WI 上均为低信号或中等信号，MRI 增强后无明显强化。

2.结核性关节炎

(1)临床及病理表现：绝大多数关节结核(结核性关节炎)继发于肺结核。该病可累及全身各关节，以侵犯大关节为主，如髋关节、膝关节及脊椎。单关节发病常见，亦有多关节结核病例的报道。关节结核可发生于各年龄阶段，多见于儿童和青少年。与化脓性关节炎不同，该病病程缓慢，通常表现为慢性疼痛和关节肿胀，而炎症反应体征并不明显，因此常耽误诊断。病理学改变：滑膜充血、水肿和增厚；关节软骨破坏；骨质破坏。

（2）影像学表现：

1）X线表现：影像学上，可根据首发感染灶部位的不同将关节结核分为骨型和滑膜型。骨型关节结核（图5-4）的首发病灶位于干骺端或骨骺，也可由邻近干骺端或骨骺的结核感染扩散而来，该型多见于成年人。滑膜型关节结核（图5-5）是结核菌经血行感染首先侵犯滑膜引起，此型多见于儿童，且受累关节多为膝、踝关节。而无论是哪一型，最终结果是相同的，疾病晚期，骨质均会受累。在疾病早期，X线平片通常仅显示关节附近软组织肿胀及进行性骨质疏松，此时诊断比较困难。在出现明显的软骨及骨质破坏以前，关节结核的类型很难明确。当关节结核发生于承重关节，如膝、髋关节时，可出现特征性的关节边缘侵蚀，X线片表现为关节周边骨质缺损，这点与其他侵犯滑膜的疾病相似，如类风湿关节炎。在关节结核，软骨下骨质侵蚀亦可见，表现为软骨下骨板与其下的骨小梁中的边界不清的缺损，而此时关节间隙可能正常。待关节软骨破坏较多时，则关节间隙变窄，有的患者在出现大量边缘和中心骨质破坏后才表现出关节间隙狭窄，而有的患者只在轻度边缘骨质侵蚀时即可出现间隙变窄。该病通常只在继发化脓性感染时才有明显的骨质增生。关节破坏可导致关节脱位。关节结核病变愈后最终多产生纤维性强直，偶见骨性强直。

2）CT表现：CT检查除能观察到以上改变外，还可清楚显示关节囊及关节周围软组织肿胀，关节腔积液（图5-6），隐匿的骨破坏，小块的"对吻"死骨，以及冷脓肿。冷脓肿在CT上表现为低密度影，增强扫描后，脓肿边缘可强化。

3）MRI表现：MRI用于观察关节结核的病变较CT更为敏感。MRI在疾病早期即可显示关节肿胀，包括滑膜增厚，关节周围软组织和关节囊肿胀，以及极少量关节腔积液。随病程发展，MRI还可观察到关节软骨破坏，骨质破坏以及冷脓肿。

以下对关节结核影像学主要特点作一小结：①单关节发病；②软组织肿胀，骨质疏松早期轻微，但呈进行性发展；③在非关节持重面，即骨端的边缘部分出现关节面下鼠咬状骨质破坏；④关节间隙狭窄出现晚，呈非匀称性狭窄，与骨质破坏程度不同步；⑤只在继发化脓性感染时，才出现明显的骨质硬化和骨膜反应；⑥小块"对吻"死骨；⑦冷脓肿，穿破皮肤可形成窦道，亦可发生碎片状钙化；⑧关节破坏较多时，可发生病理性脱位；⑨纤维性强直。

（3）鉴别诊断：若在常见部位（如髋、膝关节处）观察到典型的影像学改变，关节结核的诊断并不十分困难，若病变的部位和表现均不具特征性，则诊断务必慎重。发现关节周围骨质疏松，边缘骨质破坏和关节间隙的轻微狭窄或不狭窄均可作为诊断本病的有利依据。而类风湿关节炎表现为骨质疏松及边缘骨质破坏，常伴有发生早且明显的关节间隙狭窄；痛风性关节炎可见边缘骨质破坏，骨间隙正常，而骨质疏松不明显或较轻微，在骨质疏松的区域，边缘性侵蚀不明显，且关节间隙仍正常。特发性软骨溶解病可见明显的骨质疏松和早期关节间隙变窄，尤以髋关节多见，偶可发生于全身其他关节。单关节发病者多考虑为感染性疾病，虽然明确感染病原体（如化脓性、结核性）尚有一定困难，但较化脓性关节炎而言，关节结核有如下特点以资鉴别：病程缓慢，骨质疏松明显，骨质硬化轻微等（表5-1），而最终确诊仍有赖于关节腔穿刺取滑囊液检查或滑膜活检。其他单关节疾病，如色素沉着绒毛结节性滑膜炎和特发性滑膜骨软骨瘤病，因与关节结核表现相似，亦应鉴别。色素沉着绒毛结节性滑膜炎的典型表现为结节状软组织肿块，关节间隙正常，无骨质疏松。而特发性滑膜骨软骨瘤病通常表现为关节腔内结构明显的钙化和骨化。

3.其他种类感染性关节炎

引起化脓性关节炎的细菌还有：布氏杆菌、沙门氏菌、大肠埃希菌、流感嗜血杆菌等。除此以外，螺旋体、真菌、病毒、立克次体、寄生虫都可以是感染性关节炎的病原体，但影像学上通常无特殊表现。

表 5-1 关节结核与化脓性关节炎的区别

区别	结核	化脓性关节炎
软组织肿胀	+	+
骨质疏松	+	-
关节间隙狭窄	出现晚	出现早
关节边缘侵蚀	+	-
骨质增生	-	+
骨性强直	-	+
病程缓慢	+	-

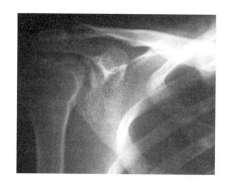

图 5-5 肩关节骨型结核的 X 线平片表现

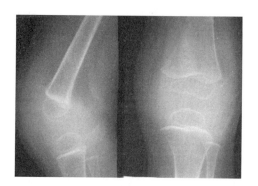

图 5-6 膝关节滑膜型结核的 X 线平片表现

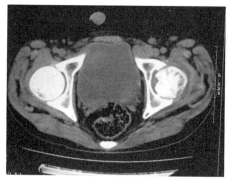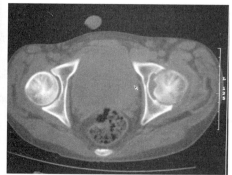

图 5-7 髋关节结核的 CT 影像表现

4. 关节创伤

关节创伤包括关节内骨折、关节脱位、半脱位、关节软骨损伤,关节囊、肌腱、肌肉及韧带撕裂伤,创伤性滑膜炎、创伤性关节积血等。X 线平片、CT、MRI 均能准确显示骨折、关节肿胀和脱位,关节创伤的诊断首选 X 线平片。此外,CT 还能发现隐匿性骨折、骨软骨小体、关节内出血、关节软骨损伤和韧带撕裂。如果体征及体格检查结果均提示有血管损伤,此时有必要行血管造影,通过造影可清楚显示出是否存在血管畸形,如大血管破裂和闭塞,动静脉窦及动脉瘤。

(1)关节软骨骨折及骨软骨骨折:

1)临床及病理表现:由于关节不正规运动所产生的剪切力、旋转力或压缩力而引起的软骨和软骨下骨质骨折。通常情况下，骨折线与关节面相平行，并可通过损伤的深度来判断骨折碎片中的软骨和骨性成分。

2）影像学表现：X线平片不能直接显示关节软骨骨折，只能提供骨折部分线索。如果发现骨折线波及骨性关节面（图5-7），甚至骨性关节面因此而错位时，应考虑关节软骨骨折的可能。关节造影可明确骨折的性质和部位，表现为关节软骨面的缺损，受损骨质中可有对比剂充盈，还可见关节内软骨与骨质小体。MRI可显示关节软骨损伤的征象如下：软骨缺损，关节内软骨小体在T2WI和脂肪抑制上的高信号区域，而正常时应为低信号（图5-8）。MRI还能发现骨髓水肿（图5-9），表现为T1WI上低信号，T2WI和脂肪抑制上高信号增强后无明显强化。

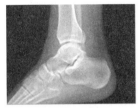
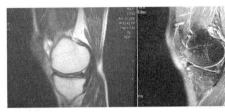
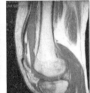
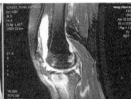

图5-8　骨折累及关节面　　　　　图5-9　半月板撕裂　　　　　图5-10　关节囊积液、骨挫伤

（2）创伤性滑膜炎和关节血肿：

1）临床及病理表现：急性创伤性滑膜炎常累及膝、肘、肩和踝关节。临床表现有疼痛，肿胀和关节功能障碍。病理改变：滑膜充血、水肿、出血、关节内积液，关节内出血还可形成关节血肿。

2）影像学表现：X线平片、CT和MRI均可显示关节及其周围软组织肿胀。除此之外，CT和MRI还有其特征性发现。CT可用于区别关节积液和血肿，关节积液在CT上表现为低密度，而血肿呈高密度病灶。渗出液在T1WI上呈低信号，T2WI上呈高信号（图5-9），急性血肿在T1WI和T2WI上均为低信号，亚急性血肿在T1WI和T2WI均为高信号，而慢性血肿在T1WI上呈低信号，T2WI上呈高信号。有时可发现血性渗出液中有一液平面，其上层为血浆，下层是血液的细胞成分，两者在CT和MRI上均有不同表现。MRI还能显示滑膜的增厚。

（3）肌腱及韧带损伤：

1）临床及病理表现：肌腱及韧带损伤可分为完全撕裂与不完全撕裂两种。临床症状有疼痛、压痛、局部肿胀和功能障碍。

2）影像学表现：单纯肌腱及韧带损伤在普通X线平片上无阳性改变，应力X线摄影可发现患侧关节活动度大于健侧。MRI能直接显示肌腱和韧带的损伤，表现为关节肿胀，边缘不规则，撕裂的肌腱和韧带在T2WI和脂肪抑制上呈高信号，还可并发骨髓水肿。

5. 类风湿关节炎

（1）临床及病理表现：类风湿关节炎（RA）是以侵犯滑膜为主的全身性非化脓性炎症反应的结缔组织疾病。流行病学显示本病发生率0.3%～1.5%，且多见于年轻女性。RA以主要侵犯手足小关节为特征，易受累关节有近端指间关节、掌指关节和腕关节。全身症状有疲劳、厌食、消瘦，精神不振，局部表现为疼痛、晨僵、关节肿胀和关节脱位或半脱位等。实验室检查：类风湿因子阳性，血沉增快，C-反应蛋白增高。主要病理变化有滑膜的非特异性炎症，关节内渗出，血管翳形成，关节软骨及软骨下骨质破坏，晚期可以关节强直。

（2）影像学表现：

1）X线表现：X线征象的出现明显滞后于临床症状，而从症状出现直到影像学发现异常需要多久也是未知的。RA是一个多发的，关节对称性受累的疾病，X线早期表现为关节周围软组织肿胀，肿胀是由关节渗出和滑膜炎引起的，多呈梭形。局部骨质疏松为该病的特征性表现，常起始于关节附近。随疾病进展，关节软骨发生不可逆破坏，关节间隙进一步缩小，关节下骨皮质轮廓模糊甚至消失，可只发生在病灶处，亦可呈弥漫性。在缺乏关节软骨的地方，即关节边缘极易发生骨侵蚀，边缘模糊，无硬化带形成，机械性压迫可能是影响侵蚀的发生部位及进展的重要原因。骨膜反应少见。病情进一步严重时，可出现弥漫性骨质疏松，最终将导致关节半脱位、挛缩和骨性强直。骨性强直多发生于腕骨和腕关节，而在掌指关节和指间关节却不常见。因关节力学变化，可继发伴骨赘及增生硬化的骨性关节炎。受累关节可形成滑膜囊肿，引起软组织不均匀肿胀，若发生于膝关节，可形成巨大囊肿，并伸及附近软组织中。关节造影可清楚显示滑膜囊肿。80%以上的晚期 RA 病例均侵及颈椎，有些病例中颈椎也可以是唯一的发病部位。椎间隙和骨突关节均可受累，最常见的影像学表现是骨质疏松，关节面侵蚀和椎间隙变窄，常可并发一个或多个关节半脱位。枢椎齿突若受侵犯，可表现为椎管容积减小，圆钝的突起变尖，造成枢椎齿突与寰锥前弓的间隙增宽。切勿将类风湿引起的颈椎病变与进行性上行性脊椎炎相混淆，后者可以是类风湿源性，但多认为是由强直性脊柱炎引起。类风湿关节炎的重要 X 线表现(图 5-10)有：关节间隙均匀变窄，边缘侵蚀和关节周围骨质疏松。长期皮质类固醇治疗可引起一系列并发症，如消化性溃疡，Cushing 综合征等。Cushing 综合征还可引起骨质疏松和病理性骨折，后者多发生于脊柱。

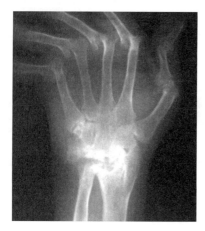

图 5-11　类风湿关节炎的 X 线表现

2)CT 表现：CT 对 RA 诊断价值大。CT 在平片尚无阳性发现时，即可显示骨侵蚀，尤其是解剖复杂部位，如骶髂关节和脊柱的病变；还可显示软组织肿胀，关节积液，关节旁肿块，如类风湿结节和滑膜恶性肿瘤。类风湿结节可小至数毫米，大的亦可超过 5 厘米，经静脉碘剂造影后，CT 扫描有强化，显示为软组织密度肿块，而滑膜恶性肿瘤经造影后无强化，表现为低密度病变。

3)MRI 表现：MRI 对于显示 RA 病变优于普通 X 线平片。虽然对于 RA 诊断无特异性，但它仍有利于其早期诊断。MRI 易于显示骨侵蚀，关节内结构异常（软骨损伤，关节积液，肌腱和韧带病变），可评估类风湿关节炎的活动性和治疗效果，观察滑膜炎症和滑膜囊肿的程度，以及类风湿结节。增强 MRI 可用于区别滑膜液和血管翳，静脉注射钆剂后，渗出液在 T1WI 上仍表现为低信号影，而血管翳则有明显强化。类风湿结节在 T1WI 上为低信号，T2WI 上为高信号。静脉注射钆剂后有强化，该表现与软组织肿瘤相似。此外，对于发现 RA 并发症，如骨缺血坏死，MRI 亦优于 X 线平片。

6.强直性脊柱炎

(1)临床及病理表现：强直性脊柱炎(AS)是一种以脊柱慢性炎症为主的疾病，多先侵犯骶髂关节和下腰椎，然后上行发展累及高位椎骨。AS 的病因不明，致病因素可能有遗传、免疫、感染和环境因素等，发病率约 0.1%，发病年龄多在 15~35 岁，AS 好发于男性的传统观点通过基因检测得到了修正，目前认为 AS 与性别没有明显关系，但女性症状更轻。主要临床表现为腰背痛和晨僵。实验室检查：类风湿因子阴性，血沉增快，C-反应蛋白增多，90%强直性脊柱炎患者血清 HLA-B27 抗原阳性。AS 关节滑膜的病理学改变与 RA 类似，但血管翳较少见，除此外还可见软骨下骨质硬化和骨膜反应，而这些改变在 RA 并不突出。

(2)影像学表现：AS 早期 X 线检查可能只显示单侧骶髂关节病变，常见为髂骨侧，数月或数年后可观察到另一侧骶髂关节亦受累。双侧对称性发病是 AS 的一个重要特征，可用于与其他侵犯骶髂关节的疾病相鉴别。最早的 X 线表现包括关节边缘模糊和骨质疏松，逐渐可发展为关节面侵蚀和关节周围硬化。由于髂骨软骨较骶骨软骨薄弱，因此病变较早易累及髂骨。2~5 年后，病变可发展为骨性强直，最终关节间隙完全消失。AS 坐骨结节和耻骨联合受累常见。

脊柱亦可发生 AS 相类似的变化，但这种改变并非与前述改变绝对一致。关节间隙变窄，并可发生椎间关节、胸肋关节融合，椎体可因破坏而呈"方椎"。晚期可发生脊椎韧带骨化，形成竹节状脊柱(图 5-11)。骨质疏松常见，很少发生椎骨脱位。

　　若病程缓慢进展，还可累及其他关节，如髋、肩、手、腕、膝、下颌关节，其影像学表现与 RA 类似，但较 RA 而言，AS 骨质疏松和关节间隙狭窄相对轻微，而骨质破坏、硬化和骨性强直则更明显。

　　AS 的诊断主要依靠临床病史，HLA-B27 抗原测定和特征性 X 线表现。诊断困难时，可选用 CT 和 MRI 检查。CT 能清楚显示骶髂、胸肋关节和椎间关节的病变(图 5-12)。MRI 则易于显示韧带病变，椎管狭窄，对评价 AS 的活动性和并发症有价值。

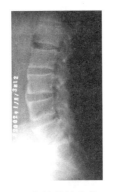

图 5-12　强直性脊柱炎的 X 线表现

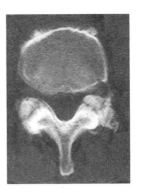

图 5-13　强直性脊柱炎的 CT 表现

7. 退行性关节病

　　(1)临床及病理表现：退行性关节病是一种常见的关节疾病，是以关节软骨退变为特征的非炎症性病变。本病分原发性(特发性)和继发性两大类。前者指不明原因导致的关节变性，后者则是其他已存在的疾病，如外伤后所引起的退变。近日有人提出另一种分类方法，即异常作用力作用于正常关节引起的退行性关节病和正常作用力作用于异常关节引起的退行性关节病。导致关节退变原因多种多样，包括年龄、职业、遗传、炎症、外伤、发育不良等。这些因素使得关节内结构很难正常承受生理压力而发生变性。其基本病理改变为软骨退变，显微镜下可见病灶组织肿胀，关节软骨面纤维化，进一步发展，可发生软骨表层撕裂、剥脱。通常认为理化因素是造成软骨退变的始发原因，该病常见症状为疼痛，受累关节运动受限，但无关节肿胀和全身症状。

　　(2)影像学表现：X 线早期改变为关节边缘骨质增厚、突起，由于关节软骨变薄引起关节间隙不规则狭窄，多发生在承重大关节，最终可见边缘骨赘形成(图 5-13)。晚期可出现软骨下囊变，关节周围和关节内钙化及半脱位，但骨质疏松不常见。CT 和 MRI 对诊断脊椎关节的退行性关节病有很大价值。

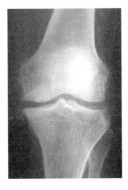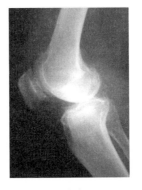

图 5-14　退行性关节病的 X 线表现

8. 痛风性关节炎

　　(1)临床及病理表现：痛风是由嘌呤代谢障碍引起的全身性疾病，其突出的生化特征为高尿酸血症，可能是由于尿酸的过度产生或肾排泄泌尿酸减少，也可能是两者共同作用的结果。习惯上把痛风分为两型：原发性痛风，是由于遗传性代谢障碍导致的较隐匿的高尿酸血症；继发性痛风，是由其他疾病引起的高尿酸血症。痛风主要侵犯关节、肾脏和心脏。当尿酸结晶沉积在关节内、关节周围、腱鞘、滑膜囊以及皮下脂肪组织中时，则可引起痛风性关节炎。痛风性关节炎患病率男性远高于女性，且多发生于50岁后男性和绝经后妇女。临床上主要表现为关节红肿、疼痛和压痛，疾病早期多为单关节发病。痛风性关节炎好发于下肢关节，尤以跖趾关节和跗骨间关节为多。病理学改变包括：多形核白细胞浸润引起滑膜非特异性炎症反应，软骨非特异的变性，尿酸可穿透软骨并沉积在软骨下或更深层骨质中，引起骨质囊性缺失（骨侵蚀）。

（2）影像学表现：影像学表现与病理学改变是一致的，疾病早期，对痛风患者关节行X线平片检查，绝大多数患者X线片无阳性发现或仅有受累关节的非特异性软组织肿胀，因此X线平片表现无异常时，不能排除痛风性关节炎的可能。数年后，影像学表现可异常，主要表现（图5-14）为软组织肿胀、骨质破坏、关节间隙变窄和钙化。若发现软组织异常的结节样突出，则说明软组织内有尿酸沉积，而RA的结节多为对称性，可资鉴别。据报道，痛风患者中约有40%发生了骨质破坏，呈圆形或椭圆形缺损，且多位于骨的长轴上，病变突出于骨边缘，深入软组织中，并形成痛风性结节，这是痛风性关节炎的特征性改变，可与类风湿关节炎的凹陷样骨质破坏相鉴别。CT和MRI均可用于痛风性关节炎的辅助诊断，尤其在显示解剖复杂部位的骨质破坏均较X线平片好。CT可发现类似钙化点的散在的尿酸盐沉积，MRI可显示软组织、滑膜、软骨和骨的受累程度。

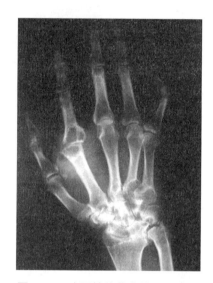

图5-15　痛风性关节炎的X线表现

9.关节及相关结构肿瘤

（1）临床及病理表现：关节及相关结构肿瘤虽不常见，但其重要性不容忽视。若对于恶性肿瘤的诊断不及时，治疗不恰当，其后果可能不堪设想。此类疾病分两种类型：良性肿瘤和恶性肿瘤。常见良性肿瘤有：腱鞘囊肿，滑膜囊肿，腱鞘巨细胞瘤，纤维瘤等。原发性恶性肿瘤以滑膜肉瘤、软骨肉瘤、纤维肉瘤多见，而其他部位的恶性肿瘤也可能侵犯关节。

（2）影像学表现：X线平片对诊断该病价值不大。CT和MRI可鉴别囊性和实质性病变，显示肿瘤的大小、外形，肿瘤与其周围组织的关系，可显示X线平片无法发现的病变，诊断价值较大。

（陈柱，蔡晔雨，孙双婧，彭书慧，肖恩华，谭利华）

Chapter 5

Joint

Section 1 Method of examination

The joints of body can be classified as three types: Fibrous joints or synarthroses, cartilaginous joints or amphiarthroses, and synovial joints. The synovial joint is a movable articulation, such as the articulation of arms and legs. This kind of articulation includes three parts: capitulum, articular-cartilage and joint capsule. The bony articular surface of the capitulum is covered with hyaline cartilage. The hyaline cartilage can protect the bony articular surface; but it cannot regeneration when the hyaline cartilage has been destructed. There are various radiographic examinations to evaluate the joint diseases. The essential and most common method is plain film. Computed tomography, magnetic resonance imaging, and digital subtraction angiography were used wide and wide. The purposes of radiographic examinations of joints are detecting the joint disease, determining the extent and severity of the lesions, assessing the activity of joint disease, choosing the appropriate methods of treatments, evaluating the therapeutic efficacy, and finding the complications. Establishing the etiology diagnosis of joint diseases must combine with clinic manifestations and laboratory parameters.

1. X-ray examination

(1) Plain film: Fluoroscopy is seldom used. Plain film is the first choice to evaluate the joint diseases in routine work. It is the foundation of other imaging examinations. Bone substance, because of its calcium content and its high density differ from the surrounding soft tissue and thus imaged on a film is full of contrast and detail. This is the advantage of plain film. The joint capsule, the ligament and the articular cartilage, because of lack of natural contrast, are invisible on a plain film, and this is the disadvantage of it. The basic principle for plain film of joint is the same of skeletal radiography.

(2) Digital subtraction angiography: Digital subtraction angiography is applied to diagnosis the tumors and vascular abnormalities. It is an invasive examination. It is used uncommon in joint disorders.

(3) Arthrography: Arthrography is an examination by injection negative or positive contrast media into the articular cavity to display the intra-articular structures. It is an invasive examination, too. It was often used to evaluate the joint diseases before, since CT and MRI are applied to study the joint disorders widely. Now it has replaced by CT and MRI gradually.

2. CT examination

Computed Tomography is animportant tool to diagnosis the joint diseases. It is a quick, accurate, and un-invasive method. The important characteristics of CT, such as cross-sectional display, excellent contrast resolution, and the ability to allow the measurement of specific attenuation values, enable CT gain the obvious advantage over plain film in joint diseases diagnosis. So that CT was used widely in following cases: the lesions located in complex anatomy region, and the lesions were more difficult to be detected by plain film. The scan method includes plain scanning, enhanced scanning, and CT arthrography. Plain CT means the scanning without intravenous contrast medium. Enhanced CT indicated the scanning with intravenous injection of iodinated contrast medium. There are two main purposes of enhanced CT. One is to elevate density difference between the lesion and normal tissue in order to discover the lesion. The other is to know the characteristics of enhancement in order to diagnose accurately. CT arthrography implies the scanning after arthrography. The trans-axial scanning and reformation are used most commonly. The CT scanning parameters of joint is the same of skeleton. All images should be observed separately at window and center settings appropriate for visualization of both bone and soft tissues.

3. MRI examination

MRI can reveal the normal structure of joint, such as capitulum, bony articular surface, articular-cartilage, joint capsule, tendon, ligament, and fat tissue and soft tissue around the joint. It also can detect the pathologic tissues, such as masses, edema, joint effusion, hemorrhage, and traumatic and degenerative tissues. It is able to show the early changes of lesions. So that MRI plays an important and unique role in diagnosis of joint diseases. Using surface coils can increase the signal-noise ratio. MRI is a multi-parameter imaging examination. Spin echo or fast spin echo sequences with T1 and T2 weighting and fat-suppressed sequences are common sequences. MRI is a multi-plane imaging examination. According to the diagnostic require the trans-axial, coronal, sagittal and oblique scanning may be selected. The use of intravenous injection of gadolinium-enhanced MR imaging for the joint lesions can increase the accuracy of diagnosis, know the characteristics of blood supply of the lesions.

Section 2   Normal appearances

1. The articular capitulum and articular-cartilage

The cortex of thearticular capitulum forms the bony articular surface. It is affluent in calcium content. So it reveals as smooth and regular linear high-density shadow on plain film(Figure 5-1-2) and CT imaging, and present thin low signal zone on all sequences in MR imaging. The medulla of the articular capitulum abounds with fat tissue. It reveal as high signal intensity on both T1WI and T2WI. The articular-cartilage who covered the bony articular surface is invisible on a plain film and CT. It shows as 1-6 mm middle signal arc on both T1WI and T2WI, and high signal arc on fat suppression sequence. The epiphysis is a mass of chondral bone. It consists of varying amount of ossified element and non-ossified cartilage. The proportion is depending on the size of the ossified center. The imaging manifestations of non-ossified epiphysis are the same of the articular cartilage.

2. The joint capsule, the ligament and the articular discs

The joint capsule, the ligament and the articular discs in some joints are the main structure to maintain the stability and integrality of joint. They consist of fibrous tissues. The joint capsule and the ligament are invisible on a plain film. They reveal as soft tissue density on CT imaging, and they reveal as low signal all sequences in MR imaging.

3. The joint space

Thejoint space reveals as low density space between the opposite capitulum on the plain film(Figure 5-1-2) and CT imaging. It includes the veritable anatomical cavity, the articular-cartilage and a little synovia. Because of incomplete ossification of epiphyseal cartilage in children, the joint space is wider than that in adults on plain film and CT. MRI can distinguish the veritable anatomical cavity, the articular-cartilage and a little synovia. The synovia may display thin low signal area on T1WI imaging, and thin high signal area on T2WI imaging.

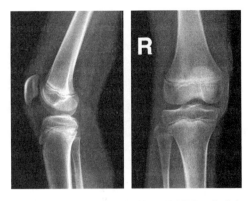

Figure 5-1　Plain film of normal children's joint.

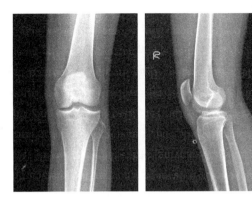

Figure 5-2　Plain film of normal adult joint.

Section 3　Basic pathological changes

There areseveral common radiologic signs in joint diseases. We can gain a lot of diagnostic information by analyzing these radiologic signs. These radiologic signs include destruction of joint, changes of joint space, swelling of the joint, ankylosis of joint, and dislocation. They may occur alone or in combination when there are joint disorders.

1. Destruction of joint

Destruction of joint indicates the articular-cartilage and the sub-chondral bone have been invaded or replaced by pathologic tissue. When the articular-cartilage was involved, the joint space would narrow. When the bony articular surface and the sub-bony articular surface were involved, there would be defect or destruction of the bony articular surface and sub-bony articular surface. It shows low-density areas where lose bone structure inside on the plain film and CT (Figure 5-3). On MRI image the spongy bone destruction reveals as the high signal of normal marrow has been replaced by low signal or mixed signal of pathological tissue; and the cortex destruction reveals as the low signal of the normal cortex has been replaced by high or mixed signal of pathological tissue. Destruction of joint is the important evidence to diagnose joint diseases. The initial involved sites may be different according to different etiology. For example, the destruction of joint occurs first at points of maximum weight bearing or stress in the pyogenic arthritis cases, but it occurs first at points of non-weight bearing or stress in the tuberculous arthritis. CT can reveal the occult or minute bone destruction more sensitive than plain film; and MRI is superior to CT.

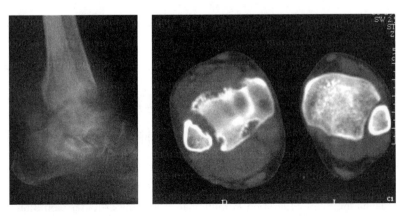

Figure 5-3　Plain film and CT manifestation of joint destruction.

2. Changes of joint space

Thelarge intra-articular effusion may lead to an increase in the width of the joint space. The narrowed joint space indicated the destruction of articular-cartilage. It allows considerable accuracy in radiologic diagnosis of joint diseases, according to its location, distribution, and pattern of erosion. It may occur in following conditions commonly: pyogenic arthritis, tuberculosis arthritis, degenerative arthritis, and rheumatoid arthritis, et al. The slight change of joint space is difficult to be found, unless comparing with the normal joint on the other side.

3. Swelling of the joint

Swelling of the joint may be caused by articular inflammation, trauma, and hemorrhage, and so on. The hyperaemia of synovial membrane, the swelling of the periarticular soft tissues and joint capsule, and the intra-articular effusion and hemorrhage are the pathologic foundation of the sign. When there is swelling of the joint, a good X-ray film of joint may reveal the increase density of the surrounding soft tissue of the joint (Figure 5-4), the loss of definition or displacement of the fat line in the soft tissue. CT and MRI are more sensitive to show this sign than plain film. The swelling of the peri-articular soft tissues and joint capsule show the enlargement of the contour, decreased of the density, and displacement of the fat line in the soft tissue on CT (Figure 5-4). The intra-articular effusion reveals as hydro-density imaging in the intro-articular on CT. When it complicated hemorrhage or pus collection, the density of the lesion would be heightened, the CT attenuation values of acute hematoma may range between 60 and 80HU approximately. MRI can show not only the thickness of the joint capsule, but also the abnormal signal: swelling of the joint revealing as low signal lesion on T1WI and high signal lesion on T2WI with no enhancement after enhanced MRI; joint effusion revealing as low signal lesion on T1WI and high signal lesion on T2WI with no enhancement after enhanced MRI; The acute hematoma shows low signal on both T1WI and T2WI; sub-acute hematoma shows high signal on both T1WI and T2WI; chronic hematoma shows low signal on T1WI and high signal on T2WI. Sometimes a fluid level is noted between two components of the bloody joint effusion. The upper component is serum and the lower component relates to the cellular components of blood, and each of the two components has different CT and MRI findings. The abscess reveals as low-density area with rim enhancement after enhanced CT. It shows low signal lesion on T1WI, and high signal lesion on T2WI with rim enhancement after intravenous administration of a gadolinium contrast agent. The rim of enhancement about abscesses represents the peripheral, cellular inflammatory zone, and the central non-enhancing region indicates the necrotic tissue.

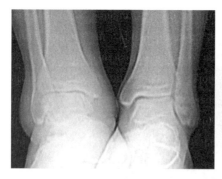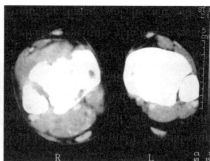

Figure 5-4   plain film and CT of joint swelling.

4. Ankylosis of joint

Ankylosis of join is the sequent of destruction of joint. It may be classified as bony ankylosis and fibrous ankylosis. The former means the total obliteration of joint space, and the articular capitulums were crossed by bony trabeculations. It can be seen commonly in pyogenic arthritis. The bony ankylosis can be discovered by plain film easy. The fibrous ankylosis indicated the joint space crossed by fibrous tissue. It can be seen commonly in tuberculosis arthritis. Fibrous ankylosis cannot be detectable in X-ray film only. We must combine the clinic information to obtain the right diagnosis.

5. Dislocation

The changes of thelocation of the opposite articular capitulum of joints are called dislocation. It means the loss of continuity at the joint. It may be complete or incomplete, the later named as sub-luxation. The causes of dislocations may divide into trauma, congenital and pathological. Any joint disease that can bring on destruction of the joint will result in dislocation. We can diagnose the dislocation according to the plain film generally, but some occult dislocation cannot be found unless comparison the healthy joint to the ill joint. CT may detect some dislocation of more complex anatomy region easier than plain film. MRI not only displays the dislocation, also can display the complications of dislocation, such as intra-articular hemorrhage, ligament injury, and tendon tear.

Section 4 Diagnosis of common diseases

The joint diseases remain greatquantity. There is no union classification of it. According to the etiology classification, arthropathy may be classified as infectious, degenerative, immune, traumatic, congenital, metabolic, and tumorous diseases. The common joint diseases were introduced as follows.

1. Pyogenic arthritis

(1) Clinical and pathological manifestations: Thepyogenic arthritis is a severe acute joint disorder. It is an infectious inflammation of joint. The staphylococcus aureus, alpha or beta hemolytic streptococci, gonococcui, and pneumococci are the most common infecting organism. It affected the joint by three principal routes usually: Hemotogenous spread of infection, spread from a contiguous source of infection, direct implantation. The pyogenic arthritis may occur at any age, although it predominates in the young. The weight bearing joints, such as the hip or the knee joints are affected most commonly. Mono-articular involvement is the major pattern. Poly-articular occurs in 20 percent of cases approximately. The onset of acute pyogenic arthritis is usually sudden. Fever and chills are the common systemic symptom. Redness, swelling, heat, and pain of the involved joint are typical local clinic manifestation. Leukocytosis, positive blood or joint effusion, elevated erythrocyte sedimentation rates and C-reactive protein levels are important laboratory parameters of pyogenic arthritis. Pathological changes include the synovial membrane hyperaemia, edema, exudation, and thickness. The increased amounts of intra-articular extravasate are produced. This kind of extravasate contains large numbers of leukocytes, fibrin, and proteolytic ferment. The proteolytic ferment results in the articular cartilage destruction rapidly. With further accumulation of fluid and hypertrophied synovium, the capsule becomes distended, surrounding soft tissue edema is evident, and osseous erosions ensue. Bony ankylosis can eventually occur.

(2) Imaging manifestations

1) X-ray findings: Radiographic abnormalities parallel the pathologic changes in pyogenic arthritis. In the early stage, radiological changes may be minimal and escape from detection even there are marked symptoms and signs clinically. By careful observation one may discover some changes within the first several days: such as the soft tissue density around the joint increases; the fascial planes or bursal fat pads displace(especially in the knee or ankle). The inflammatory effusion may lead to an increase in the width of the joint space. Later the destruction of articular cartilage and narrowing of the joint space occur first at points of maximum weight bearing or stress. Bone changes become evident two weeks later after the onset of the disease. The sites of the bone destruction locate at maximum weight bearing areas also. These are distinct from those of tuberculosis arthritis. A sequestrum may occasionally develop. Infrequently, gas formation may occur within a joint and surrounding soft tissue. Dislocation

and sub-luxation result from the destruction of the joint capsule. The periarticular calcification sometimes appears several weeks after onset of the infection. Bony ankylosis ensues if the articular cartilage is entirely destroyed. Vigorous antibiotic therapy modifies the course of disease.

2）CT findings: The advantage of CT to evaluate the pyogenic arthritis are as followings: ①In the early stage, CT can find the changes of soft tissue more sensitive; ②Joint effusions may be detected by CT when routine radiographs are normal; ③Delineation of the osseous and soft tissue extent of the disease process; ④Reveal the slight bone destructions, sequestrum, and the lesions located in the complex anatomy site those may not be evident on plain film radiography; ⑤The detection of gas which is a reliable diagnostic sign of the pyogenic arthritis; 6）CT scanning allows the detection of intra-articular fragments complicating septic arthritis.

3）MRI findings: MRI is the most sensitive imaging diagnostic method to evaluate the pyogenic arthritis. MRI is superior to CT to reveal the changes of soft tissue and the lesions of the joint capsule, the articular cartilage, and the ligament. It is possible to diagnosis the pyogenic arthritis in early stage by MRI. It can describe the range of inflammation involved accurately. The specificity of the MRI findings in case of pyogenic arthritis is limited. The edema of soft tissue and medulla presents low signal intensity lesions on T1WI, high signal intensity lesions on T2WI and on fat suppression sequence, and with no enhancement after enhanced MRI. The bone destruction demonstrates hypo-intensity focus on T1WI, hyper-intensity focus on T2WI and on fat suppression sequence, and with enhancement after enhanced MRI. The signal intensity of focus is not uniformity. The border is not clear. MRI is capable of notes the abscess and sequestrum also. The abscess reveals as low signal lesion on T1WI, and high signal lesion on T2WI with rim enhancement after enhanced MRI. Sequestra appear as regions of low to intermediate signal intensity on both T1WI and T2WI, and do not show enhancement of signal intensity after enhanced MRI.

2. Tuberculosis arthritis

（1）Clinical and pathological manifestations: In the majority of cases of joint tuberculosis, pulmonary lesions are also present. Tuberculous arthritis most typically affect large joint such as the hip, the knee and the spine, although any joint may be involved. It is generally mono-articular involvement. But poly-articular tuberculosis has also been reported. Tuberculous arthritis can affected persons of all ages, although it was usually encountered in children and young adult. Clinically, it often runs a chronic course as compared with that of pyogenic arthritis. The patient often complains of chronic pain and swelling of the joint with minimal signs of inflammation. Delay in diagnosis is frequent. Pathological changes include the synovial membrane hyperaemia, edema, and thickness; cartilaginous destruction; and osseous erosion.

（2）Imaging manifestations

1）X-ray findings: Radiologically, tuberculosis of joint may be classified according to their primary site of infection: Osseous type and synovial type. The primary focus of the osseous type (Figure 5 - 4) lies in the metaphysis or epiphysis or it may be a secondary extension of tuberculous infection from the adjacent metaphysis or epiphysis. More commonly occurs in adult. The initial focus of the synovial type (Figure 5 - 5) appears in the synovial membrane due to hemotogenous infection. This type occurs often in children and frequently the knee of ankle joint is affected. No matter the types, the end results are the same, since the later type, bone always almost involved later on. In the early stage, there often shows little change on plain film except for some soft tissue swelling around the affected joint and progressive osteoporosis and render the early diagnosis more difficult. The infectious nature of the process may be obscured until osseous and cartilagious destruction becomes evident. Marginal erosions are especially characteristic of tuberculosis in weight-bearing articulations, such as the hip, knee. They produce corner defects simulating the erosions of other synovial processes, such as rheumatoid arthritis. Sub-chondral osseous erosions are also encountered in tuberculosis arthritis. They appear as poorly defined gaps in the sub-chondral bone plate and subjacent trabeculae that may be apparent at a stage when the articular space is well preserved. Narrowing of the joint space duo to extensive destruction of cartilage always occurs. In some patients, diminution in this space is a late finding that occurs after marginal and central erosions of large size have appeared. In other persons, loss of the space can be appreciated at a time when only small marginal osseous defects are apparent. Bony proliferation is not generally unless a secondary pyogenic infection. Dislocation may occur duo to the destruction of joint. The eventual result in tuberculous arthritis is usually fibrous ankylosis of the joint. Bony ankylosis is occasionally seen.

2) CT findings: CT can detect these abnormalities also, furthermore, CT can detect the swellings of the joint capsule, the soft tissue rounding the joint, the intra-articular effusion(Figure 5-6), the occult destruction, small "kissing sequestrum", and the cold abscess. The cold abscess reveal as low-density area with rim enhancement after enhanced CT.

3) MRI findings: MR imaging is more sensitive than CT in evaluating abnormalities of tuberculosis arthritis. In the early stage, MRI can find the swelling of the joint easy, including the thickness of synovial membrane, the swelling of the periarticular soft tissues and joint capsule, and the tiny intra-articular effusion. As procedure development, MRI can find the destruction of articular-cartilage, the osseous erosions, and the cold abscess.

Cardinal radiological features of tuberculosis arthritis may be summarized as following: ① Monoarticular involvement; ② Soft tissue swelling and slight but progressive osteoporosis; ③ Marginal, mouse-eaten like subarticular bone erosion, occurs in the non weight-bearing articccular surface; ④Uneven narrowing of joint space and appears late and do not parallel to the degree of the bone destruction; ⑤ Absence of bone sclerosis and periosteal reaction, unless secondary infection supervences; ⑥small "kissing sequestrum" may present; ⑦Cold abscess formation with sinus tract and calcified debris; ⑧Pathologic dislocation occurs when there is extensive destruction of the joint; ⑨Fibrous ankylosis.

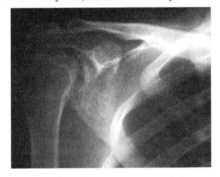

Figure 5-5　Plain film findings of bony tuberculosis of shoulder joint.

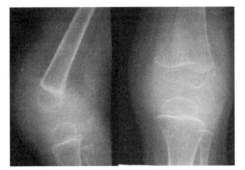

Figure 5-6　Plain film findings of synovial tuberculosis of the knee.

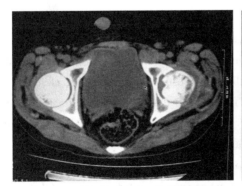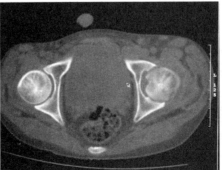

Figure 5-7　CT findings of tuberculosis of the hip.

（3）Differential diagnosis: the diagnosis of tuberculosis arthritis is not generally difficult when classic radiographic feature in typical locations, such as the knee, hip. With unusual feature or in atypical locations, the diagnosis can be more troublesome. The appearance of peri-articular osteoporosis, marginal erosions, and absent or mild joint space narrowing is most helpful in the accurate diagnosis of the disease. In rheumatoid arthritis, osteoporosis and marginal erosions are accompanied by early and significant loss of articular space. In gout, osteoporosis is mild or absent, although marginal erosions and preservation of interosseous space can be observed. In regional osteoporosis, marginal osseous defects are not apparent, and the joint space is maintained. In idiopathic chondrolysis, osteoporosis and early joint space loss are evident, especially in the hip, although they occasionally occur in other locations as well. A monarticular process must be regard as infection until proved otherwise. Although it may be difficult to define the nature of the infective agents (e. g., pyogenic, tuberculosis), slow progression of disease, significant osteoporosis, and mild sclerosis are more prominent in tuberculosis than in pyogenic arthritis(Table 5-1). Accurate diagnosis mandates synovial fluid aspiration or synovial membrane biopsy, however. Other monarticular processes, such as pigmented villonodular synovitisand idiopathic synovial osteochondromatosis, can also simulate tuberculosis arthritis. In pigmented villonodular synovitis, a nodular soft tissue mass, preservation of joint space, and absence of osteoporosis are typical; in idiopathic synovial osteochondromatosis, calcified and ossified intra-articular bodies are commonly evident.

Table 5-1   Comparison of tuberculosis and pyogenic arthritis

Differential	Tuberculosis arthritis	Pyogenic arthritis
Soft tissue swelling	+	+
Osteoporosis	+	−
Joint space loss	Late	Early
Marginal erosions	+	+
Bony proliferation	−	+
Bony ankylosis	−	+
Slow progression	+	−

3. Other forms of infectious arthritis

The other of pyogenic arthritis includes Brucellosis arthritis, Salmonella arthritis, coli arthritis, hemophilus infuenzae arthritis. The other infecting organisms may be spirochete, fungal, viral, rickettsial, mycoplasmal, parasite. The radiolographic findings are non-special.

4. Trauma of joint

The trauma of joint includes intra-articular fracture, dislocation, subluxation, articular cartilage injury, and capsular, tendon, muscular, and ligament tears, traumatic synovitis, traumatic hemarthrosis. The plain film is well suited to the evaluation of joint injury. Because it can discover most fracture, swelling of joint, and dislocation accurately. CT and MRI can do it also. Furthermore, CT is able to detect the occult fracture, osteocartilaginous bodies, and intra-articular hemorrhage. MRI has unique value in the assessment of joint injury. It is capable of reveal marrow edema, intra-articular hemorrhage, articular cartilage injury, and tear of ligament. When the signs and physical examination provide evidence of vascular injury, angiography is necessary. It may help us find vascular abnormalities, such as disruption and occlusion of major vessels, arteriovenous fistulae, and aneurysms.

（1）Chondral and osteochondral fractures

1）Clinical and pathological manifestations: The shearing, rotational, or impaction forces generated by abnormal joint motion may produce fractures of cartilage and underlying bone. In general, the fracture line parallels the joint surface, and it is the depth of the lesion that defines the cartilaginous and osseous components of the fragment.

2）Imaging manifestations: Plain film can find no direct sign of chondral fracture, but it can provide a clue to chondral fracture. If the fracture line involves the bony joint surface (Figure 5-7), especially the bony joint surfaces were staggered, the chondral fracture should be considered. Arthrography with or without CT may be used to define the nature and location of the fracture more accurately; defects in the cartilaginous surface, contrast filling of an osseous excavation, and intra-articular chondral and osseous bodies may be recognized. MRI can find following signs of damaged articular cartilage directly: The chondral defect, the chondral intra-articular bodies, high signal areas in the normal low signal articular cartilage on T2-weighted sequences and fat suppression sequences(Figure 5-8). Sometimes the marrow edema may be complicated, and MRI can detect it easy. It reveal as low signal lesion on T1WI, high signal lesion on T2WI and fat suppression sequences with no enhancement after enhanced MRI.

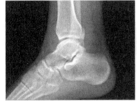 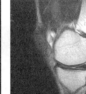 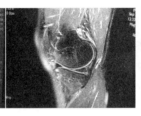 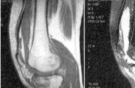 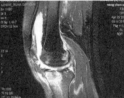

Figure 5-8　Fracture involving articular surface.

Figure 5-9　Meniscus tear.

Figure 5-10　Joint capsule effusion and bone contusion.

（2）Traumatic synovitis and hemarthrosis

1）Clinical and pathological manifestations: The acute traumatic synovitis usually affected the knee, elbow, shoulder, and ankle. The common manifestations are pain, swelling, and malfunction of the involved joint. Pathologic changes include the synovial membrane hyperaemia, swelling, hemorrhage, and intra-articular effusion. The intra-articular hemorrhage can form articular hematoma.

2）Imaging manifestations: Plain film, CT, and MRI can indicate swelling of the joint and surrounding soft tissues. Besides, CT and MRI document characteristic findings. CT can distinguish effusion from the hematoma of joint easy. The effusion shows low-density focus, and the acute hematoma shows high-density focus. The effusion shows low signal on T1WI and high signal on T2WI (Figure 5-9). The acute hematoma shows low signal on both T1WI and T2WI; sub-acute hematoma shows high signal on both T1WI and T2WI; chronic hematoma shows low signal on T1WI and high signal on T2WI. Sometimes a fluid level is noted between two components of the bloody joint effusion. The upper component is serum and the lower component relates to the cellular components of blood, and each of the two has different CT and MRI findings. MRI can show the thickness and enhanced synovial membrane.

（3）Tendon and ligament injuries

1）Clinical and pathological manifestations: Tendon and ligament injuries may be classified as complete tear and incomplete tear. The clinic manifestations of tendon and ligament injuries are pain, tenderness, local swelling, and malfunction.

2）Imaging manifestations: Pure tendon and ligament injuries show no positive finding on routine plain film.

Stress radiography discovers the movement of the damaged joint exceeds the healthy one. MRI is capable of revealing the tendon and ligament injuries directly. The abnormal signs include: the contour enlargement, the irregular edge, high signal areas in ruptured tendon and ligament on T2-weighted sequences and fat suppression sequences. The marrow edema may be complicated.

5. Rheumatoid arthritis

(1) Clinical and pathological manifestations: Therheumatoid arthritis (RA) is a systemic non-pyogenic inflammatory disease of connective tissue which locally involves the synovial membrane. The epidemiological data shows the incidence of the disease approximately 0.3% ~ 1.5%. Yong women are more commonly affected. The rheumatoid arthritis most typically affect the small joint of the hand and foot; the proximal inter-phalangeal joints, the metacarpophalangeal joints, and the wrists are the favorite sites, but practically any joint may be affected. The systemic symptom includes fatigue, anorexia, weight loss, malaise; the local manifestations include pain, morning stiffness, swelling, and dislocation or subluxation. Rheumatoid factor, elevated erythrocyte sedimentation rates and C-reactive protein levels are important laboratory parameters of rheumatoid arthritis. The pathologic abnormalities of rheumatoid arthritis are synovial inflammation, intra-articular effusion, pannus formation, destructions of cartilage and subchondral bone, and ankylosis.

(2) Imaging manifestations

1) X-ray findings: Roentgenologic findings may lag considerable behind the clinical symptoms, and a long interval between the onset of symptoms and the appearance of roentgenologic changes is not unusual. In general there is multiple and symmetric joint involvement. The earliest roentgenographic change is periarticular soft tissue swelling duo to joint effusion and synovitis; although usually fusiform, the swelling may occasionally appear lobulated. Regional osteoporosis is characteristic and initially juxta-articular. As the disease progress, irreversible erosion of the articular cartilage results in uniform joint space narrowing. The sub-articular bony cortex losses its sharp outline and disappears, either focally or diffusely. Erosion of bone tends to occur, especially at the edges of the joint, where articular cartilage is absent. The erosion has poorly defined edges without a sclerotic rim. Mechanical stress may play a role in the location and development of

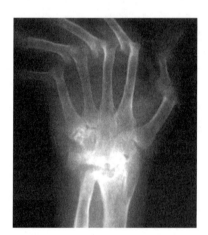

Figure 5-11　X-ray findings of rheumatoid arthritis.

the erosion. Periosteal reaction is very infrequent. With progression, diffuse osteoporosis become apparent, and eventually subluxation, contractures, and bony ankylosis may develop. Bony ankylosis is most frequent in the wrist and carpal bones. It is uncommon in the metacarpophalangeal and interphalangeal joint. Secondary changes of osteoarthritis with spurring and sclerosis may develop because of altered joint mechanics. Synovial cysts often develop in an affected joint, causing disproportionate soft tissue swelling. Around the knee, the cysts may become huge, extending into the soft tissue well beyond the joint boundaries. Synovial cysts are best demonstrated by arthrography. Cervical spine involvement occurs in over 80 per cent of well-advanced cases. Occasionally this may be the only area affected. Both the disc space and the apophyseal joints may be involved. Osteoporosis, eroded or blurred facets, and disc space narrowing are the most common findings. Subluxation of one or more joints is not an uncommon complication. The odontoid process may show erosive changes, volume decrease, and pointing of its normally rounded upper border. The space between the odontoid and anterior arch of the atlas may be widened. Cervical spine involvement in the rheumatoid patient should not be confused with progressive ascending spondylitis of the entire spine, which may sometimes be of rheumatoid origin but is a separate entity. It is considered under ankylosing spondylitis. The most significant and frequent findings in a rheumatoid joint are uniform narrowing of the joint space, marginal erosions, and periarticular osteoporosis (Figure 5-10). Prolonged corticosteroid therapy may result in a number of complications, some of which can be detected radiographically. Among these is peptic ulcer. A cushing syndrome can also develop with resultant osteoporosis and pathologic fracture, the latter occurring most frequently in the spine.

2)CT findings: CT plays an important role in diagnosis of rheumatoid arthritis. When the plain film shows no positive findings, CT can demonstrate the bone erosions, especially when the lesion located in complex anatomy region, such as sacroiliac joint and spine; swelling of soft tissue; the articular effusion; the para-articular masses, such as rheumatoid nodes and synovial cysts. Rheumatoid nodes vary in size from a few millimeters to over 5 cm. CT reveals as a soft density mass with enhanced after intravenous administration of iodinated contrast medium. Synovial cyst reveals as a hydro-density lesion with no enhancement after intravenous administration of iodinated contrast medium.

3)MRI findings: MRI is superior to plain radiographs to show the abnormities of rheumatoid arthritis. It may permit an earlier diagnosis of RA, though MRI findings of rheumatoid arthritis were diagnostically nonspecific. Magnetic resonance imaging (MRI) can demonstrate bone erosions, the intra-articular structures abnormalities (cartilage injury, articular effusion, tendon, ligament), the activity of rheumatoid arthritis and therapeutic effect, the extent of inflammatory synovial membrane and synovial cyst, rheumatoid nodes. Enhanced MRI can make difference between synovial fluid and pannus. After the intravenous injection of a gadolinium-containing agent, the effusion remains of low signal intensity on T1WI images, and the pannus demonstrates enhancement with increased signal intensity. Rheumatoid nodes show low signal intensity in T1WI and high signal intensity in T2WI, and the nodes may show enhancement of signal intensity after the intravenous administration of a gadolinium-containing agent. The appearance of a rheumatoid node may resemble that of a soft tissue tumor. Furthermore, the complication of rheumatoid arthritis, such as ischemic necrosis of bone, can be detected far more easily by MRI than by plain film.

6. Ankylosing spondylitis

(1)Clinical and pathological manifestations: Ankylosing spondylitis is a chronic inflammatory disorder affected the axial skeleton. The disease almost always begins in both sacroiliac joint and lower lumbar spine, eventually extending to higher levels of the vertebral column. The etiology remains un-know. Etiologic factors may include heredity, immune, infection, and environmental factors, etc. The incidence of this disease is estimated approximately 0.1%. The onset of ankylosing spondylitis occurs between 15~35 years. The traditional assumption that ankylosing spondylitis predominantly affects men has been revised by genetic tests, stating that there is no clear gender preference. However, women usually display a milder form of the disease. The main clinic manifestations may be low back pain and stiffness. The laboratory parameters indicates rheumatoid factor is negative, elevated erythrocyte sedimentation rates and C-reactive protein levels are elevated, and 90% of the patient with ankylosing spondylitis may be positive for antigen HLA-B$_{27}$. The pathologic changes of synovial joint alteration in ankylosing spondylitis are similar to that in rheumatoid arthritis, but severe pannus formation is less frequent. Additional pathologic feature relate to subchondral bone sclerosis and periosteal elevation. This change is not prominent in rheumatoid arthritis.

(2)Imaging manifestations

The earliest roentgenographic signs locate in unilateral sacroiliac joints, especially in the ilium. Several months or years latter, the opposite sacroiliac joints would be involved. This symmetric pattern is an important sign in ankylosing spondylitis and may permit its differentiation from other disorders that affect the sarcoiliac joint. The initial roentgenographic findings include blurring of the articular edges of the joints and osteoporosis. Subsequently superficial erosion and periarticular sclerosis may develop. Because the iliac cartilage is thinner than that of the sacrum, the lesions of ilium develop early and obviously. Ultimately, bone ankylosis ensues, generally within two to five years. Complete disappearance of the joint space eventually occurs. Erosion of the ischial tuberosity and symphysis pubis is frequent.

A similar progress takes place in the spine, although this usually is not uniform. There isjoint space narrowing and fusion of the apophyseal and costovertebral joints; The vertebral bodies become squared, with sharp corners. Later, there is calcification in the spinal ligaments; this, plus the squared vertebral bodies, gives rise to the bamboo spine (Figure 5-11). General spinal osteoporosis is frequent. Dislocation of the spine is not an uncommon complication.

In longstanding cases, involvement of peripheral joints, such as the hips, shoulders, hands, wrists, knees, and temporomandibular joints, may occur. The radiographic changes are similar to those seen in rheumatoid arthritis, but then the osteoporosis and joint space narrowing may be relative slight, and the bone erosion, sclerosis and bony ankylosis can be relative severe in ankylosing spondylitis than this in rheumatoid arthritis.

Ankylosing spondylitis is diagnosed by the clinical presentations, antigen HLA-B$_{27}$ identification, and characteristic plain radiographic findings. When the diagnosis difficulty is encountered. CT and MRI may be used to overcome the problem. CT can detect the lesions of sacroiliac, costovertebral, and apophyseal joint easy and accurately(Figure 5-12). The advantage of MRI is to evaluate the abnormities of ligaments, the spinal canal stenosis, and the activity and the complications of ankylosing spondylitis.

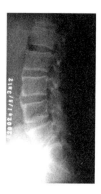 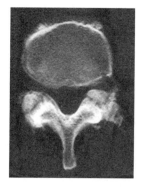

Figure 5-12　X-ray findings of ankylosing spondylitis.

Figure 5-13　CT findings of ankylosing spondylitis.

7. Degenerative joint disease

(1)Clinical and pathological manifestations: Degenerative joint disease is the frequent articular affliction. It is caused by the degeneration of articular cartilage. It is not a real inflammatory disease. Traditionally, degenerative joint disease has been classified into primary (idiopathic)and secondary types. The former has been regarded as a process in which articular degeneration occurs in the absence of any obvious underlying abnormality, whereas the latter has been regarded as articular degeneration that is produced by alteration from a preexisting affliction, such as the trauma. Recently, someone has suggested another classification: abnormal concentration of force on normal joint and normal concentration of force on abnormal joint. Many diverse factors appear to be important in the causation of degenerative joint disease. These factors include age, sex, occupation and activity, heredity, inflammation, trauma, minor mechanical disturbance, dysplasia. These factors create a situation in which the intra-articular structures can no longer resist the physical forces. The basic pathologic change of the disease is cartilaginous degeneration. On microscopic examination, focal swelling and fibrillation of the cartilaginous surface progress to extensive splitting and cracking of superficial and deeper layer of the cartilage. Physical and chemical factors are believed to be the initial factor of cartilaginous degeneration. The common manifestations are pain and disability of the ill joint, without swelling and systemic symptom.

(2)Imaging manifestations: The earliest roentgenologic changes are sharpening and thickening of the articular margins of the bones. Later, thinning of the articular cartilage causes irregular narrowing of the joint space. These changes are most marked at points of stress or weight bearing. Marginal osteophytes subsequently develop (Figure 5-13). In advanced disease, cystic rarefaction in the bone, periarticular and intra-articular calcification, and even subluxation can appear. Local osteoporosis does not occur usually. The spine degeneration can evaluate accurately by CT and MRI.

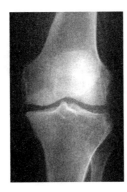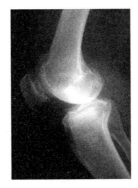

Figure 5-14   X-ray findings of degenerative arthropathy

8. Gouty arthritis

(1)Clinical and pathological manifestations: The Gouty is a systemic disease result from obstacle of purine metabolism. The biochemical hallmark of the disease is hyperuricemia, which may develop as a result of an excessive rate of production of uric acid, a decrease in renal excretion of uric acid, or a combination of two. Traditionally, gout can be classified into two types: primary gout, in which the underlying hyperuricemia is the result of an inborn error of metabolism, and secondary gout, in which the hyperuricemia is a consequence of any of a number of other disorders. The main involved organs are joints, kidney, and heart. Gouty arthritis is the sequel of urate crystal settling in intra-articular and periarticular locations, the tendon sheaths, synovial bursae, and the subcutaneous fat tissue. It occurs far more commonly in men than women. The first attack of gouty arthritis appears during the fifth decade of life in men and in the postmenopausal period in women. The main clinic manifestations are red, swollen, pain and tenderness of the affected joints. Early in the course of gouty arthritis the disorder is usually monoarticular. Gouty arthritis has a predilection for the joints of the lower extremity, particularly the first metatarsophalangeal and intertarsal joint. The pathologic changes include synovial membrane nonspecific inflammatory reaction with polymorphonuclear leukocytic infiltration, nonspecific cartilaginous degeneration, and urates penetrating cartilage and depositing in subchondral and deeper osseous areas. This deposition causes cystic defects within the bone(bone erosion).

(2) Imaging manifestations: The radiographic features of gouty arthritisaccorded with the aforementioned pathologic changes. In the early stage, plain film will show no positive findings of the joint or merely a nonspecific soft tissue swelling of the affected joint in a great percentage of patients with clinic evidence of gout. So negative findings on plain film cannot exclude the possibility of gouty arthritis. Several years latter, the detecting radiographic abnormalities may occur. The main features (Figure 5-14) consist of soft tissue swelling, bone erosion, joint space narrowing, and calcification. Eccentric nodular soft tissue prominence stands for soft tissue

deposition of urates. This change of soft tissue differentiates from the symmetrical sign of rheumatoid arthritis. It is reported that in about 40 per cent of patient with gouty erosions of bone. This lesion is generally round or oval and oriented in the long axis of the bone. The signs overhanging margin, extends outward in the soft tissue, apparently covering the tophaceous nodule are the characteristic of gouty erosions of bone. It differs from the pocketed bone erosion in rheumatoid arthritis. CT and MRI are useful in diagnosis the gouty arthritis, especially when the lesions located in complex regions, both CT and MRI can find the bone erosion easier than plain film. CT reveals tophaceous deposits with attenuation values similar to those of calcifications. MRI allows visualization of the extent of soft tissue, synovial, cartilage, and bone involvement.

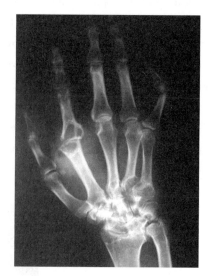

Figure 5-15　X-ray findings of gouty arthritis.

9. Tumors of joints and related structures

（1）Clinical and pathological manifestations：

Tumors of joints and related structures are not common disorder, but they are important. Especially when the malignant tumors of joints and related structures occur, if the diagnosis and treatment are notproper and timely, it may result in severe consequence. The joints and related structures can be classified as three types：benign tumor and malignant tumor. The common benign tumors include cyst of the tendon sheath, synovial cyst, giant cell tumor of the tendon sheath, and fibroma. The synovial sarcoma, chondrosarcoma, and fibrosarcoma are the common primary malignant tumors. The malignant tumors of other sites may involve the joints.

（2）Imaging manifestations

The diagnostic value of plain film is limited. CT and MRI canconfirm the cystic or substantiality content of the tumors, can draw the outline of the tumors, can judge the relation between the tumor its surrounding, can find some lesions that plain film cannot detect. So CT and MRI play important role in diagnosis of tumor of joints and related structures.

（Chen Zhu, Cai Yanyu, Sun Shanjin, Peng Shuhui, Xiao Enhua, Tan Lihua）

胸 部

　　胸部包括肺及纵隔、心脏与大血管、乳腺。胸部疾病常见且种类繁多，影像检查在胸部疾病的诊断中具有重要价值。X 线检查是胸部疾病诊断的基本方法，可观察双肺、纵隔、胸膜病变，随访复查可对肺部病变进行动态观察，了解术后改变，观察肺循环情况，乳腺 X 线摄影对乳腺钙化检出率高，已成为乳腺疾病的主要影像学检查技术。但对肺内细微病灶易漏诊，不能直接显示心腔和血管内病变，对病变定位与定性诊断均有一定难度。CT 检查易于发现胸部病变及显示病变特征，对病变定位与定性诊断优于 X 线检查，已成为肺及纵隔疾病的主要检查方法，健康体检常见低辐射剂量扫描，CT 冠状动脉血管成像在急诊胸痛诊断中起决定作用。CT 不作为乳腺的常规检查方法。MRI 常用于检查纵隔和乳腺病变，也用于肺内肿块性病变定性，是评价心脏功能和心肌病变的重要方法。但难以显示肺的细微结构，显示病变的钙化也不敏感，检查时间长，不适合于急诊患者。

Part 3

Chest

The chest includes lung and mediastinum, heart and great vessels, mammary gland. Chest diseases are common and varied. Imaging examination is of great value in the diagnosis of chest diseases. X-ray examination is a basic method for the diagnosis of chest diseases. It can observe the pathological changes of both lungs, mediastinum and Pleura, dynamically observe the pathological changes of lungs by follow-up examination, understand the postoperative changes and observe the pulmonary circulation. The mammography has become the main imaging technique for breast diseases because of its high detection rate of breast calcification. However, it is easy to miss the diagnosis of small pulmonary lesions, can not directly show the cardiac cavity and intravascular lesions, and it is difficult to locate and qualitatively diagnose the lesions. CT examination is easy to find and show the characteristics of the chest lesions, and it is superior to x-ray in the localization and qualitative diagnosis of the lesions. It has become the main examination method for lung and mediastinal diseases, CT coronary angiography plays a decisive role in the diagnosis of emergency chest pain. CT is not a routine examination of the breast. MRI is often used to examine mediastinal and breast lesions, but also used in the characterization of pulmonary masses, is an important method to evaluate cardiac function and myocardial lesions. However, it is difficult to show the fine structure of the lung, and the calcification of the lesion is not sensitive, and the examination time is long, so it is not suitable for emergency patients.

第六章

胸部影像诊断

肺内空气为其提供了良好的影像自然对比，X线透视能发现大多数的肺部病变。但是X线表现仅能反映病变的大体病理改变，而不能反映其组织学改变。因胸部X线平片经济简便，故应用广泛，是胸部疾病诊断的基本方法。CT检查较X线平片更易于发现胸部病变和显示病变的特征，这是因为其密度分辨率高于X线平片，故CT已成为呼吸系统疾病诊断的重要手段。同样的异常表现可以在不同疾病中出现，同一疾病也可因发展阶段不同或类型不同而有不同的表现。故影像表现必须密切结合临床进行全面合理的分析，才能对疾病作出正确的诊断。

第一节 检查方法

胸部的影像学检查方法有透视、胸部X线平片、高千伏摄片、支气管造影、肺动脉造影、CT、磁共振成像等，可根据情况由简到繁选择不同的检查方法。

1. 透视

透视在检查过程中可产生实时图像并可自由转动体位，但检查时间相对较长，X线曝光量比X线平片高。对于怀疑支气管异物或开放性气胸的患者，透视下应该仔细观察呼吸过程中的纵隔移动，其在胸部主要用于评估疾病所致的膈肌运动异常。

2. X线平片

胸部X线平片是呼吸系统病变的基本检查方法，能显示大于5 mm的结节病灶，摄片常用的体位有以下几种。

（1）后前位：是常规检查位置，患者取立位，胸前壁贴近片盒，X线自后方射入。双臂处于使肩胛骨尽量向前向外拉的位置，以使肩胛骨从肺野中移开。胸部后前位片应包括全部肺野、胸廓、肋膈角和下颈部（图6-1）。

（2）侧位：常用于确定病变在肺或纵隔内的位置，并显示侧面病变的形态。患者侧位，患侧尽可能贴近片盒，有利于清晰地显示患侧病变（图6-2）。

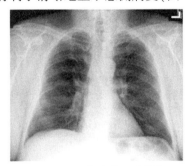

图6-1 正常胸片：后前位

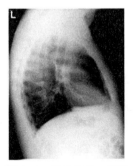

图6-2 正常胸片：侧位

（3）前后位：适用于不能站立的患者，可取仰卧位，X线自前方射入。

（4）前弓位：用于显示肺尖部及与锁骨、肋骨重叠的病变（图6-3）。

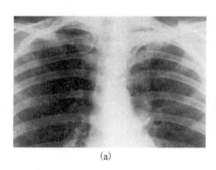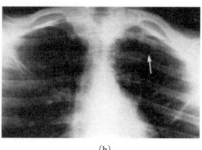

(a)   (b)

（a）正位：左肺尖模糊的阴影大部分被第1肋骨和锁骨遮挡。（b）前弓位：锁骨和第1肋骨的阴影往上移位，显示出左肺尖部病灶为厚壁空洞（箭头），提示活动性肺结核。

图6-3 前弓位影像

3.高千伏摄影

应用高电压（大于或等于120 kV）摄片，其对尘肺具有较好的诊断价值。

4.支气管造影

支气管造影是通过向气管、支气管直接注入对比剂而显示支气管树（图6-4）。现在已基本被CT取代，特别是高分辨CT取代，故而极少使用。常用的对比剂为丙碘酮水悬浮液。滴注对比剂的方法包括从口或鼻插入导管或环甲膜直接穿刺。在吸气时注入对比剂直到支气管黏膜被对比剂覆盖。支气管造影最常用的适应证是咯血，常用于计划手术的支气管扩张患者，可明确支气管扩张的诊断并显示病变的部位和范围，并可一定程度上帮助排除肺癌诊断。

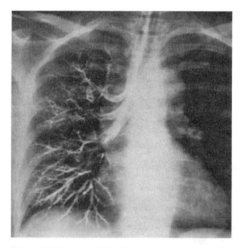

多余的支气管、支气管造影图片，显示多余支气管起源于右肺下叶支气管，它供给右肺上叶的尖段和后段，正常的右上叶支气管出现在正常的位置。

图6-4 支气管造影影像

5.肺动脉造影

肺血管造影是通过向主肺动脉或其大的分支直接注射对比剂而清晰地显示管腔改变、血管扭曲或结构破坏（图6-5）。肺动脉造影需要在透视下行肘前或股静脉插管直至心脏，是显示肺动脉栓塞的特有方法，现在已很少用于评价肺癌的可手术性，但仍是显示肺动静脉畸形及变异的最佳方法。

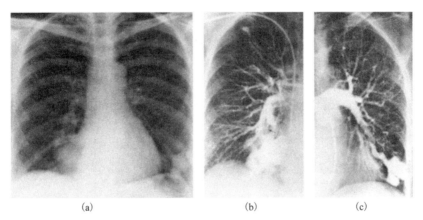

(a)肺动静脉瘘常规片显示双肺下叶有分叶状阴影，左侧病变有一根大血管向肺门延伸；(b)右肺动脉造影片，早期显示右肺下叶的肿块由扩张弯曲的血管组成，并可见引流静脉(箭头)，上叶区可见导管影；(c)左肺动脉造影片。

图 6-5　肺动脉造影影像

6.计算机断层扫描(CT)

CT 扫描是呼吸系统病变的常用检查方法，胸部 CT 扫描可更准确地描述可疑病灶的位置、轮廓、范围和组织成分，从而确定多数胸部肿瘤和肺部病变的性质和范围。常采用 5 mm 层厚连续扫描整个肺部，扫描时需屏气。观察肺和纵隔时采用不同的窗宽和窗位，显示纵隔结构采用较窄的窗宽(如 300Hu)和大约软组织密度的窗位(如 30~50Hu)，显示肺、胸膜和纵隔轮廓采用较宽的窗宽(如 1000~2000Hu)和低于 0 的窗位，通常位于-600 至-800Hu 之间。

高分辨 CT(HRCT)是检查肺部弥漫性病变的有效方法。通过优化成像和重建参数以尽可能高的空间分辨率显示肺部解剖结构。高分辨 CT 相关的技术包括采用薄层扫描、高空间频率算法或骨算法重建，大矩阵小视野，增加电压或电流。大多数扫描机可采用的最薄，准直宽度为 0.5~2 mm(图 6-6)。

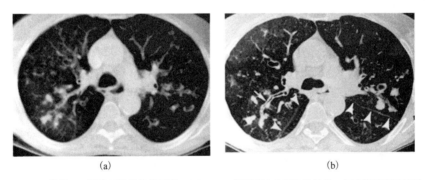

(a)5 mm 常规 CT 显示双肺斑片状阴影；(b)HRCT 能看到(a)所示的异常，支气管扩张且壁增厚(箭头)，腔内充满黏液，周边见斑片状浸润灶，囊状支气管扩张显示更加清楚，同时还可显示斜裂(箭头)，这些在(a)中都无法检测。

图 6-6　常规 CT 和高分辨率 CT 扫描对比

静脉注射对比剂有助于区分纵隔和肺门的血管结构和淋巴结，以及肺内结节性病变的鉴别诊断(图6-7)。经肘前静脉用手或高压注射器推注大约 100 mL 含碘(300 mg/mL)的溶液，进行连续扫描或单一层面扫描(动态扫描)。

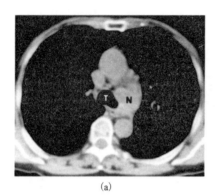
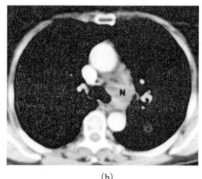

(a)　　　　　　　　　　　　(b)

(a)主动脉肺动脉窗可见软组织密度肿块(N)，左主支气管远端受压变扁(T)；(b)增强扫描示主动脉弓下淋巴结(N)明显增大，未见明显强化。

图6-7　静脉注射对比剂

多平面重组(图6-8)、最大密度投影[图6-9(a)]、容积再现[图6-9(b)]等后处理技术在呼吸系统疾病诊断中广泛运用。

目前低剂量CT对于肺癌高危人群的初筛起到了重要的作用。

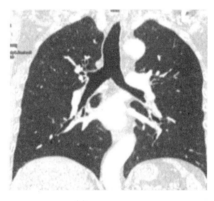
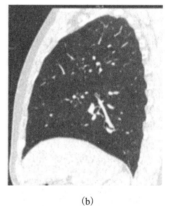

(a)　　　　　　　　　　　　(b)

图6-8　胸部多平面重组

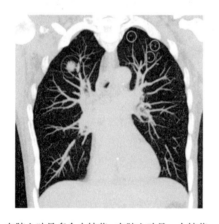
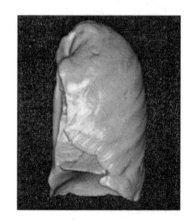

左肺上叶见多个小结节，右肺上叶见一大结节。

图6-9　(a)胸部最大密度投影　　　**图6-9　(b)左肺容积再现**

7.磁共振成像(MRI)

目前 MRI 在肺部的应用价值有限。由于肺实质内含有大量气体,磁共振信号强度极低,大大地影响了 MRI 在肺部的应用。

MRI 对血流有很高的对比分辨率和灵敏度,故可用于评价肿瘤侵犯纵隔和大血管情况,还可用于检查胸部血管其他病变,评价肺和纵隔纤维化等。

MRI 具有直接多平面成像的优点,矢状位和冠状位是横断位图像常用的补充。因 MRI 具有任意方向成像的能力,对于评价血管结构和胸壁病变等有独特的价值。

胸部 MRI 检查一般采用自旋回波(SE)及快速自旋回波(FSE)序列(图 6-10)。T1 加权图像可极好地显示解剖结构,特别是纵隔,明亮的脂肪信号与中等软组织信号形成良好的对比,如淋巴结和黑色信号的血管。T2 加权图像对组织的水含量灵敏度高,更助于显示软组织病理改变。常用呼吸门控及心电门控技术和屏气扫描以减少呼吸和心跳引起的假影。血管内注射钆剂增强的 T1 图像有助于诊断血管疾病或肺结节病灶,还可确定胸壁或纵隔肿瘤侵犯的范围,以及肺内炎性病变的范围。

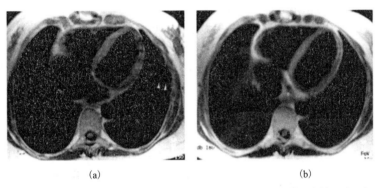

(a) (b)

(a)心脏常规自旋回波 T1 加权成像,箭头所示为运动假影。(b)快速自旋回波,由于采集速度快,呼吸运动假影被消除。

图 6-10 胸部 MRI 检查采用自旋回波及快速自旋回波序列

8.超声

超声为区别胸腔积液和胸膜增厚或胸壁肿瘤提供了一种简单可靠的技术,特别是对于肿瘤和积液共存或包裹性胸腔积液。超声是确定胸水引流时引流管放置位置非常有用的工具。对怀疑膈下感染的患者,超声检查因便宜、无创而被广泛应用。由于脊柱、肋骨和肺内气体影响超声的传导,故超声对诊断肺部病变价值不大。

9.核医学

核医学通过应用放射性核素及其标记物进行肺灌注显像、肺通气显像等方法,对血管病变及肺部肿瘤及其骨转移的诊断价值较高,其中对肺栓塞的临床诊断价值较高。正电子发射计算机断层成像可以较准确地评价肺癌的纵隔淋巴结转移及远处转移。

第二节 正常表现

1.正常 X 线解剖

(1)胸壁:

1)软组织:软组织在胸 X 线平片上形成的阴影,不要误诊为肺部病变。

①胸锁乳突肌:表现为两肺尖内侧的边缘清晰,密度均匀的阴影。两侧胸锁乳突肌影不对称时勿误认为病变。

②胸大肌：表现为两侧肺野中外带扇形均匀密度影，外缘清晰，一般右侧较明显，不可误认为病变。

③女性乳房及乳头：女性乳房可表现为两肺下野的下缘清楚，上缘不清的半圆形阴影。乳头影常见于第 5 前肋间隙处、基本对称的结节状致密影，年龄较大的女性多见，有时亦见于成年男性。

2）骨骼和软骨：

①肋骨：肋骨细长，前端和后端呈弓形，起于胸椎两侧，通过肋软骨与胸骨相连。肋骨常见的先天性变异有颈肋、叉状肋和肋骨联合等（图 6-11）。

②肋软骨：肋软骨在钙化前不显影，20 岁以后第 1 肋软骨首先钙化，随年龄增长，其他肋软骨由下而上逐条发生钙化，表现为两侧基本对称的不规则的斑片状致密影。

③锁骨：锁骨的内侧端和脊柱是评价胸片投照位置是否旋转的重要标志。锁骨内端下缘的菱形窝，肋锁韧带附着处，骨皮质有时边缘不规则，呈凹陷样改变，勿误认为骨质破坏。

④肩胛骨：肩胛骨的内缘可与肺野外带重迭，勿误认为胸膜增厚。勿误认肩胛下角的二次骨化中心为骨折。

⑤胸骨：侧位显示好，在后前位片上因重迭而显示不清，只有胸骨柄边缘有时可见，易误认为纵隔增宽。

⑥胸椎：胸椎的横突影可突出于纵隔影之外，勿误认为增大的淋巴结。

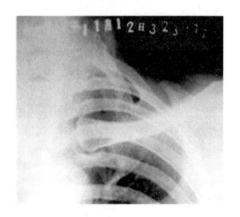

前后位 X 线显示第 1、第 2 肋骨前端融合。

图 6-11 肋骨融合

（2）纵隔：位于胸骨之后，胸椎之前，两肺之间。纵隔内主要的结构有心脏、大血管、气管、支气管、食管、淋巴组织、神经、胸腺、脂肪和结缔组织等。

通常按照侧位胸片将纵隔分为前、中、后及上、中、下九个区（图 6-12）。前纵隔为胸骨之后，心脏前缘、升主动脉和气管之前的狭长三角区；中纵隔相当于心、主动脉弓、气管和肺门的位置；食管前壁为中、后纵隔的分界，后纵隔位于食管和胸椎之间。胸骨柄、体交界处至第 4 胸椎下缘间连线和肺门下缘的水平线（约为第 8 胸椎下缘）将纵隔分为上、中、下三部分。

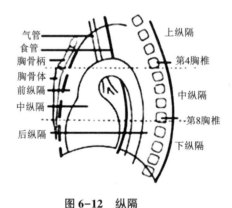

图 6-12 纵隔

（3）膈：左右半膈在后前位胸片上均表现为光滑的向上凸起的曲线。膈外侧起自肋骨形成的光滑的锐角，称为肋膈角。膈内侧与心脏形成心膈角。多数膈顶位于中肺野约第 5 或第 6 前肋间水平。右膈较左膈高约 1.5 cm。正常膈运动幅度为 1~3 cm，深呼吸时可达 3~6 cm。

（4）胸膜：肺表面覆盖着脏层胸膜，邻近纵隔、胸壁及膈表面衬有壁层胸膜。一般肺周胸膜不显影，但正常的叶间胸膜与 X 线相切时可显影。水平裂在约 70% 的胸 X 线平片上可见（图 6-13），斜裂有时可见于侧位片（图 6-14），但在后前位片上不显影。正常情况下表现为线状阴影。

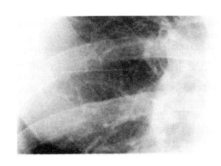

后前位胸片显示水平裂(箭头)为水平线。

图 6-13　正常水平裂

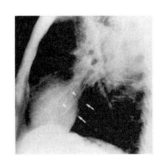

侧位胸片显示两个斜裂。两个斜裂均可见双线。

图 6-14　正常斜裂

(5)气管和支气管：气管和支气管表现为暗带状阴影。胸平片上，气管可见于上胸椎重叠处，在第5或第6胸椎水平处分为左右主支气管，正常分叉角度为60°~85°，不超过90°。右主支气管较左侧垂直。右主支气管分为上、中、下叶支气管，左主支气管分为上、下叶支气管。叶支气管进一步分为段支气管，经过6~20级分支后，成为不含软骨的细支气管。

(6)肺：

1)肺叶和肺野：肺野和肺叶并不对应。肺野的名称是为了描述方便，分别在第2、第4肋骨前端画水平线，将肺野分为上、中、下三野。另划二条虚构的线将肺野纵行分三等分，称为内、中、外三区(图6-15)。

解剖上肺叶按叶间裂划分。左肺由斜裂分为上、下二叶，右肺由斜裂和水平裂分为上、中、下三叶。双侧斜裂解剖相似，起自第5胸椎处向前下斜行，止于膈肌距前肋膈角后方的0~3cm处，中间经过肺门。水平裂自右肺门处向前和侧面水平散开直达胸壁。肺叶在后前位胸片上前后重迭，侧位片上无重迭。通常只有部分叶间裂可见。

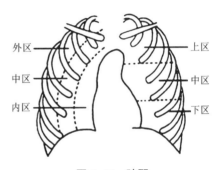

图 6-15　肺野

有时可见其他肺叶，最常见的是奇叶，约占不足人口的1%，系因奇静脉位置异常所致(图6-16)。下副叶有时见于下叶的内和前基底段(图6-17)，其叶间裂自膈向上向内斜行达肺门。

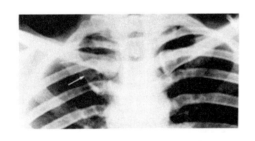

右肺上野可见轮廓清晰的曲线影(箭头)代表奇静脉裂。

图 6-16　右肺上叶

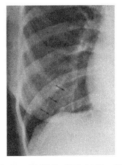

细的、界限分明的斜线(箭头)表示纤维分隔，它将近基底部与下叶的其余部分隔开。

图 6-17　下副叶

肺叶可分为 2-5 个肺段,各有其单独的支气管,肺段的名称与相应的支气管一致。肺段由许多肺小叶组成,肺小叶的直径约 1 cm。

2)肺门:肺门影由肺动脉、静脉,支气管,淋巴组织,神经及结缔组织组成。通常双侧密度和大小相近,左肺门较右侧高 1~2 cm。右下肺动脉干宽度不超过 15 mm,左肺门的高度约为 24 mm。肺门的形状主要是左侧或右侧大血管的投影。右肺门角是由右上肺静脉和右下肺动脉形成的钝角。左上肺门由左肺动脉弓组成,表现为半圆形阴影,勿误认为肿块。

3)肺纹理:肺纹理是肺血管分支形成的线状阴影,自肺门向外放射分布,逐渐变细,消失于距肺边缘约 2 cm 处。肺纹理由肺动脉、静脉及淋巴管组成。

4)肺实质和肺间质:肺组织由肺实质和肺间质组成。肺实质是呼吸功能的基本单位,包括肺泡和肺泡壁。肺间质是支气管树和血管周围、肺泡囊间隔及胸膜下由弹性和胶原纤维结缔组织所组成的支架。肺间质病变的 X 线表现和肺实质病变有明显的差别。

2.胸部正常 CT 解剖

因脂肪、肌肉、骨骼和肺实质间存在明显的密度差,CT 横断面图像可准确显示极佳的胸部解剖细节,提供独特有用的诊断信息,直接影响患者的处理和预后。事实上,详细掌握正常的解剖结构和变异有助于准确地鉴别异常。8 个有代表性的横断面图像,按顺序提供了正常胸部的主要解剖结构和之间的关系。

(1)胸腔入口层面[图 6-18(a)]:相当于胸骨切迹水平,气管居中线紧邻椎体,食管位于中线偏左。通常可见位于气管前方和侧面的 5 条主要的纵隔血管。包括主动脉弓的三条主要分支(头臂干、左颈总动脉和左锁骨下动脉)和两条头臂静脉。

(2)胸锁关节层面[图 6-18(b)]:该层面以包含位于三条动脉前面的两条锁骨下静脉为特征,三条动脉通常位于气管前方。

(3)主动脉弓层面[图 6-18(c)]:主动脉弓常起自第二肋软骨上缘位置向左后方斜行,在大约第 4 胸椎水平处变为降主动脉。主动脉弓前部位于气管前方,紧贴上腔静脉内前侧,中间位于气管的左侧,而后部正好位于食管的左侧。

(4)主肺动脉窗层面[图 6-18(d)]:解剖上,主肺动脉窗包括主动脉弓头侧和左肺动脉远侧边缘之间的区域。主肺动脉窗内包含气管远端、位于主动脉弓下方、降主动脉内方和左肺动脉上方不同程度的纵隔脂肪和少数小淋巴结。

(5)左肺动脉层面[图 6-18(e)]:主肺动脉向后延伸,左肺动脉位于气管隆突左侧面横跨左主支气管。左肺动脉后部侧面可见左上肺静脉。

(6)主或右肺动脉层面[图 6-18(f)]:右肺动脉自主肺动脉右侧向后方延伸,走行于上腔静脉后方,中间段支气管前方。

(7)左心房层面[图 6-18(g)]:左心房前方为主动脉根部和右心房,后方是奇静脉、食管和降主动脉。主动脉根部位于主肺动脉和右心室流出道的右前方。

(8)心室层面[图 6-18(h)]:右心室位于左心室右方和前方,为心脏前面的重要部分。由斜行的室间隔和左心室分开。

3.特殊的解剖结构

(1)气管与支气管:

气管位于食管的前方稍偏右侧,是软骨膜性管道,正常的气管壁较薄。老年人,尤其是女性,气管的环状软骨可发生钙化,气管的横断面形态变异较大,通常环状软骨下方为圆形,邻近气管隆突时变为卵圆形,中间可为马蹄形,但儿童的均呈圆形。

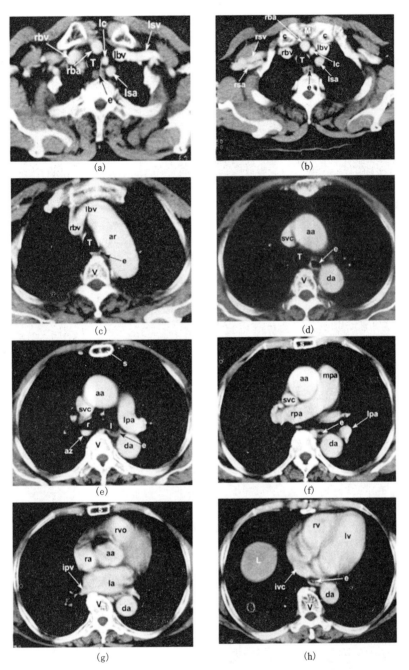

纵隔：(a)胸廓平面；(b)胸锁关节水平；(c)主动脉弓水平；(d)主肺动脉窗水平；(e)。左肺动脉水平；(f)主肺动脉和右肺动脉水平；(g)左心房水平；(h)心室水平。

Rbv：右头臂静脉；rba：右头臂动脉；lc：左颈动脉；lsa：左锁骨下动脉；lsv：左锁骨下静脉；lbv：左头臂静脉；T：气管；e：食道；rsa：左锁骨下动脉；rsv：右锁骨下静脉；c：肋软骨；m：胸骨柄；lc：左颈总动脉；ar：主动脉弓；v：椎体；svc：上腔静脉；aa：升主动脉；da：降主动脉；az：奇静脉；r：右主支气管；l：左主支气管；lpa：左肺动脉；rpa：右肺动脉；mpa：肺动脉主干；ipv：下肺静脉；rvo：右心室锁骨流出道；ra：右心房；la：左心房；L：肝脏；rv：右心室；lv：左心室。

图 6-18　胸部正常 CT 解剖

支气管的 CT 表现与管径大小、走行方向密切相关。起始端水平的支气管在轴位 CT 图像上易显示，如右上叶支气管(及其前段、后段支气管)，左上叶支气管(及其前段支气管)，中叶支气管(及其内侧段和/或外侧段支气管)，双下叶背段支气管。垂直走行的支气管可见于横断面图像，包括右上肺尖段支气管，左上肺尖上段支气管，中间段支气管，和双下叶支气管近端(背段支气管开口之后)。斜行的支气管最难显示，如舌叶支气管(包括上舌叶和下舌叶)及基底段支气管。主要的支气管开口如图 6-19。

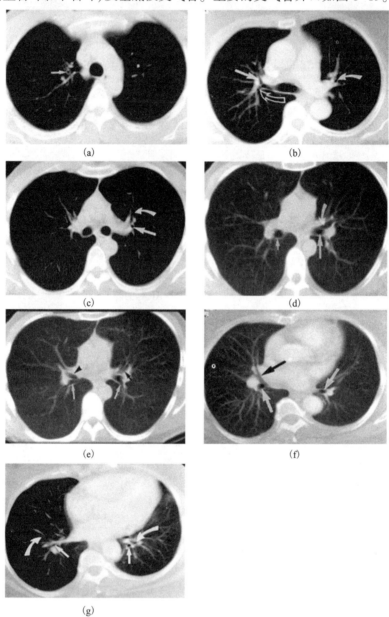

(a)主动脉弓(气管远端)水平：右上肺尖段支气管(箭头)；(b)隆突水平：图示尖后支气管(实弓箭头)；右上叶前段(直箭头)及后段(弯箭头)；(c)左肺动脉水平：支气管尖后段(直箭头)的垂直走行和前段的水平走行；(d)右肺动脉水平：可见中间段支气管(小箭头)，后壁较薄；左侧可见左上叶(弯箭头)和下叶(直箭头)分叉；(e)稍微下一点平面，左侧为舌段(黑色箭头)；右侧(箭头)可见右肺中叶支气管起；注意双肺支气管的起源(白色箭头)；(f)左心房水平：右中叶支气管(黑色箭头)位于右下叶支气管(白色箭头)前；左肺下叶支气管(白色箭头)；(g)节段支气管：弯曲箭头显示两侧的外基底节；注意后基底段支气管(直箭头)。

图 6-19　节段支气管

（2）肺实质：正常情况下，除了胸膜下 3~5 mm 宽的乏血管透亮区外，血管可见于肺周各个方向。肺实质外周 2~3 cm 范围内的支气管不显示。理解次级肺小叶结构对 HRCT 上认识和分类肺实质异常有重要的意义。次级肺小叶的大小范围为 6~25 mm 直径，呈多边形。小叶中心动脉（直径约 1 mm）和细支气管（直径约 2 mm）进入小叶核心。数条小叶静脉可见于小叶间隔，但小叶间隔的厚度小于 1 mm，正常情况下极少显示。

（3）胸膜：胸膜为双层浆膜，正常情况下在 CT 上不显示。斜裂在检查时表现为肺实质内模糊的无血管的透亮带（图 6-20），是因为肺叶周边的血管尖端变细所致。薄层扫描，特别是高分辨 CT（HRCT），斜裂可显示为线状影（图 6-21）。水平裂的方向位于 CT 层面时表现为右侧中肺野的相对少血管的透亮区。奇裂表现为 T4 或 T5 椎体外侧与右头臂静脉或上腔静脉间的前后走行的弧线，凸向外侧。

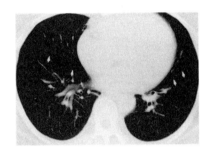

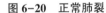

CT 显示肺裂为相对低血供的透光带（箭头）。

图 6-20　正常肺裂

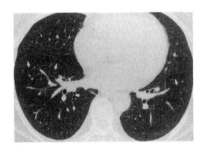

高分辨率 CT 显示肺裂为线状影（箭头）。

图 6-21　正常肺裂

（4）肺门：CT 图像可清晰显示肺门的主要肺动、静脉，气管和主支气管，包括大多数肺段支气管开口。了解基本的解剖关系有利于 CT 诊断淋巴结增大和定位支气管阻塞性病变。增强 CT 螺旋扫描时，正常的支气管肺（肺门）淋巴结一般可见。肺门的其他结构如淋巴管，神经丛和疏松结缔组织被结缔组织包裹，在 CT 上不能区分。

（5）纵隔淋巴结：CT 能可靠地显示纵隔淋巴结，正常的淋巴结呈圆形或卵圆形，能见于 90% 的患者，以中纵隔多见。按 CT 标准，直径 1 cm 以下的淋巴结被认为正常，尽管可能包含有显微镜下病变。

（6）胸腺：认识 CT 图像上正常胸腺大小、形状和密度的变化对避免误诊为纵隔异常肿块非常重要。青春期前，两叶结构的胸腺填充大血管前的中上纵隔的大部分位置。左叶比右叶稍大，且位置较高。大多数残留的胸腺融合呈箭头状或三角形状。20 岁前每叶胸腺的最大厚度不超过 1.8 cm，20 岁以后胸腺的最厚为 1.3 cm，尽管大多数正常胸腺厚度小于 0.8 cm。儿童和青少年的胸腺密度和胸壁肌肉相似，通常 40 岁后接近脂肪密度。

（7）膈：膈由中心腱和向四周叶状散开的肌肉组成。前膈多表现为相对光滑，轻微波浪状的弓形软组织影，向后凹并通过中线。后部和尾部，特别是膈肌脚，较顶部垂直，CT 上易于识别。右侧膈肌脚较厚，起自腰 1~3 椎体，左侧膈肌脚较薄，起源于腰 1-2 椎体。

4. 正常 MRI 表现

MRI 基于组织的磁信号强度的不同提供形态学的区别。因为血管腔内流动的血液无信号，和高信号强度的纵隔其他结构比较，纵隔和肺门血管结构在 T1 权重图像上易于显示。其他充气结构如气管、支气管和肺实质内质子密度极低，缺乏信号，表现为低信号。肌肉、淋巴结和塌陷的食管表现为中等信号强度。骨髓内含有丰富的脂肪，表现为特征性的高信号，然而骨皮质内质子密度低，表现为低信号。长 T1 的胸腺在 T1 加权图像上表现为相对低信号，可与高信号的纵隔脂肪区别，由于脂肪浸润，T1 时间随年龄逐渐减小，T2 弛豫时间和脂肪重叠且不随年龄变化。

第三节　基本病变

基本病变分为肺、支气管和胸膜病变。

1.肺部基本病变的X线和CT表现

（1）实变：实变在病理上为肺泡内的气体被脓、水、血、细胞或其他物质代替。常见于肺部感染、水肿、出血、肺炎型肺腺癌及肺泡蛋白沉着症等（图6-22～图6-23）。

病变早期或吸收阶段，病变没有完全填充肺泡腔，表现为不能完全掩盖肺血管的磨玻璃样密度影，当肺泡腔内的气体完全被取代时，表现为掩盖肺血管的实变影。实变影中可见空气支气管征。通常病变肺体积无明显缩小。

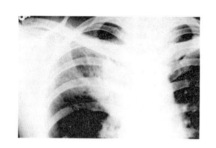

肺炎，胸部X光片显示右上肺野模糊不清。

图6-22　实变

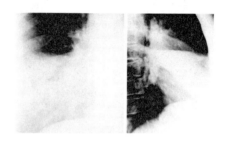

肺炎，在胸部后前位和侧位片上，右中叶大片均匀密度增高影，而没有肺体积的缩小。

图6-23　实变

（2）结节与肿块病变：病理上，多数肺部结节或肿块性病变为肿瘤、肉芽肿或结核瘤。多发结节与肿块常为转移瘤。其中直径≤3 cm者称为结节（图6-24），而>3 cm者称为肿块（图6-25）。结节根据大小又可以细分为大结节（≤3 cm）、小结节（≤1 cm）及粟粒结节（≤0.5 cm）。

影像学表现为：①形状为圆形、卵圆形或不规则形；②密度较高且均匀；③周围被肺组织包绕；④边缘清晰。良恶性的判断主要根据病变的形态特征、密度（如钙化、脂肪或强化）和生长速度。

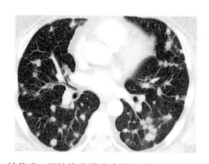

转移瘤，两肺均弥漫分布随机结节，大小不等，部分结节边缘有分叶及毛刺。

图6-24　肺结节

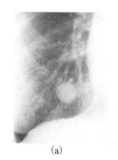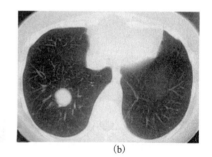

(a)　　　　　　　　　(b)

（a）局部后前位胸片显示边界清晰的右下叶肿块；（b）CT扫描（肺窗）显示界限清楚的肿块。

图6-25　肺肿块孤立性纤维瘤

（3）空洞与空腔性病变：空洞性病变由肺部病变坏死物经支气管排出形成。常见于肺脓肿、肺结核和肺癌（图6-26）。空腔性病变是肺内生理腔隙的病理性扩大，常见于肺大疱、肺囊肿及肺气囊等（图6-27）。

空洞影像学表现为：①环形薄壁或厚壁的透亮区；②内壁可光滑或不规则；③空洞内可见气液平面。

壁厚小于 3 mm 的空洞称为薄壁空洞，大于 3 mm 的空洞称为厚壁空洞。厚壁空洞常见于肺脓肿、鳞状细胞癌、韦格氏肉芽肿等。薄壁空洞最多见于肺结核。肺癌空洞的内壁不规则呈结节状，肺脓肿空洞的内壁毛糙。肺结核空洞多常见于上叶尖后段和下叶背段。肺癌可发生于任何部位，上叶多见。多数气液平面由肺脓肿引起，恶性和结核空洞中罕见。

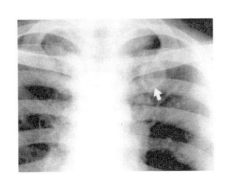
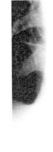

胸片显示左肺尖一个薄壁空洞（箭头），内壁光滑。可见卫星病灶。

图 6-26 空洞结核

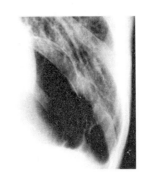

后前位胸片显示左下视野多个大小不等的肺大疱。

图 6-27 肺空腔肺大疱

肺大疱和肺囊肿为空腔，大小不等，壁常很薄，厚度通常≤1 mm。其 X 线表现和薄壁空洞相似，勿误认为空洞。

肺大疱由肺泡破裂并相通而成，肺大疱的壁由塌陷的肺组织形成。肺囊肿由先天性因素或寄生虫感染引起，囊肿壁清楚，由上皮或纤维组织构成。

（4）纤维化病变：许多肺部疾病可引起肺纤维化。纤维化代表纤维组织，以成纤维细胞增生或无细胞的致密胶原组织为特征。纤维化病变分为局限性和弥漫性两类。

X 线征象与病程有关。局限性纤维化多为肺部慢性感染的后果，表现为高密度的平行或放射状的线状阴影，厚度不等。

弥漫性纤维化表现为广泛分布的不规则线状影、网状影或蜂窝状阴影。常见于尘肺、结缔组织病和特发性肺纤维化（图 6-28~图 6-29）。

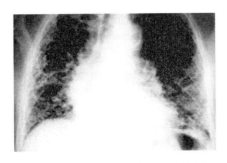
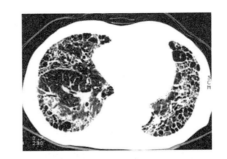

胸片显示双侧网结状间质浸润，以下肺为主。

图 6-28 肺纤维化病变，特发性肺纤维化

HRCT 显示弥漫不规则线性影，网状影和胸膜下蜂窝影。

图 6-29 纤维化病变，特发性肺纤维化

（5）钙化病变：钙化病变通常代表疾病的痊愈过程，是评价肺部疾病的重要征象，常提示良性病变。

钙化可表现为斑点状、小结节状、"蛋壳状""爆米花状"或弧形致密影。其中"蛋壳状""爆米花状"或弧形钙化为典型良性钙化（图 6-30）。

（6）间质性病变：主要侵犯肺结缔组织的疾病称为间质性病变。可表现为小叶间隔线（kerley A 线和 B 线）、磨玻璃影、网状影或网结状阴影。严重的间质性病变可表现为"蜂窝状"阴影。间质性病变常见于尘肺、癌性淋巴管炎（图 6-31）、结节病和间质性肺炎。CT，特别是 HRCT 对诊断间质性病变有重要的价值。

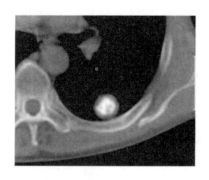

CT扫描显示左肺下叶一个界限清楚的 2 cm 结节,伴"爆米花状"钙化。

图 6-30 肺钙化(错构瘤)

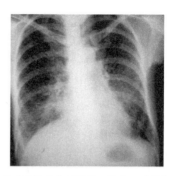

患者乳腺癌的癌性淋巴管炎。后前位胸片显示双肺小叶间隔线影。主要右侧肺下积液。

图 6-31 肺间质病变

2. 支气管基本病变的 X 线和 CT 表现

支气管阻塞常由肿瘤、异物、狭窄或渗出物等引起。支气管阻塞可导致阻塞性肺气肿(不完全阻塞)、阻塞性肺不张(完全阻塞)和阻塞性肺炎。

(1)阻塞性肺气肿:以肺泡腔的持久性扩大为特征,并伴有肺泡壁的破坏。可细分为弥漫性肺气肿、局限性肺气肿和大泡性肺气肿。

1)弥漫性阻塞性肺气肿:弥漫性阻塞性肺气肿常为慢性支气管炎、哮喘和气管肿瘤的并发症。X 线表现为双肺透亮度增高,胸腔体积增大,肋骨走行变平,侧位上胸腔前后径增大,膈肌低平,肺纹理稀疏,心影狭长位于过度膨胀的双肺之间。

2)局限性肺气肿:如主支气管、叶支气管或段支气管发生不完全阻塞,肺气肿局限于受累的解剖部位(图 6-32)。X 线胸片表现为受累部位透亮度增高,肺纹理稀疏,纵隔可向对侧移位。透视下纵隔呼气时偏离正常位置,吸气时回到正常位置,称为纵隔摆动。

3)大泡性肺气肿:当支气管或细支气管不完全阻塞时,可形成大泡性肺气肿。X 线表现和薄壁空洞相似,但通常难以显示完整的壁。

肺气肿的 CT 表现为无壁透亮区,肺血管变细、扭曲,肺密度下降(图 6-33)。CT 能提供关于肺气肿严重程度和分布的有用信息,发现胸平片不能显示的不被怀疑的伴随情况如支气管扩张,或隐匿的支气管肺癌。

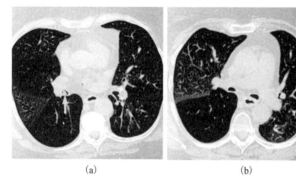

(a)CT 示中间段支气管息肉样肿块(箭头);(b)呼气相扫描显示右肺下叶明显的透亮区域。支气管镜检查发现一块菜花样物质并抽吸取出。

图 6-32 肺气肿局限于受累的解剖部位

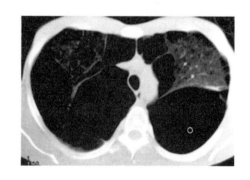

间隔旁肺气肿患者的胸部 CT 显示多发肺大泡。

图 6-33 肺大泡性肺气肿

(2)阻塞性肺不张：

支气管完全阻塞可导致阻塞性肺不张。肺不张表示肺或部分肺膨胀不全，可分为阻塞性肺不张、瘢痕性肺不张和压迫性肺不张三类。由于不张的肺组织含气量较正常肺组织少，故 X 线表现为均匀的不透 X 线阴影。阴影的外形和位置与萎陷的肺叶及萎陷的程度有关。

1）一侧性肺不张的 X 线表现：患侧肺均匀致密，患侧膈肌抬高，纵隔向患侧移位，患侧肋间隙变窄，对侧代偿性肺气肿（图 6-34）。

2）肺叶不张的 X 线表现：罹患肺叶表现为三角形致密影，尖端指向肺门，基底部朝外，肺门和纵隔向患部移位。邻近肺叶可出现代偿性肺气肿。

右中肺不张的 X 线表现（图 6-35）：后前位表现为右心缘旁区片状致密影，右心缘模糊。侧位表现为右中肺三角形致密影，尖端位于肺门，基底靠胸骨。前弓位表现为右心旁区三角形致密影，尖端在外，基底靠心缘。

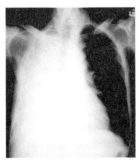

右全肺。PA 胸片显示右侧胸腔均匀密度增高，纵隔向右移位，左肺代偿性肺气肿。

图 6-34 肺不张

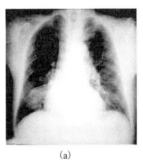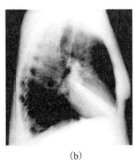

(a)　　　　　　　　　(b)

(a)后前位片显示右侧心旁区密度增高影，边界不清；(b)侧位片显示右肺中叶三角形密度增高影，尖端指向肺门。

图 6-35 肺不张（右中叶）

CT 有助于阐明继发于肺萎陷的平片的发现和指示其原因并确定阻塞性肿块的范围。肺不张的胸片上可见的直接征象（叶间裂移位、患侧胸腔缩小、血管和支气管聚集）和间接征象（纵隔摆动、肺门移位、通气不足、代偿性通气过度、患侧膈肌抬高）均适用于 CT。体积缩小的肺叶通常外缘接触胸壁，中心位于肺门，在 CT 上形成楔形阴影，而在传统 X 线片上不一定显示。

3. 胸膜基本病变的 X 线和 CT 表现

(1)胸腔积液：是最常见胸膜病理改变。正常的胸膜腔包含少量的液体以提供润滑。当液体的产生速度增加（如心力衰竭）或吸收障碍（如肿瘤阻塞淋巴管）时可发展为胸腔积液。根据胸腔积液的分布及游离或包裹，可分为游离性胸腔积液、包裹性胸腔积液、叶间积液和肺底积液。

1）游离性胸腔积液：根据积液量的多少，进一步分为大量、中量和少量游离性胸腔积液，X 线表现如下：

①中量游离积液：患者直立时，液体聚集在胸膜腔的下部，肋膈角和患侧膈肌不清，游离积液的上缘呈弧形。弧形的形成是由于液体的重力、肺膨胀的阻力、胸膜腔的毛细管吸引力、X 线切线位穿过液体层（液体弧形包绕在肺的周围），外侧区的液体较厚。因而在前后位上形成外侧最高、曲面向上的弧形（图 6-36）。

②大量游离积液：大量游离积液阴影和中量游离积液相似，但肺门不清，纵隔向对侧移位。

③少量游离积液：当肋膈角不清而膈肌未完全被液体掩盖时，胸膜腔内的液体少于 300 毫升，称为少量游离积液。仅表现为肋膈角变钝。

2）包裹性胸腔积液：是由于脏、壁层胸膜粘连所致。积液局限于胸腔的某一部位。表现为均匀密度的半圆形或梭形阴影，宽基底靠胸壁，向内侧突出，边缘清楚锐利。

3)叶间积液：液体聚集于叶间裂，表现为位于叶间裂部位的梭形阴影，长轴为受累的叶间裂线，阴影的双侧靠肺，边缘清楚(图6-37)。

侧位是判断叶间裂积液必要的体位，其他体位有时有用。

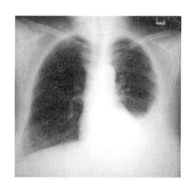

后前位片显示左下肺野均匀密度增高影。肋膈角和膈肌被掩盖模糊。液体的上缘呈外高内低的弧线。

图6-36 胸腔积液

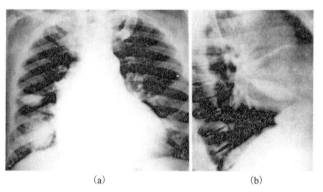

(a)   (b)

(a)右肺可见两个阴影。上方的轮廓分明，呈梭形，水平方向。下方的呈圆形；(b)侧位片很好地显示了每个叶间的积液。

图6-37 肺叶间积液

4)肺下积液：当患者直立时，积液位于肺与膈肌之间，肺漂于积液之上。阴影和膈肌抬高相似，但改变患者体位时积液可自由移动，这是确诊肺下积液一个简便明了的方法(图6-38)。

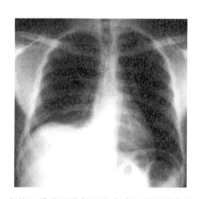

它的X线表现类似于患者直立时后前位胸片上的膈面升高。

图6-38 右侧肺下积液

CT适用于估计积液的部位和量，并显示胸片不能发现的积液。仰卧位，可移动的积液首先聚集于胸腔的后内侧(图6-39)。随着积液量的增加，液体沿胸膜腔向外侧延伸，肺远离胸壁。胸腔积液常引起一定程度的压迫性肺不张。大量胸腔积液常引起下叶不张，不张的肺叶向上移位(图6-40)。

CT也能确定局限性胸腔积液的位置和区分积液和胸膜肿瘤或肺实质病变。局限性胸腔积液横断面呈典型的凸镜状。位于叶间裂积液由于粘连可表现为"假瘤"，与肺内肿瘤相仿。

多数胸腔积液，无论漏出性或渗出性，其密度与水的密度相近。高密度的积液总是渗出液，近似或高于软组织密度的胸腔积液提示血胸。

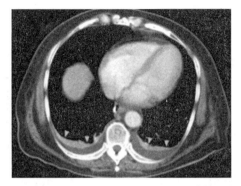

胸部对比增强 CT 显示特征性的不张肺组织的强化（箭头），患者有两侧少量胸膜积液。

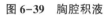

图 6-39 胸腔积液

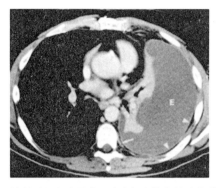

不张的肺组织有强化。胸壁与液体交界处的增亮线（箭头）表示胸膜壁层，它被丰富的胸膜外脂肪与胸壁分离开来。

图 6-40 大胸腔积液（E）伴压缩性肺不张

（2）气胸：空气进入胸膜腔有二种途径，一是壁层胸膜破裂，由外伤引起，气体通过胸部的伤口渗漏进胸膜腔。二是脏层胸膜破裂，常无穿通伤，称为自发性气胸。

气胸是空气积聚于肺和胸壁之间的胸膜腔。肺组织压缩，形成高透亮区，内无肺纹理。覆盖于萎陷的肺表面的脏层胸膜形成清楚锐利的边缘（图 6-41）。如胸膜腔大量积气时，肺显著的向肺门塌陷，纵隔向对侧移位。

CT 有助于鉴别传统放射检查值得怀疑的大肺大疱和气胸。也有助于发现初次自发性气胸患者的肺大疱和气肿性病变，以手术切除避免再发。

（3）液气胸：

当胸膜腔包含气体和液体时，称为液气胸。液气胸的特征性表现为胸膜腔内的气液平面（图 6-42）。气液平面可横贯胸腔，除非胸膜粘连引起气体和液体包裹。

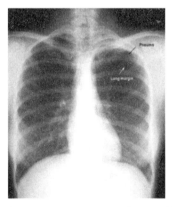

注意高度透亮区，在上肺野外带没有血管纹理。压缩的肺边缘清楚。

图 6-41 自发性气胸

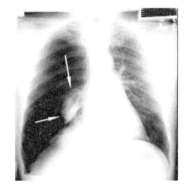

胸片显示右侧胸腔无血管纹理，呈高透亮区，纵隔左移，右肺肺不张（箭头）。由于全心输出转移至左侧，所以左侧肺野模糊。注意近右肋膈角处的小液平。

图 6-42 肺液气胸

（4）胸膜增厚、粘连、钙化：胸膜肥厚可局限或弥漫，通常由炎症或感染引起。胸膜增厚在后前位胸片上表现为沿胸壁的带状阴影，或下胸部的模糊高密度影。如胸膜增厚广泛而严重，可表现为肋间隙变窄，纵隔向患侧移位。壁层、脏层胸膜间粘连并不显影，除非有明显的胸膜增厚。有时胸膜粘连影响膈肌的形状，膈肌抬高而不再光滑。胸膜钙化表现为沿胸壁的垂直线状或带状高密度影或沿膈肌的线状高密度影（图 6-43）。

CT 能清晰显示胸膜肥厚和钙化的范围和特征，对显示局灶性胸膜斑，尤其是累及纵隔和椎旁胸膜的胸膜斑(图 6-44)，较传统放射学检查有更高的敏感性。

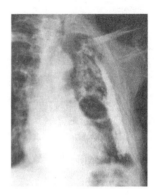

结核性胸膜炎后可出现广泛胸膜钙化，呈平行
胸壁的带状密度，左肺可见地理样阴影。钙化
的不规则分布是由于肺内空洞透亮区所导致。

图 6-43　胸膜钙化

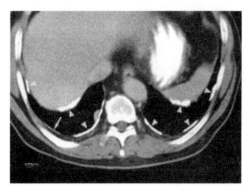

可见广泛钙化的胸膜斑块，相对对称，累及后侧胸膜，也
累及两侧膈面胸膜(箭头)。还可见小的非钙化斑块(箭)。

图 6-44　石棉相关胸膜斑

4. 基本病变 MRI 表现

目前 MRI 在肺部的临床应用价值有限，主要用于评价肺肿瘤和血管病变等。肺部肿瘤在 SE 序列为长 T2。T1 加权图像上为长 T1，和低信号的肺组织对比较差。肺门肿块和血管及支气管壁容易区分。亦可见肺门肿块的其他征象包括支气管阻塞和移位。肿瘤的 T2 弛豫时间较不张或实变的肺组织短，因而在 T2 权重图像上区分肺门旁的肿块和不张及实变的肺组织是可行的，然而在 T1 权重图像上难以区分。

第四节　常见疾病诊断

1. 肺部病变

(1)肺炎：肺炎是肺部感染导致的实变，X 线检查对病变的诊断和治疗有重要的作用。肺炎的分类方法有两种：一种是按解剖部位分为大叶性肺炎、小叶性肺炎和间质性肺炎三类，另一种是按病原学分类。后者对 X 线诊断无实用价值。

1)大叶性肺炎：

①临床与病理表现：大叶性肺炎多为肺炎双球菌致病。起病急，最初的症状为突然高热(高达39.5℃)，寒战，胸痛，起病 24 小时内或病程内可无咳嗽。数天后可出现咳铁锈色痰，为大叶性肺炎的典型临床特征。大叶性肺炎的基本病理改变为肺实质的急性炎性渗出。

②影像表现：大叶性叶炎可根据 X 线表现分为三期，即充血期、实变期、消散期。

充血期(起病约 24 小时)：病理上大叶性肺炎早期为炎性水肿。多数肺泡内仍充气，往往无明显 X 线改变，或表现为病变区肺纹理增多，或出现模糊的淡薄阴影。

实变期：感染病变区的肺泡内空气被渗出液取代。X 线表现为肺野大片状密度均匀的致密影，肺叶体积无缩小，空气支气管征常见(图 6-45)，这是由于肺泡内的空气被渗出物取代而支气管内的空气未被取代而保持开放，含气的支气管与周围不含气的肺实质产生对比，从而形成空气支气管征。致密阴影的边缘模糊不清，当病变的一侧邻近叶间裂时，该侧边缘则清晰锐利。例如上肺叶前段的下缘界限为水平裂，表现为锐利、平直的水平线(图 6-46)。右肺中叶大叶性肺炎可出现类似表现，即上缘清晰、锐利，下缘模糊。不同的肺叶实变有不同的形状，如肺段仅部分受累，阴影可表现为圆形和肿瘤相似(图 6-47)。根据临床病史和数日内阴影大小的快速改变可以作出明确的诊断。

消散期：肺泡内渗出物通过淋巴管吸收，此时肺泡内又充以气体。故实变影变为散在阴影。大约在起病后 2 周病灶完全吸收。病变区许多小支气管阻塞引起的肺膨张不全可表现为斑片状阴影和血管集聚。若仅上叶的后段受累,实变范围内存在局部透光区,易诊断为空洞,可误诊为化脓性肺炎或肺结核(图 6-48)。但随后的照片显示病灶如快速吸收,则可提示大叶性肺炎的诊断。

标准胸 X 线片是评价大叶性肺炎的基本检查,CT 有助于分析复杂的病例,其表现和胸 X 线平片所见相似,可更好地显示实变区的空气支气管征(图 6-49)。

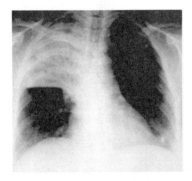

右上叶实变表现为大片均匀密度增高影,下缘锐利,其内可见支气管气象。

图 6-45 右上叶大叶性肺炎

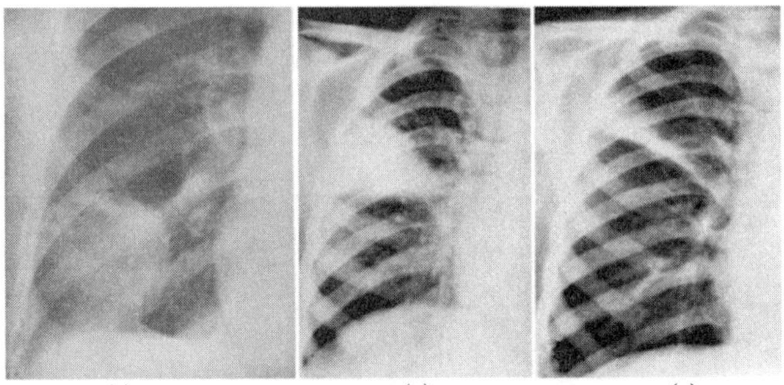

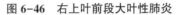

(a) (b) (c)

(a)右上肺前段近腋部的大部分实变,病变下缘被水平裂清楚勾画出来;(b)吸收过程中,由于小气道被渗出物阻塞导致部分肺不张,水平裂上抬;(c)病变完全吸收后,右上肺恢复正常,水平裂复位(箭),表明该肺叶完全复张。

图 6-46 右上叶前段大叶性肺炎

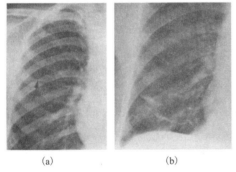

(a) (b)

(a)右下肺叶外基段肺炎类似肿瘤;(b)治疗一周后病变缩小为散在盘状肺不张。

图 6-47 大叶性肺炎

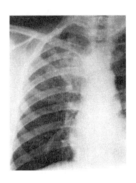

右上肺不规则阴影看起来像结核。虽然临床诊断大叶性肺炎很明确,但是影像上不进行前后系列图像的对比是不能轻易做出诊断的。

图 6-48 大叶性肺炎消散期

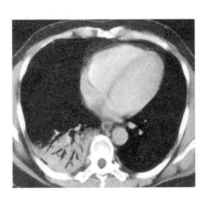

CT 显示右下肺实变及支气管气象。

图 6-49 右下肺大叶性肺炎

2）小叶性肺炎（支气管肺炎）：

①临床与病理表现：小叶性肺炎最重要的病原菌为链球菌、葡萄球菌、肺炎双球菌、肺炎克雷白杆菌、绿脓杆菌和流感嗜血杆菌等。多见于糖尿病、酗酒、气管切开、慢性支气管炎、囊性纤维化和疾病或药物所致的免疫缺陷患者。常见的临床症状为发热、咳嗽、咳脓痰和胸痛等。

②影像表现：X线表现包括肺纹理增强；中下肺野特别是心缘旁小斑片状致密阴影（图6-50）；双侧肺气肿常见；斑片状阴影融合形成大片状节段性实变；病情迁延或吸收不全可引起支气管扩张和肺纤维化。

胸平片常可作出小叶性肺炎的诊断。CT有助于显示肺实质的分布和程度，更清晰地显示空洞、纵隔淋巴结肿大及肺炎旁胸腔积液（图6-51）。

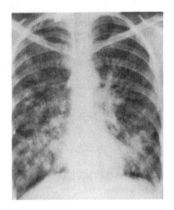
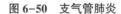

双下肺野结节状模糊影代表肺小叶实变。该患者急性起病、咳浓痰。

图6-50 支气管肺炎

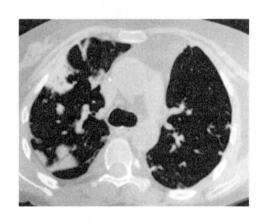

CT表现多发局灶性实变及局部支气管气象。

图6-51 支气管肺炎

3）间质性肺炎：

①临床与病理表现：间质性肺炎主要侵犯肺间质组织，包括支气管、血管束、叶间裂、小叶间和小叶内间隔。可由病毒或细菌感染所致，常继发于麻疹、百日咳或流感等急性感染性疾病。

②影像表现：间质性肺炎的X线表现（图6-52）包括两肺条状、网状、结节状或网结状阴影，边缘清晰，以中下肺野多见；双侧肺气肿常见；由于血管和支气管周围炎症及淋巴结炎，肺门阴影可能增大，密度增高。

CT，特别是HRCT可显示间质性肺炎的早期改变，易于发现间隔增厚、网状或结节影。

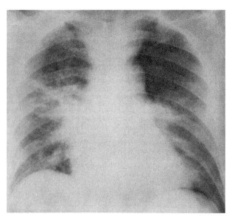

右上肺从肺门向外延伸的不规则浸润性病变，其中斜行线条状密度增高影是由于小气道阻塞所致的局限性肺不张。左上肺由于肺大泡导致透亮度增高。

图6-52 病毒性间质性肺炎

4)过敏性肺炎：

①临床与病理表现：过敏性肺炎又称外源性变应性肺泡炎，是环境中的有机粉末引起的免疫反应。农民肺和嗜鸟肺是两种常见的类型。过敏性肺炎有急性型、亚急性型和慢性型。急性者在暴露于抗原后4~6小时出现症状，咳嗽、呼吸困难、发热、寒战和不适是急性发作的特点。亚急性或慢性型过敏性肺炎的症状逐渐加重，包括咳嗽、劳力性呼吸困难、不适、食欲下降和体重减轻。

②影像表现：X线表现为弥漫性气腔实变。数日内变化结节或网结状为亚急性型特征性表现。病变以下肺野为重。慢性型最常见的影像学异常为小叶中心结节、线状致密影和肺野密度增高。

急性过敏性肺炎表现为气腔病变，在HRCT上常表现为毛玻璃影和小叶中心分布的模糊小结节影，代表肉芽肿或细支气管炎(图6-53)。线状致密影表示肺纤维化。慢性型HRCT显示模糊的小叶中心结节和弥漫性肺周纤维化伴肺基质的相对缺乏(图6-54)。HRCT对肺间质病变的评价优于胸X线平片。

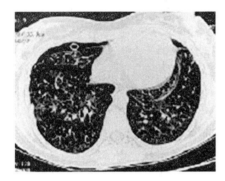

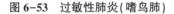

1 mm层厚HRCT显示双肺野弥漫分布的磨玻璃影以及小结节、间质增厚、少量气胸。

图6-53 过敏性肺炎(嗜鸟肺)

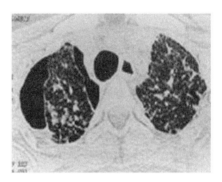

HRCT显示右侧持续存在的气胸。双肺明显见到弥漫磨玻璃影及结节灶、间质增厚。

图6-54 慢性过敏性肺炎(嗜鸟肺)

(2)肺脓肿：

1)临床与病理表现：所有肺炎的临床表现包括高热和胸痛等都可出现。一旦发生肺坏死并和支气管形成交通，咳嗽伴大量痰便是其显著的特征，多为脓臭痰，有时痰中带血。可出现大咯血。

2)影像表现：

①急性期：肺脓肿开始为坏疽性支气管肺炎，影像学表现和大叶性肺炎相似，肺内阴影多呈叶或段分布，但可见多发的致密影；

②亚急性期：亚急性期为起病后6周至3个月，脓肿壁纤维化已形成，通常表现为：(a)单个或多个脓肿空洞，当空气进入时可出现液平[图6-55(a)，(b)]。(b)厚壁空洞周围常有渗出性病灶，偶而脓肿和支气管尚未建立交通时，充满液体的脓肿可表现为密度均匀的圆形实性阴影，和肺部肿瘤的表现一致；

③慢性期：病程在3个月以上为慢性期，表现为单个或多个不规则多房空洞，空洞旁或空洞壁可见纤维化病灶，胸膜增厚常见。

(3)肺结核：1998年，中华结核病学会制定了新的结核病分类法，将结核病分为以下5类：原发性肺结核(Ⅰ型)；血行播散性肺结核(Ⅱ型)；继发性肺结核(Ⅲ型)；结核性胸膜炎(Ⅳ型)；其他肺外结核(Ⅴ型)。

1)原发性肺结核(Ⅰ型)：

①临床与病理表现：原发性肺结核为初次感染结核杆菌所致。最常见于儿童，可见于青年。常引起轻微身体不适或无特别症状。轻微症状常包括体重下降、食欲减退、不适、低热和盗汗，可出现或不出现咳嗽。

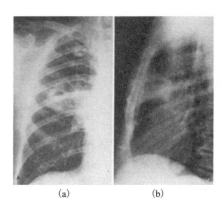

(a)

(b)

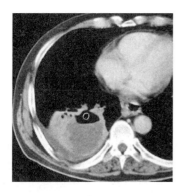

(a)右侧第四前肋水平肺野内阴影,其内见气液平面,表明病变内有空洞。(b)侧位显示空洞位于右上肺前段。

图 6-55(a)　肺脓肿 X 线表现

不规则厚壁包绕着气体和液体,该空洞壁有强化,其中央是坏死,邻近肺组织有实变和不张,胸膜腔有少许积液。

图 6-55(b)　右肺下叶肺脓肿 CT 表现

②原发性肺结核的 X 线表现为原发综合征和肺门淋巴结核两种形式。原发综合征包括肺部原发结核病灶、淋巴管炎和胸内淋巴结炎。

X 线表现为肺内渗出性病变,可见于肺的任何部位,合并同侧的肺门或纵隔淋巴结增大,可有或无胸腔积液(图 6-56)。典型者可见条索状阴影自渗出灶引向增大的胸内淋巴结,为淋巴管炎的表现。但在胸片上这种征象常不可见。

肺门淋巴结结核(胸内淋巴结结核):原发病灶常很快吸收,胸片上仍显示胸内淋巴结增大,称为肺门或胸内淋巴结结核。增大的淋巴结边缘可清楚或也可模糊,分别称为肿块型或炎症型。

CT 可有助于明确胸片上不确定的肺实质浸润和淋巴结增大[图 6-57(a)、(b)]。原发感染可伴有纵隔淋巴结增大和胸腔积液,有些病例胸部可仅表现为淋巴结增大。结核侵犯淋巴结常出现中央坏死区,在 CT 上为低密度,尤其在增强后其边缘强化时中央坏死可显示更明显。

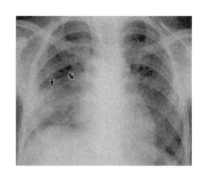

胸片显示右中肺实变(直箭)及右肺门淋巴结肿大(弯箭)。

图 6-56　原发性肺结核导致肺实变

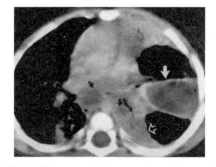

横断位增强 CT 显示肺内空洞(实心白箭)和增大坏死的隆突下淋巴结(黑箭),伴有左下肺不张(空心箭)。

图 6-57(a)　原发性肺结核的肺实质改变及淋巴结病变

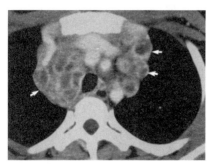

横断位增强 CT 显示肿大的淋巴结周边强化,中央为低密度坏死。

图 6-57(b)　纵隔淋巴结肿大

③原发性肺结核的预后:原发病灶和增大的淋巴结完全吸收而不留痕迹;原发病灶和增大的淋巴结可钙化;纤维和肉芽组织包裹病灶形成结节;患者抵抗力低下时,原发病灶可发生干酪坏死,坏死物经支气管排出后形成空洞,可发生支气管或血行播散。

2)血行播散型肺结核(Ⅱ型):根据症状和X线表现,血行播散型肺结核可分为二型:

①急性血行播散型肺结核(急性粟粒型肺结核):临床上急性粟粒型肺结核症状无特异性,起病急,如无结核性脑膜炎表现为发热疾病的症状。呼吸系统的症状不常见,咳嗽和呼吸困难可见于进展的病例。X线表现[图6-58(a)、(b)]:早期无改变。起病两周后出现肺部改变,表现为大量边缘清楚的针尖样致密影,大小、密度一致,分布均匀。结节直径常为1~2 mm。

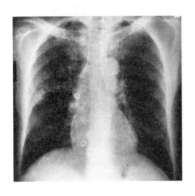

这些结节均匀地分布在其他肺野。在许多粟粒型肺结核病例中,可能看不到原发灶。

图6-58(a) 双肺分布着数不清的粟粒结节,除了肺底部

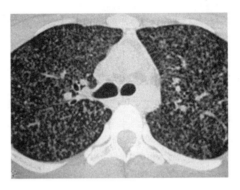

HRCT肺窗显示随机分布的大量细小结节。

图6-58(b) 粟粒型肺结核

②亚急性及慢性血行播散型肺结核:临床与病理表现:临床症状一般为亚急性或慢性,包括发热、不适、盗汗和体重减轻等。发热是其常见的特征,通常为低热。X线表现(图6-59):两肺大量的结节阴影,大小、密度和分布不均,故其X线表现和急性粟粒型肺结核不同。

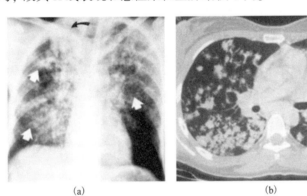

(a)胸片显示双上肺及右中肺聚集的结节及线样密度增高影(白箭),伴随肺尖胸膜增厚(黑箭);(b)横断位CT显示双肺弥漫分布不规则线状、结节状密度增高影,局部见空洞(箭头)。

图6-59 亚急性及慢性血行播散型肺结核

3)继发性肺结核(Ⅲ型):

①临床与病理表现:继发性肺结核是肺结核中最常见的类型,主要发生于成人。多为潜在的原发感染病灶重新活动或外源性再感染所致。不同的患者临床表现各异。许多X线诊断的患者可能否认有任何症状。常见的症状为低热、乏力、体重下降、盗汗、咳嗽、咳黏液痰和咯血。

②X线表现(图6-60):胸片可出现多种基本病变的X线表现,如渗出、增殖结节、纤维化、钙化和空洞,这些病变可同时见于同一患者胸片;病灶好发于上叶肺尖和锁骨下区肺野及下叶背段;渗出和空洞代表病灶有活动性;Ⅲ型肺结核有时表现为结核球或干酪性肺炎或慢性纤维空洞肺结核。

CT 有助于评价肺实质侵犯，卫星灶和支气管播散。空洞在 CT 上显示最佳[图 6-61(a)，(b)]，空洞的外壁可增厚和不规则，而内壁常光滑。可见液气平面。CT 显示支气管播散常表现为外周分布的腺泡阴影和大小不同的结节，细支气管黏液栓形成树芽征，病灶可见于整个双肺。

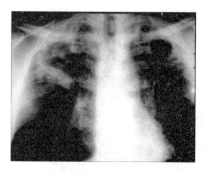

胸片显示双上肺部分肺段有密度偏高、形态不规则的实变区及厚壁空洞，左上肺空洞内可见气液平面。

图 6-60　继发性肺结核

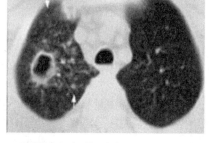

CT 显示右上肺不规则厚壁空洞，周边有条状密度增高影及小结节（箭头）。

图 6-61(a)　结核空洞

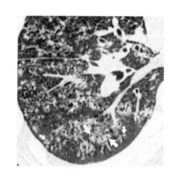

横断位 CT 显示支气管扩张及粘液栓，支气管壁增厚（直箭）、粘液栓、树芽征（弯箭）。

图 6-61(b)　结核支气管播散

4）结核瘤：干酪病灶被纤维组织包裹形成结核球，结核球直径大于 1.5 cm。

X 线表现（图 6-62）：结核球有典型特征，呈圆形或椭圆形高密度阴影，边缘清楚，好发于上叶。大约 75% 的结核球可出现钙化。周边卫星灶或多发结核球并不少见。结核球可长期保持稳定。结核球空洞非常少见，如出现提示病变重新活动。

结核球在 CT 上表现为圆形结节影，周围常伴有卫星病灶。

干酪性肺炎：多发生于抵抗力差的患者，特效的抗结核治疗引进以后，干酪性肺炎变得少见。患者常有持续高热、咳嗽和呼吸困难，痰量常较多，还可有不同程度咯血和体重下降。多为慢性病程。

X 线表现和大叶性肺炎相似，以上叶多见，但常见多发空洞及双下肺野支气管播散灶。支气管播散灶表现为许多小斑片状模糊阴影。

慢性纤维空洞肺结核：过去为肺结核的一个类型，大多数患者痰检结核分支杆菌为阳性。临床表现为反复低热、咳黏液痰、咯血、胸痛、乏力、体重下降、盗汗和厌食。部分患者可无明显的症状。

影像学表现（图 6-63）：纤维空洞，空洞外形不规则，空洞内壁光滑，壁密度较高；大量纤维病灶，由于纤维收缩，常使肺门上提，纵隔向患侧移位，肺纹理垂直向下呈垂柳状；常见下肺野的支气管播散。

5）结核性胸膜炎（Ⅳ型）：多数结核性胸膜炎可引起胸腔积液，也可不出现胸腔积液。胸部 X 线检查常显示患侧膈肌升高，活动度下降，可见胸膜增厚，以 CT 显示为佳。部分无胸腔积液患者，胸部 X 线检查可以表现正常。胸膜粘连和增厚者，可引起胸廓畸形。胸腔积液的 X 线表现在以前的章节中已经提到，CT 能清晰地显示胸腔积液和胸膜增厚（图 6-64）。

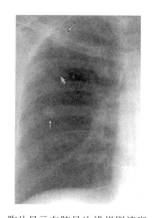

胸片显示右肺见边缘规则清晰的结节，结合结核病史，符合结核瘤。

图 6-62　结核瘤

MRI 对评价肺结核的价值有限。偶而有助于评价结核的并发症，如脓胸的胸壁侵犯程度。

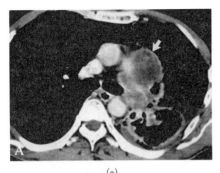 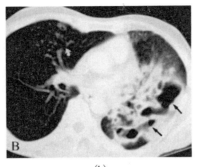

(a)增强CT纵隔窗显示淋巴结增大并中央坏死,呈低密度(箭);(b)CT肺窗显示左上肺轮廓不清的空洞沿着支气管延伸。

图6-63 慢性纤维空洞型肺结核

增强CT显示右侧大量胸水,胸膜不均匀增厚、强化。

图6-64 胸水

(5)肺部肿瘤

1)良性肿瘤:肺部良性肿瘤少见,多为脂肪瘤、血管瘤、纤维瘤和神经鞘瘤。上述肿瘤许多实际上为错构瘤。良性肿瘤特征性表现为边缘清楚,密度均匀的圆形或卵圆形阴影。有利于和大多数支气管肺癌鉴别,但不能和周围型肺腺癌或孤立性转移瘤区别。

错构瘤远较其他肺部良性肿瘤常见。起源于支气管壁的黏膜下纤维结缔组织。由结缔组织、软骨巢、成熟脂肪细胞和不同数量的骨、血管和平滑肌等混合而构成。严格来说,错构瘤是发育畸形而不是肿瘤。影像表现通常为肺内边缘锐利、密度均匀的圆形或浅分叶结节状阴影。多数错构瘤的大小为1~3 cm。瘤内如显示爆米花状钙化可基本上确诊为错构瘤。CT图像上有时可见脂肪密度(图6-65)。

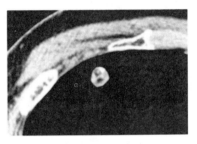

1 mm 层厚的CT扫描显示右上肺直径约1 cm的圆形结节,其内含有钙化及脂肪。

图6-65 错构瘤

2)原发性支气管肺癌:

①临床与病理表现:原发性支气管肺癌起源于支气管上皮、腺体或肺泡上皮。发病率近年逐步上升。肺癌的组织学类型分为鳞状细胞癌、腺癌(包括肺泡细胞癌)和未分化癌,未分化癌可分为小细胞(燕麦细胞)和各种大细胞癌。在特定的病例中可出现多种细胞类型共存。鳞状细胞癌和燕麦细胞癌最常见。多发性原发肺癌非常少见。

临床表现与肺癌的组织学类型、发生部位和发展程度有关。早期肺癌可无症状或体征。随着病变的发展,可出现咳嗽、咯血、咳痰、呼吸困难和喘鸣等症状。支气管阻塞可导致远端感染。肿瘤蔓延至胸膜时可引起胸腔积液、胸膜炎和胸痛(侵犯壁层胸膜)。肿瘤侵犯纵隔可表现为:左喉返神经麻痹;上腔静脉阻塞;吞咽困难;膈神经麻痹;肺尖肿瘤侵犯臂丛和交感神经节(肺上沟瘤)可引起Horner综合征。肺癌细胞可产生激素样生物活性物质(通常为肽),引起的综合征可分为内分泌和神经肌肉综合征两类。

②影像学表现:原发性肺癌按肺癌的发生部位可分为中央型、周围型和弥漫型。

中央型:发生于主支气管、肺叶支气管及肺段支气管的肺癌,位于肺门部位,称为中央型。中央型肺癌的表现分为肿瘤本身的征象和气道阻塞继发的征象,又称直接征象和间接征象。

直接征象:肺门肿块在胸片上表现为肺门增大,密度增高[图6-66(a)],为来自肺中央的原发肺癌或其转移侵犯肺门淋巴结导致其增大所致。早期在胸片上可仅表现为肺门密度增高甚至正常。肿瘤侵犯支气管腔有时可在平片上显示,常伴有肺叶或全肺不张。肺门体层或高千伏摄片可显示肿瘤旁的支气管不规则狭窄。经常会有支气管腔显示完全阻塞,但却无肺塌陷的情况出现。

CT能清晰地显示支气管异常和肺门肿块[图6-66(b)、(c)]。支气管异常包括不规则狭窄,阻塞,腔内结节和支气管壁增厚。肺门肿瘤表现为边缘清楚、外缘光滑或分叶的肿块,位于某一支气管的附近。

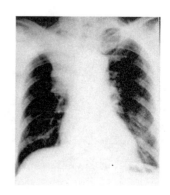

正位胸片显示右肺门肿块及右上肺不张,其下缘显示横"S"征。

图 6-66(a) 中央型肺癌

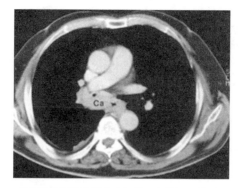

肺门肿块包绕并阻塞支气管、直接侵犯纵隔,局部胸膜增厚表明胸膜转移。

图 6-66(b) 中央型肺癌

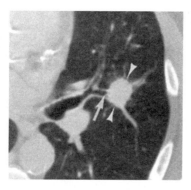

CT 显示舌叶支气管(箭)一直径 2 cm 的不规则结节(箭头),支气管纤维镜灌洗证实为鳞状细胞癌。

图 6-66(c) 支气管肺癌

间接征象:主要支气管阻塞可引起肺段或肺叶通气减少而产生肺不张和/或分泌物不能排出而产生实变。上叶肺不张和肺门肿块可形成横"S"征(图 6-67),表现为肺不张的肺门侧有密度增高的肿块突向肺不张阴影的边缘,为中央型肺癌的特征性表现。继发感染引起肺炎很常见。肺不张/实变可呈段或叶甚至一侧全肺分布。局限性肺气肿可能为肺癌的早期征象。

周围型:肿块位于周围肺野时,称为周围型肺癌。X 线表现为肺部外周肿块[图 6-68(a)]。形状呈类球形或卵圆形,可有分叶。传统的断层摄片及 CT 可很好显示病变的边缘,常有

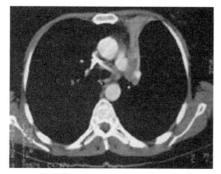

52 岁女性,肺癌位于左主支气管,导致左上叶不张。

图 6-67 支气管肺癌

分叶、凹陷和毛刺。肿瘤的边缘可清楚、毛糙或模糊。可伴有胸膜尾征,表现为肿瘤和胸膜之间的线形阴影[图 6-68(b)],以腺癌多见。

肿块较大时可出现空洞[图 6-68(c)],癌性空洞的特点为空洞的内壁常不规则,空洞多为偏心性。空洞常见于鳞状细胞癌。

通过比较以前的照片判定可疑为肺癌的病灶的生长速度对诊断非常有帮助。周围性肺癌的倍增时间为 30~490 天(平均 120 天),很少有病例超出此范围。因此肿块生长速度过慢或过快常提示其他诊断。

弥漫型:当肺癌灶散布于肺野时,称为弥漫型。弥漫型肺癌仅为细支气管肺泡癌。表现为一叶、数叶及两肺多发的斑片状阴影,大小不等,也可为单个斑片状阴影,有的仅仅表现为整个肺叶实变,且可包含充气支气管征。还可见间隔线(Kerley A 线和 B 线)和胸腔积液。形态有时与肺水肿或广泛分布的支气管肺炎相似。

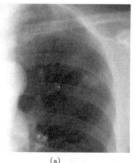

(a) (b)

(a)正位胸片显示左上肺轮廓不规则的密度增高影;(b)2 mm 层厚 CT 显示左上肺直径约 2 cm 不规则浸润性结节灶,具有支气管肺癌的典型特征,外科手术后证实为腺癌。

图 6-68(a) 支气管肺癌

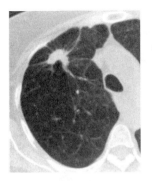

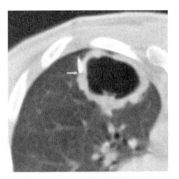

男性患者，右上肺腺癌边缘有毛刺及
胸膜尾征，有小叶中央型肺气肿。

图 6-68(b) 支气管肺癌

CT 显示右下肺不规则厚壁空洞，CT 引导下活
检(俯卧位)证实针尖位于病变壁上，切片证
实为鳞癌。

图 6-68(c) 支气管肺癌

③肿瘤扩散：肺癌可局部侵犯、经淋巴管扩散至肺门和纵隔淋巴结及经血行远处扩散至包括胸部在内的其他结构。

肺门和纵隔淋巴结转移：表现为肺门或纵隔淋巴结增大。CT 和 MRI 检查对显示纵隔淋巴结肿大有很高的敏感性。应当认识到正常大小的淋巴结也可能包含显微镜下肿瘤转移灶，故根据 CT 上淋巴结的大小来判断是否存在淋巴结转移总是有局限性。一般认为，肺门淋巴结直径超过 1 cm，纵隔淋巴结直径超过 1.5 cm 为异常(图 6-69)。

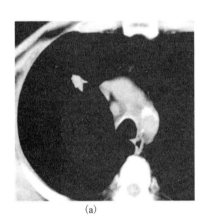

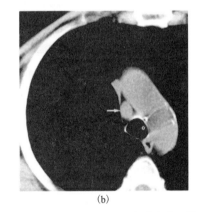

(a) (b)

(a)CT 见右上肺直径约 1.7 cm 不规则结节；(b)下部层面见直径约 2 cm 的增大淋巴结
(箭)，证实为低分化鳞癌。

图 6-69 支气管肺癌

纵隔侵犯：肺癌可直接侵犯纵隔。平片或传统体层摄片难以区分肿瘤接触胸膜时是否侵犯纵隔胸膜及纵隔，增强 CT 和 MRI 能提供侵犯的证据(图 6-70)。当心包受侵时偶可见心包积液。

胸膜受累：可见胸腔积液和胸膜肿块。但即使有恶性胸腔积液时胸膜肿块也非常少见。

胸壁侵犯：周围型肺癌可通过胸膜侵犯胸壁。平片可见肋骨或椎体破坏。CT 和 MRI 能更好地发现软组织受侵(图 6-71)。

膈神经受累：由于增大的纵隔淋巴结或肿块压迫膈神经引起一侧膈肌麻痹，胸部 X 线检查可显示膈肌麻痹而抬高。

3)肺部转移瘤：肺部转移瘤多来自绒癌、乳腺癌、肝癌、胃癌和前列腺癌等。肺转移瘤的基本征象为单个或多个分散的结节。多数转移瘤呈圆形、边缘清楚。部分可出现边缘不规则浸润。极少数可表现为以

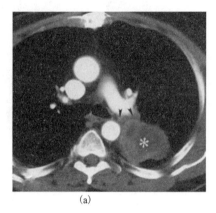 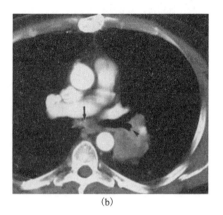

(a)   (b)

(a)左肺动脉平面 CT 显示肿瘤内局限性坏死(＊),肿瘤前缘侵犯纵隔及左肺动脉后缘(箭头);(b)右肺动脉干平面 CT 显示病变累及左肺门及左上肺尖后段支气管(箭头),隆突下淋巴结肿大(箭头)。

图 6-70 鳞癌

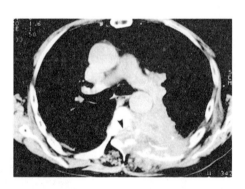

CT 见病变邻近肋骨及椎体破坏,肿瘤累及左后胸壁,左下肺背段不张。

图 6-71 鳞癌累及胸壁

间质转移为主(癌性淋巴管炎)。虽然结节多为边界清楚的球形,但也可以表现为任何形状或偶而出现非常不规则的边缘。边缘不规则的转移瘤多来自腺癌。

典型的肺转移瘤常表现为肺内多发圆形或卵圆形结节,边缘清晰,大小不等[图 6-72(a)]。偶而可表现为无数的粟粒状结节影而和粟粒性肺结核相似,并可见起自肺门或胸内肿大淋巴结的放射状线条阴影[图 6-72(b)]。

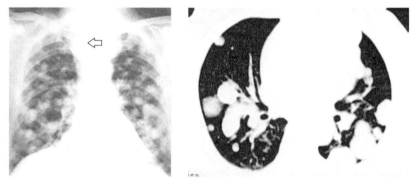

双肺多发结节灶,正位胸片显示上纵隔增宽(箭),证实为原发灶来自甲状腺的恶性肿瘤。

图 6-72(a) 转移瘤(结节型)

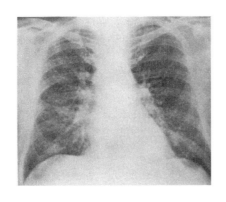

原发灶位于胰腺，双肺见多发微小结节灶，气管旁见肿大淋巴结。

图 6-72(b) 粟粒状转移瘤

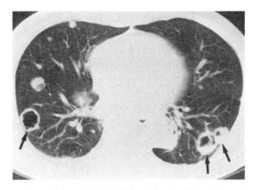

73 岁老年男性，左主支气管鳞癌伴空洞样转移灶形成，CT 显示双肺多发结节灶，双下肺见散在空洞结节，且空洞壁不规则。

图 6-72(c) 转移癌

孤立性转移可作为无已知原发肿瘤的患者的表现，当病史和体格检查排除肺外原发肿瘤时，转移瘤仍是无症状肺结节患者要考虑到的一个罕见的原因，约占无症状孤立性肺结节的 2%~3%。

空洞偶而可见，是鳞状细胞癌转移的特征性表现[图 6-72(c)]。

除骨肉瘤和软骨肉瘤转移外，钙化非常少见[图 6-72(d)]。即使原发肿瘤有钙化，如乳腺癌和结肠癌，肺内转移瘤钙化也非常罕见。

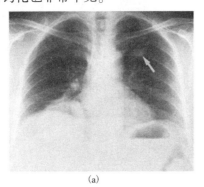

(a)胸片见双肺多发结节灶，左上叶一病灶内见局部钙化(箭)；(b)增强 CT 清晰显示病灶内钙化(箭)，病理组织检查证实转移灶内局部钙化。

图 6-72(e) 骨肉瘤钙化转移

肺部转移瘤的生长速度差别较大，部分转移瘤如绒癌和骨肉瘤转移可呈爆炸式生长，倍增时间可少于 30 天，另外一些转移瘤如甲状腺癌转移可长时间保持大小不变。

癌性淋巴管炎是转移瘤的一种形式，为肺部淋巴管受侵，并被恶性肿瘤细胞阻塞所致。可单侧或双侧出现。患者可出现呼吸困难，单侧受累时无或很少有肺部症状。肺部淋巴管扩散最常见于来自乳腺、肺、胃、结肠、前列腺和胰腺的腺癌。支气管肺癌是引起单侧癌性淋巴管的最常见的原因。肺内淋巴管转移的机制有：部分病例可能为肺门淋巴结的肿瘤向周围放射状浸润。另外部分病例可能为肿瘤最初经血行传播，侵犯肺内淋巴管，肿瘤再向肺门方向浸润，最初肺门淋巴结并未受累。胸

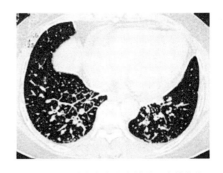

CT 显示肺间质内高密度线样影及小结节灶。

图 6-72(e) 乳腺癌肺淋巴道转移

部 X 线表现为广泛分布的 2~3 mm 大小的边缘模糊的结节影，肺间质广泛增厚。胸膜下水肿可引起叶间裂增厚。胸腔积液常见，但多为少量。CT 表现包括支气管血管束不均匀增厚和小叶间隔的增厚，常呈多角形

［图6-72(e)］。随着病程进展，可见更多的结节组成网状，形成的小结节连接成增厚的线状阴影，是特征性表现，或称"珍珠链"状表现。

2.支气管疾病

(1)支气管扩张：

1)临床与病理表现：支气管扩张是指支气管腔不可逆转的扩张，病理上根据支气管扩张的程度分为三型：柱状扩张；静脉曲张型扩张；囊状扩张。特征性的临床表现为持续性的咳嗽和咳痰，常有较多量的脓痰。反复咯血、肺炎及胸膜炎的病史相对常见。

2)影像表现：通常支气管扩张的胸部X线平片表现可无特异性，除非病变严重。扩张的支气管轮廓常因周围渗出及纤维病灶而模糊不清［图6-73(a)］。扩张的支气管有时可见液平。以前常用支气管造影来明确诊断和评价手术前患者。

各型支气管扩张在CT上均有特征性表现。对疑诊患者，可采用1~2 mm层厚扫描。高分辨CT具有足够的敏感性和特异性以确定或排除支气管扩张的诊断，总的准确性约为95%。高分辨CT主要的征象是支气管管腔的扩张，常伴有支气壁增厚。扩张的支气管和伴行的肺动脉形成"印戒征"［图6-73(b)］。严重的囊状支气管扩张可见大的椭圆形高密度影或厚壁透光区，代表扩张的支气管腔内充满粘液或空气。由于潴留的分泌物位于囊性结构中，有时可见液气平面。

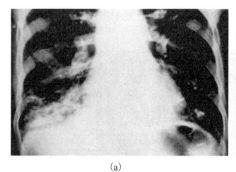

(a)

(b)

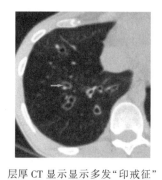

层厚CT显示显示多发"印戒征"（箭头），这是由于肺动脉紧邻扩张而又光滑的支气管壁所致。

(a)右下肺见渗出性病变；(b)支气管造影显示左下肺支气管柱状扩张，右下肺基底部支气管囊状扩张。

图6-73(a)　双下肺支扩

图6-73(b)　柱状支扩

(2)支气管异物：

1)临床与病理表现：异物吸入多见于幼儿或儿童。常见的症状为咳嗽、呼吸困难和发绀等。

2)影像表现：对于不透X线的异物诊断简单。如果是透X线异物，平片不能发现而只能显示支气管阻塞的继发改变。异物常位于主支气管或下叶支气管并常引起下叶完全阻塞形成肺不张或上叶不完全阻塞形成肺气肿。

CT可发现和定位支气管腔内的异物(图6-74)，但明确诊断通常需要结合病史。

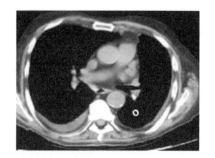

CT显示左肺下叶支气管高密度物体，右侧胸腔意外见到少量胸水。

图6-74　呼吸道异物（牙齿）

3.纵隔疾病

(1)纵隔脂肪沉积症：纵隔脂肪沉积症是一种正常脂肪组织的异常堆积，导致纵隔增宽，常为特发性。最为常见的原因是肥胖、使用糖皮质激素、柯兴综合征。在正位胸片上，可见纵隔增宽，尤其是上纵隔。侧位胸片上于前纵隔可见模糊阴影。CT扫描能够辨别纵隔脂肪沉积症与其他原因引起的纵隔增宽，CT上显示纵隔脂肪沉积为密度均匀的脂肪组成,密度同皮下脂肪(图6-75)。T1加权MR图显示为均一的高信号强度。脂肪沉积主要在前纵隔,导致纵隔侧缘呈弧形。其他常受累的区域包括心隔角、膈脚后、脊柱旁。

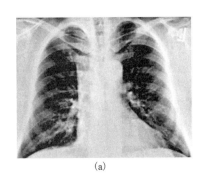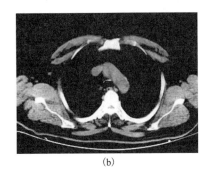

(a)　　　　　　　　　　　　　　　　(b)

(a)正位胸片显示上纵隔增宽;(b)CT见沉积的脂肪向周围突出包绕上腔静脉及主动脉弓。

图6-75　纵隔脂肪沉积症

(2)支气管囊肿:

1)临床与病理表现:支气管囊肿是由于气管支气管树腹侧异常发育所致。囊壁为呼吸上皮细胞,可包含有软骨、粘液腺和平滑肌。起源于纵隔的支气管囊肿被认为是早期的气管支气管树异常分枝所致,而不是肺实质。大多数纵隔支气管囊肿位于气道旁,最为常见的是气管隆突和气管右侧区域。绝大多数囊肿为液体充填,也可见气体,表明来自气管支气管树。患者多无症状,少数患者有呼吸困难、胸痛和吞咽困难。

2)影像表现:胸片上支气管囊肿表现为圆形、边缘光滑的肿块,可导致邻近气道移位和狭窄,可见气液平面。囊壁钙化不常见。CT显示囊肿呈边缘清晰、无强化、密度均匀的圆形肿块,大约50%的支气管囊肿CT值在液体CT值范围内(0~20 Hu),其余的CT值常超过20 Hu,提示囊肿内钙和蛋白质等物质的含量高,或先前有过出血(图6-76)。高密度囊肿与实性肿块难以区别,确诊需用超声或穿刺活检。近来应用MR评估支气管囊肿。囊肿由于含不同物质,在T1加权像上可表现为不同的信号强度。T2加权常显示出特征性的高信号,为大多数纵隔囊肿共有的征像。

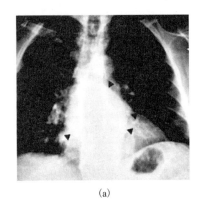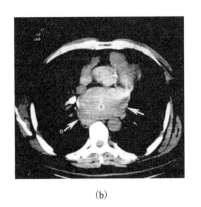

(a)　　　　　　　　　　　　　　　　(b)

(a)正位胸片见巨大的隆突下肿块(箭头);(b)CT见中纵隔边界清楚的卵圆形肿块(箭),CT值为25HU,提示其内有蛋白质或出血。

图6-76　支气管囊肿

(3)神经管原肠囊肿:神经管原肠囊肿是由于内胚层和脊索的分离异常,导致与脑脊膜的持久连接和脊椎骨化中心的正常融合打断而形成。大约一半的病例有脊椎异常,包括半椎体和蝴蝶椎。常发生在后纵隔。该囊肿的影像表现类似其他前肠囊肿,但结合椎体异常可提示本病。

（4）心包囊肿：

1）临床与病理表现：心包囊肿并不常见，是由胚胎发育过程中心包的一部分异常发育发展而来，囊肿的包膜由单一的间皮细胞层构成，大多数囊肿内含清亮的渗漏液。本病偶发咳嗽、胸痛，尤其在囊肿发生扭转或出血时。70%的囊肿位于右心膈角，20%位于左心膈角。其余的位于不同的部位，包括后纵隔。

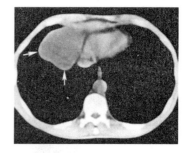

CT 见右侧心膈角病变（箭头），密度较高，提示可能既往有出血。

图 6-77 心包囊肿

2）影像表现：胸片上的典型的表现是心膈角处边缘清晰、锐利的肿块，与膈和心缘相邻。CT 扫描表现为边缘清晰、无强化的病灶，CT 值为液体密度（0~20 HU）。囊肿常形状各异。如有出血可呈高密度囊肿（图 6-77），如病灶位于典型部位，超声有助于确诊。单纯的心包囊肿在 MR T1 加权图上为低信号，T2 加权图上为高信号。

（5）胸腺囊肿：

1）临床与病理表现：先天性胸腺囊肿被认为来源于第三咽囊的管状残余，囊壁由单层鳞状或立方上皮细胞够成。囊肿可以发生于从下鄂到膈面沿胸腺咽管走行的任何区域。囊肿常常偶然被发现。出血时可引发症状。获得性胸腺囊肿与霍杰金病、胸部的钝性损伤、放射治疗、开胸手术相关，偶尔与重症肌无力有关。

2）影像表现：胸片上显示前纵隔边缘清楚的肿块，与胸腺瘤难以鉴别。超声有助于确定病变为囊性。CT 表现与其他纵隔囊肿相似。囊肿出血可致囊肿迅速增大，密度也高于水（图 6-78）。简单的囊肿在 MR T1 加权图上为低信号，T2 加权图上为高信号。囊肿出血在 T1 加权像上信号可呈高信号。

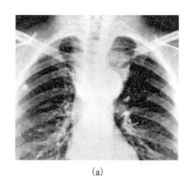
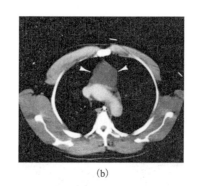

(a)   (b)

（a）正位胸片显示上纵隔肿块，主动脉弓轮廓完整；（b）CT 见主动脉弓前缘水样密度肿块（箭头）。

图 6-78 胸腺囊肿

（6）纵隔原发性实性肿瘤：纵隔原发实性肿瘤有很多种，如神经源性肿瘤、胸腺瘤、淋巴瘤等。

1）神经源性肿瘤：

①临床与病理表现：神经源性肿瘤是后纵隔肿块最为常见的原因，主要位于脊椎旁沟，也可发自纵隔其他间隙、胸壁，偶见于肺实质。病理上，这类肿瘤能划分成三组：神经鞘源性肿瘤包括神经纤维瘤，神经鞘瘤；神经节细胞源性肿瘤包括神经节细胞瘤，神经节母细胞瘤，神经母细胞瘤；副神经节源性肿瘤包括化学感受器瘤，嗜铬细胞瘤。

粗略估计，起源于胸部的神经源性肿瘤 70%是良性。通常发生于 40 岁以下年轻人。男女发病率相同。患者常常无症状，但可以导致诸如根性疼痛和神经衰弱等症状。肿瘤向椎管内延伸可产生束带样压榨症状。起源于外周神经的肿瘤趋向于圆形，起源于交感神经链的肿瘤常常呈纺锥形。

②影像表现：在胸部 X 线片上，神经源性肿瘤表现为圆形、边缘清晰锐利、密度均匀的肿块。受累及的肋骨表现为边缘硬化，则提示为良性肿瘤。骨质破坏或累及多根肋骨常提示恶性肿瘤。所有的神经源性肿瘤均可出现钙化。

　　CT 上，神经源性肿瘤典型表现为密度均匀的软组织密度病灶，多种肿瘤可有低密度的脂肪组织或囊变（图 6-79）。由于肿瘤血管形成，经静脉注射对比剂后可见肿瘤强化。脊椎受累最适宜运用 MRI 作评估。多平面重建图像有助于显示沿脊柱长轴方向生长的肿瘤。神经孔的增宽常常与神经鞘瘤相关。椎体受侵犯常常与交感神经肿瘤相关。一般良性肿瘤密度均匀，边缘清楚。相反，恶性肿瘤密度不均匀，边界不规则。在 MR 图像上，神经源性肿瘤表现为信号均匀，边界清晰的肿块，在 T1 加权图上信号强度明显高于骨胳肌，在 T2 图像上信号强度明显增高。用钆增强扫描，均质和非均质的肿瘤都有强化，非均质肿瘤的强化取决于组织构成，如血管成份的多少和有无囊变等。

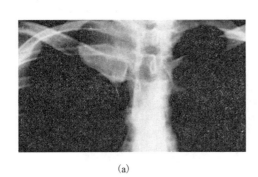 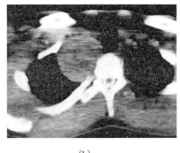

（a）　　　　　　　　　　　　　　　（b）

（a）正位胸片显示已被证实的右上纵隔神经鞘瘤；（b）CT 显示右肺尖被神经鞘瘤压迫移位。

图 6-79　低密度的脂肪组织或囊变

　　2）胸腺瘤：

　　①临床与病理表现：胸腺瘤来源于胸腺上皮组织，为胸腺肿块性病变最常见的原因，位于前纵隔。胸腺瘤由胸腺上皮细胞和不同数量的反应性淋巴细胞组成，囊变常见，完全囊变则罕见。大多为良性，约 30% 有纤维包膜，亦可为侵袭性，常突出到包膜外。

　　胸腺瘤发生于 40~60 岁人群，男女比例相等。20 岁以下发病罕见。偶尔在健康人的胸片中被发现。也可见于其他病症的患者，如重症肌无力。约 50% 的胸腺瘤患者患有重症肌无力，15% 的重症肌无力患者患有胸腺瘤。

　　②影像表现：胸部平片上，胸腺瘤表现为圆形、分叶状的位于前纵隔的肿块，侧位常表现为胸骨后清晰的间隙中有一边缘清楚的肿块。有时，肿瘤位置偏低，位于心脏的左或右缘，偶尔低到心膈角处。有时肿瘤太小（1 cm），平片无法发现，只有 CT 扫描可以发现。CT 上良性或侵袭性胸腺瘤可见钙化灶，良性胸腺瘤表现为圆形或椭圆形肿块，位于血管前间隙。亦可见于前纵隔从胸廓入口至膈肌的任何一处。侵袭性胸腺瘤典型的表现为沿胸膜区生长的不规则肿块（图 6-80）。

　　3）畸胎瘤：畸胎瘤通常为良性。25% 的畸胎瘤 X 线平片可显示有骨或牙齿及外周的钙化。畸胎瘤分三类：依赖皮肤（表皮样）、皮肤和其附器（表皮）、两或三胚层的派生组织（畸胎样）各自占优的情况分类。在图 6-81 上，肿瘤从膈延伸至胸廓入口，主要的大血管位置大部分被长长的肿瘤占据，为少见征像。极少数畸胎瘤位于后纵隔。

　　4）纵隔甲状腺肿：当甲状腺肿块下降至胸腔时，通常进入血管前间隙（图 6-82）。甲状腺肿的 CT 表现有其特征性：通常能显示其为颈部甲状腺的解剖上的延续；点状钙化和密度不均匀也为常见特征；注射对比剂后，出现延时强化。因为胸廓入口平面不再被血管分隔为血管前和后间隙，增大延长的甲状腺也可能经胸廓入口向后滑动进入血管后间隙。

　　5）淋巴瘤：霍杰金和非霍杰金淋巴瘤常常累及胸部。67% 霍杰金氏病累及胸内淋巴结，其中有 46% 累及前纵隔。43% 的非霍杰金氏淋巴瘤累及胸内淋巴结，只有 13% 累及前纵隔。胸内淋巴瘤的放射学常表现为较大的位于前或中纵隔的软组织肿块，可将大血管、气管向后推移。CT 增强如显示肿块局部密度减低，提示有坏死。淋巴瘤也可表现为单个的或分散的淋巴结肿大，但最常表现为大的融合肿块(图6-83)。

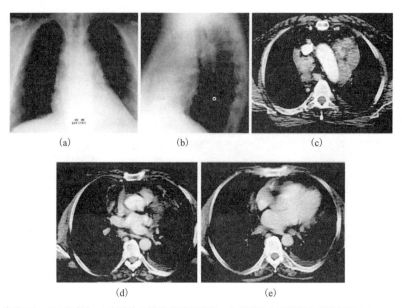

胸片(a)、(b)患者自12岁时检查就发现纵隔增宽,考虑肿块位于纵隔血管前间隙(c)~(e)增强CT见纵隔肿块有脂肪和其他软组织成分,肿块局部延伸至上腔静脉后缘及气管右前缘,沿着主动脉延伸至膈肌平面,病理证实为伴有淋巴结集合增生的良性胸腺脂肪瘤。

图6-80　侵袭性胸腺瘤典型的表现

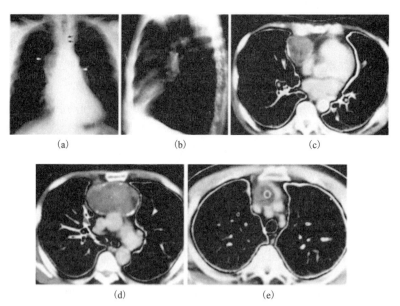

(a)、(b)巨大肿块压迫双肺尖(箭头),气管受压后移,提示肿块位于其前方;肿块边缘与肺野分界清晰,提示肿块位于纵隔,箭头指示的是胸膜;(c)~(e)肿块下至膈肌平面,上至胸廓入口,位于血管前间隙,其内见钙化、脂肪、水样密度物质,推测为皮样囊肿。

图6-81　畸胎瘤从膈延伸至胸廓入口

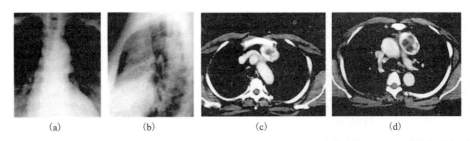

48岁女性正位胸片见纵隔肿块,正侧位(a)、(b)胸片上,正位显示主肺动脉窗附近见边界清楚的肿块,侧位见气管前缘轻微受压移位,从而确定肿块位于纵隔血管前间隙。增强CT(c)、(d)见血管前肿块周边明显强化,起初并没有考虑甲状腺病变而是考虑富血管性肿瘤如副神经节瘤、血管瘤,术后诊断为甲状腺肿。

图6-82　当甲状腺肿块下降至胸腔时,进入血管前间隙

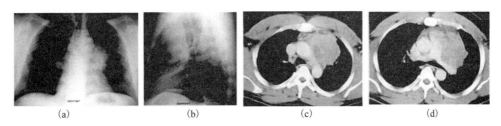

正侧位胸片(a)、(b)显示左前纵隔巨大肿块,气管受压后移。增强CT(c)、(d)显示病变位于纵隔血管前间隙,局部见密度减低区提示有坏死,左肺动脉干受压变窄,肿块确诊为大B细胞型恶性淋巴瘤。

图6-83　分散的淋巴结肿大,但仍表现为融合的肿块

4.胸膜疾病

胸膜肿瘤少见,最常见的胸膜的良性肿瘤为脂肪瘤和纤维瘤。最常见的侵犯胸膜的恶性肿瘤为转移瘤,原发于胸膜的恶性肿瘤,如间皮瘤,在胸膜恶性肿瘤中占比不足5%。如胸膜增厚超过1cm,出现播散性胸膜结节,纵隔胸膜受累等均提示为胸膜恶性病变。但明确诊断常需要进行细胞学或组织学检查。

(1)恶性胸膜间皮瘤:

1)临床与病理表现:胸膜间皮瘤是一种起源于胸膜的恶性肿瘤,通常有接触石棉的职业史。病理上可分为上皮型、纤维型和混合型。临床症状出现较晚,可包括胸痛、呼吸困难、咳嗽、虚弱乏力和体重下降等。

2)影像表现:恶性胸膜间皮瘤影像学表现为类圆形或轻度分叶状肿块,边缘光滑锐利,可随体位及呼吸运动而移动。肿块可偶见于叶间裂,需要和叶间裂积液鉴别。CT和MRI可显示肿块形态、范围和胸腔积液。病变也可呈不规则弥漫性结节状胸膜增厚或胸壁和肺之间的团块影(图6-84)。恶性胸膜间皮瘤在T1WI上呈中等信号,T2WI呈稍高信号,而包裹性胸腔积液T2WI呈高信号。

CT和MRI较平片能更好的显示肿瘤在胸膜表面、纵隔、横膈或胸壁的范围。肿瘤侵犯胸壁表现为胸壁脂肪层消失或胸壁出现结节灶。

(2)胸膜转移瘤:

胸膜转移瘤通常同时侵犯壁层和脏层胸膜,多伴有胸腔积液,多数胸膜转移瘤来源于肺癌、乳腺癌和淋巴瘤。

胸膜表面渗出引起的胸腔积液是多数转移瘤的首要表现。CT可显示被胸腔积液掩盖的胸膜结节,常呈比较小的扁豆状软组织结节影,与胸壁呈钝角相交(图6-85)。增强检查肿瘤的软组织成分常常强化,这有助于区别相邻的无强化的胸腔积液。另外,CT还可发现纵隔淋巴结增大、肺部结节、肋骨病变、皮下肿块等,有助于胸膜转移瘤的诊断。

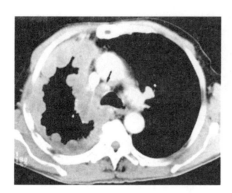

可见环状轻度强化的胸膜增厚结节包绕右肺，右肺体积减小，气管隆突旁淋巴结肿大(箭头)。

图 6-84 恶性胸膜间皮瘤

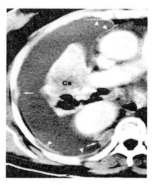

大量胸水旁见小的胸膜结节(箭)及不张的右肺，增强显示胸膜壁的异常强化(箭头)。

图 6-85 支气管肺癌胸膜转移并胸水形成

(尚全良，陈娟，尹芝兰，郭茜，肖恩华，罗建光)

Chapter 6

Radiology of thorax

The air in lung tissues gives good contrast. So most of the diseases affecting the lungs can be detected by X-rays. X-ray features are reflection of gross pathological changes only. It cannot reflect the histological changes. Because chest plain film is economical and simple, it is widely used and the basic method for the diagnosis of chest diseases. CT scan is easy to detect and display the features of chest lesions, and its density resolution is higher than X-ray plain film, which is an important means for the diagnosis of respiratory diseases. The same abnormal manifestations can occur in different diseases, and the same disease can have different abnormal manifestations depending on different stages or types of development. So precise diagnosis depends upon the proper analysis of imagine features together with clinical findings.

Section 1 Method of examination

There are fluoroscopy, simple chest filming, high K. V. radiography, bronchography, pulmonary angiography, computed tomography and magnetic resonance imaging etc. According to the patient's condition to choose methods that is from simple to complex.

1. Fluoroscopy

The advantages of fluoroscopy are real-time imaging and the freedom to freely position the X-ray field during examination. However, due to the length of the fluoroscopic examinations, the exposure rate is much higher than in common radiography. Otherwise, the fluoroscopic image suffers from inferior spatial resolution and a high noise level when compared to common radiographs. For these seasons, it is rarely used. Patients suspected of bronchial foreign bodies or open pneumothorax, the mediastinal movement during breathing should be carefully observed, which is mainly used in the chest to assess the abnormal mediastinal flutter caused by disease.

2. Simple chest filming

As a basic examination of respiratory system disease, it can demonstrate little node lesions large than 5 mm. Its commonly position is used as following:

(1) P-A position is ordinary routine examinations position. The patient is placed in the erect position with the anterior portion of the chest in contact with the cassette and the X-ray travels through the patient from behind forward. The arms should be placed in such a position that the scapulae are drawn forward and outward, so that they are removed from the pulmonary field. A P-A position film should included all lung field, thoracic wall, costophrenic angle and inferior part of neck (Figure 6-1).

(2) Lateral position is usually used to locate lesions within lung or mediastinum, and to show the lateral forms

of lesions. In placing the patient in position for the lateral position, it is important to have the side involved by the lesion as close to the cassette as possible. This produces clearer definition of the shadows on the affected side (Figure 6-2).

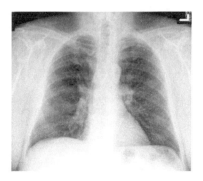
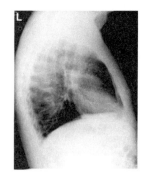

Figure 6-1   Normal chest: P-A position.   **Figure 6-2   Normal chest: lateral. position.**

(3) A-P position is usually used in those patients unable standing, who keep supine position and X-ray is projected fromanterior position.

(4) Lordotic position is used todemonstrate lesions located in apex of lung or the position overlapped with collarbone or lobs (Figure 6-3).

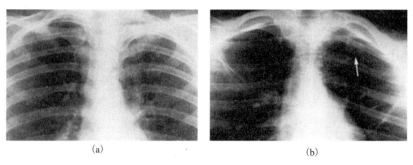

(a)   (b)

(a) On the frontal projection, there is an indistinct shadow at the left apex, mostly hidden by the first rib and the clavicle.

(b) On lordotic view, the shadows of the clavicle and first rib are displaced upward, exposing the lesion in the posterior portion of the upper lobe. This contains a thick-walled cavity (arrow), representing an active tuberculous lesion.

Figure 6-3   Use of lordotic position

3. High K. V. radiography

Radiography is obtained with high kilovoltage (above 120 kV). It has better diagnostic value for pneumoconiosis.

4. Bronchography

Bronchography shows the bronchial tree by instillation of contrast medium directly into the trachea or bronchi (Figure 6-4). It is now rarely performed, has nearly completely superseded by CT, and especially high resolution CT. The most commonly used contrast medium for bronchography is an aqueous suspension of propyliodone (Dionosil). Several techniques exist for instillation of the contrast medium, including a catheter introduced through the nostril or the mouth, and a direct needle puncture of the crico-thyroid membrane etc. Even coating of the bronchial mucosa is accomplished by injection of the contrast medium during inspiration. The most common indication for bronchography is haemoptysis. Bronchography is performed to definite a diagnosis of bronchiectasis and the extent and site of bronchiectasis if surgical treatment is contemplated, or to exclude a diagnosis of carcinoma.

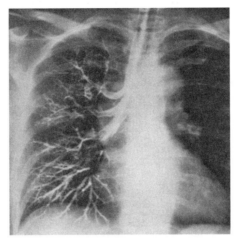

supernumerary bronchus. The bronchogram shows an anomalous bronchus arising from the lower trachea. It supplies the apical and posterior segments of the right upper lobe. The normal right upper lobe bronchus arises in its usual position.

Figure 6-4　Bronchography

5. Pulmonary angiography

Pulmonary angiography can clearly show lumen changes, vascular distortion or structural damage by injecting contrast agent directly into the main pulmonary artery or its large branches (Figure 6-5). It requires the passage of a catheter from an antecubital or femoral vein through the heart under fluoroscopic control. Pulmonary angiography is the most specific method for the demonstration of pulmonary emboli. Similarly pulmonary angiography is now seldom required in the assessment for operability of patients with bronchial cancer. It remains the best and most appropriate technique for the demonstration of pulmonary arteriovenous malformations and pulmonary varices.

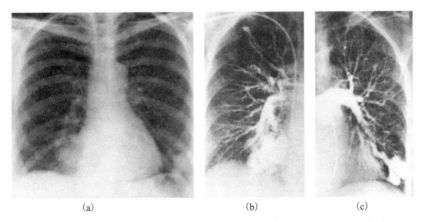

(a)　　　　　　　　　(b)　　　　　　　　　(c)

Pulmonary arteriovenous fistula. (a) The conventional film shows a lobulated density in the lower part of each lung. A large blood vessel extends from the mass on the left side toward the hilum. (b) Right pulmonary arteriogram. An early film shows the mass in the lower lobe to be composed of dilated, tortuous vessels. The vein (arrow) draining the lesion is opacified. A small fistula is seen in the upper lobe. (c) Left pulmonary arteriogram.

Figure 6-5　Pulmonary angiography

6. Computed tomography

CT scan is the commonly method in respiratory system. Chest CT can characterize the nature and extent of most thoracic tumors and lung diseases, by providing more precise characterization of the size, contour, extent, and tissue composition of the suspicious lesion. Contiguous 5 mm thick sections are usually obtained with the breath held at total lung capacity. Separate window widths and centers are needed to view the lungs and the mediastinum. The mediastinal structures are best demonstrated with a narrow window e. g. 300 and a center approximately that of soft tissue, e. g. 30 to 50HU. The lungs, pleura and mediastinal contour are best demonstrated with a wide window e. g. 1000 to 2000HU and a center of less than 0, usual between −600 to −800HU.

High-resolution CT (HRCT) has become established as a useful technique for the detection and characterization of diffuse lung disease. It is based on optimized imaging and reconstruction parameters to demonstrate lung anatomy with the greatest possible spatial resolution. The essential technical features of HRCT include the use of thin collimation, data reconstruction with a high-spatial-frequency sharp or bone algorithm, small pixel size derived from the use of a large image matrix and small FOV, and the use of increased kVp or mA. The thinnest collimation available on most scanners is 0. 5 to 2 mm(Figure 6−6).

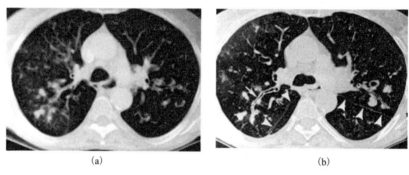

(a) Standard CT image obtained with 5−mm collimation demonstrates patchy areas of opacity in both lungs. (b) High-resolution image obtained at the same level as A. Bronchial dilatation and wall thickening (arrow), mucous −filled bronchi, and patchy infiltrates are more clearly recognized in this patient with cystic bronchiectasis. Note also the superior pleural margins of the oblique fissures (arrowheads), not detectable in a.

Figure 6−6　Comparison of conventional and high−resolution thin section technique

Intravenous contrast medium injection helps identify vascular structures and lymph nodes in the mediastinum and hila and also differentially diagnose lung nodule diseases(Figure 6−7). Approximately 100 ml of iodinated solution of 300mgI/ml are injected manually or with a power injection via the antecubital vein, and then scans the regions of interest continuously or scans at a single level (dynamic scanning).

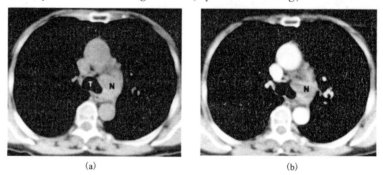

(a) Soft-tissue density mass (N) is seen in the aortopulmonary window, flattening the left side of the distal trachea (T). (b) Scan after administration of contrast material demonstrates no notable enhancement of markedly enlarged subaortic lymph nodes (N).

Figure 6−7　Intravenous administration of contrast material

In recent years, post-processing techniques such as multi-planar reformation (Figure 6 - 8), maximum intensity projection[Figure 6 - 9(a)], volume rendering[Figure 6 - 9(b)] have been rapidly developed in the diagnosis of respiratory diseases.

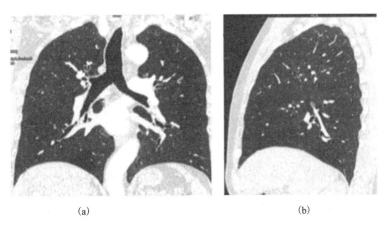

(a)   (b)

Figure 6-8 MPR image of the Chest

Low dose CT plays an important role in the initial screening of lung cancer high risk population.

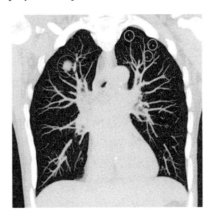

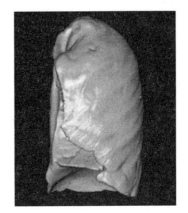

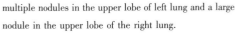

multiple nodules in the upper lobe of left lung and a large
nodule in the upper lobe of the right lung.

Figure 6-9(a) Chest MIP image shows   **Figure 6-9(b) VR image of left chest**

7. Magnetic resonance imaging

Magnetic resonance imaging currently has limited clinical value in lung. The poor signal potential of the aerated lung parenchyma is perhaps the most significant obstacle to successful MRI of this organ.

Because of its high contrast resolution and sensitivity to flowing blood, it may be utilized to assess extent of tumor invasion into the mediastinum and great vessels, to study possible vascular lesions in the chest, and in the assessment of pulmonary or mediastinal lesions in which fibrosis is a consideration.

An advantage of MRI is its direct multiplanar imaging capabilities. Sagittal and coronal images are the common supplements to transaxial images, MRI in any orientation is possible. This may be particularly helpful, especially in the assessment of vascular structures, the chest wall disease etc.

For chest MRI, SE and FSE sequence is usually used (Figure 6-10). T1-weighted images are excellent for depiction of anatomy. This is especially true in the mediastinum where the bright signal of fat provides excellent contrast between intermediate signal soft-tissue structures, such as lymph nodes, and the black signal void of vascular structures. Because of its sensitivity to the increased water content of tissue, T2-weighted imaging will help further characterize pathologic soft-tissue findings. To reduce artifacts caused by both respiratory and cardiac motion, breath-holding techniques are necessary to use, and respiratory gating and cardiac gating are frequently used. Intravascular gadolinium chelates have been used with T1-weighted images to diagnose lung vascular disease or lung nodule, to determine the extent of chest wall or mediastinal tumor invasion, or to study the extent of inflammatory or infectious lesions.

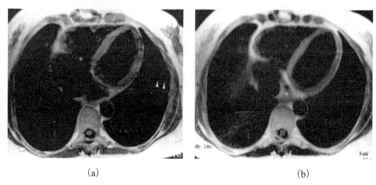

(a)   (b)

(a) Conventional transaxial T1-weighted spin-echo (SE) image of the heart. Arrowheads mark respiratory motion artifact. (b) On a FSE (TR 1000 msec; TE 43 msec) image, because of the speed of acquisition respiratory motion artifact is eliminated.

Figure 6-10

8. Ultrasound

Ultrasound provides a simple and reliable technique for distinguishing between pleural fluid and pleural thickening or tumor. Particularly when tumor and fluid coexist or the pleural fluid is localized. Ultrasound is a very valuable tool in detecting the placement of chest drainage tubes. If subphrenic infection is suspected ultrasonic examination is an inexpensive, noninvasive, widely available and sensitive technique for establishing the diagnosis. However, it is without more value in diagnosis of lung disease due to spine, ribs and intrapulmonary gases affecting ultrasound transmission.

9. Nuclear medicine

Nuclear medicine has high diagnostic value for vascular lesions, pulmonary tumors and bone metastases by using radionuclides and their markers to conduct pulmonary perfusion imaging and pulmonary ventilation imaging, among which pulmonary embolism is the main aspect of clinical application. Positron emission tomography can accurately diagnose lung cancer, mediastinal lymph node metastasis and distant metastasis.

Section 2　Normal appearances

1. Normal X-ray anatomy

(1) Soft tissue: Some soft tissues can be seen on the chest film and appear as opaque shadows. They should not be mistaken for pulmonary lesions.

①Sternocleidomastoid muscle: It shows as opaque shadows with well-indicate foreign border and homogeneous density inside of both apexes. Don't mistake it for lesions when both sides of shadows of sternocleidomastoid muscle aren't symmetry.

②Pectoralis major muscle: It appears as fan-like shadows with homogeneous density in middle and outer zones. The outside border is well-defined. The right side is obvious in general. Don't mistake it for lesions.

③The breast and nipple in females: Female breast can appear as semicircle shadows with well-defined lower margin and ill-defined upper margin locating at both lower lung fields. Nipples shadow are usually seen at 5th anterior intercostal space as essentially symmetrical nodule opaque. They are commonly found in older female, and occasionally in an adult male.

(2) Bones and cartilages

①Ribs: The ribs are long and thin. The front and back ends are arched. They start from both sides of the thoracic vertebrae and connect with the sternum through costal cartilage. Common congenital abnormalities of ribs are cervical rib, bifurcation of rib, and fusion of rib (figure 6-11) etc.

②Costal cartilages: They are invisible except when they become calcified. The first costal cartilage characteristically calcifies first of all in the early twenties. Other costal cartilages calcify gradually one by one upward from the lowest along with the addition of age. They appear as irregular patchy opacities, and they are essentially symmetrical.

③ Clavicle: The medial clavicular ends are important landmarks used together with the spine in assessing patient rotation on a radiograph. The rhomboid fossa is an inferomedial cortical

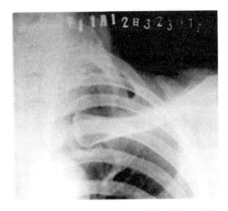

The PA view film demonstrates the fusion of the anterior ends of the first and second ribs.

Figure 6-11 Fusion of rib

irregularity related to the attachment of the costoclavicular ligament, it may be quite irregular and deeply excavated, don't mistake it for an erosive arthropathy.

④Scapula: The inner margin of the scapula may be overlapping with the outer zone of the lung. Don't confuse it with pleural thickening. The secondary ossification center of subscapularis cornu should not be mistaken for bone fracture.

⑤Sternum: This is well displayed in a lateral radiograph but inconspicuous on a frontal projection overlapping in which only the manubrium margins are sometimes visible and the source of confusing shadows may mimic mediastinal widening.

⑥Thoracic spine: Shadows of the transverse process of thoracic spines may be prominent out of the border of the shadow of the mediastinum. Don't mistake it for enlarged lymph nodes.

(3) Mediastinum

The mediastinum lies behind the sternum, in front of the thoracic spines, and between two sides of the lungs. The mainstructures of mediastinum include heart, large arteries and veins, trachea, bronchi, esophagus, lymph tissues, nerves, thymus, fat and associated areolar tissue etc.

Mediastinum is usually divided into anterior, middle, posterior, and superior, middle, and inferior regions according to lateral chest radiographs (Figure 6 - 12). The anterior mediastinum is along and narrow triangular zone behind the sternum and in front of the heart,

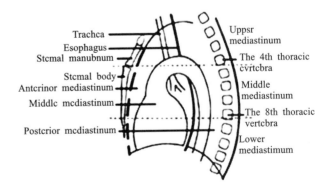

The sketch shows the mediastinum zones.

Figure 6-12 Mediastinum

ascending aorta, and trachea. The site of the middle mediastinum is equal to the site of the heart, aorta arch, trachea and hilum. The anterior wall of the esophagus is the boundary of middle and posterior mediastinum. The posterior mediastinum lies between oesophagus and thoracic spine. The upper, middle and lower mediastinum are divided by a line between the junction of the sternal manubrium and sternal body and the inferior margin of the fourth thoracic vertebra and horizontal line via the inferior margin of the hilum (the inferior margin of the eighth thoracic vertebra).

(4) Diaphragm

Each hemidiaphragm is normally represented on the PA chest film by a smooth curved line convex upwards. The lateral origin of the diaphragm onto the ribs is represented by the lateral costophrenic recess, a sharply defined acute angle, called costophrenic angle. The medial origin of the diaphragm onto the heart forms an angle called cardiophrenic angle. In most people the top of diaphragm in the mid-lung field lies at the level of the 5th or 6th anterior rib interspace. The right hemidiaphragm is higher than the left. This difference in height on the PA film is usually about 1.5 cm. The range of normal diaphragmatic movement is 1.0 cm to 3.0 cm, or 3 cm to 6 cm while deeply inhaling and exhaling.

(5) Pleura

The lung is covered with visceral pleura and the adjacent surfaces of the mediastinum, chest wall and diaphragm are lined by parietal pleura. The normal pleura around the periphery of the lung is invisible, but the normal interlobar fissure may be seen on chest film when it is tangential to the X-ray beam. The horizontal fissure is seen in about 70% of chest film (Figure 6-13). The oblique fissure sometimes is seen on the lateral chest film (Figure 6-14). It is invisible on P-A view. Normally, they appear as a hairline shadow.

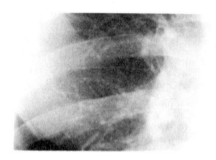

PA chest film shows the horizontal fissure (arrow) as a horizontal line.

Figure 6-13   Normal horizontal fissures

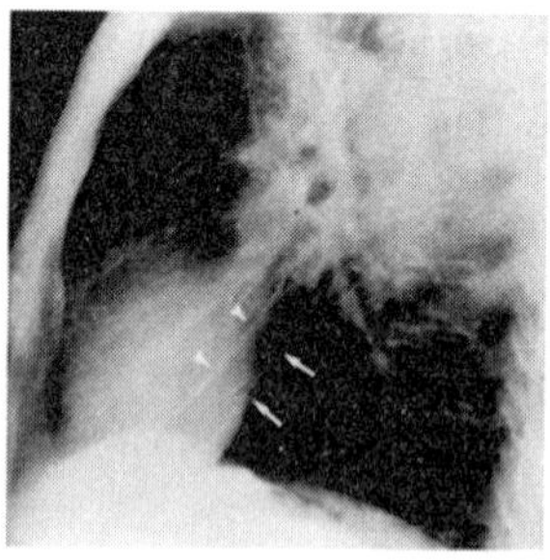

Note that both fissures are seen as double lines and that the left fissure (arrows) is behind the right fissure (arrowheads).

Figure 6-14   Normal major fissures. Lateral chest film demonstrates the two major fissures

(6) Trachea and bronchi

They are shown as a dark band. The trachea is seen superimposed on the upper vertebrae at P-A view chest film and divides into right and left main bronchus at the level of 5th or 6th thoracic spine.

The bifurcating angle is referred to as carina, which is normally about 60-85 degrees, but never exceeds 90 degrees. The course of the right main bronchus is more vertical than that of the left main bronchus. The right main bronchus subdivides into upper, middle and lower lobe bronchi, and the left right main bronchus subdivides into upper and lower lobe bronchi.

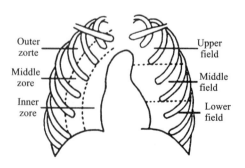

The lung is divided to three fields and three zones.

Figure 6-15   Lung fields

Farther, lobe bronchi divide into segmental bronchi and the segmental bronchi divide into smaller and smaller divisions until after 6 to 20 divisions which no longer contain cartilage in the walls and become bronchioles.

（7）Lungs

1）The lung lobes and lung fields

The lung fields do not correspond to actuarial lung lobes. The name of the lung field is usually for descriptive purpose, which is divided into an upper, middle and lower lung fields on each of the lung by horizontal lines between the anterior ends of the second and fourth ribs. The lung field is also divided longitudinally into 3 equal zones by drawing two imaginary lines. That is the inner, middle and outer zone（Figure 6-15）.

Anatomically each lung lobe is divided by interlobar fissue. There are two lobes on the left that is the upper and lower, which are separated by the oblique fissure and three on the right that is the upper, middle and lower lobes, which are separated by oblique and horizontal fissures. The oblique fissure has similar anatomy on the two sides. It runs obliquely forwards and downwards from approximately the fifth thoracic vertebra to contact the diaphragm 0 to 3 cm behind the anterior costophrenic angle, passing through the hilum. The horizontal fissure fans out forwards and laterally from the right hilum in a horizontal direction to reach the chest wall. There is an overlap of the lobes on P-A view chest film. Nonoverlap of the lobes is on lateral chest film. Usually only part of any fissure is seen.

Occasionally other fissures are present. The commonest is the so-called 'azygos lobe fissure' （Figure 6-16） seen in less than 1% of the population. It results from the abnormal position of the azygos vein. An inferior accessory fissure （figure 6-17）is sometimes seen in the lower lobe separation of the medial and anterior basal segments. This fissure runs obliquely upward and medially toward the hilum from the diaphragm.

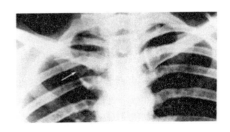

The sharply defined, curvilinear shadow （arrows） in the right upper lobe represents the azygos fissure.

Figure 6-16　Azygos lobe

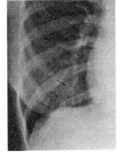

The thin, sharply demarcated, oblique line （arrows） represents a fibrous septum which separates the mesial basal segment from the remainder of the lower lobe.

Figure 6-17　Inferior accessory lobe

Each lobe divides into 2 to 5 segments, and each segment has their own bronchi. Their names are same to the name of bronchi. The pulmonary segment is composed of many pulmonary lobules, the diameter of which is about 1 cm.

2）The hilum of the lung

The composite hilar shadows include arteries, veins, bronchi, lymph tissues, nerves, and associated areolar tissue. In general the hila are equally dense and approximately the same size. The left hilum is higher than the right with 1 to 2 cm. The width of the right low artery does not exceed 15 mm. The height of left upper hilum is about 24 mm. The shape of the hilar shadow is the projection of the right and left large pulmonary arteries and veins. Right hilar angle is an obtuse angle between right upper pulmonary vein and right lower pulmonary artery. The upper left hilum is made up of left pulmonary artery arch, which appears as a semicircle shadow similar to a knob. Don't confuse it with a mass.

3）The lung markings

The lung marking is a linear shadow formed by pulmonary vascular branches, radiating outward from the hilum of lung, gradually thinning, and disappearing about 2 cm away from the edge of lung. The lung marking is composed of pulmonary artery, vein and lymphatic vessel.

4）Pulmonary parenchyma and interstitial tissue

The lung tissue is composed of parenchymatous tissue and interstitial tissue. The pulmonary parenchyma is the respiratory functional basic unit, including pulmonary alveoli and alveolar wall. The interstitial tissue is that portion of pulmonary framework composed of elastic and collagenous connective tissues that surround the bronchial tree, vessels, is between the alveolar sacs and under the pleura. The X-ray features of the diseases that affect the interstitial tissue are quite different from that of parenchymatous tissue.

2. Normal CT thoracic anatomy

The cross-sectional CT images display the fine anatomic detail of the thorax with great precision, and often yield unique and useful diagnostic information directly affecting the management or prognosis of the patient. This is due in large part to the fact that striking density differences exist between fat, muscle, skeletal structures, and lung parenchyma. As a fact, accurate identification of abnormalities will depend on a detailed knowledge of normal anatomy as well as an awareness of the wide range of anatomic variants that can exist. A brief introduction to thoracic anatomy based on eight representative transaxial images of the chest will be presented. This series of eight basic levels provides an orderly demonstration of the major structures in the chest and their associations.

（1）Thoracic inlet level［Figure 6-18（a）］: At about the level of the sternal notch, the trachea is typically midline and may be close to the adjacent vertebral body. The esophagus usually lies slightly to the left of the midline. Five major mediastinal vessels are usually noted anterior and lateral to the trachea. They include the three major branches of the aortic arch (the brachiocephalic, left common carotid, and left subclavian arteries) and the two brachiocephalic veins.

（2）Sternoclavicular joint level［Figure 6-18（b）］: This level typically contains two brachiocephalic veins anterior to three arteries usually positioned just anterior to the trachea.

（3）Aortic arch level［Figure 6-18（c）］: The aortic arch usually arises paralleling the superior border of the right second costal cartilage and after an oblique course extends posteriorly and to the left, becoming the descending aorta approximately at the level of the fourth thoracic vertebra. The anterior portion of the arch lies in front of the trachea and is intimately related to the anteromedial aspect of the superior vena cava. The midportion of the arch lies just to the left of trachea. Its posterior portion is just lateral to the esophagus.

（4）Aortopulmonary window level［Figure 6-18（d）］: Anatomically, this area comprises the region between the aortic arch cephalad and the left pulmonary artery as its caudal margin. The aortopulmonary window region contains the distal trachea, variable amounts of mediastinal fat just beneath to the arch medial to the descending aorta and above the left pulmonary artery, and a few small lymph nodes.

（5）Left pulmonary artery level［Figure 6-18（e）］: The posterior extension of the main pulmonary artery, the left pulmonary artery lies just to the left and lateral to the carina as it crosses over the left main stem bronchus. The left superior pulmonary vein often is visible lateral to the posterior portion of the left pulmonary artery.

（6）Main and right pulmonary artery level［Figure 6-18（f）］: The right pulmonary artery extends posteriorly and to the right of the main pulmonary artery, coursing behind the superior vena cava and anterior to the bronchus intermedius.

（7）Left atrium level［Figure 6-18（g）］: The left atrium lies between the aortic root and right atrium anteriorly, and the azygos vein, esophagus, and descending aorta posteriorly. The inferior pulmonary veins course into its posterolateral aspects. The aortic root lies to the right and posterior to the main pulmonary artery and right ventricular outflow tract.

（8）Cardiac ventricles level［Figure 6-18（h）］：The right ventricle both anterior and to the right of the left ventricle represents a significant portion of the heart's anterior surface. It is separated from the left ventricle by the obliquely oriented interventricular septum.

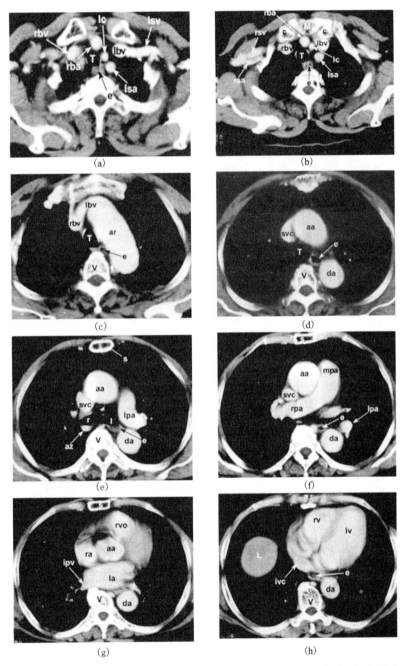

（a）Thoracic inlet level；（b）Sternoclavicular joint level；（c）Aortic arch level；（d）Aortopulmonary window level；（e）Left pulmonary artery level；（f）Main and right pulmonary artery level；（g）Left atrium level；（g）Cardiac ventricles level. rbv, right brachiocephalic veins；rba, right brachiocephalic artery；lc, left carotid artery；lsa, left subclavian artery；lsv, left subclavian vein；lbv, left brachiocephalic veins；T, trachea；e, esophagus；rsa, left subclavian artery；rsv, right subclavian vein；c, costal cartilage；m, manubrium；lc, left common carotid arteries；ar, aortic arch；v, vertebral body；svc, superior vena cava；aa, ascending aorta；da, descending aorta；az, azygos vein；r, right principal bronchus；l, left principal bronchus；lpa, left pulmonary artery；rpa, right pulmonary artery；mpa, main pulmonary artery；ipv, inferior pulmonary vein；rvo, right ventricle clavicles outflow tract；ra, right atrium；la, left atrium；L, liver；rv, right ventricle；lv, left ventricle.

Figure 6-18　Normal CT anatomy：mediastinum

3. Specific Anatomic Structures

（1）Trachea and bronchi

The trachea lies anterior or slightly to the right of the esophagus. The trachea is a cartilaginous and membranous tube. The normal tracheal wall is relatively thin. The ring cartilages may be irregularly calcified in the elderly, especially in women. The cross-sectional shape of the trachea varies greatly. It is usually round below the cricoid cartilage, oval when adjacent to the tracheal carina, and horseshoe shape in the middle. But in children, it is round.

The CT appearance of bronchi is closely associated with its size and direction. The origin and proximal portion of the horizontally coursing bronchi are routinely imaged on the transaxial CT sections. These include the right upper lobe bronchus (as well as its anterior and posterior segmental branches), the left upper lobe bronchus (and its anterior segment), the middle lobe bronchus (and generally some portion of both the medial and lateral segmental branches), and the superior segments of both lower lobes. The vertical bronchi is seen in cross-section. These include the apical segmental bronchus of the right upper lobe, the apical posterior segmental bronchus of the left upper lobe, the bronchus intermedius, and the proximal portions of both lower lobe bronchi (after the origin of the superior segments). The most difficult bronchi to recognize are those that course obliquely. These are the lingular bronchus (including the superior and inferior segments), as well as the basilar segmental bronchi. The origin of main bronchi appears as following(Figure 6-19).

（2）Parenchyma

Typically, vessels will be seen to the periphery on the lung images but there is almost always a small subpleural radiolucent zone, 3 to 5 mm in width, devoid of vessels. The bronchi, in distinction, normally are not seen in the outer 2 to 3 cm of the lung parenchyma. Understanding the anatomy of the secondary lobule is crucial to the recognition and categorization of pulmonary parenchymal abnormalities on HRCT. The secondary lobule varies in size from 6 to 25 mm in diameter and can appearpolygon shape. The centrilobular artery (about 1 mm in diameter) and the bronchiole (about 2 mm in diameter) enter at the central apex. Several perilobular veins are present in the septa, but the septa themselves are less than 1 mm in thickness and rarely seen normally.

（3）Pleura

The pleura is a double serous membrane which is not visible on CT under normal circumstances. The major fissures, with wider collimation, appear as somewhat indistinct broad lucent bands within the pulmonary parenchyma (Figure 6-20). They appear to be avascular because of the diminutive tapering of the pulmonary vessels in the most peripheral portions of the lobes. On thin sections, especially on HRCT, the major fissures are seen as lines (Figure 6-21). The orientation of thehorizontal fissure at the level sectioned determines the pattern of the lucent zone of relative paucity of vessels, in the right midlung field. Azygos fissure appears as a laterally convex curved line, extending from the right brachiocephalic vein or superior vena cava anteriorly to a posterior position alongside the lateral aspect of the T4 or T5 vertebra.

（4）Pulmonary Hila

CT images of pulmonary hila can clearly demonstrate the major pulmonary arteries and veins and the trachea and major bronchi, including most of the segmental orifices. Understanding the basic anatomic relationships facilitates CT diagnosis of hilar lymph node enlargement, and can permit the CT localization of bronchial obstructing lesions. Normal bronchopulmonary (hilar) lymph nodes are commonly seen on contrast enhanced helical scans. Other structures in the hilum such as lymphatic vessels, nerve plexi, and areolar tissue, all within a connective tissue envelope, are not defined on CT images.

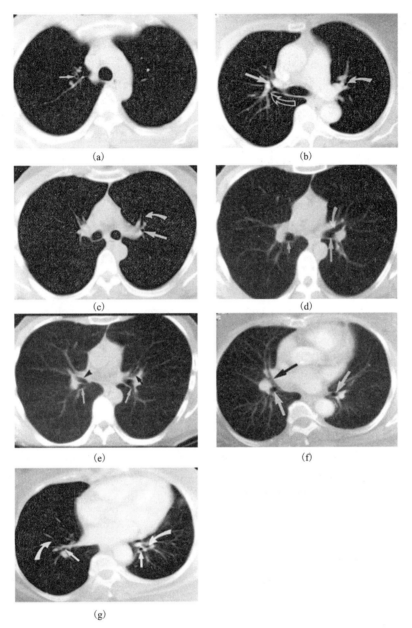

(a) Aortic arch (and distal trachea) level. The apical segmental bronchus (arrow) of the right upper lobe is seen; (b) Carina level. The apical posterior segmental bronchus is demonstrated (solid curved arrow). Anterior segment of the right upper lobe (straight arrow) and posterior segment branch (curved arrow) are also seen; (c) Left pulmonary artery level. The cephalad course of the apicoposterior segmental bronchus (straight arrow) and horizontal course of the anterior segment are depicted at this level; (d) Right pulmonary artery level. The bronchus intermedius (small arrow) is seen, with its thin posterior wall. On the left, the bifurcation of the left upper lobe (curved arrow) and lower lobe (straight arrow) are visible; (e) Slightly lower level. On the left, the lingular segment (black arrow) is seen. The origin of the middle lobe bronchus is seen on the right (arrowhead). Note the origins of the superior segment bronchi bilaterally (white arrows); (f) Left atrium level. The right middle lobe bronchus (black arrow) is seen anterior to the right lower lobe bronchus (white arrow). The left lower lobe bronchus is also demonstrated (white arrow); (g) Segmental bronchi. Curved arrows demonstrate the lateral basal segments bilaterally. Note the posterobasal segment bronchi (straight arrows).

Figure 6-19 Segmental bronchi

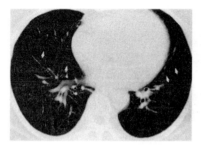

CT scan shows the major fissures as lucent bands of relative hypovascularity (arrows).

Figure 6-20　Normal major fissures

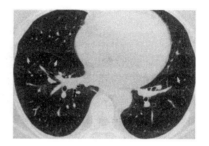

High-resolution CT scans show the major fissures as lines (arrows).

Figure 6-21　Normal major fissures

（5）Mediastinal lymph nodes

CT can show mediastinal lymph nodes well. Normal lymph nodes, usually oval or round in shape, soft-tissue densities, can be seen in up to 90% of patients, especially in the middle mediastinum. Lymph nodes less than 1 cm in cross-sectional diameter are considered normal by CT criteria, although such a normal size node may be involved with microscopic disease.

（6）Thymus

It is very important to recognize the changes of normal thymus size, shape and density on CT images to avoid misdiagnosis as mediastinal abnormal mass. Prior to puberty, this bilobed structure fills most of the anterosuperior mediastinum in front of the great vessels. The left lobe is usually slightly larger and situated slightly higher than the right lobe. In most of the remainder the lobes are confluent and the thymus assumes an arrowhead (or triangular) configuration. The maximum thickness of either lobe is 1.8 cm prior to age 20; thereafter, 1.3 cm is a maximal thickness although most normal lobes are less than 0.8 cm in width. In the pediatric and adolescent age group the density of the thymus is similar to that of the chest wall muscles. Usually after the age of 40 the organ approaches pure fat in attenuation value.

（7）Diaphragm

It is composed of a central tendon and peripheral leaf-like muscle extensions bilaterally. The anterior diaphragm most often appears as a relatively smooth, slightly undulating, soft-tissue arc, concave posteriorly and continuous across the midline. The posterior and caudal portion of the diaphragm, especially the crural part, which is oriented more vertically than the dome, is generally well defined on CT. The thicker right diaphragmatic crus arises from the first three lumbar vertebrae; the left crus is smaller and originates from the first two lumbar vertebrae.

4. Normal MRI appears

MRI provides morphologic distinctions based on magnetic tissue signal intensity differences. Mediastinal and hilar vascular structures are easily visible on T1-weighted images because the moving blood in their lumen produces no signal, in comparison to the higher signal intensity of other mediastinal structures. Those structures that are air-filled, such as the trachea, bronchi and pulmonary parenchyma, also are devoid of signal because of extremely low proton density. Muscle, mediastinal lymph nodes, and the collapsed esophagus are of intermediate signal intensity. The bones show characteristic high signal intensity in the marrow due to the abundance of fat, whereas the cortical regions are of low signal intensity due to low proton density. Thymus shows the relatively lower intensity and distinction from higher intensity mediastinal fat on T1-weighted images because of the long T1 of the thymus. The progressive decrease in T1 with advancing age reflects the fatty infiltration. The T2 relaxation times of the thymus do not change with age and overlap with those of fat.

Section 3　Basic pathological changes

It is divided into diseases of lung, the bronchus and the pleura.

1. X-ray and CT findings of basic pulmonary lesions

（1）Consolidation lesion

Consolidation lesion, in this situation, pathologically, the air within the acinus is replaced by fluid, blood, pus, cells, or other substances. It commonly occurs in infection, edema and hemorrhage of lungs, and less commonly occurs in pneumonia-type lung adenocarcinoma and alveolar proteinosis（Figure 6-22, 23）.

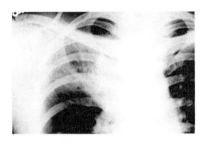

Pneumonia. Chest radiograph shows ill-defined opacities in the right upper field.

Figure 6-22　Consolidation lesion

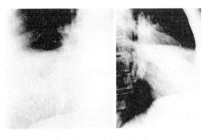

Pneumonia. On PA and lateral chest images, a large homogenous density opacity lies in the right middle lobe without loss of lung volume.

Figure 6-23　Consolidation

In the early stage or resorption stage of the lesion, the lesion do not completely fill the acinus, which shows as ground glass opacity that it could not completely cover of the pulmonary blood vessels. When the air in the acinus is completely replaced, it appears as a consolidation shadow covering the pulmonary blood vessels. Air bronchograms may be seen in consolidation opacity. As a general rule, there is no significant loss of lung volume in consolidation.

（2）Nodule and mass lesion

Pathologically, most of the pulmonary nodule and mass lesions are tumor, granuloma or tuberculoma. Multiple nodules or masses are often due to metastatic tumor. Among them, those with a diameter of ≤3 cm are called nodules（Figure 6-24）, and those with a diameter of >3 cm are called masses（Figure 6-25）. Nodules can be subdivided into large nodules（≤3 cm）, small nodules（≤1 cm）and miliary nodules（≤0.5 cm）according to their size.

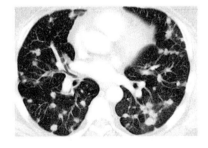

Metastasis tumor. Both lungs are diffusely distributed with random nodules, varying in size, some nodules are lobulated and spiculated.

Figure 6-24　Nodule lesion

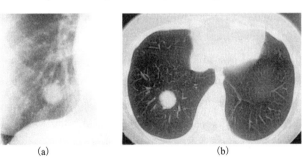

(a)　　　　　　(b)

（a）Localized posteroanterior chest radiograph shows a well-defined right lower lobe mass; （b）CT scan（lung windowing）shows a nonspecific, well-circumscribed mass.

Figure 6-25　Mass lesion: Solitary fibrous tumor

The nodule or mass lesion usually appears as: 1) Round, oval or irregular in shape. 2) Homogeneous and high in density. 3) Surrounded by lung tissue. 4) The border of the mass lesion usually is well-defined. The judgment of benign or malignant is mainly based on morphologic characteristics, density (i. e., calcium, fat, or contrast-enhancement), and growth rate.

(3) Cavitary and air containing space lesion

The cavitary lesion is formed as result of the expulsion of necrotic material into the bronchus. It is often seen in pulmonary abscess, tuberculosis and carcinoma (Figure 6-26). The air containing space lesions are pathological enlargement of physiological spaces in the lungs, which are common in lung bullae, lung cysts and lung air sacs (Figure 6-27).

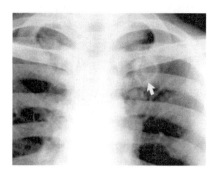

Chest film shows a thin walled cavity (arrow) with smooth lining in the apex of left lung. Satellite lesions also are seen.

Figure 6-26　Cavity lesion, tuberculosis

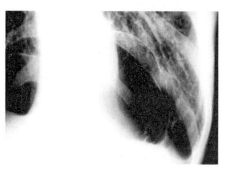

Bullae. PA view chest film demonstrates multiple bullae with various sizes in the left lower field.

Figure 6-27　Air containing space

The cavity appears as: 1) A radiolucent shadow with a definite thin or thick ring wall. 2) The inner lining may be smooth or irregular. 3) There may be an air-fluid level in the cavity. If the thickness of the wall of the cavity is less than 3 mm, it is termed the cavity of thin wall. If the thickness of the wall of the cavity is more than 3 mm, it is termed the cavity of thick wall. Thick-walled cavities are usually seen in lung abscess, squamous cell lung cancer, Wegners granulomatosis, etc. Thin-walled cavities are most commonly seen in tuberculosis. The lining of wall is irregular and nodular in lung cancer or shaggy in lung abscess. Tuberculous cavities are common in superior segments of upper and lower lobes. Lung cancer can occur in any segment and be seen more in the upper lobes. Most common cause for air fluid level is lung abscess. Air fluid levels can rarely be seen in malignancy and in tuberculous cavities.

Bulla and cyst are intrapulmonary air containing space varying in size and the wall is usually very thin. The thickness of the wall is usually less than 1 mm. The radiologic appearance is like a thin-walled cavity. It should not be mistaken as cavities.

The bulla is formed due to rupture of alveolar wall and communicated with each other. So the wall of the bulla is formed by atelectatic tissue. The cyst is formed by congenital cause or by some parasitic infection. The wall of the cyst is well-defined lined by epithelium or fibrous tissue.

(4) Fibrotic lesion

A number of lung diseases result in pulmonary fibrosis. Fibrosis can represent cellular fibrous tissue characterized by fibroblast proliferation or dense acellular collagenous tissue. Fibrotic lesion is divided into two types of local and diffuse fibrosis. The radiologic signs depend upon the process of disease. Local fibrosis usually is the end result of chronic pulmonary infection. It appears as a few or numerous irregular parallel or radiating linear shadows of varying thickness. They are high in density.

Diffuse fibrosis appears as widespread irregular linear shadows or reticular shadow or honeycomb shadows. It is often seen in pneumoconiosis, connective tissue diseases or idiopathic pulmonary fibrosis (Figure 6-28, 29).

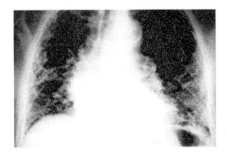

Idiopathic pulmonary fibrosis. Chest film demonstrates bilateral reticular and nodular interstitial infiltrates with lower fields predominance.

Figure 6-28　Fibrotic lesions

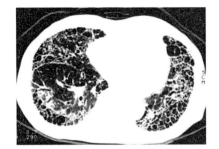

Idiopathic pulmonary fibrosis. HRCT shows widespread irregular linear shadows, reticular shadow and subpleural honeycomb shadows.

Figure 6-29　Fibrotic lesions

(5) Calcific lesion

Calcific lesion usually represents the healing process of a disease. It is an important sign to the assessment of pulmonary disease, indicating its benignity.

Calcification may appear as tiny spots or small nodules or egg-shell-like or popcorn-like or arc shadows. It is very high in density. Among them, eggshell, popcorn, or arc-shaped calcifications are typical benign calcifications (Figure 6-30).

(6) Interstitial lesion

Diseases that invade primarily the pulmonary connective tissue are called interstitial lesion. It may appear as widespread of: interlobular lines (kerley A and B lines), ground glass opacity, reticular shadows, and reticulo-nodular shadows. If the interstitial lesion is severe, it may appear as a honeycomb-like shadow. The interstitial lesion is often seen in pneumoconiosis, lymphangiitis carcinomas (Figure 6-31), sarcoidosis and interstitial pneumonia. CT, especially HRCT play an important role in diagnosis of interstitial lesion.

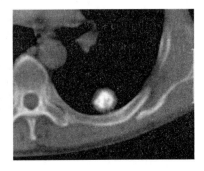

Hamartoma. CT scan demonstrates popcorn-like calcification within a well-circumscribed 2 cm left lower lobe nodule.

Figure 6-30　Calcific lesion

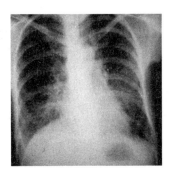

Lymphangitic metastasis of breast cancer. PA plain film demonstrates interlobular lines shadows in both lungs. Note infrapulmonary effusion on right.

Figure 6-31　Interstitial lesion

2. X-ray and CT findings of basic bronchial lesions

Obstruction of the bronchus is usually caused by tumor, foreign body, narrow, or exudation etc. Obstruction of the bronchus may results in obstructive emphysema (incomplete obstruction), obstructive atelectasis (complete obstruction) and obstructive pneumonia.

(1) Obstructive emphysema

Obstructive emphysema is characterized by permanent enlargement of alveoli and is accompanied by destruction of alveolar walls. It is subdivided into diffuse emphysema, localized emphysema, and bullous emphysema.

1) Diffuse obstructive emphysema

Diffuse obstructive emphysema is usually a complication of chronic bronchitis, asthma and tracheal tumors. Its X-ray features as follows: Lucency of both lungs, size of the thoracic cavity, and the diameter of the anterior-posterior of the thoracic cavity on lateral view increase. The ribs become more horizontal. The diaphragm appear depression and flattening. Lung markings appear thinner than normal. Heart shadow appearslong and narrow between the hyperinflated lungs on both sides.

2) Localized emphysema

If the incomplete obstruction occurs in the main bronchus, lobar or segmental bronchus, the emphysema will be localized to the affected anatomic area (Figure 6-32). The features on chest plain film as follows: Lucency of the affected region increases. Lung markings appear as thinner of the involved area. The mediastinum may shift to the unaffected. The mediastinum deviates from the normal position during expiration and return to the normal position during inspiration on fluoroscopy. This is called the pendular movement of the mediastinum.

3) The bullous emphysema

When incomplete obstruction of the bronchus or bronchiolus, the bullous emphysema can be formed. The X-ray features are similar to a cavity of thin wall. But the whole wall usually cannot be observed.

The CT features of emphysema include lucency areas without visible walls, pruning of pulmonary vessels, pulmonary vessel distortion, and decreased lung density gradients (Figure 6-33). Computed tomography provides helpful information regarding the severity and distribution of emphysema, and may disclose unsuspected concomitant conditions such as bronchiectasis, or an occult bronchogenic carcinoma not detected on the plain chest radiograph.

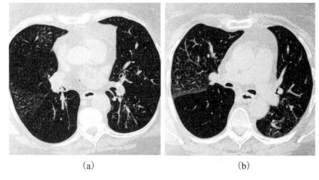

(a)   (b)

(a) CT demonstrates a polypoid mass (arrow) in the bronchus intermedius; (b) Scan obtained in expiration demonstrates marked lucency areas in the right lower lobe. An aspirated piece of cauliflower was found at bronchoscopy and removed.

Figure 6-32   Obstructive emphysema

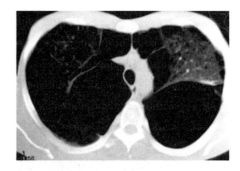

CT in a patient with paraseptal emphysema shows multiple large bulla.

Figure 6-33   Bullous emphysema

（2）Obstructive atelectasis

Complete obstruction of the bronchus results in obstructive atelectasis. Atelectasis means incomplete expansion of the lung or of a portion of the lung. It is divided into 3 forms of obstructive atelectasis, cicatrization atelectasis and compressed atelectasis. The atelectatic lung contains less air than normal lung, so the X-ray feature is a homogenous radiopaque shadow. The shape and position of the shadow depends on the degree of collapse and which lobe or lobes collapse.

1）X-ray features of atelectasis of an entire lung（Figure 6-34）: The affected side presents homogeneous opacity with elevation of hemidiaphragm. Mediastinum displace to the affected side. The intercostals spaces on the affected side become narrowing. Compensatory emphysema on the opposite side lung appears.

2）X-ray features of lobar atelectasis: The affected lobe appears as a dense triangular shadow. The apex of the triangular shadow is at the hilum and its base is at the outside. The hilum and mediastinum displace to the affected area. Compensatory emphysema in the adjacent lobe appears.

X-ray features of the right middle lobar atelectasis（Figure 6-35）: On P-A view, there is opacity at the right paracardiac area, and the right border of the heart is hazy. On lateral view, there is an opaque triangular shadow on the area of the right middle lobe, its apex is at the hilum and its base is against the sternum. On lordotic view, there is an opaque triangular shadow at the right paracardiac area, its apex is at the outside, and its base is against the heart border.

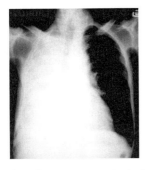

PA chest film shows homogeneous opacity in the right side, mediastinum displaced to right and compensatory emphysema of the left lung.

Figure 6-34　Atelectasis of the entire right lung

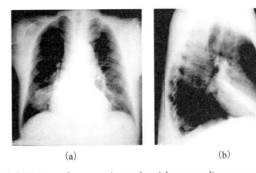

(a)　　　　　　　　(b)

(a) PA view shows opacity at the right paracardiac area with ill-defind border; (b) lateral view shows triangular shadow on the area of the right middle lobe and apex at the hilum.

Figure 6-35　Atelectasis of right middle lobe

CT is often helpful in clarifying that the plain film findings are secondary to collapse, and furthermore may suggest the cause and determine the extent of any obstructing mass. Both the direct（fissural displacement, decreased size of hemithorax, vascular/bronchial crowding）and indirect（mediastinal shift, hilar displacement, hypoaeration, compensatory hyperaeration, elevation of hemidiaphragm）signs of collapse seen on plain chest radiographs can be applied to CT. The lobes lose volume while generally maintaining contact with the chest wall peripherally and the hilum centrally, resulting in a wedge shape on CT, which is not always apparent on conventional radiograph.

3. X-ray and CT findings of basic pleural lesions

（1）Pleural effusion

Pleural effusions are the most common pleural pathology. The pleural space normally contains a small amount of pleural fluid, which provides lubrication. Pleural effusions develop when the rate of fluid production is increased, such as in heart failure, or when resorption is impaired, such as in lymphatic obstruction by tumor. According to the distribution of pleural effusion and it is free or encysted. It can be divided into pleural free fluid, pleural encysted fluid, interlobar fluid and infrapulmonary fluid.

1) Free pleural effusion: According to the amount of effusion, it can be further divided into large, medium and small amount of free pleural effusion

① Moderate amount of free fluid

When the patient is erect, the fluid collects at the lower portion of the pleural cavity. The costophrenic angles and hemidiaphragm are obscured. The upper border of the shadow of the free fluid is concave.

The concave border is formed due to the influence of fluid gravity, the resistance of the lung to expansion, the capillary attraction of the pleural cavity, the X-ray pass tangentially through the layer of fluid (as it curves around the lung) because lateral area of the fluid is more thicker than the other areas. So there is a curve of free fluid that is highest at the outside and the concave face is upward on P-A view (Figure 6-36).

② Large amount of free fluid

The shadow of large amount of free fluid is similar with the middle amount fluid. But the hilum of the lung is obscured and there is displacement of mediastinum to the opposite side.

③ Small amount of free fluid

When the costophrenic angle is obscured, while the hemidiaphragm have not been obscured entirely by the fluid, in this situation, we call the small amount free fluid. If the fluid in the pleural cavity is less than 300cc, it only shows blunting of the costophrenic angle.

2) Pleural encysted fluid

Encapsulated pleural effusion is caused by adhesion of visceral and parietal pleura. The fluid is localized in the pleural cavity. It appears as a homogeneous semicircular or fusiform shadow with a wide base against the chest wall and a convex inner, sharply defined border.

3) Interlobar pleural effusion

The fluid collects in the interlobar fissure, it appears as a fusiform-shaped shadow (Figure 6-37). The long axis is the involved interlobar fissure line. The shadow is close to the lung on both sides and the edge is clear (Figure 6-37).

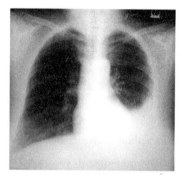

PA view shows homogenous density in left lower filed. Costophrenic angle and hemidiaphragm are obscured. The upper border of liquid is a curve with high outside and low medial.

Figure 6-36   Pleural effusion

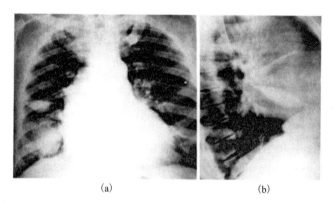

(a)   (b)

(a) Two shadows are seen in the right lung. The upper is sharply outlined and fusiform in shape and is oriented horizontally. The lower shadow is round in shape;
(b) The collection of fluid in each fissure is well demonstrated in the lateral view.

Figure 6-37   Interlobar effusion

Lateral position is the necessary position to judge the effusion of interlobar fissure, and other positions are sometimes useful.

4) Infrapulmonary pleural effusion

The fluid is situated between the lung and hemidiaphragm, when the patient is erect. The lung floats on the fluid. The shadow is similar to an elevated hemidiaphragm (Figure 6-38). But the fluid is free to move with change in the position of the patient. It provides a definite method for confirming the diagnosis of infrapulmonary effusion.

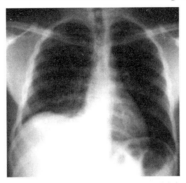

Its X-ray appearance is similar to an elevated hemidiaphragm on PA chest film while patient is erect.

Figure 6-38　The right infrapulmonary pleural effusion

CT is well suited to evaluating the location and size of fluid collections, and may demonstrate a pleural effusion not detected on radiographs. In the supine position, mobile pleural fluid initially collects in the posteromedial hemithorax (Figure 6-39). As an effusion increases in size, it conforms to the pleural space and may extend laterally, displacing lung away from the thoracic wall. Pleural effusions usually cause at least some compressive atelectasis of the underlying lung. Large pleural effusions usually result in lower lobe collapse with upward displacement of the collapsed lobe (Figure 6-40).

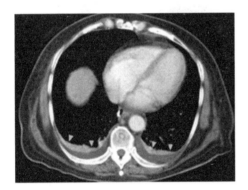

Contrast-enhanced CT examination of the thorax shows the characteristic enhancement of atelectatic lung (arrowheads) in this patient with small bilateral pleural effusions.

Figure 6-39　Pleural effusion

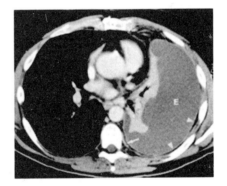

The atelectatic lung is enhanced. The thin line of enhancement at the interface of the chest wall and fluid (arrowheads) represents the parietal pleura separated from the thoracic wall by abundant extrapleural fat.

Figure 6-40　Large pleural effusion (E) with compressive atelectasis

CT also can identify localized pleural fluid in nondependent locations and distinguish pleural fluid collections from pleural masses or true lung parenchymal lesions. Localized collections are typically lenticular in cross section. Fluid localized within a fissure due to adhesions may produce a "pseudotumor," which can simulate an intrapulmonary mass.

Most pleural effusions, whether transudative or exudative, have a homogeneous, near-water attenuation. Higher density effusions are almost always exudates. Pleural fluid having attenuation similar to or higher than soft tissue is suggestive of a hemothorax.

(2) Pneumothorax

There are 2 ways of the air entering the pleural cavity. One is the rupture of the parietal pleural, due to trauma, when there is a wound to the chest, air leaks into the pleural cavity. The other is the rupture of the visceral pleura, usually occurs with no penetrating wound, called spontaneous pneumothorax.

Pneumothorax is due to air accumulating in the pleural cavity between the lung and the chest wall. In this situation, the lung is compressed, creating a zone of high radiolucency, devoid of lung markings in this zone. The sharply defined border of the visceral pleura over the collapsed lung can always be recognized (Figure 6-41). If large amount air is in the pleural cavity, the lung remarkable collapsed to the hilum. The mediastinum is displaced to the opposite site.

CT may be useful in differentiating a large bulla from a pneumothorax suspected on a conventional radiograph. CT also may be useful in detecting bullae and emphysematous lesions in patients with primary spontaneous pneumothorax, which may warrant resection to prevent recurrences.

(3)Hydropneumothorax

When the pleural cavity contains air and fluid, it is termed hydropneumothorax.

Thecharacteristic appears of the hydropneumothorax are with an air-fluid level in the pleural cavity (Figure 6-42). The air-fluid level extends across the entire hemi-thorax unless the air and fluid are encysted due to adhesion of pleura.

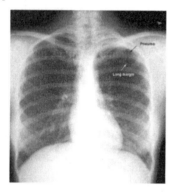

Note the high radiolucency, no vascular markings in the upper field outer zone. Lung margin is well defined.

Figure 6-41 Spontaneous Pneumothorax

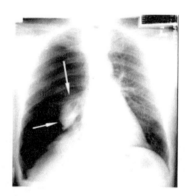

Chest film demonstrates the no vascular markings high radiolucency on right, shift of mediastinum to left, atelectatic right lung (arrow), increased haziness on left due to diversion of entire cardiac output. Note the Small fluid level near costophrenic angle.

Figure 6-42 Hydropneumothorax

(4)Pleural thickening, adhesion and calcification

Pleural thickening may be focal or diffuse, and is usually the result of a inflammatory or infectious process. The pleural thickening appears as an opaque shadow. The shape is usually a band-like, along the chest wall or a faint opaque hazy shadow on the lower portion of the chest on P-A view (Figur6-43). If the thickened pleura are severe and extensive, it can appear as narrow intercostals spaces, and displacement of the mediastinum to the affected side. Pleural adhesion between the visceral and parietal pleural does not cast a shadow unless they are associated with marked pleural thickening. Sometimes, the pleural adhesion affects the shape of the diaphragm. It becomes elevated and is not smooth. Pleural calcification appears as a high dense vertical line or high dense band-like shadow along the chest wall, or high dense linear shadow along the diaphragm.

CT can clearly demonstrate the extent and characteristics of the pleural thickening and calcification. CT is more sensitive than conventional radiography in demonstrating focal pleural plaques (Figure 6-44), especially in depicting involvement of the mediastinal and paravertebral pleura.

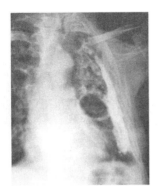

The extensive pleural calcification followed a tuberculosis pleurisy appears band-like density paralleling the chest wall, and geographic type shadow in left lung. Irregularities in the distribution of the calcium are responsible for the lucent areas resembling cavities in the lung.

Figure 6-43 Pleural calcification

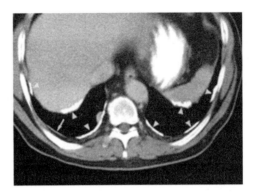

Extensively calcified pleural plaques are seen, relatively symmetric, involving the posterior paraspiral pleura as well as the pleura along both hemidiaphragmatic surfaces (arrowheads). A small, noncalcified plaque (arrows) is also present.

Figure 6-44 Asbestos-related pleural plaques

4. MRI findings of basic lesions

MRI currently has limited clinical value in lung. It is mainly utilized to assess pulmonary tumor and vascular lesions, etc.

Pulmonary tumors are recognized by their increased T2 on SE scans. These are usually not well seen on T1WI images as their long T1 produces little contrast with the low signal of lung. Hilar masses are readily distinguished from blood vessels and bronchial walls. Other signs of hilar masses may also be seen, including bronchial obstruction and displacement. The T2 relaxation time of tumor is relatively short in comparison with of collapsed or consolidated lung tissue, so distinguishing parahilar masses from collapsed and consolidated lung isfeasible on T2WI images, however it is difficult on T1WI images.

Section 4 Diagnosis of common diseases

1. The Disease of Lung

(1)Pneumonia

Pneumonia is consolidation caused by pulmonary infection. X-ray examination plays an important role in the diagnosis and treatment of the disease. There are two kinds of classification methods of pneumonia: one is divided into lobar pneumonia, lobular pneumonia and interstitial pneumonia according to anatomical location, the other is classified according to etiology. The latter has no practical value in X-ray diagnosis.

1)Lobar pneumonia

①The clinical and pathological manifestations: Lobar pneumonia is usually caused by pneumococcus. The onset is usually sudden. The initial symptoms are due to rapid development of high pyrexia (up to 39.5℃), which may induce a rigor, pleuritic pain. Cough may be absent during the first 24 hours or the whole course of the illness. After a few days sputum, which often has a characteristic rusty color, becomes a conspicuous feature. The basic pathologic lesion is acute inflammatory exudation of the pulmonary parenchyma.

②Imaging manifestations: lobar pneumonia can be divided into three stages according to X-ray findings.

The congestive stage (it is about 24 hours after onset.): Pathologically, the early stage of lobar pneumonia consists of inflammatory edema. It may be no X-ray changes, or with an increase of lung markings or with a faint shadow in the inflammatory area because many of the alveoli are still aerated.

The consolidation stage: At this stage, the air in the alveoli is replaced by exudates at the infected area. The X-ray feature is a large homogenous radiopaque shadow in the lung field, usually, there is no volume loss and air bronchogram is common (Figure 6-45). Because the air in the alveoli is replaced by exudates, while the air in the bronchus is not displaced and remain patent. This produces contrast between the air in the bronchial tree and the surrounding airless parenchyma. Borders of the shadow are ill-defined. If the border abuts against a fissure, it must appear as a sharply defined margin. For example, the lower border of a consolidated anterior segment of the right upper lobe, which is limited by the horizontal fissure, appears as a sharp, straight, horizontal line (Figure 6-46). Similarly, the right middle lobar pneumonia, the upper border of the shadow must be sharp and the lower border must be ill-

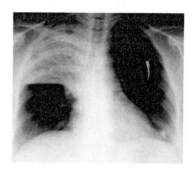

The right upper lobe consolidated appears as a large homogenous radiopaque shadow with a sharp lower border. Air bronchogram is seen.

Figure 6-45 Lobar pneumonia of right upper lobe

defined. The shape of consolidation of different lobes is different, if only one portion of a segment is involved, the shadow may be round and simulate a neoplasm (Figure 6-47). The clinical history and the rapid change in the size and appearance of the shadow within a few days make the diagnosis quite clear.

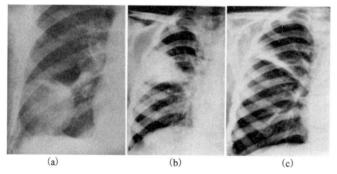

(a)   (b)   (c)

(a) the consolidation involves most of the axillary portion of the anterior segment of the right upper lobe. The inferior border of the consolidated lung is bounded by the horizontal fissure; (b) During resolution, the anterior segment has become partially atelectatic because of plugging of many of the small bronchi by exudates. The horizontal fissure is elevated; (c) After complete resolution, the right upper lobe appears normal. The horizontal fissure (arrow) has returned to its normal position, indicating that the lobe has completely reexpanded.

Figure 6-46 Lobar Pneumonia Anterior segment, right upper lobe.

Resolution stage: At the stage, the alveolar exudates are absorbed through the lymphatics and alveoli are filled with air. So the shadow of consolidation becomes scatter. Complete resorption of the lesion usually takes about 2 weeks after onset. In some cases, resorption may be delayed up to one or two moths. The shadows of lesions are mottled and the blood vessels are usually drawn together because of the atelectasis due to obstruction of many of the smaller bronchi. When only the posterior segment of an upper lobe is involved, the presence of localized areas of aeration within the consolidated region, looking like cavitation, may lead to a mistaken diagnosis of suppurative bronchopneumonia or tuberculosis (Figure 6-48). Subsequent films show rapid resolution, that can suggest the diagnosis of lobar pneumonia.

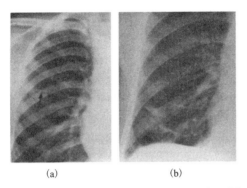

(a)　　　　　　(b)

（a）The sharply demarcated, round shadow in the lateral basal segment of the right lower lobe resembles a tumor; （b）A week later all that remains of the lesion are several areas of discoid atelectasis.

Figure 6-47　Lobar pneumonia

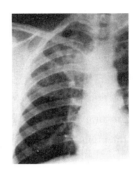

The irregular shadows in the right upper lobe look like a tuberculous lesion. Although the diagnosis of resolving pneumonia may be quite evident clinically, it cannot be made radiologically without serial films.

Figure 6-48　Lobar Pneumonia：Stage of resolution

Standard chest radiography is the primary technique for evaluating lobar pneumonia. CT can be helpful in complex cases. The findings are similar to those seen with plain film. Air bronchograms are well demonstrated within areas of consolidation (Figure 6-49).

2）Lobular pneumonia (bronchopneumonia)

① The clinical and pathological manifestations：Lobular pneumonia is often caused by streptococcus, staphylococcus, pneumococcus, klebsiella pneumoniae, pseudomonas aeruginosa and haemophilus influenzae etc. They are usually only cause pulmonary infection in patients with a predisposing factor such as diabetes, alcoholism, tracheostomy, chronic bronchitis, bronchiectasis, cystic fibrosis and immune-deficiency states due to disease or drugs. The common symptoms are fever, cough, purulent sputum and pleuritic pain etc.

② Imaging manifestations：

X-ray findings included intensification of lung markings. Small patchy opaque shadows are seen in the middle and lower lung fields especially nearby the heart border (Figure 6-50). Emphysema of the both lungs is usually visible. Confluence of these patchy opacities may produce segmental large area of consolidation. Delayed or incomplete resolution may result in bronchiectasis and fibrosis.

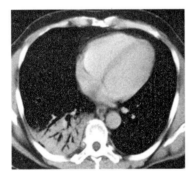

CT shows right lower lobe pulmonary consolidation with air bronchograms.

Figure 6-49　Lobar pneumonia of right lower lobe

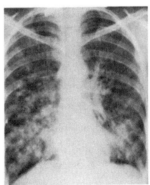

The poorly demarcated nodular shadows in the lower half of each lung represent areas of lobular consolidation. The patient was acutely ill and expectorating purulent sputum.

Figure 6-50　Lobular pneumonia

The diagnosis of lobular pneumonia usually can be made on plain chest film. CT is more helpful to demonstrate the distribution and severity of pulmonary consolidation, presence of cavitation, mediastinal lymphadenopathy, or a parapneumonic effusion more clearly(Figure 6-51).

3)Interstitial pneumonia

① The clinical and pathological manifestations: Interstitial pneumonia involves mainly the interstitial tissue of lungs, including the bronchovascular bundles, fissures, interlobular and intralobular septa. It may be caused by viral or bacterial infection, and usually secondary toacute infective diseases such as measles, pertussis or influenza etc.

② Imaging manifestations:

The X-ray features of interstitial pneumonia (Figure 6-52): There are fine streak-like, net-like, nodular or nod-reticular shadows in the both lung fields, mainly in the middle and lower lung field. Emphysema of both lungs is usually seen. Possibly there is enlargement and increase in density of the hilar shadow. This is due to perivascular and peribronchial inflammation and lymphadenitis.

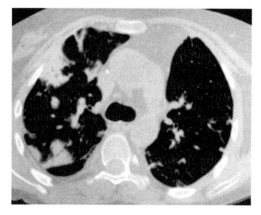

CT demonstrates multifocal areas of consolidation and air bronchograms.

Figure 6-51 Lobular pneumonia

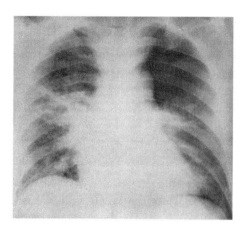

Fine and coarse interstitial infiltrations extend outward from the lung roots. In the lower part of the right upper lobe there is an oblique linear streak, representing a focal area of atelectasis due to plugging of a bronchus by secretion. The area of radiolucency in the left upper lobe is caused by a large bulla.

Figure 6-52 Interstitial infiltrations in viral pneumonia

CT, especially HRCT can depict the early sign of interstitial pneumonia. It may present as thickened septa, regional reticulation or nodules.

4)Hypersensitivity pneumonia

① The clinical and pathological manifestations: This entity, also referred to as extrinsic allergic alveolitis, is an immunologically mediated response to organic dust in the environment. Farmer's lung and bird fancier's lung are two commonly recognized types. Hypersensitivity pneumonitis may occur in acute, subacute, or chronic form. Symptoms of acute hypersensitivity pneumonia typically occur 4-6 hours after antigen exposure. Cough, dyspnea, fever, chills and malaise characterize the acute episodes. Of subacute or chronic form, symptoms develop more gradually and include cough, dyspnea on exertion, malaise, anorexia, and weight loss.

② Imaging manifestations:

Radiographic findings are variable with diffuse air-space consolidation. Within days, the radiographic findings change to the nodular or reticulonodular pattern characteristic of the subacute form. They are more severe in the lower zones of the lung. The most common radiographic abnormalities of chronic form are centrilobular nodules, linear opacities, and an increase in lung density.

Acute hypersensitivity pneumonitis presents as airspace disease, usually with areas of ground-glass attenuation and small ill-defined centilobular nodular opacities representing granulomas or bronchiolitis on HRCT (Figure 6-53). Linear opacities usually indicate fibrosis. In chronic hypersensitivity pneumonitis, HRCT demonstrates indistinct centrilobular nodular opacities and diffuse peripheral pulmonary fibrosis with relative sparing of the lung bases (Figure 6 - 54). HRCT provides superior assessment of the interstitial lung disease than plain chest radiography.

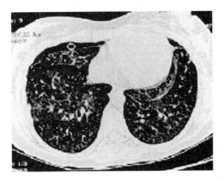

HRCT scan with 1-mm-thick axial images. Diffuse ground glass opacification through both lung fields is noted. Nodular opacities, a thickened interstitium, and pneumothorax present.

Figure 6-53 Hypersensitivity pneumonitis (bird fancier's lung)

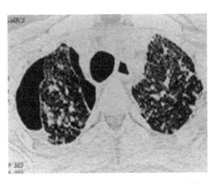

The image of HRCT depicts a persistent right pneumothorax. Diffuse ground glass opacification through both lung fields is noted. Nodular opacities, a thickened interstitium are more prominent.

Figure 6-54 Chronic hypersensitivity pneumonitis (bird fancier's lung)

(2) Lung abscess

1) The clinical and pathological manifestations: All the symptoms of pneumonia including high pyrexia and pleuritic pain may be present. Pulmonary necrosis communicates with a bronchus, which leads to cough and copious amounts of sputum. It is the most conspicuous feature. The sputum is often foul smelling and blood-stained. Massive haemoptysis may occur.

2) Imaging manifestations:

Acute stage: The lung abscess begins as an area of gangrenous bronchopneumonia. Radiological features are similar to lobar pneumonia, pulmonary shadowing which is usually lobar or segmental, but multiple pulmonary opacities may be seen.

Subacute stage: The subacute stage is arbitrarily defined as the period between 6 weeks and 3 months after the onset of infection. During this period fibrosis of the wall becomes established. It usually appears as①A cavity or multiple abscess cavities with air-fluid level [Figure 6-55(a), (b)]as air enters these foci. ②The cavity with thick wall surrounded by exudative lesion. In occasional cases, the abscess does not establish an adequate bronchial communication. It remains as a solid round shadow of uniform density. The pus-filled abscess has the appearance of a pulmonary neoplasm.

Chronic stage: After 3 months, the abscess is considered to be chronic. There are one or more irregular cavities and with multiloculation, some fibrotic lesions nearby the cavity or in the cavitary wall. Thickened pleura are usually seen.

Hematogenous lung abscess: Multiple abscesses are found in both lungs.

(3) Pulmonary tuberculosis

In 1998, the Chinese Antituberculous Association adapted a new classification of pulmonary tuberculosis. It has been divided into 5 types as follows: Primary tuberculosis (Type Ⅰ); Hematogenous pulmonary tuberculosis (Type Ⅱ); Secondary pulmonary tuberculosis (Type Ⅲ); Tuberculous pleuritis (Type Ⅳ); Extrapulmonary tuberculosis (Type Ⅴ)

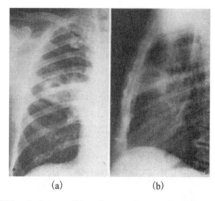

(a)　　　　　　(b)

(a)The shadow overlying the anterior portion of the fourth rib contains an air-fluid level, indicating that it represents a cavity; (b) The later view shows the cavity within the anterior segmet of the upper lobe.

Figure 6-55(a)　Lung abscess

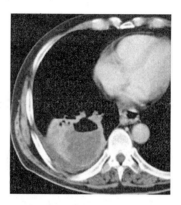

thick irregular wall surrounds a low-density center containing air and fluid. The cavity appears peripheral enhancement and central necrosis. There is some adjacent pulmonary consolidation and atelectasis present as well as a small pleural effusion.

Figure 6-55(b)　Lung abscess in the right lower lobe.

1) Primary tuberculosis (Type Ⅰ)

① The clinical and pathological manifestations: The first infection with the tubercle bacillus results in 'primary tuberculosis'. It is most often encountered in children, usually young people. It frequently produces little constitutional upset and it has no specific symptoms. Symptoms are slight include loss of weight and appetite, malaise, pyrexia, night sweat and cough which may or may not be productive.

② Imaging manifestations: Two forms of X-ray features are primary complex tuberculosis and hilar tuberculous lymphadenitis.

Primary complex tuberculosis: The combination of the primary pulmonary tuberculous focus, lymphangitis and intrathoracic lymphadenitis is known as the primary complex tuberculosis. It occurs chiefly in children.

Its X-ray appears as an exudative lesion in any portion of the lung field and combined with the ipsilateral enlargement of hilar lymph nodes or mediastinal lymph nodes, and/or pleural effusion (Figure 6-56). Typically, there are streaky shadows leading from the exudative lesion to the enlarged intrathoracic lymph nodes. It represents the lymphangitis. But this manifestation is often invisible on chest film.

Hilar tuberculous lymphadenitis (intrathoracic tuberculous lymphadenitis): The primary focus is usually absorbed quickly. The intratheracic lymph nodes remain enlarged and visible on chest film. This manifestation is known as hilar tuberculosis or intrathoracic

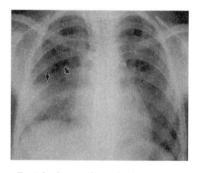

Frontal chest radiograph demonstrates consolidation in the right middle lobe (straight arrow) with right hilar adenopathy (curved arrow).

Figure 6-56　Consolidation in primary tuberculosis

tuberculous lymphadenitis. The margin of the enlarge lymph nodes may be clear or hazy. Maybe, It is known as the type of tumor or the type of inflammation, respectively.

CT helps confirm the presence of an ill-defined parenchymal infiltrate, as well as lymphadenopathy[Figure 6-57(a), (b)]. Mediastinal lymphadenopathy and pleural effusions may accompany the primary infection and in some cases adenopathy may be the only intrathoracic manifestation. The involved lymph nodes in patients with tuberculosis often demonstrate central areas of necrosis, which are low in attenuation on CT, especially on post-contrast-enhanced scan with peripheral rim enhancement.

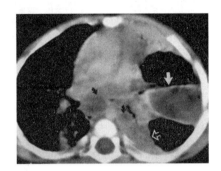

Axial contrast enhanced computed tomographic (CT) scan demonstrates a parenchymal lung cavity (solid white arrow) with enlarged necrotic subcarinal lymph nodes (black arrows). There is accompanying collapse of the left lower lobe (open arrow).

Figure 6-57(a)　Pulmonary parenchymal changes and lymphadenopathy in primary tuberculosis.

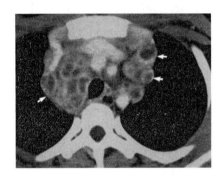

Axial contrast-enhanced CT scan demonstrates multiple enlarged mediastinal lymph nodes with central areas of low attenuation and peripheral enhancement (arrows).

Figure 6-57(b)　Mediastinal tuberculous adenopathy

③Prognosis of the primary tuberculosis: Both the primary focus and enlargement of lymph nodes may completely be absorbed and leave no trace. The primary focus and enlargement of lymph nodes may calcify. c. Fibrous or granulation tissues will encapsulate the lesion and form a well circumscribed nodule. When the patient's resistance is lowered, caseation may take place within the primary focus and the necrotic material can be extruded into the bronchus resulting in formation of a cavity. Bronchogenic or hematogenous dissemination may take place.

2) Hematogenous pulmonary tuberculosis (Type II)

According to the symptoms and X-ray features, the hematogenous pulmonary tuberculosis is divided into 2 types.

①Acute hematogenous disseminated tuberculosis (Acute miliary pulmonary tuberculosis)

The clinical and pathological manifestations: There are no specific symptoms of miliary pulmonary tuberculosis. The onset of the disease is sudden and symptoms are those of any febrile illness unless tuberculous meningitis also develops. Respiratory symptoms are uncommon, but cough and breathlessness may develop in advanced cases.

X-ray features[Figure 6-58(a), (b)]: No changes are found in the early stage. About 2 weeks after onset, it will begin to show changes in both lungs. There are a lot of fine, pin-point mottling opacities, and with the same size, the same density and homogenous distribution. These are varying up to 1-2 mm in diameter.

②Subacute or chronic hematogenous pulmonary tuberculosis

The clinical and pathological manifestations: Symptoms are generally subacute or chronic and include pyrexia, malaise, night sweats and loss of weight etc. Pyrexia is a usual feature but often low grade.

X-ray features(Figure 6-59): There are a lot of nodular shadows in both lung fields. The shadows are not uniform in size, in density and in distribution. So the X-ray features are different with acute miliary tuberculosis.

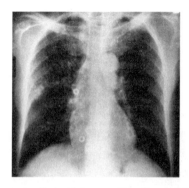

Both lungs are studded with innumerable miliary nodules. These are distributed uniformly throughout the lungs with the exception of the extreme bases. In most cases of miliary tuberculosis, the primary lesion is not visible.

Figure 6-58(a)   Miliary tuberculosis

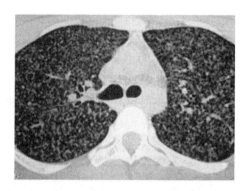

High-resolution CT scan obtained with lung windowing demonstrates numerous fine, discrete nodules bilaterally in a random distribution.

Figure 6-58(b)   Miliary tuberculosis

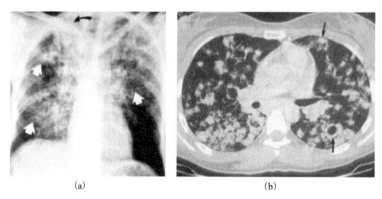

(a)   (b)

(a)Chest film shows clumped nodular and linear areas of increased opacity in both upper lobes and in the right middle lobe (white arrows). There is accompanying apical pleural thickening (black arrow); (b)Axial CT scan demonstrates bilateral diffuse, coarse, linear, and nodular areas of increased attenuation with cavitation (arrows).

Figure 6-59   X-ray features

3）Secondary pulmonary tuberculosis (Type Ⅲ)

①The clinical and pathological manifestations: Secondary pulmonary tuberculosis is the most common type of pulmonary tuberculosis and occurs chiefly in adults. It may result from reactivation of a latent focus of a primary infection or exogenous reinfection. Symptoms vary in different patients. Many patients diagnosed by X-ray may deny any symptoms. The common symptoms are low pyrexia, lassitude, weight loss, night sweats, cough productive of mucoid sputum and haemoptysis.

②X-ray findings(Figure 6-60): It usually presents simultaneously multiple basic X-ray features on the chest film. For example, exudation, proliferation, fibrosis, calcification and cavitation. These lesions may be seen on a patient chest film at the same time. The site of predilection of the lesion is at the apex and subclavicular region of the upper lobe and the superior segment of the lower lobe. The lesions of exudation and cavity represent the active lesion. The type Ⅲ T. B. may sometimes manifest in the form of tuberculoma or caseous pneumonia or chronic fibro-cavitary pulmonary tuberculosis.

CT scans may be helpful in evaluating parenchymal involvement, satellite lesions, and bronchogenic spread of infection. Cavitation is best demonstrated on CT scans [Figure 6-61(a), (b)]. The outer wall of the cavity tends to be thick walled and irregular, whereas the inner wall tends to be smooth. An air-fluid level may be identified.

The bronchogenic spread of tuberculosis is recognized on CT scans by the presence of acinar shadows and nodules of varying sizes in a peribronchial distribution. Mucoid impaction of branching bronchioles results in 'tree-in-bud' sign. The lesions are seen throughout both lungs.

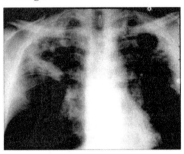

Chest film demonstrates patchy, ill-defined segmental consolidation of the upper lobes of both lungs, a thick-walled cavity with smooth inner margins and a short air-fluid level in the left upper lobe.

Figure 6-60 Infiltrative pulmonary tuberculosis

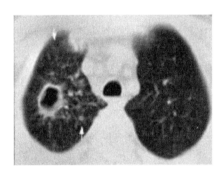

CT scan obtained with the pulmonary window setting in the right upper lobe shows an irregular, thick-walled cavity with some increased markings around it. A nearby nodule is also shown (arrow).

Figure 6-61(a) Cavity of pulmonary tuberculosis

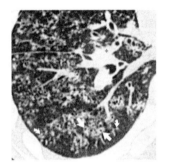

Axial CT scan shows severe changes of bronchiolar dilatation and impaction. Bronchiolar wall thickening (straight arrows) and mucoid impaction of contiguous branching bronchioles produce a tree-in-bud appearance (curved arrows).

Figure 6-61(b) Endobronchial spread of tuberculosis

Tuberculoma

The tuberculoma is formed by fibrous tissue encysted caseous lesion. The size is larger than 1.5 cm in diameter.

X-ray findings(Figure 6-62): The tuberculoma appears typically as a round or oval opaque shadow with well-defined margin and high density typically in the upper lobes. There may be calcific lesion in it. About 75% tuberculomas appear as calcification. "Satellite" lesions or multiple tuberculomas are not uncommon. These lesions are generally stable for long periods of time. Cavitation is extremely rare with tuberculomas and suggests reactivation of disease.

Tuberculomas can be identified on CT scans as rounded nodules that usually have surrounding associated satellite lesions.

Caseous pneumonia

The caseous pneumonia occurs in poor health patient. It is less seen than before because of the introduction of specific antituberculous treatment. The patient is usually with high fever for a long time, cough and expiration, with a lot of sputum, haemoptysis of varying amount and weight loss. The course of the disease is chronic.

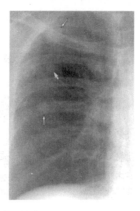

Frontal radiograph of the right lung demonstrates well-defined nodules (arrows), findings that are consistent with tuberculomas.

Figure 6-62　Tuberculomas in primary tuberculosis

X-ray findings are similar to lobar pneumonia commonly in the upper lobe, but multiple cavities usually seen in it and usually with bronchogenic disseminated focus in both low fields. The bronchogenic disseminated focus appear as a lot of small ill-defined patchy opaque shadows.

Chronic fibro-cavitary pulmonary tuberculosis

As a type of pulmonary tuberculosis in the past, in most of the cases, examination of the tubercle bacille in the sputum is positive. Symptoms are repeated episodes of low pyrexia, cough productive of mucoid sputum and haemoptysis, chest pain, lassitude, weight loss, night sweats and appetite etc. Some patients may be without marked symptoms.

Image features(Figure 6-63): With Fibrotic cavity: The shape of the cavity is irregular and the cavitary wall is smooth and high density. With many fibrotic lesions, in association with the shrinking process due to fibrosis, there will be elevation of the hilum and displacement of the mediastinum to the affected side. The lung markings become straightened and appear asweeping willow. Usually with bronchogenic dissemination to the lower lung fields.

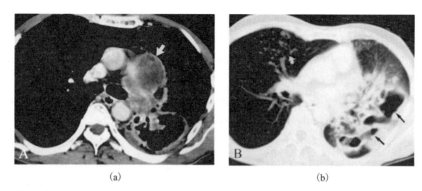

(a)　　　　　　　(b)

(a) Axial contrast-enhanced CT scan obtained with mediastinal windowing demonstrates an enlarged mediastinal lymph node with a central area of low attenuation (arrow); (b) Axial CT scan obtained with lung windowing demonstrates ill-defined cavities (black arrows) accompanied by endobronchial spread in the left upper lobe (white arrow).

Figure 6-63　Chronic fibro-cavitary pulmonary tuberculosis

4)Tuberculous pleuritis (Type Ⅳ)

Tuberculous pleuritis often leads topleural effusion. However, pleuritis without an effusion may occur. In such a situation, chest radiographs may show diaphragmatic elevation, reduction in diaphragmatic excursion. Pleural thickening may also be present, better depicted on CT. In some cases of pleuritis without effusion, the chest radiograph may be normal. Other features include pleural adhesion and thickening, which can result in malformation of chest cage. The X-ray features of the pleural effusion have been mentioned in the previous section. CT can demonstrate pleural effusion and thickened pleura clearly (Figure 6-64).

MRI is of limited value in the evaluation of patients with pulmonary tuberculosis. Occasionally, MRI is helpful in evaluating the complications of tuberculosis, such as the extent of thoracic wall involvement with empyema.

(4) Pulmonary tumor

1) Benign tumors

Benign tumors of the lung are extremely rare and consist of lipoma, hemangioma, fibroma and neurinoma. Actually, some of these may really be hamartoma. They are characterized by their sharp circumscription and the homogeneity of the round or oval shadow. While these characteristics serve to differentiate them from most cases of bronchogenic carcinoma, they cannot be distinguished radiologically from the peripheral form of bronchia adenoma or a solitary metastasis.

The hamartoma is by far the most common benign tumor of the lung. Hamartoma originate in the submucosal fibrous connective tissue of the bronchial wall. They contain mixtures of connective tissue, nests of cartilage and mature fat cells, variable amounts of bone, vessels and smooth muscles. Strictly speaking, they are malformations rather than neoplasms. Radiologically, the hamartoma usually appears as a sharply circumscribed, round or slightly lobulated homogeneous density with in the lung. Most hamartomas are 1 - 3 cm in size. A hamartoma can be diagnosed with a considerable degree of certainty when "Popcorn-like" calcification is seen within a hamartoma. Fatty tissue density may be seen in hamartoma on CT images (Figure 6-65).

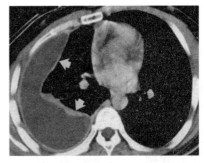

Axial contrast-enhanced CT scan demonstrates a large, right-sided pleural effusion. The enhancing pleura are uniformly thickened (arrows).

Figure 6-64 Pleural effusion

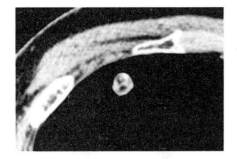

1-mm thick CT scan demonstrates both fat and calcification within a well-circumscribed 1 cm nodule of right upper lobe.

Figure 6-65 Hamartoma

2) Primary bronchogenic carcinoma

① The clinical and pathological manifestations: Primary bronchogenic carcinoma arises from the bronchial epithelium, bronchial glands and epithelium of the alveolus. The incidence of the carcinoma is now steadily increasing. Bronchogenic carcinoma is usually classifiedhistologically into squamous cell carcinoma, adenocarcinoma (including alveolar cell carcinoma) and the undifferentiated carcinomas which are divided into small cell (oat cell) and various large cell types. The distinction between these groups is not always clear in a given case and more than one kind of cell type may coexist. Squamous cell carcinoma and oat cell carcinoma is the commonest. Multiple primary tumors are very occasionally seen.

The clinical features are very variable correlated with the histological type, site, and degree of development of the carcinoma. There may be no signs or symptoms in the early stage. Along with the development of the lesion, cough, haemoptysis, sputum, breathlessness and stridor etc may be occurred. Obstruction of the bronchus often leads to distal infection. Spread to the pleura may cause pleural effusion, pleuritic pain and chest wall pain (spread beyond the parietal pleura). Tumor invasion of mediastinum can present as: Left recurrent laryngeal nerve palsy; Superior vena caval obstruction; Dysphagia; Phrenic nerve paralysis; Apical tumors involving brachial plexus and sympathetic ganglia ('Pancoast' tumors) cause Horner's syndrome. The cells of the bronchial tumor can produce biologically active hormone-like substances (usually peptides). These syndromes can be conveniently divided into two groups, endocrine and neuro-muscular.

②Imaging manifestations: The primary lung carcinoma is generally divided into central type, peripheral type and diffuse type by radiologist according to the site of carcinoma.

The central type: When the carcinoma originated from main bronchi, lobar bronchi orsegmental bronchi and located in the area of hilum. It is called central type. The signs of a central tumor can be thought of as the signs of a central tumor itself and the signs of airway obstruction as a consequence of the tumor. They are so called direct signs and indirect signs.

The direct signs: A hilar mass on the chest film, commonly presents as unilateral hilar enlargement and increased density of the hilum [Figure 6-66(a)]. It may be due to the primary carcinoma which has arisen centrally, or to enlargement of hilar lymph nodes from metastatic involvement. In the early stage, it may only appears increased density of the hilum even normal on plain chest film. Encroachment of tumor on the bronchial lumen is occasionally identifiable on a plain film and when visualized is usually accompanied by lobar or lung atelectasis. Hilar tomogram or high KV chest film may reveal an irregular narrowing of the bronchus by the tumor. Frequently the lumen appears completely obstructed, even in those cases where no lobar collapse is present.

CT scans can demonstrate the abnormality of bronchi and the hilar mass clearly [Figure 6-66(a), (c)]. The abnormality of bronchi includes irregular stenosis, obstruction, intralumen nodule and thickening wall of bronchi. The hilar tumor appears as a mass near a certain bronchi usually with clear, smooth and lobulate border.

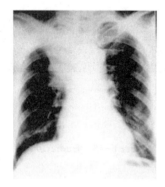

The PA view chest film shows the right hilar mass and the right upper lobe atelectasis. Its lower margin appears as transverse 'S' sign.

Figure 6-66(a)   Central carcinoma

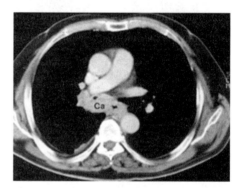

The hilar mass surround and obstruct the bronchus intermedius. It invades the mediastinum directly. The localized thickened pleura suggest the pleural metastase.

Figure 6-66(b)   Central carcinoma (Ca)

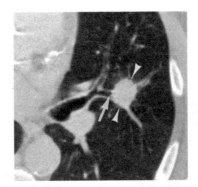

CT demonstrates a 2-cm spiculated mass (arrowheads) arising from a lingular bronchus (arrow). Bronchoscopic washings in this patient were positive for squamous cell carcinoma.

Figure 6-66(c) Bronchogenic carcinoma

The indirect signs: Obstruction to a major bronchus leads to atelectasis due to reduced ventilation of the affected segments or lobes and/or consolidation due to the inability to evacuate secretions. The superior lobar atelectasis and hilar tumor form "Transverse s" sign (Figure 6-67), which appears as the process and increased density near hilum of the shadow of atelectasis due to hilar tumor, it is thecharacteristic appears of central lung cancer. Secondary infection resulting in pneumonia is common. The collapse/consolidation may be segmental or lobar even an entire lung. Localized obstructive emphysema may be the early sign of the carcinoma.

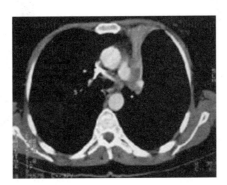

A 52-year-old woman with a bronchogenic carcinoma of the left mainstem bronchus and resultant left upper lobe atelectasis.

Figure 6-67 Bronchogenic carcinoma

The peripheral type: When the mass locates in the peripheral lung field, it is called the peripheral type of the primary lung carcinoma. The peripheral tumor is identified radiographically as a mass in the lung [Figure 6-68 (a)]. The shape of the mass is usually approximately spherical, oval and lobulated configurations. The edge of the lesion that is best revealed by conventional tomography and CT is usually lobulated, notched and spiculated infiltrating. The border of the mass may be clear, shaggy or cloudy, or with pleural tail sign, which appears as a peripheral line shadow between a peripheral located mass lesion and the pleura [Figure 6-68(b)], the pleural tail sign is commonly seen in adenocarcinoma.

There may be a cavity in a large mass [Figure 6-68(c)]. The inner wall of the cavity usually is irregular. The cavity is frequently eccentric. It is the character of the cavity of the carcinoma. The cavity is commonly seen in squamous cell carcinoma.

The rate of growth of a suspected lung cancer as assessed by comparing previous films, can be very helpful in making a diagnosis. It has been calculated that a peripheral mass to primary carcinoma of the lung doubles its volume between 30−490 days (median 120 days) with only the very occasional case showing a doubling time outside this range. Therefore slower or faster rates of growth point to an alternative diagnosis.

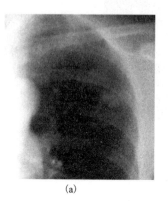
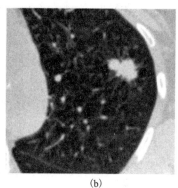

(a)   (b)

(a) Detail view from posteroanterior chest radiograph demonstrates an ill-defined left upper lobe opacity. B. A 2−mm collimated CT demonstrates a 2−cm left upper lobe mass with spiculated infiltrating margins, characteristic of a primary bronchogenic carcinoma. Surgical resection disclosed adenocarcinoma.

Figure 6−68(a)   Bronchogenic carcinoma

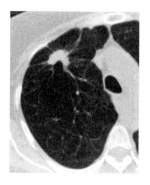
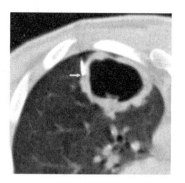

Right upper lobe adenocarcinoma with spiculated margins and associated pleural tail signs in a man with centrilobular emphysema.

    CT shows a left lower lobe cavity with irregular thick wall. CT-guided biopsy (done in the prone position) verifies needle tip (arrow) in wall of the lesion. Specimens disclosed squamous cell carcinoma.

Figure 6−68(b)   Bronchogenic carcinoma   **Figure 6−68(c)   Bronchogenic carcinoma**

The diffuse type: When the focus of the carcinoma is to be distributed in the lung fields, it is called the diffuse type. The diffuse type of primary lung carcinoma results from bronchioloalveolar carcinoma only. The diffuse form appears as some opaque mottled shadows in a lobe or multiple lobes of both lungs. The sizes of the shadows are various. The individual shadows varying from barely visible to lobar consolidation, and may contain air bronchograms. Septal lines (Kerley A and B) and a pleural effusion may be seen. The pattern may closely resemble pulmonary oedema or widespread bronchopneumonia.

③Spread of tumor

Primary carcinoma of the bronchus invades locally, spreads via lymphatics to the hilar and mediastinal lymph nodes and also spread via the blood stream to remote sites including other thoracic structures.

Hilar and mediastinal lymph node metastase: It appears as enlargement of hilar or mediastinal lymph nodes. CT and MRI are sensitive examinations for detecting mediastinal adenopathy. However it should be realized that normally-sized nodes may contain microscopic foci tumor. The accuracy of predicting the presence or absence of metastatic lymph node involvement based on size at CT will always be limited. A reasonable compromise is to regard nodes of up to 1 cm of hilar and up to 1.5 cm of mediastinum in diameter as abnormal(Figure 6-69).

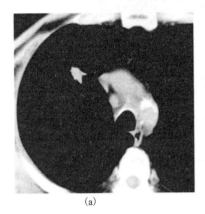 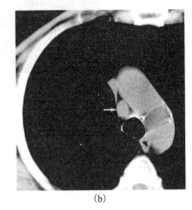

(a)　　　　　　　　　　　　　　(b)

(a)CT demonstrates an irregular 1.7-cm right upper lobe nodule;(b)On the next more caudal scan, an enlarged 2cm mediastinal lymph node (arrow) is shown, which was confirmed to contain poorly differentiated squamous cell carcinoma.

Figure 6-69　Bronchogenic carcinoma

Mediastinal invasion: Primary carcinoma can invade the mediastinum directly. It is difficult to distinguish from plain films or conventional tomography between a tumor in contact with but not transgressing the mediastinal pleura, and one that has invaded the mediastinum, enhanced CT and MRI can provide evidence of invasion (Figure 6-70). Pericardium effusion is occasionally seen when pericardium is invaded.

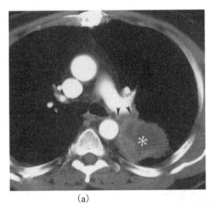 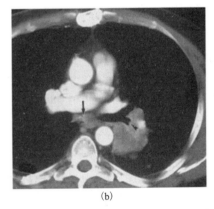

(a)　　　　　　　　　　　　　　(b)

(a) CT image obtained at the level of the left pulmonary artery shows the mass with regions of necrosis within it (*). The anterior aspect of the lesion appears to invade the mediastinum posterior to the artery (arrowheads);
(b)CT image obtained at the level of the right pulmonary artery shows involvement of the posterior left hilum with cutoff of the superior segmental bronchus (arrowhead) and subcarinal lymphadenopathy (arrow).

Figure 6-70　Squamous cell carcinoma

Pleural involvement: Pleural effusion or pleural masses is seen. Pleural masses are infrequently seen even in patients with malignant effusions.

Chest wall invasion: A peripheral lung carcinoma may cross the pleura and invade the chest wall. Rib or spinal destruction may be visible on plain films. Soft tissue invasion is best detected by CT and MRI (Figure6-71).

Phrenic nerve invasion leads to paralysis and elevation of the hemidiaphragm on the chest radiograph. It is due

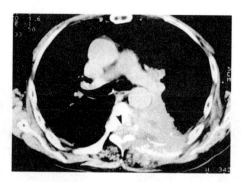

chest wall involvement. CT image shows the rib and spinal destruction, and the soft tissue tumor in the posterior chest wall. Atelectasis of the superior segment of left lower lobe also presents.

Figure 6-71　Squamous cell carcinoma

to the enlarged mediastinal lymph nodes or tumor compressing the phrenic nerve to result in the paralysis of the hemidiaphragm.

3) Pulmonary metastatic tumors

Pulmonary metastatic tumors usually come from chorioepithelioma, breast carcinoma, hepatic carcinoma, gastric carcinoma and prostatic carcinoma etc. Pulmonary metastases are usually due to haematogenous spread. The basic sign of pulmonary metastases is one or more discrete pulmonary nodules. Most lung metastases are round and well circumscribed, although some have irregular infiltrating margins. Rarely, a predominantly interstitial ("lymphangitis") pattern occurs, which will be discussed later. The nodules are usually spherical and well defined but they may be almost any shape and can occasionally have a very irregular edge. Such irregular edges are seen particularly with metastase from adenocarcinomas.

Typical pulmonary metastases usually appear as multiple round or oval nodules with clear border in the lungs, and the nodules are various in size [Figure 6-72(a)]. Occasionally, they may show innumerable miliary mottlings similar to miliary tuberculosis, and may show some linear shadows radiating from the hilum and enlargement of intrathoracic lymph nodes [Figure 6-72(b)].

A solitary metastasis may be the presenting feature of a patient without a known primary tumor. Metastasis is a rare cause for the asymptomatic pulmonary nodule, once extrathoracic primary neoplasm has been excluded by history and physical examination. It comprises 2%~3% of most series of asymptomatic solitary pulmonary nodules.

Cavitation is occasionally seen. It is a particular feature of metastases composed of squamous cell carcinoma [Figure 6-72(c)].

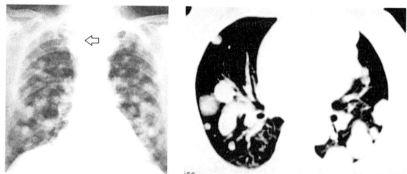

nodular type. Both lungs are studded with numerous, fairly well demarcated nodules. On the PA view chest film, the shadow in the superior mediastinum (arrow) represents a carcinoma of the thyroid which was the primary growth.

Figure 6-72(a)　Metastatic carcinoma

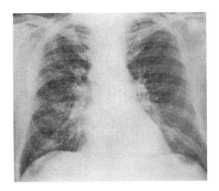

Metastatic spread from a primary carcinoma of the pancreas. Both lungs are diffusely studded with innumerable tiny nodules and there is a mass of enlarged lymph nodes in the right paratracheal region.

Figure 6-72(b)　Metastatic carcinoma, miliary form

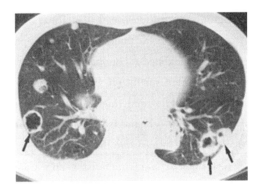

Cavitating metastasis in a 72-year-old man with a squamous cell carcinoma in the left main bronchus. Transverse CT scan shows multiple metastatic nodules in both lungs. There are several cavitating nodules (arrows) in both lower lobes. Note the irregular thickening of the cavity walls.

Figure 6-72(c)　Metastasis carcinoma

Calcification is very unusual except in osteosarcoma and chondrosarcoma [Figure 6-72(d)]. Even in those tumors whose primaries calcify e. g. breast and colon, calcification in the pulmonary metastases is very rare.

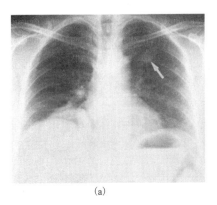
(a)

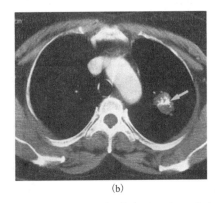
(b)

(a) Chest film shows multiple areas of nodular attenuation in both lungs. A focal calcification (arrow) is suspected in the nodule in the left upper lobe; (b) Transverse contrast-enhanced CT scan clearly shows calcification (arrow) within the nodule. Histopathologic examination of the resected mass revealed a metastatic osteosarcoma with the foci of ossification.

Figure 6-72(d)　Calcified metastasis: osteosarcoma

The rate of growth is very variable, some metastases e. g. choriocarcinoma and osteosarcoma may be explosive and double in volume in less than 30 days. Alternatively, some metastases can remain unchanged in size for a very long time e. g. thyroid carcinoma.

Carcinomatous lymphangitis is a form metastatic carcinoma in which the pulmonary lymphatics are invaded and often blocked by cords of malignant cells. It may be unilateral or bilateral. The patients are usually dyspnoeic but may have few or no pulmonary symptoms if the involvement is unilateral. Pulmonary lymphangitic spread is most frequently seen secondary to metastatic adenocarcinomas of the breast, lung, stomach, colon, prostate, and pancreas. Carcinoma of the bronchus is much the commonest cause of unilateral carcinomatous lymphangitis. Lymphatic permeation radiation from tumor in hilar lymph nodes is a probable mechanism in some cases. In others it is probable that the initial dissemination is via the blood stream and invasion of intrapulmonary lymphatics takes place with permeation of tumor towards the hila, with no initial involvement of the hilar lymph nodes. The sign on chest radiograph are a widespread ill-defined 2~3 mm nodular pattern together with widespread thickening of the pulmonary septa. The fissures may be thickened by subpleural oedema. Pleural effusions are common but are often small. CT findings include uneven thickening of bronchovascular bundles and thickening of the interstitial septa, often in a polygonal fashion [Figure 6-72(e)]. As the diseases progresses, a more nodular appearance may be seen superimposed on this reticular pattern, resulting in a characteristic appearance of small nodules connected to thickened lines, or a "beaded chain" appearance.

CT reveals interstitial linear opacities and tiny nodules in both lungs.

Figure 6-72(e)   Lymphangitic spread of breast cancer

2. The diseases of bronchi

（1）Bronchiectasis

1）The clinical and pathological manifestations: Bronchiectasis, which by definition represents irreversible dilatation of the bronchi, has been classified pathologically into three forms, depending on the severity of the bronchial dilatation: Cylindrical (tubular), Varicose, Cystic. The characteristic symptoms are continuous cough and sputum. Sputum can be copious and is frequently purulent. A history of recurrent haemoptysis, pneumonia and pleurisy is relatively common.

2）Imaging manifestations: The plain chest radiographic findings in bronchiectasis are often nonspecific, unless the disease is very advanced. Surrounding infiltrate or fibrosis, which may be obscure recognition bronchi [Figure 6-73(a)]. Dilated bronchi, sometimes with fluid levels, are seen only in gross disease. In the past, bronchography usually was performed to confirm the diagnosis and was essential in the assessment of patients for surgical treatment.

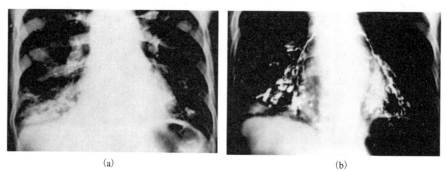

(a)   (b)

(a)There is dense infiltration of the right lower lobe; (b) The bronchogram shows cylindric dilation of the branches of the left lower lobe. The basal divisions of the right lower lobe bronchus show sacculated dilatations.

Figure 6-73(a)   Bronchiectasis of both lower lobes

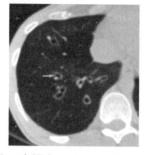

A 2-mm collimated CT demonstrates multiple examples of the signet ring sign (arrow), due to a pulmonary artery adjacent to a dilated bronchus exhibiting smooth mural thickening.

Figure 6-73(b)   Cylindrical bronchiectasis

Each of the pathologic types of bronchiectasis has a characteristic appearance on CT. When the diagnosis is respectively suspected, this can be accomplished by obtaining thinly collimated 1 – to 2-mm sections. High resolution CT is sufficiently sensitive and specific to serve as both the screening and the definitive diagnostic imaging technique in patients suspected of having bronchiectasis, and it has an overall accuracy of about 95%. The cardinal sign of bronchiectasis on HRCT is dilatation of the bronchus, which usually is accompanied by bronchial wall thickening. Dilated bronchus and concomitant pulmonary artery results in a signet ring configuration [Figure 6 –73(b)]. Large elliptical circular opacities or thick-walled lucencies can be seen in far advanced cystic bronchiectasis and represent bronchiectatic cavities filled with mucopurulent material or air. Sometimes air-fluid levels may be seen, due to retained secretions in these cystic structures.

(2)Foreign bodies

1) The clinical and pathological manifestations: Foreign bodies aspirated are usually occurred in infants and children. The common symptoms of foreign bodies include cough, dyspnea, cyanosis, etc.

2) Imaging manifestations: The diagnosis of a foreign body in a bronchus is usually quite simple when the aspirated substance is radiopaque. If the foreign body is radiolucent, it cannot be detected on films and only the effects of the bronchial obstruction may be visible. Foreign bodies are almost always located in the main or lower lobe bronchi and usually cause complete obstructive with atelectasis of the lower lobe and incomplete obstruction with emphysema of the upper lobe.

CT may detect and localize the foreign bodies intralumen of bronchi (Figure 6-74), but to make certain diagnosis usually need the history.

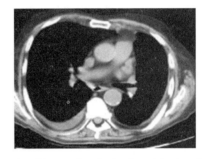

tooth. CT scan through the lower-lobe bronchi demonstrates a high-density object in the left lower-lobe bronchus (arrow). Incidentally, a small pleural effusion on the right side should be noted.

Figure 6-74　Aspiration foreign body

3. Mediastinal diaseases

(1)Mediastinal lipomatosis

Mediastinal lipomatosis is an abnormal collection of histologically benign unencapsulated fat that often results in a widened mediastinum. The condition is frequently idiopathic. The most common predisposing factors are obesity, corticosteroid administration, and Cushing syndrome. On the frontal chest radiograph, there is symmetric widening that is most marked in the upper mediastinum. The lateral radiograph may show vague opacity in the anterior mediastinum. CT scan can distinguish lipomatosis from other causes of mediastinal widening. On CT scan, lipomatosis consists of homogeneous fat density that is of similar attenuation to subcutaneous fat(Figure 6-75). MR imaging demonstrates uniform high signal intensity on T1-weighted images. Fatty accumulation occurs predominantly in the superior mediastinum and often results in convex lateral mediastinal margins. Other areas including the cardiophrenic angles, retrocrural and paraspinal regions may be affected.

(2)Bronchogenic cysts

1)The clinical and pathological manifestations: Bronchogenic cysts result from abnormal ventral budding of the tracheobronchial tree. The cyst wall is lined by respiratory epithelium and may contain cartilage, mucus-secreting glands, or smooth muscle. Bronchogenic cysts that arise in the mediastinum are thought to result from an earlier abnormality of tracheobronchial branching than those in the lung parenchyma. The majority of mediastinal bronchogenic cysts are located adjacent to the airway, most commonly in the subcarinal and right paratracheal regions. Most cysts are fluid-filled, but air may enter the lesion if a communication exists with the tracheobronchial tree. Symptoms, which occur in a minority of patients, include respiratory distress, chest pain, and dysphagia.

213

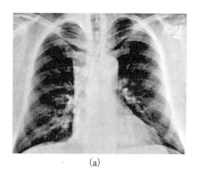
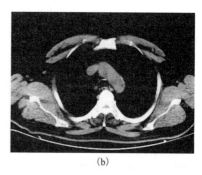

(a)　(b)

(a)Frontal radiograph demonstrates widening of the superior mediastinum; (b)CT shows extensive fat convex margins encasing the superior vena cava and aortic arch.

Figure 6-75　Mediastinal lipomatosis

2）Imaging manifestations: The chest radiograph demonstrates a round, smoothly marginated mass that may cause deviation or narrowing of the adjacent airway. An air-fluid level indicates communication with the tracheobronchial tree. Mural calcification is an uncommon radiographic finding. CT scan shows a well-defined, nonenhancing, rounded mass of homogeneous attenuation. About 50% of bronchogenic cysts have CT numbers in the fluid range (0-20 HU). The remainder have density measurements higher than 20 HU, reflecting a high content of calcium, proteinaceous material, or previous hemorrhage (Figure 6-76). High attenuation cysts may be indistinguishable from a solid mass. The diagnosis can be confirmed by ultrasound or cyst aspiration.

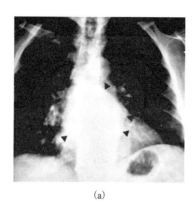
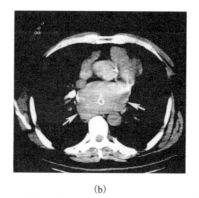

(a)　(b)

(a)Frontal radiograph demonstrates a large subcarinal mass (arrowheads); (b)CT scan shows a well-circumscribed ovoid mass in the middle mediastinum (arrows). The cyst fluid measured 25 HU, indicating proteinaceous or hemorrhagic content.

Figure 6-76　Bronchogenic cyst

More recently, MR has been used to evaluate bronchogenic cysts. The lesion demonstrates variable signal intensity on T1-weighted images because of differences of cyst content. T2-weighted images show a characteristic high signal intensity, a common feature to most mediastinal cysts.

(3)Nenrenteric cysts

Neurenteric cysts result from abnormal separation of endoderm and notochord, resulting in a persistent connection with the meninges and interruption of normal fusion of the vertebral ossification centers. About half of all cases are associated with a vertebral abnormality, including hemivertebra and butterfly vertebra. Neurenteric cysts usually occur in the posterior mediastinum. The imaging appearance of this lesion is similar to other foregut cysts, but the associated vertebral anomalies suggest the diagnosis.

(4)Pericardial cysts

1）The clinical and pathological manifestations: Pericardial cysts are uncommon developmental abnormalities that result from pinching off of a part of the pericardium during embryogenesis. The cyst is lined by a single layer of mesothelial cells, and most cysts contain clear, transudative fluid. The lesion infrequently causes symptoms of chest pain or cough, particularly if cyst torsion or hemorrhage occurs. A total of 70% of pericardial cysts are located in the right cardiophrenic angle, 20% in the left cardiophrenic angle, and the remainder in a variety of locations including the posterior mediastinum.

2）Imaging manifestations: The chest radiograph typically demonstrates a sharply marginated mass in the cardiophrenic angle that abuts the diaphragm and heart border. CT scan shows a well-defined nonenhancing lesion with attenuation numbers in the fluid range (0~20 HU). The cyst may have a pointed appearance and variable shape on sequential examinations. High attenuation numbers may be found if the cyst hemorrhages (Figure 6-77). If the lesion is in a typical location, ultrasound is useful to demonstrate its cystic nature. Uncomplicated pericardial cysts have low signal intensity on T1weighted MR images and high signal intensity on T2-weighted images.

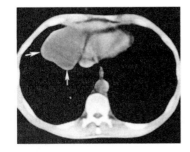

CT scan demonstrates a lesion in the right cardiophrenic angle (arrows). Relatively high attenuation of cyst contents suggests prior hemorrhage.

Figure 6-77　Pericardial cyst

（5）Thymic cysts

1）The clinical and pathological manifestations: Congenital thymic cysts are thought to arise from tubular remnants of the third pharyngeal pouch. The lesion is lined by a single layer of squamous or cuboidal epithelium. Cysts may occur anywhere along the course of the thymopharyngeal duct from the mandible to the diaphragm. The cysts are most often discovered incidentally but may cause symptoms if hemorrhage occurs. Acquired thymic cysts have been associated with Hodgkin disease, blunt trauma, radiation therapy, prior thoracotomy, and rarely, myasthenia gravis.

2）Imaging manifestations: The chest radiograph demonstrates a well-defined anterior mediastinal mass that is indistinguishable from a thymoma. Ultrasound may be useful to show the cystic character of the lesion. CT findings are similar to other mediastinal cysts (Figure 6-78). Hemorrhage into the thymic cyst may cause rapid enlargement and attenuation numbers higher than water. MR imaging of uncomplicated cysts demonstrates low signal intensity on T1-weighted images and high signal intensity on T2-weighted images. Hemorrhagic cysts show higher than normal signal intensity on T1-weighted images.

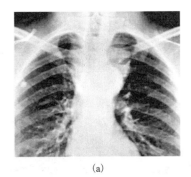
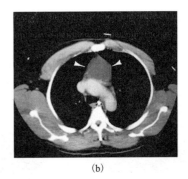

(a)　　　　　　　　(b)

（a）Frontal radiograph demonstrates a superior mediastinal mass. The silhouette of the aortic arch is intact; （b）CT scan shows a fluid density mass anterior to the proximal aortic arch (arrowheads).

Figure 6-78　Thymic cyst

（6）Primary mediastinal solid tumor

Primary mediastinal solid tumors include multitudinous kinds of tumours, such us neurogenic neoplasm, thymoma, malignant lymphoma and so on.

1）Neurogenic neoplasm

①The clinical and pathological manifestations: The most common cause of a posterior mediastinal mass, mainly in a paraspinal location. Neurogenic neoplasms may also arise in the other compartments of the mediastinum, the chest wall and occasionally the lung parenchyma. Pathologically these neoplasms can be divided into three main groups: Nerve sheath neoplasms include neurofibroma and schwannoma; Ganglion cell neoplasms include ganglioneuroma, ganglioneuroblastoma, and neuroblastoma; Paraganglionic cell neoplasms include chemodectoma and phaeochromocytoma.

Roughly 70% of neurogenic tumours arising in the chest are benign. Usually, they occur in younger patients, in the first four decades of life. Males and females are equally affected. Patients with neurogenic neoplasm are often asymptomatic, although these neoplasm may induce symptoms such as radicular pain and neurasthenia. Symptoms of cord compression may be present in case of intravertebral extension. Tumours arising from the peripheral nerves (intercostal) tend to be round in shape, and those arising from the sympathetic chains are usually fusiform with a more vertical orientation.

②Imaging manifestations: On chest radiography, neurogenic neoplasms are seen as a sharply circumscribed homogeneous mass. Rib erosion with a sclerotic border is suggestive of a benign lesion. The presence of frank bone destruction or spread to multiple rib is suggestive of malignancy. Calcification may be present in all types of neurogenic neoplasm.

On CT scans, neurogenic neoplasms typically appear as homogeneous soft tissue density although many of them have a low attenuation attributed to the lipid elements in the nerve sheaths or cystic degeneration (Figure 6-79). Due to their vascularization, they enhance after the administration of intravenous contrast medium. Spinal involvement is particularly well assessed by using MRI. Multiplanar imaging helps demonstrate the longitudinal spread of the tumour along the spine. Widening of the neural foramina is often associated with nerve sheath neoplasm. Vertebral body erosion is mostly associated with sympathetic chain tumour. Generally benign neoplasms are homogeneous with well defined margins, whereas malignant neoplasms are mostly heterogeneous with irregular margins. On MR scans, neurogenic neoplasms appear as well-defined masses of homogeneous signal intensity appearing greater than that of skeletal muscle on T1-weighted images and markedly increased on T2-weighted images. They enhance following gadolinium administration homogeneously or inhomogeneously depending on various tissue components, vascularity or cystic degeneration.

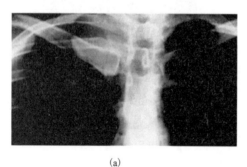 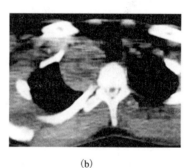

(a)   (b)

（a）PA radiograph demonstrating a proven schwannoma in the right superior paravertebral region; (b) CT scan demonstrating displacement of the medial aspect of the right lung laterally by the schwannoma.

Figure 6-79

2）Thymoma

① The clinical and pathological manifestations: Thymoma arises from thymic epithelium. It is the most common cause of a thymic mass. It presents as an anterior mediastinal mass. Thymomas are composed of thymic epithelial cells and a variable amount of reactive lymphocytes. Pathologically, cystic changes are common and rarely, the tumour may be almost totally cystic. The majority of thymomas are benign lesions confined within a fibrous capsule. About 30% of them, however, may be more aggressive and demonstrate invasion through the fibrous capsule.

Thymomas occur usually between the ages of 40 and 60 years old, in males or females equally. They are very unusual in patients under the age of 20. Thymomas generally occur as incidental findings discovered on a chest radiograph in otherwise healthy individuals. They may also occur in association with other abnormalities such as myasthenia gravis. Myasthenia gravis, is present in roughly 50% of patients with thymoma. Approximately 15% of patients with myasthenia gravis have a thymoma.

② Imaging manifestations: On the chest radiograph, thymomas are depicted as a round or lobulated mass located in the anterior mediastinum. On lateral films, they often appear as a well-defined mass in the normally clear restrosternal space. Sometimes, the tumour is situated more inferiorly adjacent to the left or right borders of the heart and occasionally as low as the cardiophrenic angle. Occasionally he tumour is too small(1 cm)to be depicted on the chest radiography, and is only detected on CT scans. Calcifications may be seen in both benign or invasive thymomas. On CT scans, benign thymomas appear as a round or oval mass located in the prevascular space of the mediastinum, or at any level from the thoracic inlet to the diaphragm within the anterior mediatinum. Invasive thymomas typicall appear as irregular masses growing along pleural surfaces(Figure 6-80).

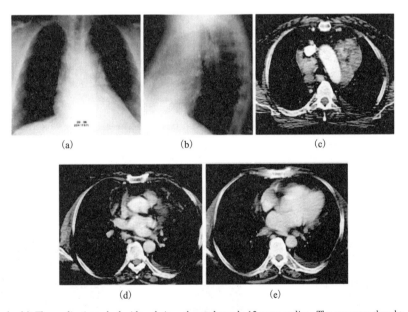

(a)   (b)   (c)

(d)   (e)

(a. b) The mediastinum had widened since the study made 12 years earlier. The mass was thought to be located in the prevascular compartment. (c to e) Contrast-enhanced CT demonstrates a mass that contains fat and soft tissue masses. Some of the masses extend posterior to the cava and anterior to the trachea on the right side. The fat and soft tissue abnormality extended from the thoracic inlet to the level of the diaphragm. Pathologic examination demonstrated adipose tissue with benign lymphoid aggregates consistent with benign thymic lipoma.

Figure 6-80　Routine chest radiography

3）Teratomas

Teratomas usually are benign. Of these tumors, 25% have radiographically demonstrable bone or teeth or a peripheral rim of calcification. The teratomas have been separated into three categories, depending on the respective preponderance of skin（epidermoid）, skin and appendages（dermoid）, and derivatives from two or more germ layers（teratoid）. In Figure 6-81, the lesion can be seen extending from the diaphragm to the thoracic inlet. There is considerable displacement of the major vessels by this long-standing mass, which was an incidental finding. Rarely, teratomas may develop in the postvascular compartment.

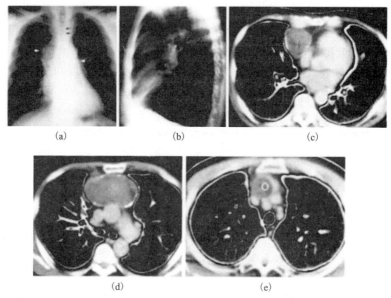

(a)　　　　　(b)　　　　　(c)

(d)　　　　　(e)

（a）（b）The trachea is displaced posteriorly, indicating the anterior position of the mass. The edges are clearly delineated, indicating that the mass resides within the mediastinum. The arrows refer to the posterior junction line.（c）~（e）. The mass extends from the diaphragm to the thoracic inlet entirely in the prevascular space. The mass contains calcium, fat, and water-dense material and was presumed to be a dermoid.

Figure 6-81　A large mass indents the medial aspect of the right

4）Mediastinal Thyroid

When thyroid masses descend into the thorax, they usually extend into the prevascular space（Figure 6-82）. The CT appearances of thyroid goiters are specific. Anatomical continuity usually can be demonstrated with the cervical thyroid. Focal calcifications and inhomogeneity are frequent features. After injecting contrast material, there is a definite prolonged rise in the CT Hounsfield number. Thyroid extensions can slide posterior to enter the postvascular space, because the prevascular and postvascular spaces are no longer separated by the vessels as the thoracic inlet is reached.

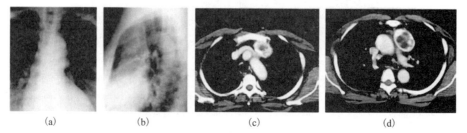

(a)　　　　　(b)　　　　　(c)　　　　　(d)

On the frontal（a）and lateral projection（b）, there is a sharply defined mass that projects in the AP window region on the frontal projection. On the lateral view, a subtle posterior displacement of the anterior wall of the trachea places the lesion in the prevascular compartment. Enhanced CT images（c~d）demonstrate the prevascular mass with significant peripheral enhancement. A thyroid lesion was not considered. Vascular tumor such as a paraganglioma or hemangioma were prime considerations. The lesion was surgically removed. It was a nodular goiter.

Figure 6-82　Chest radiograph demonstrates a mediastinal mass in this 48-year-old woman

5）Lymphomas

The thorax is frequently involved in patients with Hodgkin's and non-Hodgkin's lymphomas. The 67% patients with Hodgkin's disease have radiographic evidence of intrathoracic disease, of which 46% involve the anterior mediastinum. The 43% patients with non-Hodgkin's lymphoma have intrathoracic disease, of which only 13% involve the anterior mediastinum. The radiologic manifestations of lymphoma in the thorax demonstrate a large mass in the anterior or middle mediastinum, which may be displaces the great vessels the trachea posteriorly. Enhanced CT images show a mass reduced attenuation indicative of necrosis. Individual discrete nodes may be encountered; however, the disease frequently presents as a large conglomerate mass (Figure 6-83).

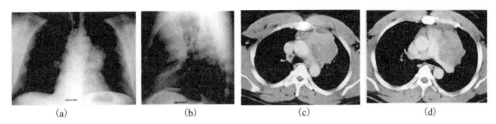

(a) (b) (c) (d)

The radiographs (a)(b) demonstrate a large mass in the left anterior mediastinum, which displaces the trachea posteriorly. Enhanced axial CT images(c)(d). show a mass in the prevascular compartment with an area of reduced attenuation indicating necrosis. The left pulmonary artery is narrowed by the mass. The mass was a malignant lymphoma of the large B-cell type.

Figure 6-83 Chest radiograph of the frontal

4. The disease of pleura

Pleural tumors

These are rare. The most common benign tumors involving the pleura are lipomas and fibrous tumors, and Metastatic disease is the most common malignant neoplasm involving the pleura. Primary pleural tumors, such as mesothelioma, account for less than 5% of malignant pleural neoplasms. Features suggesting a malignancy rather than a benign process include pleural thickening over 1 cm, disseminated pleural nodules, and mediastinal pleural involvement; definitive diagnosis usually requires cytologic or histologic analysis.

（1）Malignant mesothelioma

1）The clinical and pathological manifestations: Mesothelioma is a malignant neoplasm originating from pleural surfaces that is usually associated with occupational exposure to asbestos. The 3 primary pathologic types of mesothelioma are epithelioid, sarcomatoid, and biphasic. Clinical symptoms are typically a late finding and include chest pain, dyspnea, cough, weakness, and weight loss.

2）Imaging manifestations: The radiological findings are of a well demarcated rounded and often slightly lobulated mass which may show marked positional change with posture and respiration. They may occasionally arise in a fissure and they need be distinguished with interlobar pleural effusion. Both CT and MRI are able to demonstrate the presence and extent of the pleural mass and pleural effusion. The tumor may present as irregular diffuse nodular pleural thickening or focal masses between the lung and chest wall (Figure 6-84). Malignant mesothelioma has an intermediate signal intensity on T1-weighted MR images and slightly high signal intensity on T2-weighted images. Loculated pleural fluid presents as areas of high signal intensity with T2 weighting.

Tumor extent along the pleural surfaces and into the mediastinum, diaphragm, or chest wall can be evaluated much better with CT or MRI than plain radiography. Chest wall invasion manifests as obliteration of fat planes or chest wall nodules.

（2）Pleural metastases

Pleural metastases usually involve both the visceral and parietal pleural surfaces, and almost always cause an associated effusion. Most of pleural metastases are the result of lung and breast carcinoma and lymphoma.

Infiltration of the pleural surfaces usually results in a pleural effusion, which is the first manifestation in most cases. CT may reveal pleural-based nodules obscured by the pleural fluid. Pleural metastases usually appear as relatively small, lenticular masses having obtuse margins with the chest wall (Figure 6-85). The soft-tissue component often enhances following contrast administration, allowing or improving differentiation from any adjacent nonenhancing pleural effusion. Ancillary findings on CT, such as mediastinal lymph node enlargement, lung nodules, rib lesions, or a subcutaneous mass, support a presumptive diagnosis of pleural metastases.

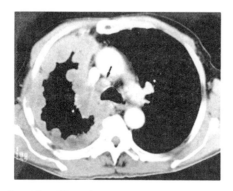

Circumferential mildly enhancing nodular pleural thickening is present, encasing the right lung. Noting diminished volume of right lung. Precarinal lymphadenopathy is seen (arrow).

Figure 6-84   Malignant mesothelioma

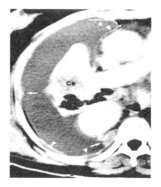

Small pleural masses (arrows) are seen in association with a large pleural effusion and atelectasis of the right lung. Note the abnormal enhancement of the entire parietal pleural surface (arrowheads).

Figure 6-85   Pleural effusion with pleural metastasis from a bronchogenic carcinoma (Ca)

(Quanliang Shang, Juan Chen, Zhilan Yin, Qian Guo, Enhua Xiao, Jiangguang Luo)

第七章

心脏与大血管

心脏是一个空腔肌性器官，位于胸腔内且被左肺和右肺包绕。它像一个斜锥，底部向右侧投影，尖端向左侧投影。目前，心脏评估多以X线为主，更深层次的心脏放射学诊断常依赖于其他放射学的技术，如计算机断层扫描（CT），磁共振成像（MRI），超声，血管造影，甚至核医学。这些检查的联合应用往往能对心脏病变进行较好的诊断。过去使用的技术如透视、体层摄影技术等，现在已经完全淘汰。本章我们重点讨论心脏及大血管的医学影像学技术应用。

第一节　检查技术

1. X线平片及血管造影检查

正常吸气状态下，站立位的全X线胸片十分重要，至少需要两个位置投照，即后前位和侧位。投照距离2米，在此距离下心脏放大最小，有时还需要另外2个斜位片进行观察。

导管造影或心血管造影是一种基于X线的对比增强技术，可显示冠状脉（简称冠脉）、大血管、心室和心房腔。检查在患者仰卧位时进行。在心血管造影中，经典的成像角度包括右前斜位（RAO）和左前斜位（LAO）。该方法不仅能评估心脏的大小、形态、功能和收缩能力，而且能够对冠脉进行选择性评估。但其禁忌证包括甲状腺功能亢进、对比剂过敏、充血性心力衰竭、凝血功能障碍等。

2. CT检查

自从多探测器的心电（ECG）门控引入CT以来，心脏的CT成像逐渐成为可能。随着技术的发展，心脏的体积测量能在一次约3 s到15 s的屏气中采集完成。从得到的数据中可以在任何RR间期重建毫米级图像，并且能够做到完全没有运动假影的产生。心脏CT的主要局限性在于患者的心率需要维持在70次/分以下。从一个完整的RR间期中重建的多期图像也能对心肌运动和功能进行评估。

高档的多探测器CT扫描仪的时间分辨率充其量为80 ms，因此明显低于心脏MRI（40~50 ms）或透视（高达20 ms）。因此，特别是在心率升高的情况下，运动假影阻碍了我们对心脏结构和冠脉的有效分析。心脏钙化很容易在非增强CT中找到。该方法在冠心病的早期诊断起着越来越重要的作用，阴性预测率大于96%。增强CT冠状动脉造影可有效评估冠状动脉血管和动脉粥样硬化斑块。空间分辨率目前为0.4 mm³。然而，CT冠状动脉造影的临床适应证仍有争议，确定的适应证范围仅限于以下方面：心包或心肌钙化、心包积液、心脏肿瘤、冠脉钙化、冠脉旁路形成、冠脉畸形等。

3. 超声检查

超声检查由于易于使用且相对价格便宜，以及没有电离辐射等优点，超声心动图已经成为目前心脏诊断的常规项目。M型、B型、多普勒和彩色多普勒超声各有不同。特殊对比剂技术的应用属于较新的范畴。

M型超声心动图能够对心脏瓣膜进行功能分析，确定心肌厚度，并在心脏周期中测量心脏大小。B型为二维成像，主要用于心脏结构的形态学评估。

多普勒超声用于评估和分析瓣膜疾病、心脏内血压和血流情况。连续波（CW）和脉冲波（PW）多普勒有一定区别。连续波多普勒超声能比较准确地分析心脏高速血流（如在瓣膜狭窄病变中），但无距离选通性能，缺乏距离分辨力。另一方面，PW多普勒超声允许自由选择深度范围，但不能精确地测量心脏高速血流。彩色多普勒超声将多普勒效应与二维成像相结合。通过应用不同的颜色编码，来显示流动血液的流动方向和速度。该方法特别用于检测和评估分流或瓣膜疾病。

在超声造影中，通过静脉注射的超声对比剂使得超声波的反射明显增强。超声对比剂由微泡组成。它尺寸为2~3 mm，约为红细胞大小的四分之一。一旦声波碰到这些微泡，它们会比正常的血液分散得更加明显。超声波以不同的速度反射回换能器，从而影响屏幕上吸光度的差异。因此，对比剂增强的区域显得更明亮，周围的结构则更容易地区分和识别。

4. MRI 检查

MRI可以通过无创且无辐射的方式对心脏结构和功能进行评估，心功能的评估包括心功能、心肌收缩力、室壁运动、灌注等方面。心脏磁共振成像过程是复杂的，扫描参数的选择往往取决于设备的不同和技术员的扫描经验。目前大多数研究使用快速梯度回波序列进行扫描。心功能和心肌收缩力的评估常使用CINE成像技术而非使用对比剂，而心脏流量的测量则需借助对比剂。除此之外，对比剂（钆）还通常用于心脏缺血、冠脉造影、心肌活力评估和灌注测量等方面。心脏MRI的时间分辨率约为50 ms，空间分辨率约为0.3 mm。目前，MRI相关的科学研究包括冠脉造影、心脏血管移植（搭桥）术的功能评价、瓣膜疾病和分流缺陷的诊断等方面。

心脏MRI的常用临床适应证如下：①先天性心脏病术前和术后复查；②先天性或获得性纵隔病变；③心脏室壁或心腔内肿块；④心包疾病；⑤炎症性心肌病；⑥缺血性心脏病心肌活性测定和心功能测定。禁忌证如下：①安装心脏起搏器患者；②植入式自动心脏复律除颤器；③由磁性材料制成的异物、假体或医用植入器材。

5. 核医学检查

核医学相关的多项技术在心脏成像中有应用。它们都是基于静脉注射的放射学核素体内裂解的原理，包括心脏闪烁扫描法、单光子发射计算机断层成像术（SPECT）、正电子成像术（PET）等。

心脏闪烁扫描法中，体内放射学物质产生的辐射会在闪烁光下发出光信号，并通过光电增强管将光信号转换为电信号。这种技术也称为伽马照相术，能记录具有较高时间分辨率的脉冲信号。

在SPECT中，几个伽马相机围绕患者旋转，从而能在各方向投影中记录不同的测量值。该技术类似于多排CT，可以进行横断位、冠状位和矢状位的图像重建。因此，避免了放射性信号在同一平面相互叠加的问题。放射性核素心室造影（锝-99 m标记红细胞）和心肌代谢活性测量即心肌灌注显像（201-氯化铊/锝-99 m），这两种方法主要用于评价心室功能。此外，在监测移植物排斥反应或诊断心肌炎等免疫成像方面该方法也少有应用。

PET主要基于电子和正电子的湮灭反应。该反应能产生光能（511 KeV），并同时产生互成相反方向的伽马光子。断层扫描装置中两个对称位置上的探测器能同时对两个光子进行记录，从而能对湮灭反应中的光子对进行定位。该技术主要应用于心肌活力的评价。

第二节　正常表现

在正常生理条件下，大约三分之二的心脏位于胸部的左侧，心脏其余部分位于胸部右侧。个人的心脏大小与其对应的拳头大小相近，重量约为250 g到350 g之间（即每千克体重对应心脏重量约为5 g）。纵向隔膜将心脏分为左半部分和右半部分，每个部分又分为心房和心室。四个心脏瓣膜充当单向阀的功能，在正常生理条件下，它们只允许顺行方向的血流通过。右室有三尖瓣和室上嵴，将肺动脉与三尖瓣环分开。

左心室具有二尖瓣，没有圆锥肌位于主动脉和二尖瓣之间，因此，主动脉瓣后瓣与二尖瓣前瓣是连续的，升主动脉位于左心室的右前方，左心室位于左后方，肺动脉干位于右心室左后方，而右心室位于右前方。这种螺旋状关系为正常大血管表现。主动脉结和降主动脉位于左侧。4个投影位置构成的心脏检查方法能准确地显示心脏和其房室的解剖关系(图7-1)。

1. 后前位胸片(PA)

从上往下，右心缘由上腔静脉、右心房构成，两者的相交处可见交角，当升主动脉扩张舒展时，升主动脉参入右心缘的组成[图7-1(a)]；左心缘由主动脉结、主肺动脉、左心室构成，主动脉结代表所观察到的主动脉弓，主动脉结下方是主肺动脉的左外侧壁，代表肺动脉段或肺动脉干(右心室流出道)。有时，在肺动脉段和左心室之间，有一小段，代表左心房耳部。在心脏收缩期，左心室向内收缩，与向外扩张的肺动脉段和主动脉结运动方向相反。相交点即是相反搏动点，为左心室的标志，降主动脉沿脊柱左缘下行，一般为高密度的心影掩盖，左侧心膈角常见一小的三角形阴影，此为心包脂肪垫。

2. 左侧位

心脏阴影位于前部膈肌上方下部胸骨之后，前缘上部由右心室漏斗部和肺动脉干前壁构成，下部由右心室(窦部)前壁构成，后上缘为左心房，后下缘由左心室构成[图7-1(b)]。食管充盈钡剂后，显示在紧贴心影后方行走。主动脉弓为一个大弓，肺动脉位于主动脉弓下方显示为一个小弓。

3. 右前斜位(RAO)

在此投照位置患者向前旋转45°，右肩贴近胶片，心脏呈斜位，从上往下，左前缘由主动脉、肺动脉段和右心室前壁构成[图7-1(c)]。左心室仅参与构成心尖前部的一小段心缘。右后心缘由上而下为左心房、右心房、下腔静脉，在此投照位置，左心房与食管关系显示最理想，食管显示光滑，位于左房后缘。左房增大，造成食管压迹和食管移位，局限性移位具有意义。心脏和前胸壁之间上宽下窄的三角形透亮影为右肺，在右后心缘和脊柱之间的含气透亮区为心后间隙。

4. 左前斜位(LAO)

患者往左旋转60°，左肩贴近胶片，心脏呈垂直状态，室间隙几乎平行于X线，心室大致可均分为前、后两半，右前心缘由右心构成，由上往下，依次为升主动脉、右房、右心室[图7-1(d)]。紧接升主动脉下方为一斜面，1/3的心右缘由右心房构成，其余部分由右心室构成。左后心缘上部由左心房构成，左房位于气管分叉下方，与左侧气管关系密切，左心室构成左心缘下部。在正常和标准位置上，左心室的后缘不应与胸椎影重叠。在此位置，主动脉弓和降主动脉显示最佳。

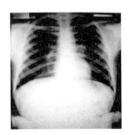 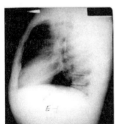 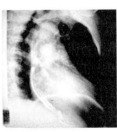 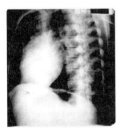

(a)正常后前位　　(b)正常左侧位　　(c)正常右前斜位　　(d)正常左前斜位

图7-1　心脏和其房室的解剖关系影像

在心脏疾病的诊断中，特别是在评价肺循环状态时，肺血管改变非常重要。应当仔细观察其血管类型、分布、并且与同侧和对侧肺血管比较。区别动脉和静脉有一定难度，一个较实用的方法是分析血管的走行方向以判断为动脉或静脉。在后前位胸片上，左、右肺动脉易于辨认，肺动脉自肺门区呈放射状向肺内扇形分布，右下肺动脉宽度15 mm左右。上肺静脉位于上肺动脉外侧，在肺门区，在下肺动脉前方交叉下行汇入左房的外上部分。下肺静脉较水平走行，汇入左房。正常情况下，肺门血管直径大，肺血管也较粗大,肺门血管直径小,肺血管也较细小;下叶血管较上叶血管明显,在正常人肺血管宽度由血流量决定,直立体位,血流量由下往上逐渐减少,肺尖几乎为零。血管直径反映了血流状态,第一前肋间内血管直径很少超过3 mm,而在膈上血管直径可达6 mm或更大。锁骨下区血管直径小于3 mm。在心脏疾病中,肺循环状态可通过肺血管类型推断,此点重要,应当牢记。肺血可以是正常、增多、减少或肺血再分配。

第三节　基本病变

放射学医生的主要作用在于通过X线平片判断心脏疾病时心脏和大血管的大小、形态、位置、肺血循环的状态。心脏大小的异常,一般来讲,可以反应心脏疾病的存在。而肺血的改变常是血流动力学变化的结果。这些分析有助于得出解剖学(形态学)的诊断或者有利于选择恰当病例进一步检查,以探讨有无外科手术治疗可能。因此,对于放射学医生,认识这些基本变化是最基本的要求。

1. 心影的改变

放射学能提供解剖方面的信息,最重要的是判断心脏是否增大,哪个(些)房室受累,左心房可准确评估,大的右心或左心(心室)具有特征性的形态可以判断,但是在双室增大的情况下,有时难以获得正确的分析。右心房大小也有时难以准确判断。均须要结合不同投照位置照片综合分析。

(1)弥漫性心脏增大:心脏向两侧增大,心脏横径明显增加,斜位上胸骨后和心后间隙变窄,食管向后均匀移位,气管分叉变平上抬。在后前位胸片,心脏横径与胸廓横径之比CTR(心胸比值)常超过55%。

(2)左心室增大:左心室构成心左缘,轻度的左心室增大不会引起心脏外形(心影)的明显变化,左心室逐渐增大后,左心缘圆隆,左下心弓延长,向左扩大,心尖位置低,向左下移位延伸至膈下,在左前斜位和侧位投照时,左心室向后凸出。根据与下腔静脉投影的关系,往后凸出的左心室易于辨认,在下腔静脉上部之处如果后凸超过2.2 cm,应当怀疑有左室扩大。如果左室进一步扩大,左侧位上左心室可与脊柱重叠。常见于高血压、主动脉瓣病变、二尖瓣关闭不全、扩张型心肌病或部分先心病(动脉导管未闭)等。

(3)右心室增大:正位胸片上,右心室增大使心尖圆钝上翘,心尖向左移位,左心缘肺动脉段突出,肺动脉段突出是诊断右室增大的一个可靠的间接征象,这是由于在右心室增大时,心脏向左旋转。在侧位胸片上,心前缘下段前凸,与胸骨后间隙模糊。常见于二尖瓣狭窄、肺动脉高压、肺源性心脏病、左向右分流的先天性心脏病等。

(4)左房增大:在侧位或右前斜位上,食管吞钡时,增大的左房在食管下1/3处形成局限压迹或压迫食管向后移位。在正位胸片,扩大的左心房在右心缘产生额外的投影,重叠于右心缘,形成双房影。由于左心房耳部扩大,在心左缘肺动脉段与左心室间形成心弓,此即所谓病理性第三弓,在左前斜位增大的左房使左主支气管上抬,增大显著时还可造成压迫,气管分叉角增宽。常见于二尖瓣病变、左心衰竭等。

(5)右房增大:右心房构成心右缘,右心房增大时心右缘膨凸或延长。右房增大有时难以判断,常见于先天性心脏病,如房间隔缺损。心右下缘往右突出,右房高度增加,达整个纵隔右缘高度的一半。此征象有参考价值。

(6)混合性心室扩大:如果某一心室增大占优势,心脏形态的改变可提示该心室的扩大。如果两个心室均等地扩大,左心室影延长,向上、外舒展,结果是后前位胸片上(左心弓延长)心室影变长,心尖上翘。

2. 心脏钙化

心脏和心包钙化的显示,放射学起着非常重要的作用,在诊断方面,有一些钙化非常有价值,这些钙化区域在高穿透透视、体层、电影影像和CT上显示良好。

瓣膜钙化:瓣膜钙化常见于二尖瓣和主动脉瓣,二尖瓣瓣膜钙化主要见于风湿性心脏病,而二尖瓣环钙化主要是由于退行性变。在年轻者,主动脉瓣钙化提示先天性主动脉二瓣化狭窄。区分二尖瓣和主动脉瓣钙化及二尖瓣和二尖瓣环钙化非常重要。

心包钙化:1/2的缩窄性心包炎患者,放射学可发现其心包钙化。此具有确诊价值。这种钙化可表现为蛋壳样钙化，沿心室膈面包绕心影，有时，侧位显示最佳。

3. 心脏疾患的肺血变化

肺血的变化与肺血管压力有良好的对应关系，当肺静脉压高于最大平均正常压力 10 mmHg，肺静脉扩张显示为上肺门外侧血管和下叶静脉扩张；如果肺静脉压接近或高于 18 mmHg，肺血的放射学表现典型，上肺静脉明显扩张，下肺静脉反而较前缩小，这种与正常肺血分布相反的情况是由于下叶血管收缩，血流再分配流入上叶，这种典型表现见于二尖瓣狭窄；当静脉压超过 25 mmHg，水肿液聚集，发生肺水肿。放射学将肺水肿分为 2 型：

间质性肺水肿：左心室衰竭前期即在左心临床衰竭前放射学所显示的征象，水肿液积聚于肺间质组织，表现为：①肺野云雾状改变——肺野密度增加，呈磨砂样改变；②肺门影扩大，结构模糊；③上肺静脉扩张；④下肺静脉收缩；⑤克氏线：为水平走行的细小短线，与胸膜垂直，紧邻外侧胸膜，常见于下肺的肋膈角区，不见于上肺，为增厚或水肿的小叶间隔。当经过恰当治疗后，静脉压恢复正常，克氏线消失。

肺泡性肺水肿：发生于急性左心衰，特征性表现为双肺野云絮状密度增高，典型者呈两侧对称分布，可表现为"蝶翼形"，偶尔表现为以肺门为中心的单侧肺野的大片高密度影（蝶翼）。这是由于水肿液进入肺泡，短时间内可迅速消失。

肺血增多（肺充血）：正常情况下，右心输出量与左心输出量相等，故体循环与肺循环血量相等，当存在左——右分流时，肺循环血流量将超过体循环血流量。当肺循环血量接近或超过保持正常肺动脉压血量 2 倍时，出现放射影像表现，当分流量大于肌性动脉所能承受的限度时，肺动脉压力因血流量过大而升高，导致肺动脉高压。肺血流量增多的变化包括：①肺动脉段（肺动脉干）和肺门血管扩张突出，搏动增强；②右下叶动脉扩张，宽度成人超过 15 mm，肺动脉轮廓清晰；③中央肺动脉扩张正比于外周肺段动脉，并延伸到上、下叶外周；④肺野清晰，与肺静脉高压表现不同。

肺动脉高压：肺动脉高压的原因可以是原发的或继发的，原发性肺动脉高压是由于动脉壁和动脉腔的异常所致，本文不与讨论。继发性肺动脉高压，继发于肺静脉高压或先天性心脏病中的左——右分流，或者继发于肺部疾病（肺源性心脏病）。

当肺动脉压力超过 30 mmHg 时，即为肺动脉高压，其压力由肺血流量和肺血管阻力之间的关系决定。放射学改变包括：①肺动脉干和相应的肺动脉扩张，透视下见肺门舞蹈；②段肺动脉变细或收缩；③右心室扩大。

肺静脉压超过 10 mmHg 表明肺静脉高压，如果压力超过 25 mmHg，发生肺水肿，放射学表现包括：①上肺静脉扩张，这同正常肺血分布相反，表明左房压力升高，上叶肺静脉的大小与肺静脉压力基本保持平行；②间质性或肺泡性肺水肿的 X 线征象；③肺野透亮度减低，磨玻璃状改变；④胸腔积液，游离性或包裹性。

肺血流量减少（肺血减少）：因为肺血管的大小与肺血流量密切相关，肺血的减少表明右心室流出量减少或梗阻，梗阻常位于肺动脉瓣或肺动脉漏斗部，如肺动脉狭窄，法鲁氏四联症。放射学表现为：肺野透亮度高，肺血管影稀少，肺门区和外周肺野内的肺血管均变细小，心腰（肺动脉段）内凹，系肺动脉干发育不良，肺血减少可以是局部的或单侧，如肺动脉栓塞。

4. 心包积液

心影扩大应当考虑到有心包积液的可能，一般而言，无特殊心型的心脏扩大，特别是无肺静脉充盈扩张时，应当考虑到心包积液的可能。

正常心包腔内含有 15~30 mL 左右的液体，300 mL 以下的心包积液，X 线平片难以发现，当液体量积聚较多时，X 线方能发现，其影像表现：①心脏影大小和形态的改变，后前位胸片上液体通常积聚于心包底部，逐渐在腔内向上扩展，这种液体的分布引起心影的对称性扩大，双侧正常心脏各房室轮廓被掩盖，呈烧瓶形心脏或球形；②心影大而主动脉结小：因为主动脉结位于心包之外，而且心包积液时，心脏排血量降低；③心影增大，而无肺静脉高压表现，肺野相对透亮，血管纹理稀疏；④上腔静脉扩张；⑤透视下，心室缘搏动减弱或无搏动,而主动脉搏动仍然正常存在。

第四节　常见疾病诊断

心脏疾患有很多分类方法,最常用的是分为2大类:先天性和获得性心脏病。先天性心脏病又进一步分为发绀型和非发绀型,对于放射学医生,解剖和生理学的知识是分析心脏疾病的基础。

1. 获得性心脏病

（1）高血压性心脏病:

1）临床与病理表现:高血压性心脏病是由于体循环高压引起的,是指收缩压持续高于140 mmHg和（或）舒张压持续高于90 mmHg。如果血压仅仅是短暂升高,高血压心脏病便不会发生。此外,中、重度高血压可以多年存在,但却无心脏扩大,心脏扩大一般在心功能衰竭之后才出现。人体对血压升高的心室反应为心肌肥厚,但心室肥厚不一定会引起心脏大小和形态改变。原发性高血压的发病基础是全身小动脉广泛性痉挛,造成周围血流阻力增高,动脉血压因此升高。此时,左心为维持正常供血承担过大的负荷,致使心肌肥厚。当左心不能代偿而出现失代偿时,会导致左心扩大,左心功能不全。临床表现为高血压引起的头昏、头痛、耳鸣、乏力等,左心衰导致呼吸困难、端坐呼吸、咯血、心绞痛等。

2）影像学表现:

①X线表现:以左心室扩大增厚和主动脉增宽延长为主。左心室扩大表现为心界向左扩大,左心缘圆钝、外凸,心尖向下、向外移位。左前斜位可见增大的左心室与脊柱影重叠。主动脉增宽延长表现为主动脉扩张、迂曲,主动脉结突出,主动脉心型。左心房也可有增大表现,严重情况下,出现全心功能不全,所有心腔出现扩张,心脏中—重度增大,心脏搏动减弱,可有心包和胸腔积液。

②CT和MRI表现:CT表现为左心室增大以及升主动脉扩张。MRI可以发现室间隔普遍均匀性增厚,左心室心腔稍缩小,但心室壁心肌信号无异常。升主动脉扩张但不累及主动脉窦。左心室腔增大时提示病变已经到达晚期,左心功能代偿不全,此时电影可见左心室壁运动减弱,二尖瓣收缩期反流。

（2）慢性风湿性心脏瓣膜疾病:在慢性风湿性心脏病中,放射诊断对瓣膜病变的诊断意义重大,因瓣膜狭窄或关闭不全引起的血流动力学变化的后果常常是产生特征性的心脏外形的改变。二尖瓣受累常见,其次为主动脉瓣,也可发生多个瓣膜同时受累。

1）二尖瓣狭窄

①临床与病理表现:二尖瓣狭窄比二尖瓣关闭不全常见,瓣膜狭窄是由于瓣缘（尖）的瘢痕和增厚所致,始于瓣膜联合区域逐渐融合,导致近瓣膜中央部分呈裂隙状,开放受限,在瘢疤组织和僵硬融合的瓣膜联合部可发生钙化。

正常二尖瓣口大小为2.3~3.5 cm^2,当瓣口面积减小到1.0~1.5 cm^{2}时,因为血液从左房向左室流出受限,而引起明显的血流动力学变化。出现左心房轻中度增大,如果合并二尖瓣关闭不全时,可以出现左心房明显扩大。应当注意的是,在没有明显血流动力学变化的轻型病例,则难以发现左房增大。二尖瓣狭窄使左心房压力升高,压力传导于肺静脉,最终引起肺静脉高压,长期反复的肺静脉高压引起肺小血管的痉挛,最终出现肺动脉高压,致使右心室增大。而左心室因排血量减少,左心室不扩大,主动脉结不突出。

当肺静脉压力超过10 mmHg时,出现间质性肺水肿和克氏（Kerleys）线,间质性肺水肿和克氏线常常见于二尖瓣狭窄合并二尖瓣关闭不全,病程终末期,可以表现为肺静脉和肺动脉高压混合存在。

②影像学表现:首先,当左心房出现增大时,X线表现可以表现为右心缘可见双房影,严重者可以出现左主支气管上抬,气管分叉角增大（图7-2）。如果出现了肺静脉高压,可以表现为间质性肺水肿和肺泡性肺水肿以及肺淤血,从而出现kerley线以及上肺静脉扩张、下肺静脉收缩,血管模糊。进一步发展可以出现肺动脉高压,表现为肺动脉段隆起,肺动脉增粗。最后出现右心室增大,表现为心尖上翘。如果合并有关闭不全,可以出现左心室增大。

CT和MRI表现:CT一般仅能展现风湿性心脏病所致继发性心脏房室大小的改变,不能显示瓣膜受损的情况。MRI 对其诊断价值较高，并以四腔心切面显示最佳，表现为左心房增大，内有缓慢的血流高信号影，左心室不大。肺动脉扩张，右心室壁肥厚，右心室亦可见扩大。电影序列还可以显示二尖瓣狭窄形态和程度，收缩期可见左心室的低信号血流束，如果继发二尖瓣关闭不全，在收缩期还可以见到血液反流信号。此外，有时可见附壁血栓形成。

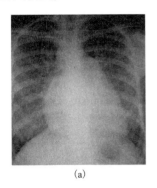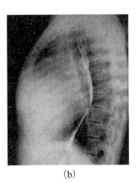

(a)　　　　　　　　　　　　　　　　(b)

(a) 正位：肺淤血，右室增大，肺动脉段突出，左心房增大，左心缘可见
病理第 3 号；(b) 二尖瓣狭窄。侧位：右室左房增大。食道下 1/3 处可
见局限左房压迹和移位。

图 7-2　二尖瓣狭窄

2) 二尖瓣关闭不全：

①临床与病理表现：由于二尖瓣叶和腱索的瘢痕和短缩，使二尖瓣不能正常关闭，此情况较二尖瓣狭窄少见，但二尖瓣狭窄和一定程度的关闭不全可同时发生。在严重情况下，左室收缩大量血流返流进入左心房，为了代偿，左心室必须扩大以容纳较多血液，同时，也会出现左心室心肌肥厚，以代偿性增加心肌收缩力，增大心输出量。最终导致左心室扩张、心肌肥厚。大多数情况下，左心房的扩张较二尖瓣狭窄更明显。

②影像学表现：影像学表现与返流量的大小和心肌状态有关。在轻型病例，返流量不大时，心脏大小和肺血的改变不明显，返流量中度—重度时，左心房明显扩大，可观察到左心房搏动。与二尖瓣狭窄时相反。左心室扩大，肺血量的变化与二尖瓣狭窄时变化相似，但当左心房扩大非常明显，起到血池作用时，肺血的改变轻微。选择性左心室造影可以量化二尖瓣返流。

(3) 慢性肺心病 (慢性肺源性心脏病)：

1) 临床与病理表现：慢性肺源性心脏病是由肺组织、肺动脉血管或胸廓的慢性病变引起肺组织结构和功能异常，致肺血管阻力增加，肺动脉压力增高，使右心扩张、肥大，伴或不伴有右心衰竭的心脏病，最常见的病因为慢性阻塞型肺疾病。此疾患肺部存在广泛的纤维化和阻塞性肺气肿，心脏病变系继发于该慢性肺实质病变，引起肺血管阻力增加，该疾患同时有呼吸功能不全和肺泡氧含量降低 (低氧血症)。肺血管阻力增加导致肺动脉高压，引起右心衰竭，表现为颈静脉怒张，肝颈静脉反流征阳性，第二心音亢进等。

2) 影像学表现：

①X 线表现：存在肺部纤维和肺气肿等慢性肺实质病变，X 线表现为双肺纹理增粗、紊乱，双肺透亮度增高。右心室增大，早期右心室轻度肥厚，X 线表现不明显难以诊断。当肺动脉段突出，搏动增强，右下肺动脉增粗时，或者出现肺动脉段突出，提示右心室增大。

②CT 和 MRI 表现：CT 上表现为双肺支气管血管束增多增粗紊乱，双肺可见多发薄壁及无壁透亮影。CT 和 MRI 上表现为主肺动脉管径增宽，宽于同层面主动脉，右心室增大，一般左心室不受影响。

(4) 心包疾病：

1) 心包积液：

①临床与病理表现：正常情况下，心包囊内有少量液体，当病变累及心包时如结核、风湿性或化脓性

感染,心包腔内液体过多,引起一定的心影改变。如果是少量心包积液,一般无特殊不适,如果是大量心包积液,可以表现气短、胸痛等。如果心包积液突然急剧增长时,心包的顺应性下降,表现为限制性的心包积液,有可能出现心包填塞。

②影像学表现:X线表现心影普遍性增大,心影搏动减弱或消失,肺野清晰,肺纹理稀少(图7-3)。

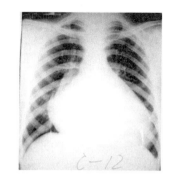

图7-3　心包积液。心影普遍性增大,肺野清晰,肺纹理稀少

2)缩窄性心包炎:

①临床与病理表现:当两层心包因粘连或者纤维化,或瘢痕而融合时,心包增厚,心脏被包裹,心脏搏动明显受限,结核是最常见的病因,其他有风湿热、外伤、结核、化脓性感染和恶性肿瘤。很多情况下,病因不明。慢性缩窄性心包炎由于常需外科治疗而得到重视。

②影像学表现:心影多不增大,甚至比正常小,也可以轻度增大。因心包增厚、粘连,心影常表现为怪异形,正常心影轮廓消失。心影搏动减弱或某些部分消失。心包钙化,是诊断该病的直接征象。

2.先天性心脏病

先天性心脏病是指胚胎发育时期(一般在胚胎发育第4~8周)由于心脏及大血管的形成障碍或发育异常而引起的解剖结构异常,或出生后应自动关闭的通道未能闭合(在胎儿属正常)的情形。为了便于放射学的评价,根据肺血、心影大小和形态的表现对先天性心脏病进行分类。左—右分流的先天性心脏病,肺血增多,而在右室流出道梗阻时,肺血则减少。肺血的评价是基础,肺血的改变必须与心脏的大小和形态改变相结合。此外,心影正常和肺血正常不能排除有先天性心脏病。因此,必须结合临床资料做出恰当的诊断。对于复杂病例,其他检查手段也不可缺少,如超声、心导管检查和心血管造影。本章仅讨论一些简单的病例。

(1)左-右分流(非发绀型)

1)房间隔缺损:房间隔缺损(ASD)是指房间隔在发育过程中没有完全封闭而形成的缺损,导致左、右心房之间异常血液交通的先天性心脏畸形。正常情况下,卵圆孔在出生后数小时或数天内即在功能上闭合,通常在6岁前完成解剖上闭合。ASD包括以下几种类型:原发孔型(Ⅰ孔型)、继发孔型(Ⅱ孔型)和其他类型,以继发孔型常见。

①临床与病理表现:房间隔缺损,不管其何种类型,在心室舒张期,因大量血液从左心房向右心房分流,导致右心的负荷增加,分流量多少同缺损的大小有关。

②影像学表现:

典型者X线表现为肺血增多,双肺门及外周血管增粗,透视下可见搏动增强(肺门舞蹈),肺动脉段膨出,右心房及右心室增大,导致心影向右向前增大,心尖向左移位(图7-4)。主动脉结细小,左室细小或增大。

CT及MRI表现:CT上直接征象为房间隔连续性中断,可显示缺损位置、大小、数量。间接征象为右心房、右心室增大、肺动脉扩张。CT检查的目的不是为了诊断房间隔缺损本身,而是成人(>50岁)外科介入治疗术前排除冠脉病变;观察有无合并其他心外畸形,如肺静脉畸形引流;诊断超声难以诊断上述特殊类型。MRI可用于鉴别房间隔缺损和卵圆孔未闭,如果单纯为了诊断ASD,通常不做MRI检查。

2)室间隔缺损:室间隔缺损(VSD)是心室间隔各部分发育不全或相互融合不良而形成心室间血流异常交通的一种先天性心脏畸形。发生率仅次于房间隔缺损(ASD),可以分为膜部室间隔缺损、嵴上型室间隔缺损以及肌部室间隔缺损。膜部或肌部50%以上的VSD是单独存在的,即不合并其他心脏缺损。

①临床与病理表现:室间隔缺损产生左向右分流,分流量取决于缺损的大小、左右心室压力差、肺血管阻力。分流较大的VSD左心负荷加重,左心房、左心室扩张,可导致动力性肺动脉高压。随着病程的进展,最终导致器质性肺动脉高压,甚至引起右向左分流,出现艾森门格综合征,患者此时

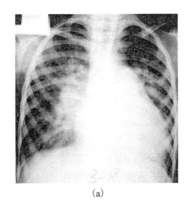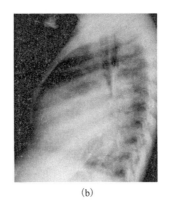

(a)后前位：心影增大，呈二尖瓣型，右室右房增大，肺动脉段突出，肺血增
多；(b)侧位：右心增大，左心室及左心房被向后推移。

图 7-4　房间隔缺损(ASD)

可出现发绀。

②影像学表现

X 线表现：小的室间隔缺损心影改变不明显，中-重度缺损者，心脏增大，并二尖瓣返流，双心室和左心房扩大，肺血增多，肺动脉段突出，可见肺门舞蹈，并且，由于肺血管阻力增加，易于导致肺动脉高压，随着年龄增大和病变的发展，肺血管阻力可超过体循环压力，而导致反向分流(右-左分流)，此时患者有发绀，影像表现为典型肺动脉高压表现。

CT 与 MRI 表现：CT 直接征象为室间隔连续性中断，并可显示室间隔缺损的部位和大小，间接征象为左心房、左心室增大，肺动脉扩张。CT 检查的目的不仅仅是为了诊断室间隔缺损本身，主要是为了诊断是否合并其他心脏畸形，主动脉瓣周病变的鉴别，如主动脉窦瘤破裂，上述特殊类型的 VSD 而超声难以诊断者。MRI 对室间隔中膜部和肌部的缺损显示较好，但是对漏斗部缺损易漏诊。

3)动脉导管未闭(PDA)

胚胎时期，左肺动脉与左锁骨下动脉开口远端的降主动脉间存在一个管道交通，它的重要功能是将大部分进入右心室的血流引流入主动脉，从而绕过尚未充气的肺，出生后，呼吸的建立和肺血管血流量的增加，该导管的功能结束，最终变为一条韧带，称之为动脉韧带。如果在出生后该管道没有自然闭合，肺动脉和主动脉之间仍保持有血管相通，形成血液异常分流的病变，是最常见的先天性心脏病之一。

①临床与病理表现：这是一种心外的左-右分流，在肺血管阻力尚未升高时，分流的方向从主动脉流向肺循环，类似于 VSD，当肺血管狭窄阻力明显升高，大于体循环压力时，则反向分流，从右-左分流，产生下半身的分界性紫绀。根据未闭动脉导管的形态，可以分为以下几种类型：漏斗型，窗型，管状型，动脉瘤型，其中以管状型最常见。

②影像学表现：

X 线表现：典型表现为肺血增多，左心室增大，左心房可以增大，主动脉结增宽，肺动脉段突出。如果出现肺动脉高压、艾森门格综合征时则表现为全心增大。

CT 和 MRI 表现：直接征象表现为主动脉弓层面可见降主动脉近端与肺动脉分叉部间的异常血管影或交通，间接征象为当 PDA 较大时可有左心负荷增大，肺动脉高压的表现，比如左心室增大，肺动脉增宽等，CT 并不作为动脉导管未闭的首选检查。MRI GRE 序列对于发现细小的动脉瘤比较敏感，狭窄的动脉瘤内高速血流呈高信号，并且能够显示血流的喷射方向，从而确定分流类型。

所有这些放射学表现，在明显的左-右分流的情况下均可出现，X 线平片上(ASD、VSD、PDA)之间存在差别(表 7-1)：

表 7-1 ASD、VSD、PDA 鉴别诊断要点

	右心房	右心室	肺动脉干	肺血	左心房	左心室	主动脉
ASD	↑	↑	↑	↑	→	→	→↓
VSD	→	→↑	↑	↑	↑	↑	→
PDA	→	→	↑	↑	→↑	→↑	↑

注：↑—增加，→—无变化，↓—减少。

(2)右-左分流(发绀型)：1)法洛氏四联症：为儿童和青少年中最常见的发绀型复杂先天性心脏病。外科手术可完全纠正，手术效果良好。该疾患由四种畸形组成：肺动脉狭窄，室间隔缺损，右心室肥厚和主动骑跨，但室间隔缺损和肺动脉狭窄具有主要的生理学意义。

①临床与病理表现：法洛氏四联症的病理生理变化主要取决于肺动脉狭窄和室间隔缺损对血流动力学的影响。由于室间隔缺损使左右心室收缩压相近，肺动脉升高更使右心室压力增高并导致心内右向左分流。动脉血氧饱和度减低，组织缺氧，临床出现发绀，肺血减少使体肺循环侧枝增加。肺血减少程度主要取决于肺动脉狭窄程度和肺动脉发育情况，狭窄越重，组织缺氧与发绀就越明显。

②影像学表现：

X 线表现(图 7-5)：两肺血减少，肺野清晰，肺门和外周血管变细小，肺动脉段凹陷，右心室圆隆，增大，同时由于右心室的漏斗部狭窄，肺动脉干变小，表现为靴型心，左心室和左心房大小正常，主动脉弓增宽，右位主动脉弓发生率为25%，手术前常须心导管和选择性心血管造影确诊，并与紫绀型先天性心脏病鉴别。

CT 和 MRI 表现：CT 和 MRI 能够清晰显示肺动脉狭窄的部位及其程度，同时可以了解有无合并其他畸形。

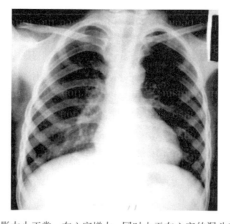

心影大小正常。右心室增大，同时由于右心室的漏斗部狭窄，肺动脉干变小，表现为"靴型"心。肺血减少，肺野清晰，肺门和外周血管变细小。左心室左心房正常。

图 7-5 法洛氏四联症(F4)

(曾牧，刘佳易，肖恩华，罗建光)

Chapter 7

Heart and great vessels

The heart is a hollow muscular organ. The heart lies like an oblique cone within the chest, surrounded by the right and left lungs. The base of the heart projects to the right, and the apex to the left. At present, any assessment of the heart by means of conventional technology will predominantly be done by chest x-ray. For any in-depth cardiac diagnosis, other, more radiological techniques such as computed tomography (CT), magnetic resonance imaging (MRI), sonography, angiography, or even nuclear medicine procedures appear preferable. Previously used techniques such as x-ray-based cinematography for motion analysis or tomography have now completely been abandoned.

Section 1　Method of examination

1. Plain film and angiography examination

It is important to taint a full chest film in normal inspiration and upright position. At least, two views should be taken, PA and lateral views, at the distance of 2 m. At this distance, the magnification is minimal. Sometimes, two oblique views also taken if necessary.

Catheter angiography orangiocardiography is an X-ray contrast-based technique that allows for the display of coronary arteries, the great vessels, and the heart chamber. Image acquisition is performed with the patient supine. Classic projections are RAO and LAO. Angiocardiography allows not only assessment of the size, form, function, and contractile response of the heart but also selective evaluation of the coronary arteries. Contraindications to angiography are the following: Hyperthyroidism, allergic reactions to contrast agents, congestive heart failure, coagulation disorders.

2. Cardiac computed tomography

Cardiac imaging by means of CT has been possible only since the introduction of electrocardiogram (ECG)-gated multidetector-row CT. With this technique, volume data sets of the heart can be acquired within a relatively short acquisition time of $3-15$ s total breath-hold. From these data, overlapping submillimeter thin slices can be reconstructed during any phase of the R-R cycle, allowing for CT images of the heart that are virtually free of motion artefacts. The main limitation is that the patient's heart rate must be low to medium-high (<70 bpm). By combining multiphase reconstructions from one complete R-R cycle, myocardial movement and function can also be evaluated.

Temporal resolution of a high-end multidetector-row CT scanner amounts to 80 msat best and therefore is distinctly lower than that of cardiac MRI ($40\sim50$ ms) or fluoroscopy (up to 20 ms). Thus, especially at elevated heart rates, motion artefacts prevent valid analysis of cardiac structures and coronary arteries. X-ray exposure is approximately in the region of that for catheter angiography. Coronary calcifications are easily detected by means of unenhanced cardiac CT. With a negative predictive value of>96%, this method plays an increasingly important role in early detection of coronary heart disease. Contrast-enhanced CT coronary angiography allows for valid assessment of the coronary vessels and atherosclerotic plaques. Spatial resolution is currently 0. 4 mm³. However, clinical indications for CT coronary angiography are still controversial, and the range of established indications is restricted to the following: Calcifications of the pericardium/myocardium, pericardial effusions, cardiac neoplasms, coronary calcifications, coronary artery bypass, coronary artery anomalies.

3. Sonography

Due to ease of use, ubiquitous availability, and the absence of ionizing radiation, echocardiography has become the standard procedure in cardiac diagnostics nowadays. A distinction is drawn between M-mode, B-mode, Doppler, and color Doppler sonography. Relatively new is the use of specific contrast agents.

M (motion)-mode echocardiography enables functional analysis of the heart valves, determination of the myocadiac thickness, and measurements of heart cavity size during the cardiac cycle. B-mode represents two-dimensional echocardiography and is mainly used for morphological assessment of cardiac structures.

Doppler sonography is used for assessment and analysis of valvular disease, intracardiac blood pressure, andflow conditions. A distinction is drawn between continuous wave (CW) and pulsed wave (PW) Doppler methods. CW Doppler sonography allows for accurate analysis of high flow rates (e. g. , in valvular stenosis), but not for a statement about the formation depth. PW Doppler sonography, on the other hand, allows for free choice of the depth range but not for exact determination of high flow rates. Color Doppler sonography combines Doppler effect with two-dimensional B-mode imaging. By the application of different color coding, flowing blood is displayed depending on flow direction and speed. This method is used in particular for detecting and assessing shunt vitiate or valvular insufficiency.

In contrast-enhanced echocardiography, the reflection of the ultrasonic waves is significantly enhanced by intravenous administration of an ultrasound contrast agent. Echo contrast agents consist of microbubbles. They have a size of 2~3 microns, which is about one-quarter the size of a red blood cell. As soon as ultrasonic waves impinge on these microbubbles, they are dispersed more than normal blood. Ultrasonic waves are reflected back to the transducer at different speeds, effecting absorbance differences on the screen. Tus, contrast-enriched regions appear brighter, and surrounding structures can be distinguished and recognized more easily.

4. Magnetic resonance imaging

MRI allows for non-invasive, radiation-exposure free evaluation of cardiac chambers, structures, and function. Assessment of cardiac function includes pump function, myocadiac contractility, wall motion, perfusion. Sufficient MR cardiac imaging is very complex, and the choice of scanning parameters is specific to the examiner and the device. Most studies nowadays are performed using fast spoiled gradient-echo sequences. Cardiac function and myocardial contractility are assessed by using cine sequences and without contrast agent; flow measurements are done by means of phase-contrast angiography; and contrast agent (gadolinium) is usually needed for ischemia diagnosis, MR coronarography, assessment of myocadiac viability, and perfusion measurements. Temporal resolution of cardiac MRI amounts to approximately 50 ms and spatial resolution to about 0. 3 mm. Still under scientific evaluation is the use of MR angiography for the coronary arteries, functional diagnostics of cardiac bypass grafts, and diagnosis of diseases of the heart valves and shunt defects.

Commonly accepted clinical indications for cardiac MRI are assessment of the following: (1)Congenital heart disease before and after surgical correction. (2)Congenital or acquired disorders of the great mediastinal vessels.

（3）Mural or intracavitary cardiac masses. （4）Peri cardiac diseases. （5）Inflammatory myocardial diseases. （6） Myocardial viability in ischemic coronary disease and myocardial function. MRI scanning is contraindicated in the presence of the following: （1）Pacemakers. （2）Implantable automatic cardioverter defibrillators （ICDs）. （3） Foreign bodies, prostheses, or medical implants made of ferromagnetic material.

5. Nuclear medicine

Several nuclear medicine procedures are used in cardiac imaging. As a basic principle, the intracorporeal disintegration of artificial intravenous radionuclides is involved. Relevant procedures include cardiac scintigraphy, single photon emission computed tomography （SPECT）, and positron emission tomography （PET）. In cardiac scintigraphy, radiation emerging from a body inducesflashes in a scintillation light, which are reinforced by means of a photomultiplier tube. This arrangement is called a gamma camera and allows recording of electrical signals with high （ms）temporal resolution.

In SPECT, several gamma cameras rotate around the patient and thus register measurement values from various projections. Similar to multidetector row CT, this technique allows reconstruction of transverse, coronal, and sagittal images. Superposition of the radioactivity-as on planar scintigrams-is thus avoided. Both procedures are primarily used for the appraisal of ventricular function （radionuclide ventriculography ［technetium-99m-marked erythrocytes］） and myocadiac metabolism activity （myocadiac perfusion scintigraphy ［201-thallium chloride/ technetium-99m］. Rather rare areas of application are immunoscintigraphic, e. g. , in the case of graft rejection or for diagnosis of myocarditis.

PET is based on the appearance of electrons and positrons at their immediate recombination （destruction radiation）under emission of light energy （511 keV）. This leads to the emission of two photons in diametrically opposing directions. A closed detector ring in the tomography device permits simultaneous registration of the two photons on two opposite （180°） detector elements and therefore allows for determination of the place of the destruction radiation. The main area of application is appraisal of myocadiac viability.

Section 2　Normal appearances

Under physiological conditions about two-thirds of the heart lies in the left side of the chest and one-third in the right. The size of the heart is quite similar to that of the individual's closed fist （total weight about 5g/kg ［250～ 350 g］）. The longitudinal septum divides the heart into left and right halves, which are each subdivided into an atrium and a chamber （ventricle）. Four cardiac valves act as "check valves", and under physiological conditions they allow bloodflow only in an antegrade direction. A distinction is made between the tricuspid and mitral valve （i. e. atrioventricular valves）located between the respective atrium and ventricle （in-flow tract）and the pulmonary and aortic valves （i. e. semilunar valves）located between the right chamber and pulmonary circulation and the left chamber and systemic circulation, respectively （outflow tract）. The right ventricle has a tricuspid valve and a crista supraventricular is separating the pulmonary from the tricuspid valve ridge. The left ventricle has a mitral valve without conical muscles, between the aortic and mitral valve rings, so that there is continuity between the posterior cusp of the aortic valve and the anterior cusp of the mitral valve. The ascending aorta lies to the right and anteriorly relative to left ventricle which is left and posterior. The pulmonary trunk is left and posterior relative to the right ventricle which is right and anterior. The spiral relationship indicates the normally related great vessels. The aortic knob and the descending aorta descend on the left. For an appreciation of the anatomic relationships of the heart and its chamber, there is examined in series consisting of 4 projections （Figure 7-1）.

1. Posterior to anteriorview （PA）

The right cardiac border form above downward is formed by the superior vena cave, the right atrium, the junction of which is indicated by a distinct angle[Figure 7-1(a)]. Only in the presence of marked elongation or dilatation of the ascending aorta does participate in the formation of the right heart border. The left border is formed by the aortic knuckle, which represents that portion of aortic arch observed and below the knob is the left lateral border of the main pulmonary artery, designated as pulmonary segment or pulmonary trunk, (outflow tract of the right ventricle). The left ventricle forms the rest part of the left cardiac border. Sometimes, between the pulmonary segment and the left ventricle, there is a small segment, it represents the left auricular appendage. The motion of the left ventricle is imparting on systole, opposite to the outward pulsation of the pulmonary segment and the aortic knuckle. This is the point of opposite pulsation which serves a landmark of the left ventricle. The descending aorta descends along the left side of the spine and often obscured by the heavy cardiac shadow. The left cardio phrenic angle is often occupied by a small triangular shadow, the epicardial fat pad.

2. Left lateral view

The cardiac shadow is situated over the anterior portion of the diaphragm, just behind the lower part of the sternum [Figure 7-1(b)]. The anterior border is formed above by the infundibulum of the right ventricle and anterior wall of the pulmonary trunk, and below by the anterior wall of the right ventricle (sinus portion), the upper posterior border is that of left atrium, the posterior inferior border is that of left ventricle. The barium-filled esophagus courses immediately posterior to the cardiac shadow. The aortic arch is recognizable as a big arch, the pulmonary artery is seen as a second small arch just below the former.

3. Right anterior oblique view (RAO)

In this projection, the patient rotates anteriorly about 45 degrees with his right shoulder against the film. The heart is positioned obliquely. The left anterior border is formed from above downward by aorta, pulmonary segment anterior wall of the right ventricle [Figure 7-1(c)]. The left ventricle contributes only a small portion to the cardiac border over the apex anteriorly. The right posterior border is formed by the left atrium above and the right atrium and inferior vena cava below. In this view, it is best to show the relationship between the left atrium and the esophagus which shows a smooth located the posterior border of the left atrium. Enlarged left atrium will indent and displace this portion of esophagus. Localized displacement is significant. The translucent triage-shaped space between the anterior chest wall and the heart is occupied by the right lung. It is wider in the upper portion than the lower portion. The air space between the right posterior border of the heart and the spine is called retrocardiac space. The gastric bubble is located away from the spine.

4. Left anterior oblique view (LAO)

Patient rotates about 60 degrees to right with his left shoulder against the film [Figure 7-1(d)]. The heart is positioned vertically, the ventricular septum is almost parallel to the plan of the film. The bulk of the heart is almost equally divided into anterior and posterior portions. The right anterior border is formed by the right heart, from above downward, the ascending aorta right atrium, and right ventricle. Just below the ascending aorta, there is a slope, about 1/3 of the right cardiac border is formed by the right atrium, the rest by the right ventricle. On the left posterior border, the left atrium is situated above, just below the bifurcation of the trachea and in close relationship with left bronchus, while the left ventricle occupies the rest of border. Under normal and standard positioning, the posterior border of the left ventricle should not overlap the shadow of the thoracic spine, the aortic arch and descending aorta are best seen in this view.

The pulmonary vessels of great importance in the diagnosis of cardiac diseases, especially in the evaluation of the status of pulmonary circulation. The vessel pattern and its distribution should be carefully inspected and comparedwith the same or the other side. The differentiation between the arteries and veins is not without difficulty, however, a useful method is by analyzing the direction of the vessels to determine whether they are arterial or venous. The right and left pulmonary arteries are readily recognizable on PA film. The pulmonary arteries radiate out from the hilar region in a fan-like appearance. The width of the right lower pulmonary artery is measurable. It is about 15 mm in width. The views on the other hand, follow a different course because the lower location of the left atrium. The upper lobe vein lies lateral to upper lobe artery and crossing in front of the descending pulmonary artery in the hilum and enters the upper and outer portion of the left atrium. The lower lobe vein assumes a more horizontal course to enter the left atrium. Usually in the normal person, large caliber hilar vessels go with large lung vessels and smaller hilar vessels with small lung vessels. The vascularity of the lower lobes is more prominent than that of the upper lobes. The width of the pulmonary vessels in normal person is depend on blood flow, in the erect position, blood flow diminishes progressively from the lower to the upper zones, being nil at the apex. As the caliber of the vest reflects the flow pattern, so that the vessels on the last. The diameter of first anterior intercostal vessels is often less than 3 mm. In diameter where as those immediately above the diaphragm may be 6 mm, or more. Vessels below the clavicles are even less than 3 mm. It is important to remember that the state of pulmonary circulation in cardiac diseases may be inferred from the pattern of pulmonary flow. Pulmonary vascularity may be normal, increased or decreased or there may be redistribution of pulmonary vascularity.

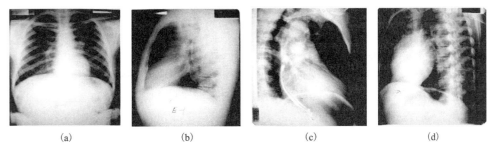

(a) Normal X-ray findings. Posterior to anteriorview (PA); (b) Normal X-ray findings. Left lateral view; (c) Normal X-ray findings. Right anterior oblique view (RAO); (d) Normal X-ray findings. Left anterior obliqueview (LAO).

Figure 7−1

Section 3 Basic pathological changes

The primary role of the radiologist is to find out from the plain film in cardiac disease the size, a shape and position of the heart and great vessels and the state of the pulmonary circulation. Abnormality in the heart size reflects the adverse effect of the cardiac lesion, while changes in the pulmonary vascularity may give some indication of the homodynamic consequence of the lesion and this aids in reaching an anatomical diagnosis or in the selection of cases for further studies with a view to possible surgical treatment. So for the radiologist, it is essential to recognize these basic changes.

1. Changed in the cardiac shadow

The radiology provides information about anatomy, the most important tasks are to determine whether the heart is enlarged and which chamber is involved. The left atrium can be quite accurately assessed, a large right heart or a left heart (ventricles) have characteristic shape, but they are often misleading in biventricular enlargement. Right atrium size is difficult to assess.

(1) Diffuse cardiac enlargement: The heart size is increased to both sides, the transverse diameter is markedly increased. The oblique view shows narrowing of both the substernal and the retrocardiac spaces, the esophagus is displaced uniformly backward, and the trachea bifurcation is sprayed. In posterior anterior chest radiographs, the

ratio of the transverse diameter of the heart to the transverse diameter of the chest(CTR)is usually over 55%.

(2) Left ventricular enlargement: The left ventricle forms the left margin of the heart. There may be no significant change in the cardiac configuration in minor degree of left ventricular enlargement. With increasing enlargement, the border of the left side of the heart becomes progressively rounded and more convex, increasing the length of the left lower cardiac curve and extend more to the left side.

The cardiac apex appears depressed extending below the level of the diaphragm. Posterior bulging of the left ventricle may be demonstrated in LAO and lateral projections. This posterior bulge of the left ventricle is best recognized in relation to the shadow of the inferior vena cava. If the bulge extends posteriorly more than 22 cm, beyond the upper portion of the inferior vena cava, left ventricular enlargement should be suspected. Further enlargement of the left ventricle may overlap the spine in left lateral view. It is commonly seen in hypertensive aortic valve disease, mitral valve insufficiency, dilated cardiomyopathy or partial congenital heart disease (patent ductus arteriosus).

(3) Right ventricular enlargement: It leads to rounding and elevation of the cardiac apex. The apex is shifted to the left. The prominence of the pulmonary artery segment of the left cardiac border serves a valuable indirect sign of right ventricular enlargement, this is due to rotation of the heart to the left in the presence of right ventricular enlargement. These findings are recognizable on PA film. On the lateral film, the anterior inferior segment of the heart is convex and the retrosternal space is blurred. It is commonly seen in mitral stenosis, pulmonary hypertension, pulmonary heart disease, congenital heart disease with left to right shunt, etc.

(4) Left atrial enlargement: The enlarged left atrium forms a localized trace in the lower 1/3 of the esophagus or compresses the esophagus backward by barium swallow on lateral or RAO view. On PA film, the right border of an enlarged left atrium may produce an extra shadow superimposed on the right cardiac border, giving a double contour.

It may form a separate arch between the pulmonary segment and the left ventricle, due to enlargement of the atrial appendage. On the left anterior oblique view, the enlarged left atrium may elevate the left main bronchus and even compressed in case of marked enlargement. The tracheal bifurcation may also be widened. It is commonly seen in mitral valve disease, left heart failure, etc.

(5) Right atrial enlargement: The right atrium forms the right margin of the heart. When the right atrium is enlarged, the right margin of the heart expands or lengthens. This sometimes is difficult to assess. It is often seen in congenital heart disease as in ASD. The right lower cardiac border bulges to right and increase the height of the right atrial. The height should be at least half as long as the total height of the right border of the mediastinum.

(6) Combined ventricular enlargement: If one ventricle to dominant, the cardiac shape may suggest enlargement of that ventricle. If both ventricles are more of less equally enlarged, the left ventricular contour is both elongated and displaced upwards and outwards. The result is often a long ventricular contour with high apex, on the PA view.

2. Cardiac Calcification

Radiology plays an important role in the recognition of cardiac and pericardium calcification. Some ofthese calcifications are most significant in the diagnosis. These calcified areas are best shown on image intensifier fluoroscopy, tomography and cine radiography.

Valvular calcification: Valvular calcifications are found in mitral and aortic valves. Calcification of valve leaflet of the mitral valve is nearly always of rheumatic origin, where as calcification of the mitral annulus is mostly due to degenerative changes. In young subject, calcification of the aortic valve is diagnostic of congenital bicuspid aortic stenosis. It is important to differentiate calcification of the mitral valve and aortic valve and also differentiation between mitral and mitral annulus, (see previous on position of cardiac valve).

Pericardial calcification: In nearly 1/2 of patient with constrictive pericarditis pericardial calcification can be demonstrated radiologically. This is of diagnostic value. The calcification appears as an eggshell type of calcification, around the cardiac border and along the diaphragmatic surface, of the ventricle. Sometimes, this is best shown on lateral film.

3. Changes in pulmonary vascularity in cardiac disease

There is remarkable well correlation between the change of pulmonary vascularity and the pulmonary pressure. When the pulmonary venous pressure is above the maximum mean normal of 10 mmHg, there is dilatation of the pulmonary veins, dilated vesselsseen in the superior lateral aspect of the hilum and lower lobe veins. If the pressure goes up near or above 18 mmHg, as in case of chronic mitral stenosis, chronic heart failure, there is distinct roentgen appearance of the pulmonary vasculature. The superior pulmonary veins become markedly dilated, the inferior pulmonary veins are smaller than usual.

This is the reversal of the normal pulmonary vascular pattern and has been explained on the bases of vasoconstriction in the lower lobes with redistribution of blood flow to the upper lobes. This pattern is so typicallyseen in mitral stenosis. As venous pressure exceeds the osmotic pressure above 25 mmHg, oedematous fluid is accumulated and pulmonary oedema develops. There are two types of pulmonary oedema observed radiologically:

Interstitial pulmonary oedema: Incipient left ventricular failure, that is radiographic visible sign before left clinical heart failure (subclinical heart failure). The oedematous fluid accumulates in the interstitial tissue of the lungs. The roentgen findings: (1) Cloudy appearance of the lung—sight increase of lung density giving a veil-like appearance. (2) Hazziness and loss of their sharp difinition of the hilar shadow. (3) Dilatation of the upper lobe veins. (4) Constriction of the lower lobe veins. (5) Kerley's line. These are thin dense straight, horizontal lines, perpendicular to and almost reaching the lateral pleural surface. They are most commonly seen in the costs phrenic angle in the lower lung but never seen in the upper lung. These are resulted from thickened or oedematous interlobular septa. They usually clear-up when the venous pressure is released after proper treatment.

Alveolar pulmonary oedema: It occurs in acute let heart failure, and is characterized by clouding of the lungs with bilateral. The typical pattern is symmetrical on both sides and can be presented as a butterfly wing. The occasional appearance is unilateral large patches of hazy density in the perihilar region (bating pattern), this is due to edema fluid getting into the air spaces. The onset of clearing may be dramatic within a short period of time.

Increased pulmonary blood flow(plethora). Normally the cardia output of the right side of the heart is equate to that of the left side, so that the systemic and pulmonary blood flows are equal. When a left to right shunt is present, the pulmonary blood flow will exceed the systemic blood flow, andradiographic manifestations will be present when the pulmonary blood flow is around or above 2:1. If the shunt is very large, the limit of dispensability of the muscular arteries is reached and the pulmonary pressure rises because of torrential flow, then hyper kinetic pulmonary hypertension develops. Basic changes of increased pulmonary blood flow includes: (1) Prominence of both hilar vessels and dilatation of the pulmonary segment (pulmonary trunk)with visible pulsation. (2) Enlargement of the right lower lobe artery, its width exceeds 15 mm in adult. The outlines of the pulmonary arteries remain clear. (3) The central arteries enlarge proportionately to the periphery segmental arteries and extends to the periphery of both the upper and lower lobes. (4) The lung fields remain clear, which differs from that of pulmonary venous hypertension.

Pulmonaryhypertension: The cause of pulmonary hypertension may be primary or secondary. Primary pulmonary hypertension is due to abnormalities involving the arterial wall or lumen and this entity will not be discussed here in this text. The secondary pulmonary hypertension is usually secondary to venous hypertension or to left right shunt as in case of congenital heart diseases, or due to diseases of the lung, (pulmonary heart disease).

When the pulmonary arterial systolic pressure exceeds 30 mmHg, it is said to have pulmonary arterial hypertension. The level of the pressure is determined by the relationship between the pulmonary blood flow and the vascular resistance. The radiologic changes include the followings: (1) Dilatation of the pulmonary trunk and control pulmonary arteries, hilar dance may be observed on fluoroscopy. (2) Tapering or constriction of the segmental pulmonary arteries. (3) Enlargement of the right ventricle.

When the pulmonary venous pressure exceeds 10 mmHg, it indicates the presence of pulmonary venous hypertension. If the pressure exceeds 25 mmHg, pulmonary oedema develops. The radiological changes include the followings: (1) Dilatation of upper lobe veins, a reversal of the normal blood flow pattern, this indicates increased left trial pressure. The size of the superior pulmonary vein is parallel to the pressure of the pulmonary vein. (2) Roentgen signs of interstitial or alveolar pulmonary oedema. (3) General haziness of the lung fields. (4) Pleural effusion, it may be either free fluid in the pleural cavity or encapsulated.

Decreased pulmonary blood flow (oligemia): Since the size of the pulmonary vessels is closely related to pulmonary flow, decreased vascularity indicates a general reduction or obstruction. Obstruction is usually at the pulmonic valve or infundibular region as in case of pulmonary stenosis, or tetra logy of Fallot. The radiological manifestations are as follows: The lung fields become unusually clear, the vascular shadows are scarce, the pulmonary vessels in hilar area and peripheral lung field become smaller. The cardiac waist becomes concave because of a hypoplastic pulmonary trunk. Decreased vascularity may be local or unilateral. This may be seen in pulmonary embolism.

4. Pericardial effusion

Pericardial effusion must be considered when evaluating an enlarged heart. In general, a large heart of nonspecific configuration, particularly in the absence of pulmonary venous engorgement, should suggest a pericardial effusion.

The pericardial sac normally contains 15－30ccof fluid and an amount below 300 cc may not be detectable radiologically. When there is sufficient amount of fluid accumulated, it becomes recognizable. The radiological manifestations are as follows: (1) Change of heart size and shape: On EA film fluid usually accumulate in the most dependent part of the pericardial sac and gradually spread upward within the sac. This distribution of fluid causes symmetrical enlargement of the cardiac shadow with obliteration of the normal cardiac curvature on both sides, giving a flask-like or globular in shape. (2) A large heart shadow with an unusual small aortic knuckle, because the later lies outside the pericardium and cardiac output is reduced with pericardial effusion. (3) A large heart with an absence of signs of pulmonary venous hypertension and shows a relatively clear, scanty vascular markings. (4) Engorgement of the superior vena cava. (5) Under fluoroscopy, the ventricular limbic pulsation is weakened or no pulsation, while the aortic pulsation still exists normally.

Section 4   Diagnosis of common diseases

There are many ways to classify cardiac disease. A popular classification used two large categories; congenital and acquired cardiac diseases. Congenital cardiac disease is further subdivided into cyanotic and non-cyanotic. For a radiologist an anatomic and physiologic approach affords an understandable and useful basis for dealing with heart diseases.

1. Acquired heart disease

(1) Hypertensive heart disease

1) Clinical and pathological manifestations: Hypertensive heart disease is due to systemic hypertension. In this

condition systolic blood pressure remains above 140 mmHg and/or diastolic blood pressure remains above 90 mmHg. Hypertension may not be followed by hypertensive heart disease if the hypertension is transient, and moderate to marked degree of hypertension may exist for years without cardiac enlargement until heart failure and dilatation ensue. Ventricles respond to load by hypertrophy, and hypertrophy of a ventricle is not likely to cause an alteration in the size and shape. The pathogenesis of primary hypertension is generalized spasm of small arteries in the whole body, causing increased vascular resistance around the blood, which the arterial blood pressure is increased as followed. The left heart takes on too much load to maintain pumping capacity, resulting in cardiac hypertrophy. When this condition cannot be compensated, it will lead to left ventricular enlargement and left ventricular dysfunction. The clinical presentation are dizziness, headache, tinnitus and fatigue caused by hypertension, and dyspnea, sitting breathing, hemoptysis, angina caused byleft ventricular failure.

2) Imaging manifestations:

①X-ray findings: Hypertensive heart disease is characterized by the enlarged and thickened left ventricle, and the widened and prolonged aorta. The left ventricular dilatation shows that there is an increase in convexity with rounding of the left cardiac border, the apex of the heart shifts downward and outward and the enlarged left ventricle extends posteriorly, often sufficiently to superimpose on the vertebral column in the left anterior oblique. Aorta widening shows aorta dilatation, tortuosity, aortic node protrusion and have an aortic configuration. The left atrium can also be enlarged. In several cases, there may be biventricular failure. All of the cardiac chambers are dilated. The heart is moderately or markedly enlarged. The cardiac pulsations become weak. There may be fluid in the pleural as well as in the pericardial sac.

② CT and MRI findings: CT findings include enlargement of the left ventricle and dilation of the ascending aorta. MRI shows that the ventricular septum is generally and homogeneously thickened, the left ventricular cavity is slightly narrowed, but there is no abnormal signal in the ventricular wall. The ascending aorta is dilated but does not involve the aortic sinus. The enlargement of the left ventricular cavity indicates that the disease has reached advanced stage and left ventricular function can not compensated completely. At this time, the motion of the left ventricular wall can be seen in the cine, and mitral systolic regurgitation also can be seen.

(2) Chronic rheumatic valvular diseases

In chronic rheumatic heart disease, the valvular lesion is of radiologic diagnostic importance. The consequenceses of hemodynamic changes following the valvular lesion either stenosis or insufficiency are most influential in producing characteristic changes in the contour of the heart. The most commonly affected valve is the mitral valve and aortic valve the next. A combined involvement of these valves may also occur

1) Mitral valve stenosis

①Clinical and pathological manifestations: Stenosis is more common than insufficiency. Stenosis of the valve is due to scarring and thickening of the valve cusps which usually begins in the region of the commissure and then follows by fusion, resulting in a slit-like opening somewhere near the central portion of the valve. Calcification may occur in the scarred tissue and rigidly fuses the commissure. The normal orifice of the mitral valve ranges from 2.3 cm^2 to 3.5 cm^2 of the body surface. When the orifice area has reduced to 1.5 to 1.0 cm^2, there is significant hemodynamic alterations because of the obstruction of the blood flow from the left atrium to the left ventricle. There will be dilatation of the left atrium, often slight or moderate, but rarely grossly enlarged in the absence of mitral insufficiency. This is the most common radiologic evidence of mitral stenosis. One should also bear in mind, that in mild case with insignificant hemodynamic changes, the left atria enlargement may not be detectable. Mitral stenosis produces pressure load on the left atrium and leads to elevation if the left atrial pressure. The high left atrial pressure is transmitted to the pulmonary vein and consequently there is rise in the pulmonary arterial pressure. Ultimately the right ventricle enlarges also. Because of the low output of the left ventricle, the left ventricle is not enlarged and the aortic knobbecome less conspicuous.

When the pulmonary venous pressure rises above 10 mmHg. There are definite changes in the pulmonary vasculature. The upper lobe veins dilate, the lower lobe veins become smaller, just reverse to the normal. When the pulmonary venous pressure exceeds 25 mmHg. Interstitial edema and kerley's line are commonly found in mitral stenosis and indicates a severe obstruction. Pulmonary arterial hypertension ultimately develops and presents a mixture of pulmonary venous and pulmonary arterial hypertension.

②Imaging manifestations:

X-ray findings (Figure 7-2): First of all, when the left atrium is enlarged, it can be manifested as double atrial shadow at the right cardiac margin. In severe cases, the left bronchial uplift can occur, and the trachea bifurcation angle increases. If pulmonary venous hypertension is present, it may present as interstitial pulmonary edema and alveolar pulmonary edema, as well as congestion of the lungs, resulting in kerley line, upper pulmonary vein dilation, lower pulmonary vein discrimination, and blurred vessels. Further development may result in pulmonary hypertension, which is characterized by pulmonary segment elevation and pulmonary artery thickening. Finally, the right ventricle appears enlarged, presenting as apical upturned. Left ventricular enlargement may occur if there is an insufficiency of closure.

CT and MRI findings: CT can only show the change of atrial size of secondary heart caused by rheumatic heart disease, and can not show valve damage. MRI is of high diagnostic value and shows the best results in the four-chamber view, showing enlargement of the left atrium, slow blood flow high signal shadow and small left ventricle. Pulmonary artery dilation, right ventricular wall hypertrophy, right ventricular enlargement is also seen. The movie sequence can also show the shape and extent of mitral stenosis, low signal flow in the left ventricle can be seen during systole, and if secondary mitral insufficiency occurs, blood reflux signals can be seen during systole. In addition, mural thrombosis is sometimes seen.

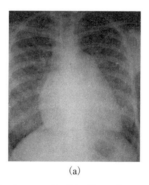 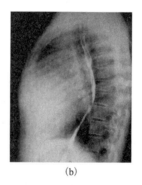

(a)   (b)

(a) Mitral valve stenosis. PA: The pulmonary venous is congested. The right ventricle enlarges with protruded of the pulmonary segment. The left atrium is dilated, there is a separate arch (The third pathological arch) between the pulmonary segment and the left ventricle; (b) Mitral valve stenosis. Lateral view: The right ventricle and the left atrium enlarge. There is a localized left atrial press and displacement on the lower third of the barium filled oesophagus.

Figure 7-2

2) Mitral valve insufficiency

①Clinical and pathological manifestations: This is due to scarring and shortening of the mitral valve leaflets and the chordae tendinae, which prevent proper closure of the valve. It is less common than mitral stenosis, bur mitral stenosis and some degree of insufficiency may co-exist. In severs case, a considerable amount of blood refluxes to the left atrium during each left ventricle systole. If the heart is to maintain its normal output, the left ventricle must dilate so as to accommodate a larger volume of blood, and hypertrophies in order to expel the blood, finally, the left ventricle hypertrophied and dilated. The left atrium in most cases, is considerably larger than those in mitral stenosis.

②Imaging manifestations: It is related to the amount of regurgitant and status of the myocardium. In mild case, it may show no apparent change in the heart size and pulmonary vasculature when the regurgitant is small. When it is moderate to severe in amount, the left atrium enlarges considerably and pulsation may be observed. The left ventricle also enlarges in contrast to mitral stenosis. The change of the pulmonary vascular pattern is similar to that of mitral stenosis, but when the left atrium enlarges considerably and serves as a blood reservoir, the change in pulmonary vascularity may be minimal. Mitral insufficiency may be studied quantitatively by selective left ventriculography.

（3）Chronic pulmonary heart disease

1）Clinical and pathological manifestations: Chronic pulmonary heart disease is caused by the pulmonary tissue, pulmonary artery vessels or thoracic chronic diseases caused by lung tissue structure and function abnormalities, resulting in increased pulmonary vascular resistance, pulmonary artery pressure, dilation and hypertrophy of the right heart, with or without right heart failure heart disease, the most common disease because of chronic obstructive pulmonary disease.

In this condition, the heart disease is caused secondarily to chronic parenchymatous disease of the lungs in which extensive fibrosis or obstructive emphysema eventually develops. Consequently, there is increased pulmonary vascular resistance as a combination result from impaired respiratory function and low oxygen content of the alveolar air(hypoxemia). Pulmonary arterial hypertension develops and leads to right heart failure.

2）Imaging manifestations:

①X-ray findings: There are chronic lung parenchymal diseases such as lung fiber and emphysema. X-ray shows thickening and disorder of lung texture, increased permeability of both lungs. The right ventricle is enlarged. The early right ventricle is slightly hypertrophic, and the X-ray findings are not obvious and difficult to diagnose. When pulmonary segment protrusion, pulsation intensification, right inferior pulmonary artery thickening, or pulmonary segment protrusion occurs, it indicates right ventricle enlargement.

②CT and MRI findings: CT shows increasing and thickening of bronchial vascular bundle of both lungs, multiple thin-walled and non-walled transparent shadows can be seen in both lungs. And CT and MRI findings show that the main pulmonary artery diameter is widened, wider than the same level aorta, right ventricle is enlarged, and the left ventricle is usually not affected except there is a heart failure.

（4）Disease of pericardium

1）Pericardial effusion

① Clinical and pathological manifestations: Normally there is small amount of fluid in the pericardial sac. But when the pericardium is involved by disease processes such as tuberculosis, rheumatic or pyogenic infections, there is excessive accumulation of fluid in the sac and produces definite change in the cardiac shadow. If it is a small amount of pericardial effusion, it generally causes no special discomfort. If it is a large amount of pericardial effusion, it can cause shortness of breath, chest pain, etc. If pericardial compliance is reduced during a sudden sharp increase, as evidenced by restrictive pericardial effusion, pericardial occlusion may occur.

②Imaging manifestations（Figure 7－3）: X-ray shows there is general enlargement of the cardiac shadow with diminished or absence of lung marking. The lung fields are clear and much of pulmonary stasis.

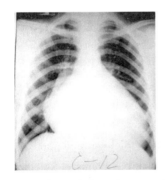

The cardiac shadow is general enlargement, the lung fields are clear and lack of pulmonary marking.

Figure 7-3　Pericardial effusion

241

2）Constrictive pericarditis

①Clinical and pathological manifestations: When the two layers of the pericardium become fused together with adhesions or fibrosis, even scarring, the pericardium thickens and the heart is enclosed in a rigid case. The heart motion is considerably restricted. Tuberculosis is proven as the common etiology agent, and other proven agents are rheumatic fever, trauma, schistosomiasis, pyogenic infection and malignant tumor. In a number of cases, the etiologic agent has disappeared and the cause becomes unknown. Chronic constrictive pericarditis has received considerable attention because it is often amenable to surgical treatment.

②Imaging manifestations: The heart size is usually not enlarged, even smaller than normal. Consequently, it should be emphasized that the heart may be slightly enlarged. The heart often shows a bizarre shape as a result of pericardial thickening and adhesions. The normal cardiac curvatures are lost. In general, cardiac pulsation is diminished or absence in some portion of the heart. Calcification in the pericardium is a sign of considerable diagnostic importance.

2. Congenital malformation of the heart

This is an error in the development of the heart, it occurs during the period between the 4th to 8th weeks of gestation. In an attempt to bring some order to the radiological evaluation of congenital malformations of the heart, a classification on the appearance of the pulmonary vasculature and of the size and configuration of the heart has been found useful. Significant hemodynamic changes, either a shunt or an obstruction will alter the appearance of pulmonary vasculature. The pulmonary vasculature may be increased in cases of left-to right shunt, and may be diminished in cases of obstruction to the outflow of the right ventricle. The evaluation of the pulmonary vasculature is essential and must be correlated with the size and configuration of the heart. A normal sized heart with normal pulmonary vasculature may not exclude the presence of congenital formation of heart. For this reason, in approaching to a probable diagnosis one must also take the clinical problems into consideration. In complex cases, other means of investigation also be indispensable, such as ultrasound, catheterization and cardio-angiographic studies. Here in this paragraph only those simple cases are presented.

（1）Left-to right shunt（acyanotic）

1）Atrial septal defect

Atrial septal defect（ASD）is a congenital heart malformation that occurs when the atrial septal is not completely closed during its development, resulting in abnormal blood traffic between the left and right atria. Normally, the foramen oval closes functionally within hours or days after birth, and usuallyanatomically before age 6. It includes the following types: Primary type（I type）, secondary type（II type）, and other types. Of them, secondary type is common.

①Clinical and pathological manifestations: Patient with an atrial septal defect, regardless of types, has a burden placed on the right side of the heart as a result of significant shunt of blood from the left atrium to the right atrium during ventricular diastole. The amount of shunt is related to the size of the defect.

②Imaging manifestations:

X-ray findings [Figure 7－4（a）, （b）]: The typical manifestations include increased pulmonary blood volume, thickening of both hilum and peripheral blood vessels, enhanced pulsation（hilum dance）under fluoroscopy, bulging of pulmonary artery segment, enlargement of right atrium and right ventricle, leading to the enlargement of cardiac shadow to the right and left shift of cardiac apex. The aortic boundary is small, the left ventricle is small or enlarged.

CT and MRI findings: The direct sign on CT is the interruption of atrial septal continuity, which can show the location, size and number of the defect. Indirect signs areenlargement of right atrium and right ventricle, pulmonary dilatation. The purpose of CT examination is not to diagnose the atrial septal defect itself, but to exclude coronary artery disease before surgical intervention in adults (> 50 years old), observe whether there are other external cardiac malformations, such as pulmonary venous malformation drainage. Diagnostic ultrasound is difficult to diagnose the above special types. MRI can be used to distinguish atrial septal defects from patent foramen oval, and is usually not performed for ASD diagnosis alone.

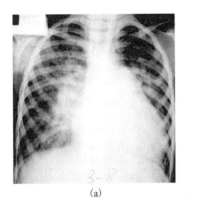 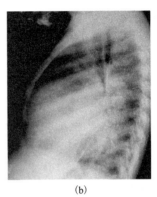

(a)　　　　　　　　　　　　　(b)

(a)PA: The heart is enlarged and has a mitral configuration. The right ventricle and the right atrium are enlarged. There is pulmonary plethora with prominence of the pulmonary trunk. Lung blood increases; (b)Lateral view: The right heart is enlarged and the left ventricle and the left atrium are pushed backward.

Figure 7-4　Atrial septal defect(ASD)

2）Ventricular septal defect

Ventricular septal defect (VSD) is a congenital heart malformation caused by ventricular septal dysplasia or malfusion. The incidence rate is secondary only to atrial septal defect (ASD), which can be divided into membranous ventricular septal defect, supracristal ventricular septal defect, and muscular ventricular septal defect. More than 50% of the VSD around the membrane or around the muscle is isolated, meaning no other heart defects.

①Clinical and pathological manifestations: Ventricular septal defects produce left-to-rightshunt, and the amount of shunt depends on the size of the defect, the difference in left and right ventricular pressure, and pulmonary vascular resistance. In VSD with large shunt, left ventricular and left atrium dilate, which can lead to dynamic pulmonary hypertension. As the disease progresses, organic pulmonary hypertension eventually leads to right-to-left shunt and Eisenmenger syndrome, in which cyanosis may occur.

②Imaging manifestations:

X-ray findings: No detectable changes exist in small defect. For moderate and large defect, the heart is enlarged and has a mitral configuration. Both ventricles and left atrium are enlarged. There is increased pulmonary vascularity, prominent pulmonary trunk and visible hilar dance. In this condition, there is particular liable to produce pulmonary hypertension caused by elevation of pulmonary vascular resistance. With time and progression of the disease process, pulmonary vascular resistance may exceed the systemic pressure, so that the shunt may be reversed (right-to left shunt). Patient becomes cyanotic, andradiologically present a typical feature of pulmonary arterial hypertension, secondary to high pulmonary vascular resistance.

CT and MRI findings: CT direct sign is ventricular septal continuity interruption, and can show the location and size of ventricular septal defect. Indirect signs are left atrium and left ventricle enlargement, pulmonary dilatation. The purpose of CT examination is not only to diagnose ventricular septal defect itself, mainly to diagnose whether with other cardiac malformations, the differentiation of lesions around aortic valve, such as the rupture of aortic sinus tumor, the above special type of VSD that ultrasound is difficult to diagnose. MRI shows the defects of the membrane and muscle in the interventricular septum well, but the defects in the funnel are easy to be missed.

3) Patent ductus arteriosus

Normally, during the fetal life, there is a duct communicating between the leftpulmonary artery and the descending aorta just distal to the origin of the subclavian artery. It carries out the vital function of delivering most of the blood entering the right ventricle to the aorta, thus bypassing the non-aerated lunge. After the onset of respiration and subsequent increase in pulmonary blood flow at the birth, this duct loses its function and finally closes to become a ligament. If the pipeline does not close naturally after birth, blood vessels still remain connected between the pulmonary artery and the aorta, resulting in abnormal blood diversion, which is one of the most common congenital heart diseases.

①Clinical and pathological manifestations: This is an extra-cardiac left-

to-right shunt. The direction of the shunt is usually from the aorta to pulmonary circulation when the pulmonary vascular resistance has not increased and similar to VSD. When there is marked increased pulmonary vascular resistance, greater than systemic, the shunt may be reversed, from right to left, creating differential cyanosis of the lower part of the body. According to the shape of the patent ductus arterioles, it can be divided into the following types, including funnel type, window type, tubular type and aneurysm type, among which the tubular type is the most common.

②Imaging manifestations:

X-ray findings: Typical manifestations include increased pulmonary blood volume, enlarged left ventricle, widened aortic junction, and prominent pulmonary artery segment. In the case of pulmonary hypertension and Eisenmenger syndrome, total enlargement of the heart is present.

CT and MRI findings: The direct sign is abnormal vascular shadows or traffic between the proximal end of the descending aorta and the bifurcation of the pulmonary artery at the level of the aortic arch. The indirect signs are left cardiac load increase and pulmonary arterial hypertension when PDA is large, such as left ventricle enlargement and pulmonary arterial broadening. CT was not the preferred examination for patent ductus arterialis. MRI GRE sequence is sensitive to the detection of small aneurysms. In narrow aneurysms, high speed blood flow shows high signal and can show the direction of blood flow injection to determine the shunt type.

All these radiologic features, however, may be seen in any cases with significant left-to-right shunt. There are differentiationsamong ASD, VSD, and PDA in the plain chest films(Table 7-1).

Table 7-1　Key points of differential diagnosis among ASD, VSD and PDA

	Right atrium	Right ventricle	Pulmo-nary trunk	pulmonary vessels	Left atrium	Left ventricles	aorta
ASD	↑	↑	↑	↑	→	→	→↓
VSD	→	→↑	↑	↑	↑	↑	→
PDA	→	→	↑	↑	→↑	→↑	↑

Note: ↑ -increase, → -no change, ↓ -decrease.

(2) Right-to-left shunt(cyanotic)

1) Tetralogy of Fallot

This is the most common form of complex cyanotic congenital malformation of heart especially in children and adolescences and is amenable to total corrective surgery with good result. This entity is defined as tetrad: Pulmonary stenosis, ventricular defect, enlargement of the right ventricle and overriding of aorta, but in fact, only the VSD and pulmonary stenosis are of physiological importance.

①Clinical and pathological manifestations: The pathophysiological changes of tetralogy of Fallot mainly depend on the influence of pulmonary stenosis and ventricular septal defect on hemodynamics. The ventricular septal defect causes the systolic pressure of the right and left ventricles to be similar, the descending pulmonary artery increases the pressure of the right ventricle and leads to right-to-left shunt in the heart. Arterial oxygen saturation decreases, tissuehypoxia, clinical cyanosis, decreased pulmonary blood flow and increased collateral branches of systemic pulmonary circulation. The degree of pulmonary blood decrease mainly depends on the degree of pulmonary stenosis and pulmonary artery development. The more severe the stenosis, the more obvious the hypoxia and cyanosis.

②Imaging manifestations:

X-ray findings (Figure 7-5): The pulmonary vascularity diminishes, and the lung fields appear clear with small hilar and peripheral vessels. Pulmonary artery segment depresses. Right ventricular is protuberance and enlarged. Due to stenosis of the infundibulum portion of the right ventricleand a small pulmonary trunk, heart shows the "boot shaped", normal left ventricle and left atrium, widened aortic arch. The right sided aortic arch occurs in about 25%. Cardiac catheterization and selective cardio-angiography are usually required to confirm the diagnosis and help to differentiate from other cyanotic congenital malformations before surgery.

CT and MRI findings: CT and MRI can clearly show the location and extent of pulmonary stenosis, and can also know whether there are other malformations.

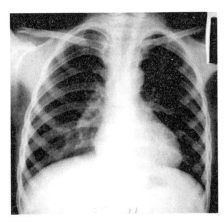

The heart is normal size. The right ventricle is enlarged. Due to stenosis of the infundibulum portion of the right ventricle and a small pulmonary trunk, heart shows the "boot shaped". Pulmonary vascularity diminishes, the lung fields appear clear with small hilar and peripheral vessels. Left ventricle and left atrium are normal.

Figure 7-5   Tetralogy of Fallot(F4)

(Mao Zeng, Jiayi Liu, Enhua Xiao, jianguang Luo)

第八章

乳腺

第一节　检查方法

1. 乳腺钼靶 X 线摄影

乳腺钼靶 X 线摄影是指用"软 X 射线"来进行乳腺摄影，是用来在健康女性人群中筛选乳腺癌病变的一种检查方法。常用来发现和诊断有症状的乳腺病变，包括乳腺肿块、乳房疼痛、乳头溢液及乳头凹陷等，或没有症状的乳腺疾病。

乳腺钼靶 X 线摄影是检测早期乳腺癌的一种非常重要的检查方法。美国癌症学会推荐 40 岁及以上女性每年需进行一次乳腺钼靶筛选检查。美国国立癌症研究院亦推荐 40 岁及以上妇女每 1~2 年进行一次乳腺钼靶摄影检查。

乳腺钼靶摄影常规投照体位采用：

（1）轴位：患者身体面向乳腺机，将照片托架高度调整至患者乳腺水平，将乳腺置于照片托架上，乳腺下部胸壁紧靠托架边缘，如图 8-1(a)，轴位摄影如图 8-1(b)、(c)。

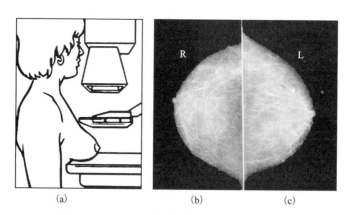

图 8-1　（a）~（c）乳腺钼靶 X 线摄影——轴位

（2）斜位：患者身体面向乳腺机，机架向对侧旋转 60°，将摄影托架高度调整至患者乳腺水平，患者患侧手上举，托架上方置于腋窝下，身体向对侧侧转 15°，将乳腺置于摄影托架上，乳腺侧部胸壁紧靠托架边缘，摄影如图 8-2(a)、(b)。

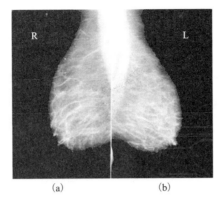

图 8-2 （a）、（b）乳腺钼靶 X 线摄影——斜位

2.乳腺超声检查

乳腺超声成像是一种利用高频超声波通过乳腺组织所产生的回波经计算机处理转换成图像并在计算机屏幕显示的成像技术。超声成像过程中不需曝露在 X 线辐射下，如图 8-3（a）、（b）。

乳腺超声检查可以帮助阐明体检或乳腺钼靶摄影所发现的可疑病变。在下列情况有一定的价值，但乳腺超声并不用于常规乳腺疾病的筛选检查：

（1）对乳腺钼靶照片上显示边界清楚的结节，可以较容易且较准确地判断是囊性或是实性病变。但有些囊肿呈中度回声时，超声较难辨别为囊肿；有些有包膜的癌瘤可呈低度回声而与囊肿相似亦难辨别。当一个病变显示为实性时，要鉴别良性和恶性常较为困难。

（2）当乳腺体检和乳腺钼靶摄影有不符合的情况时，超声有助于分析病变。如体检时发现有病变，而乳腺钼靶照片为阴性时，尤其是致密型乳房，超声常能显示有或无局灶性病变。同样，在乳腺钼靶照片发现有边界不清楚的阴影时超声可协助肯定或排除局灶性病变可能。

（3）超声有利于观察因解剖原因而不能为乳腺钼靶摄影所显示的病变。如近胸壁的肿瘤及腋窝深处的淋巴结。

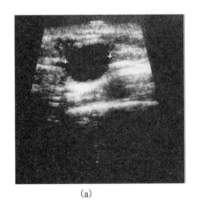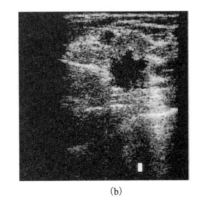

图 8-3 （a）、（b）超声检查示乳腺囊肿呈低回声、边界清楚结节影

3.影像介导乳腺活检

乳腺钼靶摄影是发现乳腺疾病极好的方法，但是在很多病例的诊断中不能凭照片所见来判断病变是良性还是恶性。影像介导乳腺活检有 2 种形式：一是细针抽吸活检（FNA），二是粗针穿刺活检（CNB）。细针或粗针活检是一种重要的检测方式，其可以通过 X 线引导（图 8-4）或通过超声导引。医生可在超声引导下

直接将穿刺针导向肿块部位进行活检。在 X 线引导下除可将穿刺针导向肿块部位进行活检外,还可以对某些有钙化而触摸不到肿块的病灶进行活检及术前定位。针吸或穿刺活检使用得当,可减少良性病变的外科活检数目,癌症患者可于手术前能得到明确诊断。

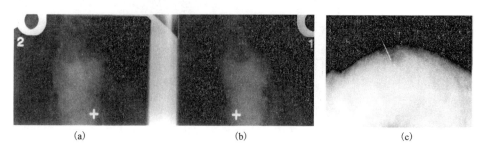

(a) (b) (c)

图 8-4 (a)、(b)乳腺 X 线病变定位;(c)乳腺 X 线引导下穿刺活检

4. 磁共振成像

磁共振成像利用磁化及无线电波替代 X 线而产生非常清晰而具有代表性的图像,目前常用的成像技术包括自旋回波(SE)、梯度回波(GE)和脂肪抑制。使用正确的技术和特制的表面线圈,乳腺磁共振成像在某些情况下是有价值的。如静脉注射对比剂(GD-DTPA)后[图 8-5(a)、(b)],动态观察增强的影像可提供重要的鉴别诊断资料。恶性肿瘤几乎总是较良性肿瘤增强快且更强化。但细胞丰富的纤维腺瘤,某些类型的增生性乳腺病和炎性病变,以及在手术后 6 个月中的手术瘢痕组织,可以显示增强影像与癌瘤相似。在手术 6 个月后,用乳腺钼靶 X 线摄影评估有困难时,乳腺 MRI 检查有一定的价值,尤其是对有硅植入物的患者,可以观察硅植入体有无破裂、漏出或邻近的恶性病变。MRI 检查对乳腺内单发或多发囊肿及乳腺内出血或血肿有独特的优点。MRI 能发现乳腺钼靶摄影不能发现的病变,但对病变良恶性的判断不如乳腺钼靶摄影,且乳腺的 MRI 由于其检查的复杂性及高费用而应用有限。

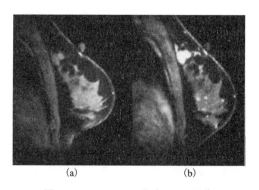

(a) (b)

图 8-5 (a)、(b)乳腺 MRI 图像

5. 数字乳腺摄影

数字乳腺摄影的图像以数字图像的形式被存储在计算机上,可以方便地以电子方式共享。虽然于传统的乳腺钼靶 X 线摄影相比其空间分辨率差,但其较高的对比度可以作为补偿,且其拥有强大的影像的算法和影像的后处理。数字技术对小钙化的定性有重要的意义。目前,数字化技术(CCD 摄像机)近乎实时的成像作立体定位活检的仪器已经显示其独特的优越性。

6. 乳腺导管造影

乳腺导管造影[图 8-6(a)、(b)]是经乳头上溢液的大导管开口注入对比剂,使导管系统显影,以诊断乳腺导管内及其周围病变的技术,特别适用于导管的病变。

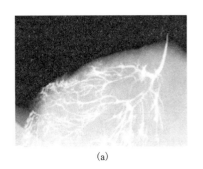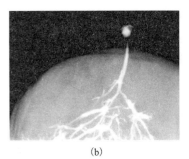

图 8-6 （a）、（b）乳腺导管造影

第二节　正常表现

女性乳腺主要是由乳叶、乳腺小叶、乳导管及间质（纤维结缔组织、脂肪组织，其间有血管、神经、淋巴管）构成（图 8-7）。乳腺小叶内的终末导管和腺泡称为终末导管小叶单位，是乳腺功能的基本单位。乳腺组织位于皮下浅筋膜浅层与深层之间，浅筋膜的浅层纤维与皮肤之间有网状束带相连，称为乳腺悬韧带，又名 Cooper 韧带。

乳腺的动脉血供有 3 个主要来源：1.胸廓内动脉的穿支，又称内乳动脉，主要供应内侧；2.腋动脉分支，如胸肩峰动脉、胸外侧动脉，供应乳腺外侧部和上部；3.肋间动脉的外侧皮支。乳腺静脉引流通常伴随动脉，主要引流至腋窝。

乳腺内有丰富的淋巴网和淋巴结，大多数淋巴管回流至腋下淋巴结。乳腺癌转移的主要途径是淋巴系统，是否发生腋下淋巴结转移对乳腺癌治疗方案的选择至关重要。

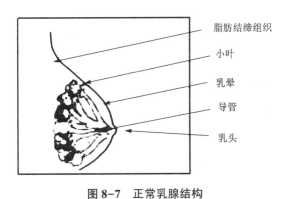

图 8-7 正常乳腺结构

第三节　基本病变

乳腺的基本病变主要有肿块、钙化、结构扭曲变形、局限性皮肤增厚凹陷、乳头回缩与漏斗征、乳腺导管异常、局限性不对称致密、血供增多、淋巴结肿大。

1.肿块

肿块为乳腺的占位性病变，分为良性及恶性肿块。

（1）X 线表现：两个不同投照体位共同确定是否存在肿块。肿块的大小对肿块良恶性的鉴别意义不大，但当临床触诊的大小大于 X 线测量时，则倾向于恶性肿块的可能性大。而肿块形状、边缘、密度及周围情况对肿块的良恶性鉴别非常重要。肿块的形状一般分为圆形、椭圆形、分叶状及不规则形,恶性程度依次递增。边界清晰、边缘光滑的肿块一般为良性病变,而边缘模糊、呈分叶状的肿块则为恶性病变的可能性大,在放大图像上观察更可靠。良性病变大多数呈等密度或低密度,密度接近正常腺体,而恶性结节大多数密度较高,含脂肪密度的肿块一般仅见于良性病变,如错构瘤、脂肪瘤等。部分肿块周围可见透亮线或透明晕,透亮线多见于良性病变,如纤维腺瘤等;透明晕多见于乳腺癌(图8-8、图8-9)。

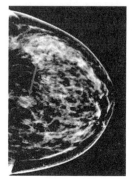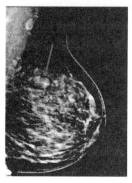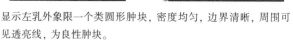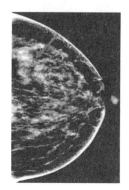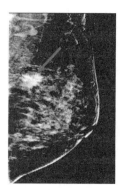

显示左乳外象限一个类圆形肿块,密度均匀,边界清晰,周围可见透亮线,为良性肿块。

图8-8　左乳的 CC 位和 MLO 位

显示左乳外上象限一个不规则形肿块,密度不均匀,边界不清,边缘呈分叶状,可见毛刺,为恶性肿块。

图8-9　左乳的 CC 位和 MLO 位

(2)MRI 表现:良性病变在平扫图像上表现为形态规则、边界清晰,恶性病变表现为形态不规则,边界不清,边缘呈分叶状、星芒状或毛刺样改变。平扫 T1WI 图像上肿块以中低信号为主,T2WI 图像上信号多变,与肿块内成分相关,肿块含纤维成分较多时呈中低信号,细胞及水含量较多时成高信号。良性病变肿块内部信号较均匀,恶性病变可出现液化、坏死、囊变、出血或纤维化改变,呈现混杂信号。动态增强扫描有助于病变的定性诊断,良性病变强化多发较均匀或呈弥漫性斑片状强化,部分病变可出现离心性强化;恶性病变强化不均匀或以边缘强化为主,多呈向心性强化。良性病变的动态增强曲线呈缓慢上升型,而恶性病变的动态增强曲线呈速升速降型,速升平台型曲线则良恶性病变均有可能(图8-10、图8-11)。

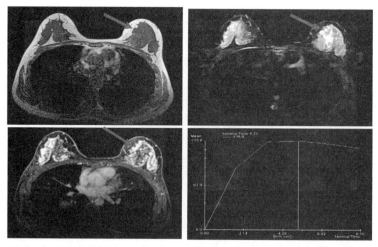

显示左乳多发类圆形肿块,呈等 T1 长 T2 信号,信号均匀,边缘清晰,增强扫描呈显著均匀强化,动态增强曲线(T1C max)呈持续型(I 型),为良性肿块。

图8-10　左乳的 MRI 图像

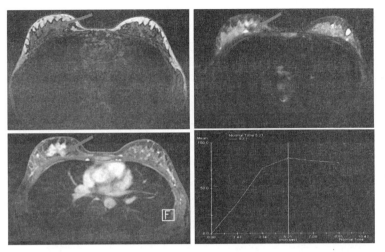

显示右乳一个较大的不规则形肿块，信号不均匀，呈等T1混杂T2信号，边缘不规则，呈明显深分叶，
有毛刺，增强扫描呈显著不均匀强化，动态增强曲线(ST-T曲线)呈平台型(II型)，为恶性肿块。

图8-11 右乳的MRI影像

2.钙化

乳腺的良恶性病变均可出现钙化，钙化的形态、分布、密度等特征有助于良恶性病变的鉴别。良性钙化多较粗大，呈爆米花样、颗粒状、圆形、条状、小环形或新月形，密度较高，散在分布；而恶性钙化多呈线状、砂粒状、叉状或杆状，大小不等，密度不均匀，常呈典型的簇状分布，钙化可位于肿块内或肿块外部。多数临床上未发现明显肿块的隐性乳腺癌，可根据钙化特点做出诊断。根据美国放射学会提出的BI-RADS分级标准，乳腺钙化可分为三种类型：典型良性、中间性(不能定性)和高度可疑恶性。X线钼靶是临床上发现和诊断钙化的主要检查方法，而超声、CT和MRI检查通常难以发现微小钙化(图8-12)。

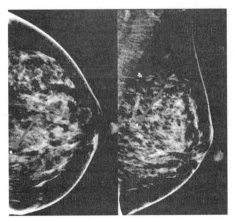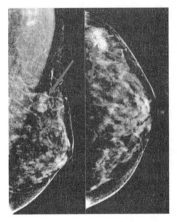

显示左乳散在分布的斑片状粗大钙化；右图为左乳的CC位和MLO位显示恶性肿块内多发沙粒
状、杆状钙化，密度不均匀，呈簇状分布。

图8-12 左图为左乳的CC位和MLO位

3.结构扭曲、变形

结构扭曲需在X线钼靶片两个不同投照体位上均显示才能确定。乳腺的良恶性病变均可出现结构扭曲、变形，良性病变如慢性炎症、脂肪坏死、活检、手术后瘢痕及放疗后可出现结构扭曲；而乳腺实质与脂

肪界面发生扭曲、变形、紊乱，但未见明显肿块时，考虑浸润性乳腺癌所致的反应性纤维增生所致。良恶性难以鉴别时需活检（图8-13）。

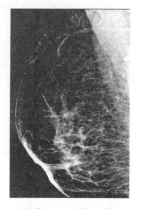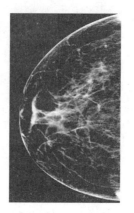

显示右乳中央区结构扭曲、变形，密度增高，邻近皮肤增厚、轻度凹陷，为术后改变所致。

图8-13 右乳的CC位和MLO位

4.局限性皮肤增厚、凹陷

乳腺炎症性疾病通常表现为弥漫性皮肤增厚，而局限性皮肤增厚、凹陷常见于恶性病变，是由于肿瘤浸润、侵犯皮肤造成皮肤局限性增厚并向肿瘤方向回缩，称为"酒窝征"。部分手术后瘢痕患者也可出现术区皮肤增厚、凹陷。

5.乳头回缩与漏斗征

乳头回缩、内陷常见于先天性乳头发育不良、乳头后方的乳腺癌浸润；"漏斗征"表现为乳头下方三角形致密影，尖端指向腺体内侧，可见于乳腺癌浸润乳晕下方腺体组织，也可见于乳晕周围炎症（图8-14、图8-15）。

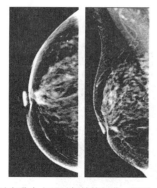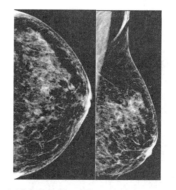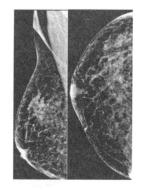

显示右乳中央区局部结构扭曲、变形，密度不均匀，呈肿块样改变，邻近皮肤增厚，乳头内陷，为恶性肿瘤浸润所致。

图8-14 右乳的CC位和MLO位

左图为左乳的CC位和MLO位显示左乳的乳头内陷；右图为右乳的CC位和MLO位显示右乳的乳头内陷。

图8-15 双侧乳腺乳头内陷

6.乳腺导管异常

乳腺导管异常表现为乳头下方乳导管增粗、边缘粗糙、密度增高，良恶性病变均可出现。主要依赖于乳腺导管造影检查，可表现为导管扩张、充盈缺损、截断、受压移位、破坏、走行僵直、排列紊乱及分支减少等（图8-16）。

7. 局限性不对称致密

诊断局限性不对称致密需与既往 X 线钼靶片或两侧乳腺进行对比时观察,若出现新发局限性致密影,尤其是当致密区在随访过程中出现进行性密度增高或范围扩大时,则需考虑浸润性癌的可能(图 8-17),建议活检。

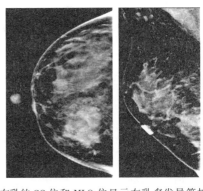 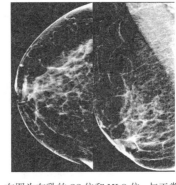 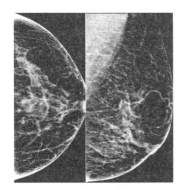

右乳的 CC 位和 MLO 位显示右乳多发导管扩张,走行迂曲。

图 8-16　患者有乳头溢液

右图为左乳的 CC 位和 MLO 位,与正常左乳对比,右乳中央区显示局限性不对称致密影,边缘模糊,密度不均匀,邻近皮肤增厚。

图 8-17　左图为右乳的 CC 位和 MLO 位

8. 血供增多

恶性肿瘤常可出现血供增加,表现为乳腺内出现增多、增粗、迂曲的异常血管影及病灶周围出现细小静脉丛(图 8-18)。

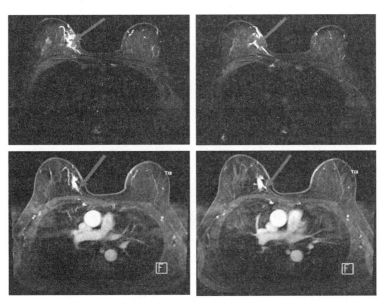

显示右乳内上象限肿块周围多发增多、增粗、迂曲的血管影,伸入肿块,提示肿块血供增多,最终病理诊断为乳腺癌。

图 8-18　上图为双乳的 MRI T2 图像,下图为增强扫描

9. 淋巴结肿大

一般呈圆形或不规则形肿大,密度增高,淋巴结门消失,恶性肿瘤或炎症均可导致淋巴结肿大(图 8-19)。

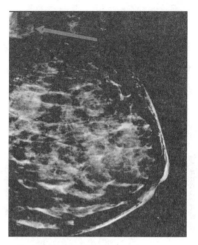

显示左侧腋窝淋巴结肿大，呈类圆形，密度
较高，淋巴结门消失，为乳腺癌淋巴结转移。

图 8-19　左乳的 MLO 位

第四节　常见疾病诊断

1.急性乳腺炎及乳腺脓肿

（1）临床与病理表现：急性乳腺炎是乳腺的急性化脓性感染，乳腺感染常见于哺乳期妇女，通常是由乳头或乳晕区正常皮肤上的常见细菌引起，腺体乳汁淤积导致感染的发生。感染发生于乳腺实质（脂肪组织），导致乳腺导管以外的乳腺实质的肿胀、乳腺导管受压，引起感染的乳房疼痛，肿胀。乳腺脓肿是乳腺炎的后期表现。急性乳腺炎通常是葡萄球菌引起的局部感染，但少数情况下链球菌可引起弥漫性感染。急性乳腺炎临床表现为发热，白细胞增高，血沉增快，乳房表现为红、肿、热、痛，病变边界不清，皮肤固定，乳头溢液（可能是脓液），腋窝淋巴结肿大、疼痛、有压痛。后期，病变的边界可能逐渐清晰，然后脓肿形成。

（2）影像表现：诊断急性乳腺炎和乳腺脓肿最可靠的方法是乳腺 X 线摄影。急性乳腺炎典型的乳腺 X 线表现为皮下小梁增粗，皮肤增厚，乳腺普遍密度增高，边界模糊的斑片状阴影。有时可表现为一个不规则的肿块影。不规则高密度病变边缘围绕火焰状阴影可提示乳腺脓肿。最初，脓肿的边缘可能是模糊的，随后逐渐变清晰。脓肿常伴有水肿及皮肤增厚（图 8-20）。腋窝淋巴结肿大也比较常见。

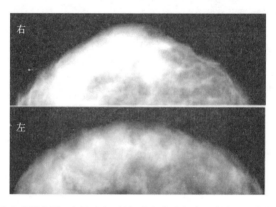

右乳外侧大片密度增高影，边界不清，局部乳房皮肤水肿、增厚。左乳未见明显异常。

图 8-20　急性乳腺炎乳腺 X 线影像

2.乳腺增生

(1)临床病理表现:乳腺增生是女性最常见的乳腺疾病。病因包括雌激素水平增高及黄体素比例不均衡。意味着乳腺小叶对激素十分敏感。依据不同的病理表现分为三种类型。1)腺性增生,是乳腺小叶增生及纤维结缔组织增生。乳腺小叶增大、扭曲,形态不规则。增生的小叶形态上类似纤维腺瘤。2)囊性增生,是乳腺小叶增生伴囊肿形成,是乳腺腺体增生的晚期表现。囊肿是由于终末导管扩张形成的。3)纤维增生,主要是乳腺的纤维组织增生。临床上,虽然乳腺增生可发生于青春期晚期至绝经期的任何年龄,但最常发生于乳腺发育正常的30~40岁女性。可发生于一侧或两侧乳腺。乳房肿胀伴肿块是最主要的症状,通常发生于月经前一周。表现为单个或多个质硬的肿块散在分布,边界模糊。大部分女性表现为局限性疼痛,症状在月经来潮前加重,经期结束后缓解或消失。

(2)影像表现

1)乳腺 X 线摄影是诊断乳腺增生最可靠的检查方法。①腺性增生。通常发生于双侧乳房,但也可以发生于一侧。病灶通常局限于乳房的某一区域,多于外上象限,也可能是弥漫性的。病变密度高,形态不规则,可表现棉花状、雪花状或肿块状,边界模糊、不规则。这些小肿块的融合可能导致结构扭曲(图8-21)。②囊性增生。表现为正常乳腺结构发生扭曲,广泛高密度影伴弥漫性囊性肿块。囊性肿块的大小不一,直径大于0.5厘米的肿块才能看到,钙化少见(图8-22)。③纤维增生。纤维增生并不常见,但可发生于年龄小于30岁的女性。病变通常发生于两侧乳房,表现为弥漫性或局灶性。弥漫性纤维增生在局部区域可表现为无肿块或钙化的均匀高密度影。三种小叶增生通常混合出现,在同一病例中往往可同时存在两种或三种小叶增生。

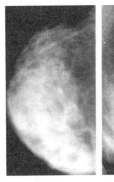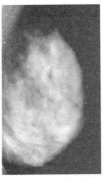

乳腺 X 线示乳腺内散在小片状密度增高影,边界模糊不清。

图8-21 乳腺腺性增生

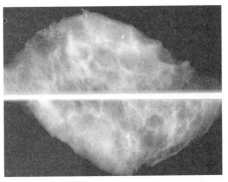

乳腺 X 线示乳腺内大小、形态不一的囊状低密度影,边界不清,伴结构扭曲。

图8-22 乳腺囊性增生

2)超声:①两侧乳房增生,乳房腺体增厚。②乳腺内部光点及回声分布不均匀,可有较多弥漫低回声区,其边界清楚或不清楚,多方位扫查低回声区缺乏球体感。③常为双乳发病,声像类似。④CDFI 示乳腺内血流无增多,低回声区结节内无血流显示。⑤乳腺囊性增生可发生于双侧乳房。超声上除乳腺小叶增生声像外,在腺体内可见多发的液性暗区。

3)乳腺导管造影:囊性小叶增生可辅以乳腺导管造影。乳导管造影时造影剂使导管显影外,部分造影剂可进入周围小囊腔内,呈密度增高小圆形或小结节状,病变范围较广泛。

(3)鉴别诊断

1)乳腺腺瘤:常见于20~25岁女性。乳腺内一个或多个圆形或卵圆形肿块,边界清楚、平滑,可推动,发展缓慢,没有症状。

2)乳腺癌:常见于40~60岁更年期前后女性。乳腺内肿块如石头般坚硬,早期可推动,进展期固定,皮肤见橘皮征,乳头内陷,腋窝淋巴结增大,淋巴结溃烂后呈菜花样、岩石般改变。从溃烂处流出伴恶臭的血性液体。早期诊断需做病理切片。腺性小叶增生极少数可发生钙化,呈细小的钙化,弥漫地分布于乳腺内,很难与乳腺癌鉴别。须结合临床,在 X 线或超声引导下细针抽吸活检。

3.乳腺纤维囊性病

（1）临床病理表现：乳腺纤维囊性病是累及乳腺组织的常见良性病变。"疾病"一词具有误导性，许多学者更喜欢使用"改变"一词。这种情况在正常的乳房中很常见，被认为是一种正常的变异。其他相关术语包括"乳腺发育不良"、"良性乳腺疾病"和"弥漫性囊性乳腺病"。病因尚不完全清楚，但是这种变化被认为与卵巢激素有关，因为这种状况通常会随着绝经期的到来而缓解，并且可能随着月经周期变化。据估计，该发病率占所有妇女的60%以上。服用避孕药的女性发病率较低。风险因素可能包括家族史和饮食（如过量的饮食脂肪和咖啡因摄入），尽管这些都是有争议的。有学者建议如果患者存在乳腺纤维囊性病变，就应该减少脂肪和咖啡因摄入。尽管最近的研究对咖啡因和脂肪在纤维囊性疾病中的作用提出了质疑。临床表现：1)乳腺组织呈高密度、不规则和凹凸不平的"鹅卵石"样改变。2)通常在外上象限更为显著。3)持续或间断出现的乳房不适。4)乳房感到饱胀、疼痛和压痛。5)月经期前压痛、肿胀。6)每次月经期后乳房不适改善。7)乳头感觉变化，瘙痒。注意：症状可能从轻微到严重。症状通常在每个月经期前达到顶峰，月经期后立即好转。

（2）影像表现：体格检查触及可移动的（非锚定的）乳房"肿块"。这些团块通常是圆形的，边界光滑，或者是橡胶状的，或者是略有波动的（形状可以改变）。致密腺体组织可能增大乳房检查的难度。由于乳腺组织致密，乳房X线检查可能难以解释。为了排除其他疾病，乳腺活检可能是必要的。用细针抽吸乳腺常用于诊断和治疗较大的囊肿。

4.乳腺纤维腺瘤

（1）临床病理表现：乳腺纤维腺瘤是最常见的乳腺良性病变，尤其是20岁左右的女性，常发生于15~35岁之间的女性。其病因是由于内分泌失调而引起。在临床上常与乳腺纤维囊性变、腺病、甚至乳腺癌等良恶性病变混淆，应慎予鉴别。病理上，纤维腺瘤是由乳腺纤维组织和腺管两种成分共同构成的良性肿瘤。切面呈灰白色或粉红色，分叶状。在组织学上，可表现为以纤维组织为主要成分，或以腺上皮为主要成分，多数肿瘤以纤维组织为主要成分。其发生与乳腺组织对雌激素的反应过强有关。临床表现：体格检查时纤维腺瘤可或不可触及，表现为卵圆形或分叶状，可活动，有弹性，边界光滑的肿块，通常为无痛性的。大小各异，通常直径小于5 cm，有钙化者坚硬，多无压痛。多位于外上象限。囊性变者可有乳头溢液，溢液可是血性或清亮-黄色液体。肿瘤生长缓慢，多为孤立性，也可多发或双侧，多发性纤维腺瘤约占10%~15%。

（2）影像表现：首选的影像学检查方法决定于患者的年龄，一般来说，如果患者触诊有明确的肿块、年龄小于30岁、或患者是孕妇者首选超声检查；如果患者触诊有明确的肿块、年龄大于30岁且不是孕妇则乳腺X线摄影和超声均有帮助；乳腺CT扫描因为射线剂量大，CT对微钙化不及钼靶敏感，且对肿块缺乏特异性，因此不作为该病首选的检查方法；乳腺MRI由于费用高，假阳性率高，亦不作为首选检查方法。

1)乳腺X线摄影：单发纤维腺瘤的主要X线征象为圆形或卵圆形肿块，密度均匀，边缘光滑（图8-23），边缘有时出现分叶或小切迹（图8-24），周围由于脂肪组织的衬托，可出现细窄的透明环，即Halo征（图8-24~25）。除新近形成的纤维腺瘤外，绝大多数纤维腺瘤均有粘液化及囊性退行性改变。40岁以上患者的纤维腺瘤偶可出现粗大钙化，提示组织坏死或退变（图8-26~27）。钙化形态多种多样，可呈环状、块状、斑点状、花边状、珊瑚状或不规则。钙化可出现在肿瘤的中心或周围部分。有时肿瘤被巨大而不规则的钙化取代，形成特异的X线征象。

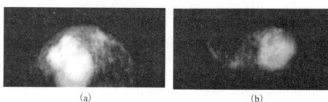

(a)   (b)

乳腺X线检查[（a)轴位,（b)侧斜位]：乳腺内可见浅分叶肿块影，边缘光整，与周围正常乳腺组织分界清楚。

图8-23 乳腺纤维腺瘤

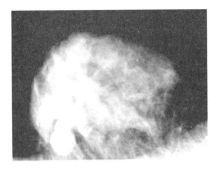

女性,32岁,发现左乳肿块1月。乳腺X线示左乳后下方见一约2×3 cm肿块,其内密度均匀,边缘见小切迹,周边与正常乳腺组织分界可见透明晕征。

图8-24　乳腺纤维腺瘤

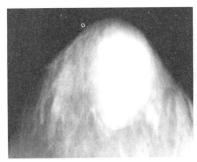
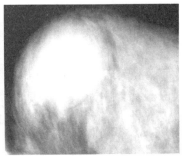

女性,29岁,发现乳房肿块1周。乳腺X线示右乳外下象限可见一约4×5 cm大小椭圆形肿块,其内密度均匀,边界清楚,外周可见与正常乳腺组织分界之透明晕征。

图8-25　乳腺纤维腺瘤

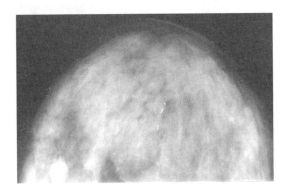

女性,40岁。乳腺X线示右乳内象限见一约1.5×2 cm大小肿块,整个瘤体见钙化。

图8-26　纤维腺瘤钙化

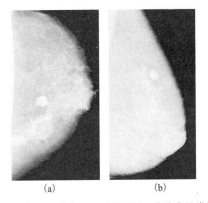

(a)　　　　　　　　(b)

乳腺X线[(a)轴位,(b)侧斜位]:乳腺内见类圆形肿块影,与周围分界清楚,可见瘤体粗大钙化。

图8-27　乳腺纤维腺瘤

2)在超声上,乳腺纤维腺瘤表现为椭圆形或圆形的均质性低回声肿块,轮廓清晰,可有浅分叶,有光滑的、薄的、有回声的包膜,回声强度不一,但分布较均匀(图8-28～29)。表现典型的纤维腺瘤能够与囊肿及乳腺癌很好地鉴别,然而,乳腺纤维囊性变伴有复杂的低回声囊肿以及部分乳腺癌可能类似纤维腺瘤,从而难以鉴别。不典型纤维腺瘤回声不均、形态不规则,难与乳腺癌鉴别。

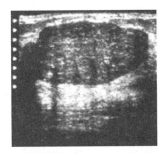

低回声肿块呈椭圆形,边缘浅分叶,表面光滑,与周围分界清楚。

图8-28　乳腺纤维腺瘤超声影像

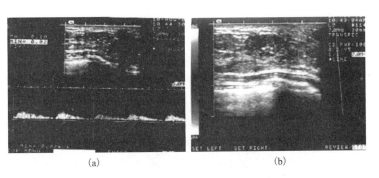

(a)　　　　　　　　　　　(b)

(a)及血流图(b)示腺瘤瘤体内可见条状血流分布。

图8-29　纤维腺瘤超声多普勒

3）CT 平扫时，纤维腺瘤多表现为边界清晰，光滑，密度均匀的卵圆形软组织肿块，CT 值高于正常乳腺腺体，且肿块常有明显强化。但由于 X 线辐射剂量增大，推广受到限制，目前国外更多改用磁共振成像检查。

4）乳腺纤维腺瘤的 MRI 表现特点多种多样，表现为光滑或有轻微分叶的圆形或卵圆形肿块。在 T1 加权像上纤维腺瘤与周围纤维腺体组织相比，呈等或低信号；而在 T2 加权像上，则多种多样，从非常低的信号到高信号均有。根据 T2 加权像及增强特点，把纤维腺瘤分为三型：Ⅰ 型：T2 加权像呈高信号，有明显强化；Ⅱ 型：T2 加权像呈等信号，有明显强化；Ⅲ 型：T2 加权像呈低信号，无强化。通过对比研究认为，T2 加权像呈高信号的肿块，具有较多的粘液样基质，有较多的基质细胞。T2 加权像呈低信号的肿块内几乎是均一的硬化组织，仅有少量基质细胞。MRI 上，无强化的内部分隔和外形分叶有助于鉴别纤维腺瘤与其他疾病。

（3）鉴别诊断

1）单纯囊肿：囊肿双侧较多，好发年龄 40 岁以上，而纤维腺瘤多发于 21~26 岁的女青年，以单发为多见。囊肿边缘清晰，多呈卵圆形，密度均匀；纤维腺瘤在脂肪较多的乳腺中呈圆形或卵圆形，边缘光滑或呈分叶状，密度均匀或不均匀。超声可鉴别囊性与实性肿块（图 8-30）。

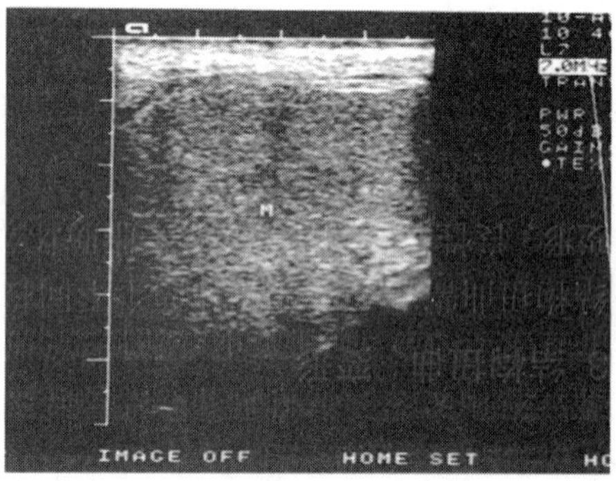

2）积乳囊肿：积乳囊肿大多发生于在哺乳期妇女，特别是患乳腺炎者，其瘤体密度较纤维腺瘤高，边缘光滑、整齐，邻近乳腺组织可出现结构扭曲或乳腺小梁增粗。

3）乳腺癌：某些乳腺癌特别是髓样癌，由于其形态规则，边缘较光滑，很难与纤维腺瘤区别。如肿块较固定，X 线测量肿块大小大于体查所示大小，则应考虑可能为恶性肿瘤，微粒钙化、肿块周边毛刺以及皮肤增厚为恶性征象。

女性，44 岁，发现右乳增大 3 月。超声见右乳巨大圆形、均匀、无回声肿块，边缘光整，边界清楚。

图 8-30 单纯囊肿

4. 乳腺癌

（1）临床病理表现：乳腺癌是起源于乳腺组织的恶性肿瘤。乳腺癌是女性最常见的恶性肿瘤，是女性第二大癌症死亡原因。因为乳腺癌的高发病率和乳腺是审美的象征，乳腺癌已成为患者及其家庭的一个重要负担。乳腺癌的病因尚未完全明确。研究发现具有乳腺癌高危因素的女性容易患乳腺癌。乳腺癌危险因素包括：1）年龄、性别，77% 新发病例和 84% 乳腺癌死亡的年龄大于 50 岁。多于 80% 的乳腺癌病例发生于 50 岁以上女性，不到 1% 乳腺癌发生于男性；2）乳腺癌基因因素和家族史，研究者发现一些有缺陷基因可能导致乳腺癌，包括 BRCA3 和 Noey2（只从家族父系遗传）；3）月经初潮过早（12 岁前）或过晚绝经（迟于 55 岁）、未生育过的女性或 30 岁后生育的女性乳腺癌的患病危险性增高；4）口服避孕药，可能增加乳腺癌危险，取决于年龄、使用时间和其他因素；5）激素替代治疗，激素替代治疗超过 5 年可增加乳腺癌危险。使用越长，危险越大；6）辐射，接触过辐射，尤其在幼年时接触过辐射，将在成年时增加乳腺癌风险；7）其他危险因素，患有子宫癌、卵巢癌、家族中有癌症史可增加患乳腺癌的危险。

病理上，乳腺癌多为来自乳腺导管或小叶上皮细胞的腺癌。OMS 分类将乳腺癌分为非浸润性癌和浸润癌。非浸润性癌由小叶原位癌和导管内癌组成。浸润癌包括浸润性导管癌、浸润性小叶癌、黏液癌、髓样癌、乳头状癌、腺样囊性癌等。

临床上，乳腺癌好发于 40 岁以上的女性。一般表现为患侧乳腺无痛性、单发肿块，好发于乳腺的外上象限。肿块质硬，表面不光滑，与周围组织分界不清，不易被推动。当肿瘤侵犯乳腺悬韧带（Cooper 韧带）出现乳头内陷。侵犯淋巴管，可引起邻近皮肤水肿，形成"橘皮样"改变。肿瘤晚期出现淋巴结转移，形成腋窝、锁骨上淋巴结肿大。乳头溢液是另一重要症状，常表现为血性溢液或脓液样。早期乳腺癌的临床表现不典型，往往发现肿块时就已经是转移的晚期患者。因此乳腺癌的早期诊断不能仅依靠临床表现。近年的研究认为在 40 岁以上"高危人群"中进行影像学筛查是乳腺癌早期诊断的关键，通过筛查可以发现一部分临床前期的原位乳腺癌。对这部分患者只要进行保留乳腺的肿块切除手术即可达到根治的效果。

乳腺癌分期(美国癌症协会)：

0 期(原位癌)：癌细胞局限于最初始发生的乳腺组织内。

1 期：肿瘤直径小于 2 cm，未累及乳腺以外的组织。

2A 期：肿瘤直径在 2~5 cm，未累及腋下淋巴结；或肿瘤直径小于 2 cm，但累及腋下淋巴结。

2B 期：肿瘤直径大于 5 cm，未累及腋下淋巴结；或直径在 2~5 cm，但累及腋下淋巴结。

3A 期：肿瘤直径小于 5 cm，腋下淋巴结转移，且淋巴结相互融合或与其他组织粘连；或癌瘤直径大于 5 cm，腋窝淋巴结转移。

3B 期：肿瘤侵犯皮肤或胸壁软组织，或胸骨旁胸壁淋巴结转移。

4 期：不管肿瘤的大小如何，肿瘤发生乳腺及胸壁以外的部位的转移，如肝脏，骨骼或肺等。

除了分期之外，许多其他因素也会影响推荐的治疗方法和可能的预后。这些可能包括癌症的精准细胞学类型和表现，癌症细胞是否对激素产生反应，以及是否存在已知能引起乳腺癌的基因。

(2)影像表现

1)乳腺 X 线检查为首选检查方法。高危人群的乳腺癌筛查或乳腺肿块的诊断先进行乳腺 X 线检查，越来越多的乳腺癌患者在临床前期就已被诊断，使乳腺癌患者得到的早期治疗，因此乳腺癌的病死率在近几年内下降了 25%。早期乳腺癌在乳腺 X 线表现为：乳腺腺体组织局部结构扭曲；微小钙化灶；或乳腺肿块。

直接征象：①肿块：乳腺癌常表现为不规则肿块或结节、其密度高于周围腺体组织或乳头的密度，边缘不清，常伴有分叶状(图 8-19~21)、毛刺状改变(图 8-21~23)。与对侧乳腺比较，乳腺组织结构不对称。当肿瘤通过乳头扩散时，可以看到肿块周围的导管不对称增厚。晚期，乳腺后间隙密度增高、模糊，胸大肌和腋窝淋巴结增大［图 8-22(a)］，代表肿瘤侵犯胸大肌以及腋窝淋巴结转移。②钙化：有 25% 的临床前期的早期乳腺癌可表现为成簇的"泥沙状"钙化(图 18-31~32)，钙化颗粒往往大小不一、直径一般在 <0.5 mm 范围内，钙化的形态不一，往往表现为多形性、尖角形或分枝形的微小钙化灶，要使用放大镜方能清晰辨认。出现这种钙化聚集时，无论是否伴有肿块都是恶性病变的征象，都必须进行活检以得到病理学诊断。

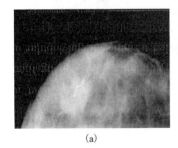
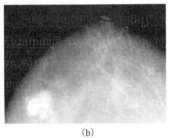
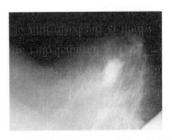

(a)　　　　　　　(b)

乳腺 X 线［(a)为轴位，(b)为侧斜位］示乳腺癌肿块呈分叶状，肿块内见沙砾状小钙化，边缘不清楚，可见毛刺征。

图 8-31 乳腺癌

乳腺 X 线示右乳外象限 3×4 cm 肿块，其内密度不均匀，边缘呈分叶状，与周围分界不清，肿块内外均可见大量的大小不等、形态不一的微小钙化灶。

图 8-32 乳腺癌

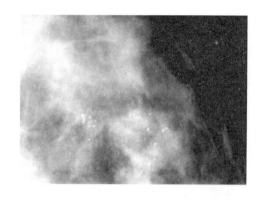

左乳外侧象限见一 2×3 cm 大小肿块,其内可见大量沙砾状、分支状钙化。

图 8-33 乳腺癌

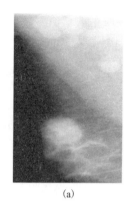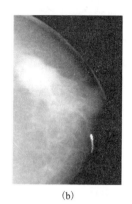

(a) (b)

(a)乳房 X 线片 CC 图;(b)MLO 图显示 1.5 cm×2 cm 的分叶状针状肿块,无钙化。图(a)显示腋窝多个肿大淋巴结。

图 8-34 乳腺癌

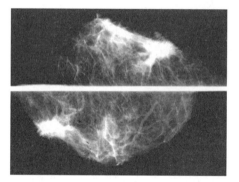

乳腺 X 线示肿块呈浸润性生长,周边可见毛刺。

图 8-35 乳腺癌

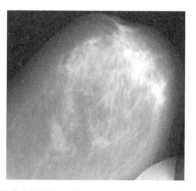

肿瘤广泛浸润,累及乳晕后方的导管,导管增厚、增粗牵拉乳头,使乳头内陷。

图 8-36 乳腺癌乳头凹陷

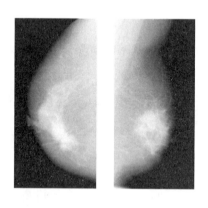

乳腺癌侵犯输乳管,乳腺 X 线示乳头凹陷。

图 8-37 乳腺癌

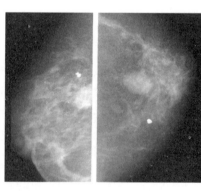

乳腺 X 线示乳腺癌浸润周围乳腺组织,其周围组织发生结构扭曲,失去正常形态。

图 8-38 乳腺癌

间接征象:①乳腺表面静脉增多、扩张通常见于生长迅速的癌及肉瘤;②水肿,表现为整个乳房密度增加;③皮肤增厚和收缩,乳线 x 线表现早于临床症状和体征的出现,提示皮肤淋巴管堵塞;④乳头内陷(图 8-24、图 8-25);⑤乳腺结构扭曲(图 8-26),肿块和增生可直接引起小叶和导管的结构扭曲;⑥乳房变形。

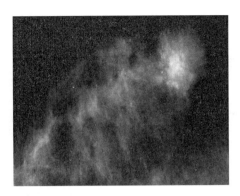

乳腺 X 线无数的微钙化主要集中在肿瘤内。

图 8-39 乳腺癌钙化

2）超声检查：超声表现为①实性肿块；②不规则肿块，边界不清，没有包膜，通常有卫星病灶；③低回声，以及不均质肿块时回声多种多样。强光点提示微钙化，对乳腺癌的诊断有重要意义。如果肿块足够大，病变内可出现坏死和液化，超声表现为无回声；④后方回声衰减；⑤同侧或对侧腋窝淋巴结肿大；⑥彩色多普勒超声（CDFI）在 CDFI 上，可能会出现肿块周边及内部血流丰富。血彩通常像一根棍子延伸到肿块内。

3）增强 MRI：MRI 不是乳腺癌的常规检查方法，但增强 MRI 可以为一些患者提供大量有用的信息。在增强 MRI 上，注入 Gd-DTPA 后肿块显著强化。乳腺癌的增强特征通常是在注射对比剂后 2 分钟内肿块立即强化，强化可持续 10 分钟以上。MRI 也可用于发现肿瘤浸润及淋巴结转移。但 MRI 不能直接显示乳腺癌早期的微钙化，因此其对乳腺疾病的作用有限。

4）影像学检查方法评估：乳房 X 线摄影因其较高的诊断符合率，被认为是乳腺癌的最佳检查方法。通过对 40 岁以上高危女性广泛调查，发现原位乳腺癌可出现微钙化。MRI 在某种程度上并不是一个传统的检查方法，但增强 MRI 对某些患者来说是非常有用的，如：①乳腺腺体致密的乳腺癌高危人群；②术后患者要求复查残留乳房；③患者植入假体。增强 MRI 通常用来区分疤痕和肿块；④多发病灶进行术前定位。超声不仅能显示肿块及其范围，还能显示腋窝淋巴结的转移情况。超声对乳腺实性肿块的诊断率可达 90%以上，近年来随着超声设备的发展，彩色多普勒超声在乳腺疾病的诊断中得到了广泛的应用，彩色多普勒超声可以定量分析肿块的血流和血流动力学变化。彩色多普勒超声有助于鉴别肿块的良恶性，恶性病变血供增加，良性肿块血供减少。但这些检查方法仍存在一些不足，如不能鉴别乳腺癌和浆细胞性乳腺炎、早期乳腺癌和纤维化等多种病变。

（3）鉴别诊断：

1）钙化：乳腺 X 线检查发现钙化灶时，需要与良性病灶的钙化鉴别.大多数的钙化是良性的，如血管钙化（图 8-40）、囊肿钙化、脂肪坏死钙化（图 8-41）、腺瘤钙化（图 8-26、图 8-27）等。钙化必须根据其形态（大小、形态和密度）、分布（分散或簇状）、和排列（线状、小叶状）来分析。良性病灶的钙化一般倾向于散在分布、呈圆形，其大小、密度较均一，表现为大颗粒状、斑片状或线状，而恶性病变的钙化倾向于大小、形态和密度不均一，多为泥沙样的不规则微小钙化灶（图 8-31、图 8-32、图 8-33、图 8-39）。在乳腺 X 线片上，钙化的范围愈大，微小浸润的可能性愈高。

2）肿块：良性病变如单纯囊肿、纤维腺瘤、乳头状瘤、血肿等的肿块常表现为边界清楚、密度相对较正常乳腺实质低的肿瘤，肿瘤周围常可见晕征，晕征即指一薄的透光带环绕肿瘤。恶性肿瘤常表现为肿块的边缘不光整，有毛刺，肿块显示的大小常较临床触摸到的肿块要小。

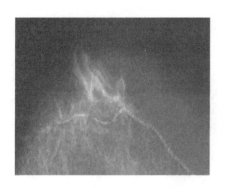

乳腺 X 线示乳腺血管钙化呈轨道样改变。

图 8-40　血管钙化

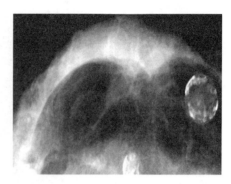

乳房自体脂肪组织充填术后，乳腺 X 线示脂肪充填区见多个圆形脂肪坏死钙化灶。

图 8-41　脂肪坏死钙化

（李艳辉，陈珊珊，肖曼君，龙孟平，肖恩华，罗建光）

Chapter 8

Breast

Section 1　Method of examination

1. Mammography

Mammography refers to "soft X-ray" mammography, and is performed to screen healthy women for signs of breast cancer. It is also used to evaluate a woman who has symptoms of breast disease such as a lump, nipple discharge, breast pain, dimpling of the skin on the breast or retraction of the nipple, or asymptomatic breast disease.

Screening mammograms are important for early breast cancer detection. The American Cancer Society recommends mammogrambe screening every year for all women aged 40 and older. The National Cancer Institute recommends mammogram be screening every 1 to 2 years for women aged 40 and older.

A screening mammogram usually takes 2 x-ray pictures (views) of each breast. 1) Axial position: The patient's body is facing the mammary gland machine. The height of the photo bracketis adjusted to the level of the patient's mammary gland. The mammary gland is placed on the photo bracket, and the lower chest wall of the mammary gland is close to the edge of the bracket, as shown in figure 8-1(a), and the axial position photo is shown in figure 8-1(b), (c).

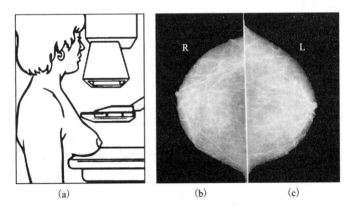

(a)　　　　(b)　　　(c)

Figure 8-1　(a) ~ (c) A view from the top(or craniocaudad-CCview)

2) Oblique position: The patient's body is facing the mammary gland machine. The frame rotates 60 degrees to the opposite side, and the height of the photo bracket is adjusted to the level of the patient's mammary gland. The patient's hand is raised on the affected side, and the upper part of the bracket is placed under the armpit. The body turns 15 degrees to the opposite side, and the mammary gland is placed on the photo bracket, and the breast wall on the side of the mammary gland is close to the edge of the bracket, as shown in Figure 8-2(a), (b).

2. Breast ultrasound

Ultrasound, also known as sonography, is an imaging method in which high-frequency sound waves are used to outline a part of the body. High-frequency sound waves are transmitted through the area of the body being studied. The sound wave echoes are picked up and translated by a computer into an image that is displayed on a computer screen. You are not exposed to radiation during this test. As shown in figure 8-3(a), (b).

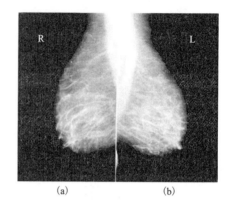

(a)　　　　(b)

Figure 8-2　(a), (b) A side view(medial lateral oblique-MLO view)

Breast ultrasound is sometimes used to evaluate breast problems that are found during a screening or diagnostic mammogram or on physical exam. It has certain value in the following cases, but breast ultrasound is not used for routine screening of breast diseases.

1) It is easier and more accurate to judge the cystic or solid lesionsfor the well-defined nodules on mammography. However, some cysts with moderate echo are difficult to be identified by ultrasound. Some encapsulated tumors may be hypoechoic and similar to cysts. When a lesion is solid, it is difficult to differentiate benign from malignant.

2) When the breast physical examination and mammography are inconsistent, ultrasound is helpful to analyze the lesions. Such as: Physical examination finds that there are lesions, and mammography is negative, especially in dense breast, ultrasound can often show with or without focal lesions. Similarly, ultrasound can help to confirm or exclude the possibility of focal lesions in mammography when there are ill defined shadows.

3) Ultrasound is helpful to observe the lesions that cannot be shown by mammography due to anatomical reasons. For example: Tumor near chest wall and lymph node deep in axilla.

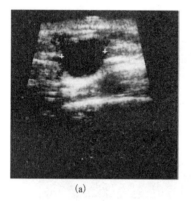
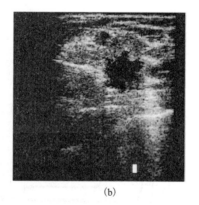

(a)　　　　　　　　　　　　　(b)

Figure 8-3　(a), (b) The ultrasonic examination shows that breast cyst shows hypoechoic and clear nodule shadow

3. Imaging-guided breast biopsy

Mammography is an excellent method to find breast diseases. But in the diagnosis of many cases, we can not judge whether the lesions are benign or malignant by the photos. There are two types of image-guided breast biopsy: Fine needle aspiration biopsy (FNAB) and core needle biopsy (CNB). Fine needle or thick needle biopsy is an important detection method, which can be guided by X-ray (Figure 8-4) or ultrasound. Under the guidance of ultrasound, the doctor can direct the needle to the mass for biopsy. Under the guidance of X-ray, the puncture needle can be guided to the mass for biopsy, and some calcified lesions that can not be touched can also be biopsied and locatedpreoperatively. Proper use of needle aspiration or needle biopsy can reduce the number of surgical biopsies of benign lesions, and cancer patients can be diagnosed before operation.

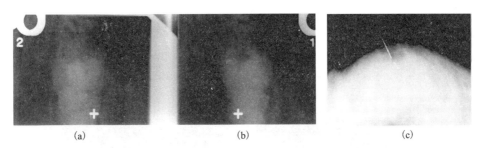

(a) (b) (c)

Figure 8-4　(a), (b) Breast lesion locating with X-ray; (c) X-ray guided breast lesion biopsy

4. Magnetic resonance imaging (MRI)

MRI uses magnetization and radio waves, instead of x-rays, to produce very detailed, cross-sectional images. Currently, spin echo (SE), gradient echo (GE) and fat suppression are commonly used imaging techniques. With the right technology and special surface coil, breast MRI is valuable in some cases. For example, after intravenous injection of Gd-DTPA [Figure 8-5(a), (b)], dynamic observation of enhanced images can provide important differential diagnosis data. Malignant tumors almost always enhance faster and more strongly than benign tumors. But fibroadenoma with rich cells, some types of proliferative breast disease and inflammatory lesions, as well as scar tissue in 6 months after surgery, can show enhanced images similar to cancer. Six months after the operation, when it is difficult to evaluate by mammography, MRI examination of the breast has certain value, especially for the patients with silicon implants, to observe whether the silicon implants have rupture, leakage or adjacent malignant lesions. MRI has unique advantages for single or multiple breast cysts, hemorrhage or hematoma. MRI can find lesions that mammography can not find, but the judgment of benign and malignant lesions is not as good as mammography, and the application of breast MRI is limited because of its complexity and high cost.

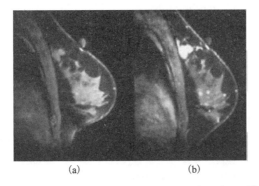

(a) (b)

Figure 8-5　(a), (b) Magnetic resonance imaging of breast

5. Digital mammograms

The image of digital mammography is stored on the computer in the form of digital image, which can be easily shared electronically. Although the spatial resolution of mammography is poor compared with the traditional mammography, its higher contrast can be used as compensation, and it has a strong image algorithm and post-processing. Digital technology is of great significance to the qualitative analysis of small calcification. At present, the digital technology (CCD camera) has shown its unique advantages by imaging in real time for stereoscopic positioning biopsy.

6. Ductogram

A ductogram[Figure 8-6(a), (b)]is a test that is sometimes helpful in determining the cause of a nipple discharge. In this x-ray procedure, a fine plastic tube is placed into the opening of the duct into the nipple. A small amount of contrast medium is injected, which outlines the shape of the duct on an x-ray image and will show whether there is a mass inside the duct.

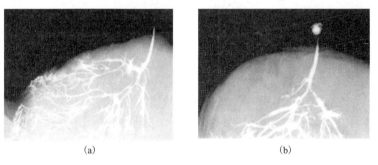

(a)   (b)

Figure 8-6   (a), (b)Image of breast ductogram

Section 2   Normal appearances

The female mammary gland is mainly composed of mammary lobe, mammary lobule, mammary duct and stroma (fibrous connective tissue, adipose tissue, with blood vessels, nerves and lymphatic vesselsamong them) (Figure 8-7). The terminal duct and acini in the lobule of mammary gland are called terminal ductal lobular unit (TDLU), which is the basic unit of breast function. The mammary gland tissue is located between the superficial and deep layers of the subcutaneous superficial fascia. The superficial fibers of the superficial fascia are connected with the skin by a reticular band, which is called the suspension ligament, also known as Cooper ligament.

The arterial blood supply of the breast has three main sources: 1. The perforator of the internal thoracic artery, also known as the internal mammary artery, mainly supplies the medial side. 2. The branches of the axillary

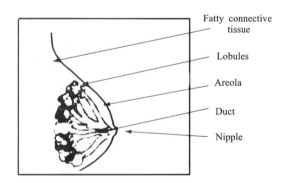

Figure 8-7   Normal breast.

artery, such as the thoracoacromial artery and the lateral thoracic artery, supply the lateral and upper part of the breast. 3. The lateral cutaneous branch of the intercostal artery. Venous drainage of the breast is usually accompanied by an artery, mainly to the axillary.

There are abundant lymphatic networks and lymph nodes in the breast, and most of the lymphatic vessels return to the axillary lymph nodes. The main way of breast cancer metastasis is lymphatic system. Whether axillary lymph node metastasis occurs or not is very important to the choice of breast cancer treatment.

Section 3　Basic pathological changes

The basic lesions on breast mainly include masses, calcification, structural distortion, localized skin thickening and depression, nipple retraction and funnel sign, abnormal breast ducts, localized asymmetry and denseness, increased blood supply and lymphadenopathy.

1. Masses

Masses are space-occupying lesions of the breast, which are divided into benign and malignant masses.

(1)X-ray findings: We need to determine whether there is a mass on the two different projection positions simultaneously. It is not significant for dividing benign and malignant tumors according to the tumors size. But when the size of the clinical palpation is larger than the X-ray measurement, the possibility of a malignant mass is high. The shape, edge, density and surrounding conditions of the mass are very important for the differentiation of benign and malignant masses. The shape of the mass is generally divided into round, oval, lobulated and irregular shapes, and the degree of malignancy increases sequentially. Masses with clear borders and smooth edges are generally benign lesions, while masses with blurry and lobulated edges are more likely to be malignant lesions. Observation on the magnified image is more reliable. Most benign lesions are iso-density or low-density which is close to that of normal glandswhile most malignant nodules have a higher density. Masses with fat density are generally only seen in benign lesionssuch as hamartomas and lipomas. Translucent lines or transparent halos can be seen around the mass. Translucent lines are more common in benign lesions such as fibroadenoma. Hyaline halo is more common in breast cancer(Figure 8-8, 9).

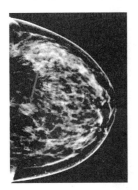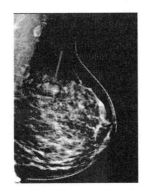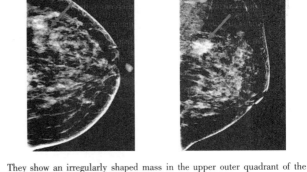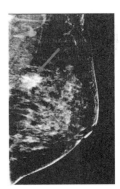

They show a round-like mass in the outer quadrant of the left breastwith uniform density, clear borders and transparent lines around it. It is a benign mass.

Figure 8-8　The CC and MLO positions of the left breast

They show an irregularly shaped mass in the upper outer quadrant of the left breast with homogeneous density, unclear borders, lobulated edges and burrs. It is a malignant mass.

Figure 8-9　The CC and MLO positions of the left breast

(2)MRI manifestations: Benign lesions show regular morphology and clear boundaries on unenhanced images while malignant lesions show irregular morphology and unclear boundaries with lobulated, star-shaped or glitch-like changes on the edge. The masses on T1WI images are mainly hypointensity and isointensitywhile the signals on the T2WI images are changeable and related to the internal components of the mass. They show isointensity and hypointensitywhen the mass contains more fibrous components. And they become high signals when the mass contains more cells and water. The internal signal of benign lesions is relatively homogeneous. The malignant

267

lesions may appear liquefaction, necrosis, cystic change, hemorrhage or fibrosis which present mixed signals. Dynamic-enhanced scanning is helpful for the qualitative diagnosis of lesions. Benign lesions often have more homogeneous enhancement or diffuse patch-like enhancement, and some lesions have eccentric enhancement. The malignant lesions have heterogeneous enhancement or mainly edge enhancement and mostly centripetal strengthening. The dynamic enhancement curve of benign lesions is a slow-rising type while the dynamic enhancement curve of a malignant lesion is a fast-rising and fast-decreasing type. And a fast-rising plateau curve is likely to be benign or malignant lesion (Figure. 8-10, -11).

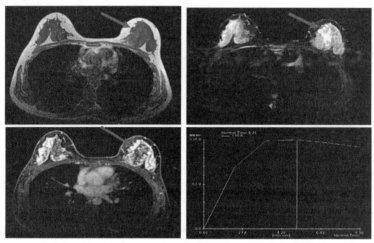

They are iso-intensity on T1WI and hyper-intensity on T2WI. The signals are homogeneous and the border are clear. They are showed significant homogeneously enhancement on enhanced scanning. The dynamic enhancement curve (T1C max) shows continuous type (type I). They are benign masses.

Figure 8-10　The MRI image of the left breast shows multiple round-like masses in the left breast

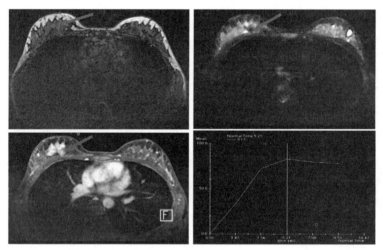

It is iso-intensity on T1WI and mixed intensity on T2WI. The border is irregular and it has obvious deep lobes with burrs. The enhanced scan shows significant heterogeneous enhancement andthe dynamic enhancement curve (ST-T curve) is a plateau type (type II). It is a malignant mass.

Figure 8-11　The MRI image of the right breast shows a large irregular-shaped mass with heterogeneous signals

2. Calcification

The calcification may present on both benign and malignant breast lesions. The morphology, distribution, density and other characteristics of calcification can be useful to distinguish benign and malignant lesions. Benign calcifications are mostly coarse, popcorn-like, granular, round, strip, small ring or crescent whichare high density and scattered distribution. The malignant calcifications are mostly linear, sand-like, fork-like or rod-like with various size, heterogeneous density and distributed in typical clusters. The malignant calcifications can be located inside or outside the mass. Most recessive breast cancers with no obvious masses can be diagnosed based on the characteristics of calcification. According to the BI-RADS grading standard proposed by the American College of Radiology, breast calcification can be divided into three types: Typical benign, intermediate (unqualified) and highly suspected malignant. X-ray mammography is the main examination method for clinical discovery and diagnosis of calcification while ultrasound, CT and MRI are usually difficult to detect micro-calcification. (Figure 8-12)

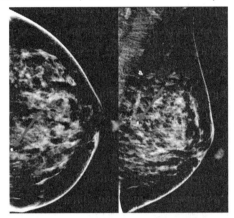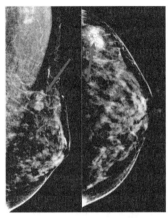

The left picture shows there are scattered large patchy calcifications in the benign mass. The right picture shows there ara multiple sand-grain and rod-shaped calcifications in the malignant mass and they are distributed in clusters.

Figure 8-12　The CC position and MLO position of the left breast

3. Structural distortion and deformation

The structural distortion must be displayed on the two different projection positions of the X-ray molybdenum target. The structural distortions and deformations may present on the benign and malignant breast lesions. The benign lesions such as chronic inflammation, fat necrosis, biopsy, post-operative scars and radiotherapy can present structural distortions. The interface between breast parenchyma and fat can be twisted, deformed, and disordered. We should consider the reactive fibrosis caused by invasive breast cancer when there were no obvious masses. Biopsy is required when it is difficult to distinguish between benign and malignant lesions (Figure 8-13).

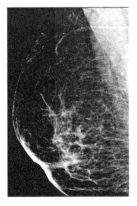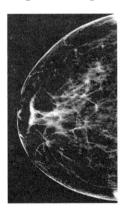

They show that the central area of the right breast is structurally distorted, deformed, increased in density and the adjacent skin thickened and slightly sunken, which is caused by postoperative changes.

Figure 8-13　The CC and MLO positions of the right breast

4. Localized thickening and sunken skin

Inflammatory diseases of the breast usually manifest as diffuse skin thickening while localized skin thickening and depression are common in malignant lesions. It will cause the localized thickening of the skin and receding toward the tumor because of the tumor infiltration and invasion of the skin which is called "dimple Levy". Some patients with scars after surgery may also have thickened and sunken skin in the surgical area.

5. Nipple retraction and funnel sign

Nipple retraction and inverted are common in congenital dysplasia of the nipple and breast cancer infiltration behind the nipple. "Funnel sign" is manifested as a triangular dense shadow below the nipple with the tip pointing to the inside of the glandwhich can be seen when breast cancer infiltrates the gland tissue below the areola. It can also be seen in inflammation around the areola (Figure 8-14, 15).

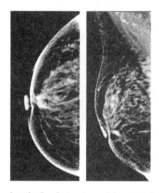 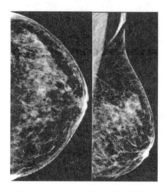 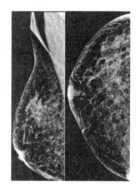

They show that the local structure of the central area of the right breast is distorted, deformed, heterogeneous density and mass-like changes. The adjacent skin is thickened and the nipple is inverted by malignant tumor infiltration.

Figure 8-14   The CC and MLO positions of the right breast

The left picture shows the CC position and MLO position of the left breast showing the inverted nipple of the left breast. The right picture shows the CC position and the MLO position of the right breast showing the inverted nipple of the right breast.

Figure 8-15   Inverted nipples on both sides of the breast

6. Abnormal breast ducts

Breast duct abnormalities are manifested as thickening, rough edges and increased density of the mammary duct below the nipple. They often happen on benign and malignant lesions. They can be manifested as duct dilation, filling defect, truncation, compression displacement, destruction, walking stiffness, disordered arrangement and reduced branching which mainly rely on mammography examination(Figure 8-16).

7. Limitations of asymmetric and dense

Diagnosis of localized asymmetry and compaction should be observed when comparing with previous X-ray mammography or bilateral breasts. We need to consider the possibility of invasive cancer if there is a new localized compaction, especially when the compact area has progressively increased or expanded during follow-up, andbiopsy is recommended (Figure 8-17).

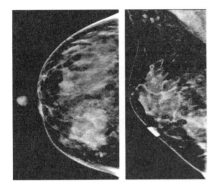
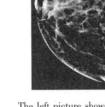
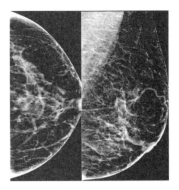

The CC and MLO positions of the right breast show multiple dilated and tortuous ducts.

The left picture shows the CC position and MLO position of the right breast and the right picture shows the CC position and MLO position of the left breast. Compared with the normal left breast, the central area of the right breast shows a localized asymmetric dense shadow with blurred edges andheterogeneous density. The adjacent skin is thickened.

Figure 8-16 The patient has nipple discharge

Figure 8-17 The CC positions and MLO position

8. Increased blood supply

Malignant tumors often have increased blood supply which manifests as increased, thickened and tortuous abnormal vascular shadows in the breast and small venous clusters around the lesion (Figure 8-18).

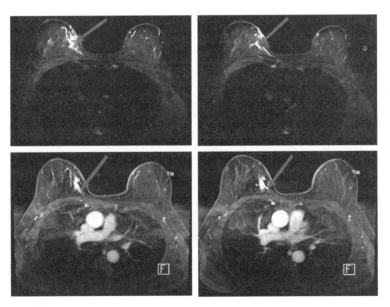

They show that there are multiple increased, thickened, tortuous vascular shadows around the mass in the upper quadrant of the right breast which extend into the mass, indicating that the blood supply of the mass is increased. And the final pathological diagnosis is breast cancer.

Figure 8-18 The upper picturesarethe T2WI images of double breasts and the lower picturesarethe enhanced scans

9. lymphadenopathy

The malignant tumor or inflammation can cause lymphadenopathy whichis generally round or irregular swelling, increased density, disappearance of lymph node hilum(Figure 8-19).

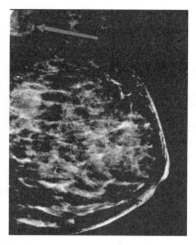

It shows that the left axillary lymph nodes are enlarged, round-shaped with high density. The lymph node hilum disappeared. It is the lymph node metastasis of breast cancer.

Figure 8-19   The MLO position of the left breast

Section 4   Diagnosis of common diseases

1. Acute mastitis and breast abscess

(1)The clinical and pathological manifestations: Acute mastitis is the acute inflammation of the breast. Breast infections usually occur in women who are breast-feeding, and it are usually caused by a common bacteria found on normal skin of the nipple or areola. The stasis of milk in the gland results in the infection. The infection takes place in the parenchyma (fatty tissue) and causes swelling of the parenchyma outside the milk ducts. This swelling compresses on the milk ducts, and the results are pain and swelling of the infected breast. Breast abscess is the advanced form of acute matitis. Acute mastitis is usually a local infection of Staphylococcus aureus. But uncommonly streptoccus may cause diffuse infection. Clinically, women present with fever, increase of white blood cell, raise of erythrocyte sedimentation rate (ESR), red、swelling、tenderness and heat in breast tissue, ill-defined margins, immobile skin, nipple discharge(may contain pus), and enlargement、pain and tenderness of axillary nodes. In advanced stage, margins of the lesion may be distinct gradually and then the abscess forms.

(2)Image manifestations:

The mostreliable method of diagnosis acute mastitis and breast abscess is mammography. Dilatation of subcutaneous trabeculum, thickening of skin, generally high density, patchy lesions with obscured margins are the typical mammography presentation of acute mastitis. Lesions can also present as an irregular mass. Flamboyancy shadow around the irregular high density should suggest breast abscess. The margin of abscess may be obscured initially and then become distinct gradually. Breast abscess is associated with edema and thickening of skin commonly (Figure 8-20). Enlargement of axillary nodes is not uncommon.

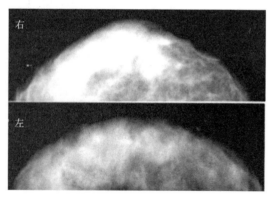

Mammographyshowslarge area of high density with unclear boundary in lateral quadrant of the right breast, accompanied by local breast skin edema, thickening. Theleftbreastisnormal.

Figure 8-20   Acute mastitis

2. Hyperplasia of mammary gland

(1) The clinical and pathological manifestations: Hyperplasia of mammary gland is the most breast disease in women. The causes include high level of estrogen and disproportion of corporin. It suggests that the lobules is very sensitive to hormone. The following three types are established according to different pathologic manifestations. 1) Glandular hyperplasia, whichis hyperplasia lobules and fibrous connective tissue. The lobules are enlarged, distorted and they become irregular. The appearance of hyperplastic lobules is similar to fibroadenomas. 2) Cystic hyperplasia, which is hyperplasia of lobules with cystogenesis, which is the advanced form of glandular hyperplasia of breast. The cysts result from the distention of terminal ducts. 3) Fibrous hyperplasia, which is hyperplasia of fibrous tissue of breast mostly. Clinically, although hyperplasia of breast present at any age between late adolescent and menopause, it is more common in women between 30 and 40 years whose mammary glands have developed normally. Onset is in both the mammae or in one. Swelling with masses typically is the main symptom which usually present at 1 week before menstruation. Single or multiple small masses are tough, obscuredand diffuse in breast. Most women present circumscribed pain that is severe usually before menstruation and relieved or stopped after menstruation.

(2) Image manifestations:

1) Mammographyis the most reliable method of diagnosis hyperplasia of breast.

①Glandular hyperplasia. Onset is usually in both mammae, but can also in one. Lesions are circumscribed in breast, usually in the outer upper quadrant, but they may be diffuse also on mammography. Density of lesions is high andappearance of the lesions may be irregular as cotton, snow or a mass. Obscured irregular margins are commonly shown on mammography. Confluence of these small masses may lead to the architecture distortion(Figure 8-21). ② Cystic hyperplasia. Architecture of normal breast is distorted and general hyperdensity with diffuse cystic masses may be shown. Size of cystic masses is variable. Only the masses more than 0.5 cm in diameter can be seen. Calcification is uncommon(Figure 8-22). ③ Fibrous hyperplasia, which is uncommon but can be seen in women younger than 30 yearsold. Lesions are commonly seenin both mammae diffusedly or locally. Diffuse fibrous hyperplasia may be shown as homogeneous hyperdensity in a circumscribed region without masses or calcification. However, lesions are often mixed having components with two or three types.

2) Breast ultrasound: ①Hyperplasia in both mammae and thickening of gland can be shown. ②Inhomogeneous internal light spots and echoes with lots of diffuse hypoechogenic, ill-defined or well-defined regions may be seen on sonography. Lesion can not be shown as a globe although multiple direction scanning. ③Hyperplasia is in both mammae with similar echogenicity. ④On colour Doppler flow imaging(CDFI), flow in the lesions doesn't increase and there is no flow through the hypoechogenic regions. ⑤Cysitic hyperplasia of breast developing in both mammae may be shown as multiple water sonolucentlesions except for the signs of glandular hyperplasia.

3) Galactography: Cystic hyperplasia may be detected by galactography. Duringgalactography, notonly the breastductcanbeshowed, some contrast agent may enter the surrounding small cysts, showing lotsof round or nodular denselesions.

(3) Differential diagnosis

1) Adenoscarcoma of breast: Adenoscarcoma of breastisusually seen in women of 20-25. One or more masses in the breast which are round or egg-shaped, distinctly-bordered, smooth, movable and developing slowly and no general symptoms.

2) Mammary cancer: Mammary canceris usually seen in women of 40-60 just before or after climacteric. Masses in the breast are as hard as stone, rough, movable in the early stage and fixed in the advanced stage. Skin dimpling, retreated nipple, enlarged and hard axillary lymph nodes which become cauliflower-like or rock-like ulcers after festering, and bloody fluid with awful smell discharged from the ulcers are seen. In the early stage,

pathological section is needed to make the diagnosis. Calcifications in glandular hyperplasia is scarce, which are weeny and diffuse in the breast. This kind of calcification is indistinguishable from the microcalcifications of breast cancer. Combination with clinical signs and imaging guided breast biopsy is very necessary.

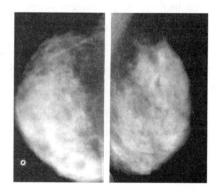

Female, 36 years old. Swelling and pain in both mammae for half one year, pain before menstruation, mass in breast for 1 month. Mammography shows diffuse patchy high densities with obscured margins.

Figure 8-21   Glandular hyperplasia

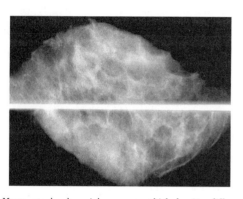

Mammography shows inhomogeneous high density, diffuse cystic low density of varying sizes and architecture distortion.

Figure 8-22   Cystic hyperplasia. Female, 48 years old

3. Fibrocystic breast disease

(1) The clinical and pathological manifestations: Fibrocysticbreast disease is described as common, benign changes involving the tissues of the breast. The term "disease" in this case is misleading, and, many providers prefer the term "change". The condition is so commonly found in normal breasts, it is believed to be a normal variant. Other related terms include "mammary dysplasia", "benign breast disease" and "diffuse cystic mastopathy". The cause is not completely understood, but the changes are believed to be associated with ovarian hormones since the condition usually subsides with menopause, and may vary in consistency during the menstrual cycle. The incidence is estimated to be over 60% of all women. Its incidence is lower in women taking oralcontraceptive. The risk factors may include family history and diet (such as excessive dietary fat, and caffeine intake), although these are controversial. Reduction of dietary fat and caffeine if you have fibrocystic breast changes has been suggested, although recent studies have questioned the role of caffeine and fat in fibrocystic disease. Clinical manifestations: 1) A dense, irregular and bumpy "cobblestone" consistency is seen in the breast tissue. 2) Usually more marked in the outer upper quadrants. 3) Breast discomfort that is persistent, or that occurs off and on (intermittent). 4) Breast(s) feel full dull, heavy pain and tenderness. 5) Premenstrual tenderness and swelling. 6) Breast discomfort improves after each menstrual period. 7) Nipple sensation changes, itching. Note: Symptoms may range from mild to severe. Symptoms typically peak just before each menstrual period, and improve immediately after the menstrual period.

(2) Image manifestations:

Physical examination reveals the presence of mobile (non-anchored) breast "masses". These masses are usually rounded, with smooth borders, and either rubbery or slightly fluctuant (changeable in shape). Dense tissue may make the breast examination more difficult to interpret. Mammography may be difficult to interpret due to dense tissue. A biopsy of the breast may be necessary to rule out other disorders. Aspiration of the breast with a fine needle is often diagnostic and therapeutic for larger cysts.

4. Fibroadenomas

（1）The clinical and pathological manifestations: Fibroadenomas are among the most common breast benign lesions, particularly in women about20yearsold. It is common in women between the age of 15 and 35. Fibroadenomas is believed to be caused by endocrine disturbance. It is requiring the consideration of fibrocystic breast disease, adenosis of breast, and even mammary carcinoma in the differentiation clinically. Pathologically, fibroadenoma is a benign tumor composed of two components: breast fibrous tissue and glandular duct. Cross section of the masses is gray or pink and macro-lobulated. Histologically, fibrous tissue or glandular epithelium may be the main component. In most tumors, fibrous tissue is the main component. Its occurrence is concerned with the excessive response of breast tissue to estrogen. Clinical manifestations: On clinical examination, fibroadenomas may be nonpalpable or palpable, oval or micro-lobulated, mobile, rubbery, smooth masses without pain. Fibroadenomas vary in size and most is smaller than 5 cm in diameter. The mass can become harder because of calcification, but without tenderness. The lesions are usually more marked in the outer upper quadrants of breast. Nipple discharge（bloody or clear-to yellow fluid）may appear since the cystis degeneration. The lesions are slow growing and always solitary. Approximately 10% ~ 15% of fibroadenomas are multiple.

（2）Image manifestations:

Thepreferred imaging method is determined by the patient's age. In general, ultrasonography（USs）is preferred if a palpable mass is found, if a patient is younger than 30 years or if the patient is pregnant. Both of mammography and US are useful if the patient has a palpable mass, is older than 30 years, and is not pregnant. Because CT has the high dose, it is less sensitive to micro calcification than molybdenum target, and it is not specific to the mass, it is not the first choice for the diagnosis of the disease. Breast MRI is not the first choice because of its high cost and high false positive rate.

1）Mammography: On mammography, solitary fibroadenoma typically appears as a smooth-margined homogeneous, oval or round mass （Figure 8-23）. Sometimes lobulation or small incisions appear on the edge （Figure 8-24）. Because of the contrast of fat tissue, a transparent thin rim may be seen around the mass （Halo's Sign）（Figure 8 - 24, 25）. Mucification and cystis degeneration may be shown in most of massesexcept for the newly formed fibroadenoma. Occasionally in the women over 40 years tumors contain coarse calcifications, which suggest infarction and involution（Figure 8-26, 27）. Appearance of calcifications may vary and be shown as ring, plague, spot, lace, coral or irregular. The calcification can appear in the center or periphery of the masses. Sometimes the lesion may be placed by a large and irregular calcification, which is specific mammographically.

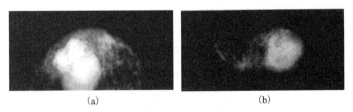

(a)　　　　　　　　　　(b)

Mammography[（a）CC view, （b）MLO view] showsoval, micro-lobulated, well-defined homogeneous mass.

Figure 8-23　Fibroadenomas

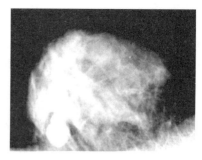

Female, 32 years old, present with a mass in the left breast for 1 month. Mammography shows a homogeneous, gentle lobulated mass with Halo's sign, 2×3 cm, in posterior lower quadrant.

Figure 8-24 Fibroadenomas

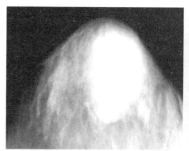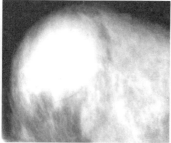

Female, 29 years old, present with a mass in the right breast for 1 week. Mammography shows a homogeneous, gentle lobulated and oval mass with Halo's sign, 4×5 cm, in the lower quadrant of the right breast.

igure 8-25 Fibroadenomas

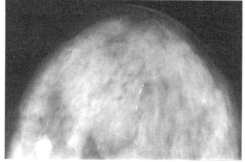

Female, 40 years old. Mammography shows a mass in inner quadrant, 1.5×2 cm. Calcifications occupied almost the whole mass.

Figure 8-26 Calcification of fibroadenomas

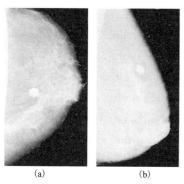

(a)   (b)

Mammography(a. CC view, b. MLO view) shows round-like and clear boundary mass with large calcification in the breast.

Figure 8-27 Fibroadenomas

2)On sonograms, fibroadenomapresentsasacircumscribed, homogeneous, oval or round, hypoechoic mass that may have gentle lobulations, a smooth, thin, echogenic capsule and variable acoustic enhancement and homogeneity(Figure 8-28, 29). Fibroadenomas often may demonstrate a typical appearance and be distinguished clearly from cysts and carcinomas. However, fibrocystic disease with complicated hypoechoic cysts and rarely, smooth carcinomas may mimic fibroadenoma. Atypical fibroadenomas, which are inhomogeneous or irregular in shape, may simulate carcinomas.

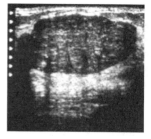

Sonogram demonstrates a hypoechoic mass with smooth partially lobulated margins that are typical of a fibroadenoma.

Figure 8-28 Fibroadenomas

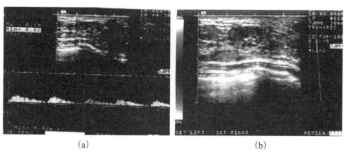

(a)   (b)

Sonography(a)and CDFI (b)show striated blood flow in the tumor.

Figure 8-29 Fibroadenomas

3) On CT, fibroadenomas appear as well-circumscribed, smooth, homogeneous, oval masses, Hounsfield number on CT of which is higher than normal gland. The masses are notable enhanced after administration of iodinated contrast. Recently, MRI has displaced this technique because of the radiation exposure of CT scan.

4) The appearance of fibroadenomas on MRI is variable. Fibroadenomas appear as smooth or gently lobulated round or oval masses. On T1WI, they are isointensity or exhibit lower intense signal than the normal gland around them. And on T2WI the signal of fibroadenomas vary from low to high. According to the signal on T2WI and the enhancement characteristics, fibroadenomas can be divided into three types. Type Ⅰ, fibroadenomas typically are high signal intensity on T2WI and may be enhanced with the administration of gadolinium-based contrast agent. Type Ⅱ, fibroadenomas are isointense signal on T2WI, and can be enhanced. Type Ⅲ, fribroadenomas are shown as hypointensity on T2WIwithout enhancement. Control study shows that masses of high intensity on T2WI contain a lot of mucoid stroma with a large percentage of stroma cel, while the hypointense masses on T2WI are almost full of homogeneous sclerosis tissue with slight stroma cell. On MRI, nonenhanced internal septa and lobulated masses may help in distinguishing fibroadenomas from other lesions.

(3) Differential Diagnosis

1) Simple cyst: Simple cyst always present in both sides of breast and are more common in women older than 40 years. Fibroadenomas are usually seen in young women between 21 and 26 years and always solitary. Cysts are typically shown as oval homogeneous lesions with smooth margin, while fibroadenomas can be round or oval, smooth or gentle lobulated, homogeneous or inhomogeneous masses. Sonography are usually used to distinguish cystic from solid mass (Figure 8-30).

2) Galactocele: Galactocele is more commonly seen in women of lactation, especially in the patients with mastitis. Its density is higher than fibroadenomas on mammography with smooth and neat edges. The existence of galactocele may cause architectural distortion and thickening of the trabecula of mammary gland.

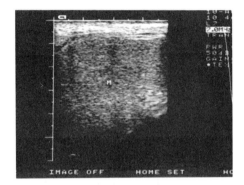

Female, 44 years old. Present with enlargement of right breast for 3 months. Sonography shows a vast homogeneous round well-defined anechoic mass.

Figure 8-30　Simple cyst

3) Breast cancer: In some patients with breast cancer, especially medullary carcinoma with a regular form and sharp margin, may be indistinguishable from fibroadenomas. A fixed mass and larger size on mammography than in physical examination should suggest the possibility a malignant tumor. Microcalcifications, spiculated masses and thickening of skin are all associated with malignant appearances.

4. Breast Cancer

(1) The clinical and pathological manifestations: Breast cancer is a malignant tumor originating from breast tissue, which is the most common malignancy and the second leading cause of death from cancer in women. Because of its high incidence and aesthetic symbolism, breast cancer has become a source of severe distress to the patient and her family. The cause of breast cancer is not completely understood. Epidemiological studies have identified many risk factors that increase the chance for a woman to develop breast cancer: 1) Age and gender — 77% of new cases and 84% of breast cancer deaths occur in women aged 50 and older. More than 80% of breast cancer cases occur in women over 50. Less than 1% of breast cancers occur in men. 2) Genetic factors and family history of breast cancer — Researchers have identified some other defective genes that may cause breast cancer, including BRCA3 and Noey2 (which is a disease inherited only from the father's side of the family). 3) Early menstruation and late Menopause — Women who started menstrual periods early (before age 12) or went through

menopause late (after age 55) are at higher risk. Also, women who have no childbearing history or who gave birth to ababy after the age of 30 have an increased risk. 4) Oral contraceptives (birth control pills) — Birth control pills may slightly increase the risk for breast cancer, depending on age, length of use, and other factors. 5) Hormone replacement therapy — Use of HRT for more than 5 years has been shown to slightly increase the risk of breast cancer and risk increases with longer use. 6) Radiation — People exposed to radiation, particularly during childhood may face an increased risk for breast cancer in adulthood. Especially at risk are those that received chest irradiation for prior cancers. 7) Additional risk factors — Some studies show previous breast, uterine, ovarian, colon cancer, and a strong history of cancer in the family may increase the risk for breast cancer.

Pathologically, generally breast cancer is a kind of adenocarcinoma which comesfrom the epithelial cells of the duct or lobules of mammary gland. According to the OMS classification, breast cancer can be divided into non-invasive carcinoma and invasive carcinoma. Non-invasive carcinoma includes lobular carcinoma in situ and intraductal carcinoma. And invasive carcinoma is consisted ofinvasive ductal carcinoma, invasive lobular carcinoma, mucinous carcinoma, medullary carcinoma, papillary carcinoma and adenoid cystic carcinoma.

Clinically, breast cancer is more common in women older than 40 years. Women may present with a painless solitary mass, which is usually more marked in the outer upper quadrants. The mass is firm to hard immovable and irregular with ill-defined borders. When the Cooper's ligament is involved in, nipple retraction may be seen. The infiltration of lymphatic vessels may cause edema of breast skin and "orange peel" appearance. In the advanced stage, because of metastasis of tumor, the enlarged axillary nodes and supraclavicular lymph nodes may beseen. Abnormal nipple discharge is another important signs, which is usually bloody or look like pus. In the initial stage, asthe symptoms and signs are always not typical clinically, some patients present in the advanced stage when seeinga doctor. Soearly diagnosisofbreastcancercannotonlydependon symptoms and signs. Recent studies believe that annually imaging screening in "high-risk population" over 40 years old is the key to early diagnosis of breast cancer, and part of pre-clinical breast cancer in situ can be found through this screening method. In this group of patients, a lumpectomy with breast conservation surgery is achieved.

Stages of Breast Cancer (from the American Joint Committee on Cancer):

STAGE 0. In Situ ("in place"): The cancerous cells are in their original location within normal breast tissue.

STAGE I. Tumor less than 2 cm in diameter with no spread beyond the breast.

STAGE IIA. Tumor 2 to 5 cm in size without spread to axillary (armpit) lymph nodes or tumor less than 2 cm in size with spread to axillary lymph nodes.

STAGE IIB. Tumor greater than 5 cm in size without spread to axillary lymph nodes or tumor 2 to 5 cm in size with spread to axillary lymph nodes.

STAGE IIIA. Tumor smaller than 5 cm in size with spread to axillary lymph nodes which are attached to each other or to other structures, or tumor larger than 5 cm in size with spread to axillary lymph nodes.

STAGE IIIB. The tumor has penetrated outside the breast to the skin of the breast or of the chest wall or has spread to lymph nodes inside the chest wall along the sternum.

STAGE IV. A tumor of any size with spread beyond the region of the breast and chest wall, such as to liver, bone, or lungs.

Many additional factors besides staging can influence the recommended treatment and the likely outcome. These can include the precise cell type andappearance of the cancer, whether the cancer cells respond to hormones, and the presence or absence of genes known to cause breast cancer.

(2) Image manifestations:

1) The most reliable and consistent method of diagnosing breast cancer is high-quality mammography.

Mammography is the first choice of breast cancer screening or diagnosis in high-risk groups. More and more breast cancer patients have been diagnosed in the pre-clinical stage, so these patients can get early treatment. As a result, the mortality rate of breast cancer has decreased by 25% in recent years. In mammography, early breast cancer may appear: Architectural distortion, microcalcification foci, or a breast mass.

Direct signs: ① Mass: Breast cancer often presents as irregular mass or nodule. Its density is higher than that of surrounding gland tissue or nipple. Its edge is unclear, and it is often accompanied by lobulated (Figure 8-19, 20, 21) and burr like changes (Figure 8-21 ~ 23). Compared with the contralateral breast, the breast tissue structure is asymmetric. When the tumor diffuses through the nipple, asymmetric thickening of the ducts around the tumor can be seen. In the late stage, the density of retromammary space is increased and blurred, and the pectoralis major and axillary lymph nodes are enlarged [Figure 8-22(a)], which represented the invasion of pectoralis major and axillary lymph node metastasis. ② Calcification: In 25% patients with preclinical carcinoma, clustered calcification can be shown (Figure 8-31 ~ 32). The size of calcification varies while the diameter is commonly less than 0.5 mm. The morphologic feature of calcification also varies. On mammography, most of calcification are shown as multiangular, sharp-angled or branched microcalcification which have to be identified clearly by magnifier sometimes. The aggregation of these microcalcification no matter with or without masses always suggests the malignancy and a biopsy have to be performed in order to make a definite diagnosis pathologically.

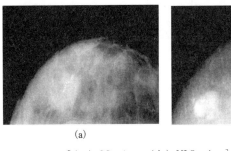
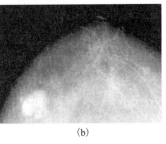

(a)　　　　　　　　(b)

Mammograms [(a) CC view, (b) MLO view] showsa lobulated ill-circumscribed mass with fine granular microcalcificationsand burr sign.

Figure 8-31　Breast cancer

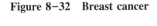

Mammogram shows a lobulated ill-circumscribed mass, and there are large amounts of microcalcifications in the mass. Those calcifications areinhomogeneous in size and form.

Figure 8-32　Breast cancer

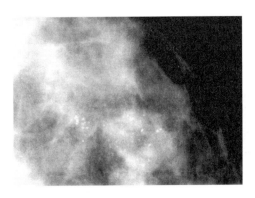

Mammogram shows a lobulatedspiculated mass measured 2×3 cm, and there are large amounts of granular or branching calcifications in the mass.

Figure 8-33　Breast cancer

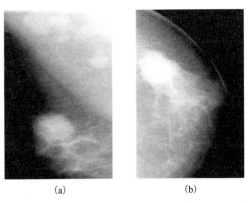

(a)　　　　　　　　(b)

Mammograms [(a) CC view, (b) MLO view] show a lobulated spiculated mass measured 1.5×2 cm, without calcifications. Figure a shows multiple enlarged axillary lymph nodes.

Figure 8-34　Breast cancer

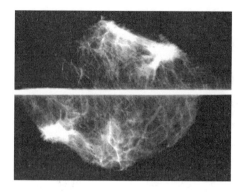

Mammograms show an invasive mass with spiculated margin.

Figure 8-35 Breast cancer

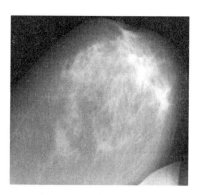

The extensive invasive tumor involves the ducts behind the areola, and the thickened ducts pull the nipple resulting in nipples retraction.

Figure 8-36 Breast cancer with nipple retraction

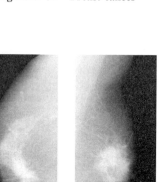

The breast cancer invades the lactation canal leading to nipple retraction in mammogram.

Figure 8-37 Breast cancer

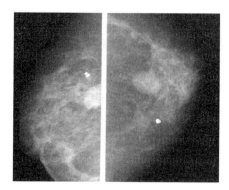

Tumor infiltrates the surrounding breast tissue resulting in architecture distortion and losing its normal shape.

Figure 8-38 Breast cancer

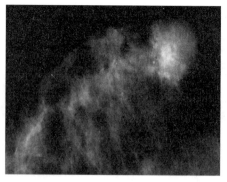

Numerous microcalcifications are concentrated in the tumor in mammogram.

Figure 8-39 Calcification of breast cancer

Indirect signs: ① Extension and increase of the vein, usually seen in carcinoma and sarcoma with high growth rate. ② Edema, shown as the density of the whole mammary gland increase generally. ③ Skin thickening and retraction, presenting on mammography before the clinical symptoms and signs, suggest the blockage of skin lymphatic vessels. ④ Nipple retraction(Figure 8-24, 25). ⑤ Architectural distortion of breast(Figure 8-26). The mass and hyperplasia may cause the architectural distortion of the lobules and ducts directly(Figure 8-26). ⑥ A change in the shape of breast.

2)Breast ultrasound: ① Solid mass. ② Irregular ill-defined mass without capsule, which usually exists with some satellite lesions. ③ Hypoechoic and inhomogeneous mass with variable amount of echo. Strong light-spots suggest the microcalcification, which is very important to the diagnosis of breast cancer. If mass is large enough, necrosis and liquefaction may be found in the lesion that is anecho on sonography. ④ Posterior acoustic attenuation. ⑤ Enlargement of axillary nodes on the same side or opposite side. ⑥ Colour Doppler Flow Imaging (CDFI): On CDFI, abundant flow in peripheral and inner region of the mass may be shown. The colour flow usually like a stick extends into the mass.

3)Enhanced MRI. MRI is not a conventional method for breast cancer, but enhanced MRI can provide a lot of useful information to some patients. On enhanced MRI, mass is marked enhanced with administration of Gd-DTPA. Enhancement characteristics of breast cancer typically is the mass can be enhanced immediately in 2 minutes after injecting the contrast medium, and the enhancement may last over 10 minutes. MRI can also be used to find the infiltration of cancer and the metastasis of lymph nodes. But MRI do not show the microcalcification in early stage of breast cancer directly, so its contribution to breast disease is limited.

4)Image analysis: Because of the high diagnosis accordance rate, mammography has been believed the most favourable method to breast cancer. By means of extensive survey to high risk women older than 40 years, microcalcification of breast carcinoma in situ may be shown. To a certain extent, MRI is not a conventional method. But enhanced MRI may be very useful to some patients, such as: ①High risk group with dense type of breast cancer. ② Patients asking for re-examination after operation remaining breast. ③ Patients implanted the prothesis. Enhanced MRI is usually used to differentiate the scar and tumor. ④ Position for multiple lesions before operation. Ultrasound can show not only the masses and their extent but also the metastasis of axillary nodes. The diagnosis correctness rate can be over 90% to the solid masses on breast sonography. Recently with the development of equipment of ultrasound, CDFI has been used widely to breast diseases. CDFI can quantitively analysis the flow and hemodynamic changes of the masses. So the capability of distinguishing benign from malignant lesions has been improved on CDFI. On CDFI, blood supply of malignant lesion increase while blood supply of benign masses decrease. But shortcomings of ultrasound still exist, for example these methods can not differentiate varieties of lesions including breast cancer and plasma cell mastitis, breast cancer in early stage and fibrosis, and so on.

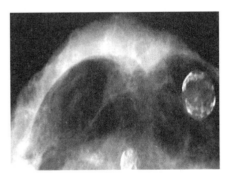

After breast autologous fat tissue filling, multiple round fat necrosis and calcification foci are observed in the fat filling area in mammogram.

Figure 8-41 Fat necrosis and calcification

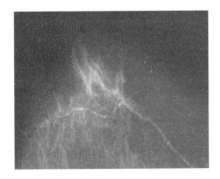

Mammogram shows a track-like change representing calcification of breast blood vessels.

Figure 8-40 Calcification of blood vessels

（3）Differential diagnosis

1）Calcification: On mammography, differential diagnosis between malignant and benign calcification has to be accomplished. The vast majority of calcification are benign, such as arterial calcification(Figure 8-40), intracystic calcifications, fat necrotic calcification(Figure 8-41) and calcification in fibroadenomas(Figure 8-26, 27). The following characteristics provide a framework for the analysis of breast calcification: Appearance (including size, form and density), distribution (diffuse or clustered) and arrangement (linear or folium), Round, diffuse calcification, homogeneous in size and density with coarse granular, mottled or linear form, are the reliable signs of benign lesions. The fine granular, irregular microcalcifications, inhomogeneous in size, form and density are commonly the reliable signs of malignant lesions(Figure 8-31, 32, 33, 39). On mammograms, the larger the extent of calcification, the higher the possibility of microinvasion.

2）Mass: The masses of benign lesions such as cyst, fibroadenomas, papilloma and hematomas are characteristically well-defined and relatively low density than normal breast parenchyma, and most often associated with Halo's sign, which is termed the thin transparent rim around the mass. However, malignant tumors often show that the edge of the tumor is not smooth and burr. The size of mass shown on mammography is often smaller than the one that is measured through physical examination.

(Yanhui Li, Shanshan Chen, Manjun Xiao, Mengping Long, Enhua Xiao, Jianguang Luo)

腹部与盆腔

　　腹部与盆腔疾病包括胃肠道、肝脏、胆系、胰腺、脾、肾上腺、泌尿系统、生殖系统疾病。疾病种类繁多，影像学检查在临床疾病诊断中起着关键作用。X 线平片能发现高密度钙化性疾病如胆结石、肾结石，用于检查急腹症中的肠梗阻和胃肠道穿孔。胃肠道钡剂造影检查是胃肠道疾病的主要影像学检查方法之一，对腔壁异常如小溃疡的检出，敏感性高，也可评估胃肠道的功能性改变，但不能评估病变的壁外延伸情况。经肝胆管造影（PTC）、T 管造影和经内镜逆行性胆管造影（ERCP）对检出和诊断这些部位的病变有一定价值。静脉性肾盂造影（IVP）、逆行肾盂造影、逆行膀胱造影、子宫输卵管造影能够反映泌尿系统疾病所致的肾盂、肾盏、输尿管和膀胱壁及其内腔改变，以及女性生殖系统疾病引起的子宫输卵管壁及其内腔改变。CT 是目前腹部与盆腔疾病最主要的影像检查技术，平扫加多期增强检查，可检出病变，并依据病变的强化方式、程度和动态变化，对病变做出定性诊断，但 CT 检查会产生辐射剂量，应适当控制。MRI 已成为腹部与盆腔疾病一种主要的影像检查技术，MRI 软组织分辨力高，加上动态增强、脂肪抑制技术、扩散加权成像（DWI）、磁共振波谱（MRS）、灌注加权成像（PWI）等功能成像，有利于病变的检出和定性诊断，MR 胆胰管成像（MRCP）和 MR 尿路成像（MRU）主要用于检查胆道和尿路梗阻，但 MRI 检查时间长，易产生伪影。

Part 4

Abdomen and pelvis

Diseases of the abdomen and pelvis include diseases of the gastrointestinal tract, liver, biliary system, pancreas, spleen, adrenal gland, urinary system and reproductive system. There are many kinds of diseases, and imaging examination plays a key role in clinical diagnosis. X-ray plain films can detect high-density calcified diseases such as gallstones and kidney stones. They are used to detect intestinal obstruction and gastrointestinal perforation in acute abdomen. Barium examination of gastrointestinal tract is one of the main imaging methods for gastrointestinal diseases. It has a high sensitivity for detecting wall abnormalities such as small ulcers, and can also assess the functional changes of the gastrointestinal tract, however, extramural extension of the lesion can not be evaluated. Transhepatic Cholangiography (PTC), T - tube cholangiography and endoscopic retrograde cholangiography (ERCP) are valuable in the detection and diagnosis of these lesions. Intravenous pyelography (IVP), retrograde pyelography, retrograde cystography and hysterosalpingography can reflect changes in the renal pelvis, calyx, ureter and bladder walls and their internal cavities due to urinary system diseases, as well as the uterine oviduct wall and its lumen change due to the female reproductive system diseases. At present, CT is the most important imaging technique in the diagnosis of abdominal and pelvic diseases. Plain scan plus multi-phase contrast - enhanced examination can detect the lesions and make a qualitative diagnosis according to the enhancement pattern, degree and dynamic changes of the lesions, but CT examination will produce radiation dose, should be properly controlled. MRI has become a major imaging technique for the diagnosis of abdominal and pelvic diseases, dynamic contrast-enhanced imaging, fat suppression technique, diffusion-weighted imaging (DWI), magnetic resonance spectroscopy (MRS), perfusion-weighted imaging (PWI) and other functional imagings are helpful for the detection and qualitative diagnosis of the lesions, MR cholangiopancreatography (MRCP) and MR urography (MRU) are mainly used to detect biliary and urinary tract obstruction, but MRI is time-consuming and easy to produce artifacts.

第九章

急腹症

第一节　急腹症检查方法

1. X 线检查

对于腹部的放射学检查有多种方法可以选用。在进行特殊检查之前 X 线平片可以对全腹部多个体位检查。腹胀、腹痛、呕吐、腹泻、腹部外伤是进行 X 线平片检查的常见病因。

2. CT 检查

CT 检查和超声一样，在评价腹壁厚度、腹膜腔、腹膜后间隙、腹腔内器官和潜在间隙方面是很好的检查技术，由于可采用标准的交叉重建方式技术使其图像比超声图像显示更清楚。对比剂在消化道中的运用成为影像检查的里程碑。静脉对比剂的应用在很多方面都有帮助，通过不同动脉期和静脉期显示病理变化来鉴别血管结构和实质性器官的强化程度。CT 在显示胰腺和腹部淋巴结方面具有独特的优越性。CT 不仅可以显示腹腔内脓肿而且可以显示脓肿准确的解剖部位和脓肿蔓延范围，对治疗方案的选定提供很大的帮助。CT 还可以判断病变累及消化道腔、消化道壁和肠系膜的范围。

第二节　正常表现

1. X 线表现

X 线平片所见的胃内气体来源主要是吞咽所致，其中部分气体通过小肠到达结肠。在一般情况下未扩张的小肠肠袢仅有少量气体。正常情况下结肠内有气体和粪渣存在且易于分辨。细菌所产生的气体被认为是结肠积气的重要来源。婴幼儿肠道内积气的情况与成人不同，正常情况下气体可以存在于整个小肠。出生后几小时整个消化道内均可见气体存在。

2. CT 表现

CT 可很好的显示腹壁厚度、腹膜腔、腹膜后间隙、腹腔内器官和潜在间隙，其正常表现详见腹部与盆腔各章节。

第三节　基本病变

1. 腹腔积气

腹腔积气又称气腹，系指腹膜腔内气体异常积聚。气腹是腹部外科手术后的自然结果，其他情况出现的气腹则为异常，常提示胃、十二指肠、结肠穿孔。站立位或侧卧位平片能显示出腹腔内的少量气体。随着体位变动，游离气体可积聚在腹腔不同的解剖区域，勾勒出肠道壁(双壁征)及腹膜韧带(镰状韧带征，脐外侧韧带征等)或上升至膈顶 (图 9-1)。

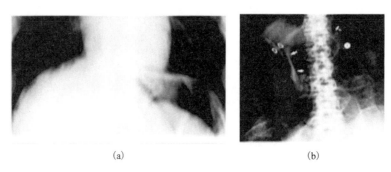

(a)   (b)

(a)、(b)仰卧位腹部片显示因游离气体勾画的镰状韧带(箭头)和"双壁"标志(箭头)。

图 9-1　腹部平片显示两侧膈下游离气体

2.腹腔积液

腹腔炎症及外伤等病因均可导致腹腔积液，表现为肾影及腰大肌影模糊，但较大量的腹腔积液才能显示出该征象，而且肠袢内积液有时与腹腔游离性积液鉴别困难。超声则能更为敏感地诊断极少量的腹盆腔游离积液或积血，它们可随患者体位变动积聚在上腹部或盆腔 (图 9-2)。

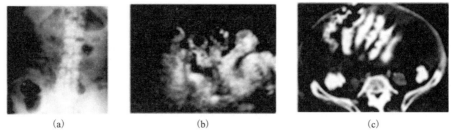

(a)   (b)   (c)

(a)平片显示许多小肠环集中聚集，但被环之间的液体隔开；(b)超声显示腹水中漂浮着增厚的肠袢；
(c)CT 显示大量腹水，小肠内充满钡剂。

图 9-2　腹水

3.胃肠道积气、积液及肠管扩张

器质性病变或肠道动力异常均可导致肠内容物无法顺利通过肠道，称为肠梗阻。腹部立卧位片是评估该疾病的常规检查方法，表现为肠道异常扩张及肠内的气-液平面。CT 能进一步寻找梗阻点位置、梗阻原因及判断有无相关并发症(缺血、肠扭转及肠套叠)等。

4.腹腔内高密度影

泌尿系结石、胆管结石、钙化或阑尾粪石均可表现为腹腔内高密度影，CT 可对其进行解剖定位。

第四节　常见疾病诊断

1.肠梗阻

(1)分类：根据病因，肠梗阻可分为机械性及非机械性(功能性)。完全性及不完全性肠梗阻分别是指肠内容物无法通过及仅部分通过梗阻点。绞窄性肠梗阻是指伴有肠道血运障碍的梗阻，如手术治疗不及时，可导致肠坏死或肠穿孔。闭袢性肠梗阻是指相邻的两个梗阻点出现在同一节段肠管中。

（2）机械性小肠梗阻：

1）临床与病理表现：对于既往有腹部手术史的患者来说，出现腹痛、腹胀、呕吐要首先考虑肠梗阻的可能。单纯性肠梗阻是指肠腔存在一个梗阻点而且无血运障碍。肠道粘连是最常见的梗阻原因，其他病因还有肠道肿瘤，腹内疝等。

2）影像学表现：梗阻发生3-5小时后，聚集在肠内的气体和液体能在腹部X线平片上显示。站立位腹部平片能显示扩张的肠袢及其内的气液平面（图9-3）。梗阻早期或不完全性肠梗阻中仅能观察少量积气、扩张的肠袢。随着时间的推移，扩张程度和扩张肠袢的数量逐渐增加。扩张的小肠往往位于腹部中央，小肠黏膜皱襞环绕肠管全周，这些特点有助于与结肠扩张鉴别。如果为完全性小肠梗阻且梗阻的时间较长，结肠内可以无气体或仅有少量气体存在。如果梗阻是不完全性的，则结肠内可见正常气体影。

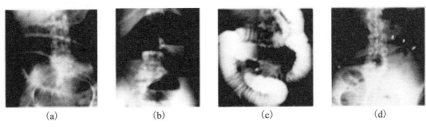

(a)　　　　　(b)　　　　　(c)　　　　　(d)

（a）仰卧位腹部平片显示梗阻伴小肠扩张；（b）站立位腹部平片显示扩张的肠袢及其内的气液平面；（c）钡剂检查显示粘连引起的梗阻部位（箭头）；（d）腹部平片显示小肠梗阻后期伴串珠征（箭头），提示肠管内积液增多、积气较少且少量气体位于黏膜皱襞间隙内。

图9-3　机械性小肠梗阻

对于空肠平面的部分性梗阻，其梗阻以上肠腔内很少能完全充满液体，在这种情况下进行稀钡检查可以显示梗阻以上肠管扩张（图9-4）。对绞窄性肠梗阻的诊断标准很多年以前就有所提及但到目前仍无金标准。现在超声、CT可以检查肠壁的增厚程度，这些方法对绞窄性肠梗阻的诊断比腹部X线平片更有价值（图9-5）。

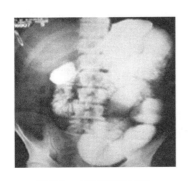

钡餐片，空肠袢明显扩张。

图9-4　粘连性不全性小肠梗阻

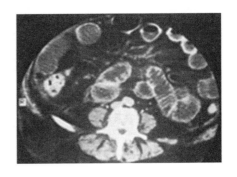

图9-5　增强CT显示小肠静脉梗塞后明显增厚的小肠壁强化减弱

（3）机械性大肠梗阻：

1）临床与病理表现：结肠梗阻最常见的病因是肿瘤，其他病因包括憩室炎，肠扭转，疝气及粪便嵌塞等。便秘和腹胀症状提示病变位于结肠。

2）影像学表现：在乙状结肠扭转时两个平行的积气扩张的肠袢起自盆腔，回盲瓣功能正常时，结肠梗阻表现为盲肠到梗阻点之间的肠管扩张（图9-6、图9-7），其内可见不同程度的积液，但积液量往往较小肠梗阻少。当回盲瓣功能不全时，结肠内的气体部分进入小肠，而结肠一定程度减压。该病的一个特征性表现是与小肠相比，结肠逐渐不成比例地显著扩张。盲肠扭转时，X线平片可在左上腹观察到充气扩张的盲肠，有时与胃泡表现相似(图9-8)，CT可见移位、积气的阑尾。紧急肠腔减压可以避免盲肠穿孔。

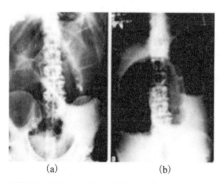

(a)近端结肠至脾曲区明显扩张。小肠内没有明显的气体，表明回盲瓣功能正常；(b)直立位片。

图9-6　乙状结肠梗阻

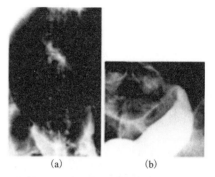

(a)乙状结肠扩张扭曲的环充满整个腹部，呈倒U形；(b)钡灌肠显示肠扭转部位有"鸟嘴"样外观。

图9-7　乙状结肠扭转

(4)绞窄性肠梗阻

1)临床与病理表现：肠道缺血是肠梗阻的一种并发症，如梗阻治疗不及时，肠道缺血的发病率及病死率较高，但临床检查及X线平片对于该病的早期识别缺乏足够的敏感度及特异度。

2)影像学表现：CT是诊断缺血的首选检查手段，表现为肠壁增厚伴强化异常，肠系膜脂肪密度增高(水肿或肠系膜血管栓塞所致)及肠壁积气(图9-9)。肠壁呈节段性环形增厚，厚度平均约8 mm，可能由水肿或出血所致。受累肠管相对正常肠壁强化减低，但当黏膜充血时，黏膜强化程度可增加。腹水也较为常见。如果梗阻没有被及时解除，缺血可进展为肠坏死，导致肠系膜甚至门静脉积气以及肠穿孔。肠扭转及肠套叠容易引起肠道缺血，需要及时手术，早期诊断非常重要。

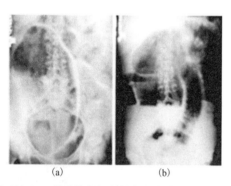

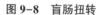

横卧(a)和直立(b)，扩张的盲肠呈椭圆形，尖端向上并向右。腹部左侧有小肠气体膨胀。在(b)图中，在中央腹部，盲肠和小肠内可见空气-液体水平，盲肠的气-液平面宽于小肠气-液平面。

图9-8　盲肠扭转

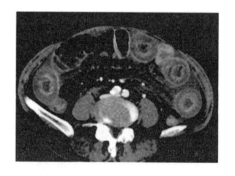

图9-9　CT表现为肠壁增厚伴异常强化，肠系膜脂肪密度增高

(5)麻痹性肠梗阻：

1)临床与病理表现：腹部手术和各种外伤可能引起肠动力的下降。甲状腺功能下降，抑制肠运动的药物和低钾血症均可形成类似肠梗阻的表现。

2)影像学表现：X线平片常常能显示小肠和结肠成比例地扩张(图9-10)。在这种情况的早期立位腹部 X 线平片显示肠管内很少液体存在，偶尔，瘫痪的患者仅引起结肠的扩张。当有机械性结肠梗阻存在时，X 线平片显示为结肠梗阻，可行肠镜或钡灌肠进一步检查。当盲肠的直径达到 12 cm 或更大时需考虑有穿孔的风险，手术或结肠镜均可用于结肠减压。

2. 腹部外伤

（1）临床与病理表现：根据外伤机制，腹部外伤可分为顿性及穿通性损伤。对于顿性损伤，脾脏是最常见的受累器官，其次是肝和肾，而在穿通性损伤中则是空腔脏器受累较常见。腹部损伤的表现和程度因损伤原因和方式而异。

（2）影像学表现：脾挫伤 CT 表现为脾脏实质内边界不清的低密度区，强化程度减低。肝、脾内出现线样低密度区提示撕裂伤。实质脏器的血肿也较常见，表现为类圆形的高密度区，可见于实质（实质内血肿）或包膜下（包膜下血肿）。应用对比剂有利于危重患者中假性动脉瘤和对比剂渗漏的诊断。对比剂渗漏表现为团状的对比剂积聚，边界不清，增强早期至晚期强化程度不变，这一征象提示活动性出血，常伴有腹腔积血，应行介入栓塞术以避免失血性休克。不同于对比剂渗漏，对比剂在假性动脉瘤中遵循血管样的强化模式。

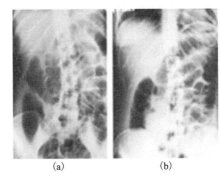

(a)　　　　　(b)

横卧(a)和直立(b)显示小肠和结肠中有大量气体。除盲肠外，液体水平不明显。

图 9-10　麻痹性肠梗阻

（颜荣华，郭焯欣，王宾，周子懿，肖恩华，刘辉）

Chapter 9

Acute abdomen

Section 1　Method of examination

1. X-ray examination

Multiple options are available for radiologic study of the abdomen. Plain films allow one to view the entire abdomen before proceeding to a more specific investigation. Abdominal distention, abdominal pain, vomiting, diarrhea, and abdominal trauma are the most common reasons for obtaining plain films.

2. CT examination

CT, like ultrasonography, is a powerful imaging technique for evaluating the abdominal walls, intraperitoneal and retroperitoneal spaces, all organs and systems, and potential spaces. Because a standard cross-sectional format is used, the images are easier to understand than those obtained by ultrasonography. The addition of contrast material to the intestinal lumen provides a marker. Intravenous contrast material is helpful in many ways. It allows identification of vascular structures and the enhancement of solid organs during different arterial and venous phases to demonstrate pathologic changes. CT excels in the evaluation of the pancreas and the abdominal lymph nodes. Intra-abdominal abscesses not only can be found, but also their exact anatomic position and extent can be defined, providing an invaluable aid in planning treatment. CT also permits study of the extent of lesions that involve the intestinal lumen, intestinal wall, and mesentery.

Section 2　Normal appearances

1. X-ray findings

Swallowed air is the source of the gas that is normally seen in the stomach. Some of that gas passes through the small bowel to the colon; it is common to see gas in limited quantities in non-distended small-bowel loops. The colon normally contains gas and feces, which can be easily recognized. Bacterial gas production has been found to be a significant source of colonic gas. The intestinal gas pattern of infants differs from that of adults in that gas is normally present throughout the small bowel. Within a few hours after birth, gas can be seen throughout the intestinal tract.

2. CT findings

CT can well display abdominal wall thickness, peritoneal cavity, retroperitoneal space, intra-abdominal organs and potential space. The normal manifestations are shown in the chapters of abdomen and pelvis.

Section 3　Basic pathologic changes

1. Pneumoperitoneum

Pneumoperitonem refers to gas accumulation in the peritoneal cavity. Although pneumoperitoneum is a natural consequence of surgical exploration of the abdomen, it is distinctly abnormal under other circumstances and usually indicates rupture of either the stomach, duodenum, or colon. Upright plain films or cross-table decubitus films can detect very small quantities of peritoneal gas. The free gas accumulate in different anatomical compartments of the peritoneal cavity with the changes of body position and can be detected on plain radiograph when gas outlines both sides of the bowel wall ("double-wall" sign), peritoneal ligament (falciform ligament sign, lateral umbilical ligament sign, etc.)or rises to accumulate underneath the diaphragm (Figure 9-1).

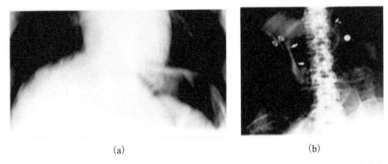

(a)　　　　　　　　　　　　　　(b)

(a), (b)Supine abdomen film shows falciform ligaments (arrows)outlined by free air and "double-wall" sign (arrowheads)from the same cause.

Figure 9-1　Upright abdomen film shows free air beneath both hemidiaphragms

2. Peritonealfluid

Causes such as abdominal inflammation and trauma can lead to seroperitoneum. In cases of massive ascites, the shadow of kidney and psoas muscle become blurred on radiograph. However, it is no longer necessary to rely on plain films to detect ascites and hemoperitoneum. Positive plain-film findings require the presence of an abundance of peritoneal fluid. Fluid-filled loops of bowel in the pelvis can beconfused with free fluid. Ultrasonography is an extremely sensitive diagnostic modality and can detect very small amounts of free fluid or blood. The free fluid accumulates in the dependent areas of the pelvis and upper abdomen and changes with the patient's position (Figure 9-2).

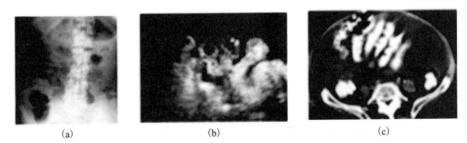

(a)　　　　　　　　　(b)　　　　　　　　　(c)

(a)Plain film shows numerous loops of small bowel collected centrally but separated by fluid between the loops; (b)Ultrasonography shows thickened bowel loops floating in ascites; (c)Computed tomographic scan shows massive ascites with barium-filled loops of small bowel.

Figure 9-2　Ascites

3. Pneumatosisintestinalis, effusion and bowel dilatation

Organic lesions or abnormal intestinal motility may causea failure of the intestinal contents to pass normally through the bowel, known as intestinal obstruction. A radiographic film of upright and supine films of the abdomen is a good routine to use in evaluating this situation, showing dilated intestinal loops and air-fluid levels. CT helps address questions regardingthe location and the cause of the obstruction, and potential complications (ischemia, volvulus, intussusception, etc.).

4. Abdominalhyperdensity

The signs can be created by urinary or biliary calculus, calcification or stercorolith. CT excels in the evaluation of their exact anatomic position.

Section 4　Diagnosis of common diseases

1. Bowel obstruction

(1)Classification: Based on the etiologies, it can be divided into mechanical or non-mechanical (functional) bowel obstruction. Complete obstruction and incomplete obstruction indicates no and partial intestinal contents passing beyond the site of obstruction. Strangulated obstruction occurs when blood flow is compromised, and intestinal necrosis and perforation may ensue when surgical management is delay. Closed-loop obstruction refers to a segment of bowel with two contiguous points of obstruction.

(2)Mechanical small-bowel obstruction

1)Clinical and pathological manifestations: Abdominal pain, distention, and vomiting occurring in a patient with a history of previous abdominal surgery direct attention to the possibility of obstruction. A radiographic film of upright and supine films of the abdomen is a good routine to use in evaluating this situation. The upright abdomen film decreases the possibility of missing perforation of the gut manifested by subdiaphragmatic air. In a simple obstruction, the intestinal lumen is occluded at a single point without any significant interference with its blood supply. Most often an adhesive band is responsible for the obstruction, although a neoplasm, or internal hernia may be the cause.

2)Imaging manifestations: Within 3 to 5 hours after the onset of an obstruction, gas and fluid accumulate proximally and can be seen on the abdominal film. On the upright film, distended bowel loops with gas-fluid levels are present (Figure 9-3). In the very early stage or if the obstruction is partial, only a few gas-distended loops may be seen. With the passage of time, the caliber and the number of visible loops increase. The small-bowel loops are distinguished from the colon by their central location in the abdomen and by characteristic small-bowel folds that are close together and extend completely around the circumference of the bowel. This is unlike the colon, where the folds are not circumferential and are widely separated. If the obstruction of the small bowel is complete and enough time has elapsed for colon evacuation, little or no gas may be present in the colon. If the bowel obstruction is incomplete, there may be a normal amount of gas in the colon.

Rarely, the obstructed bowel is entirely filled with fluid in proximal jejunal partial obstruction. In this instance the instillation of a small amount oflow density contrast material demonstrates the distended, fluid-filled small bowel (Figure 9-4). Criteria to distinguish strangulation obstruction were developed many years ago but have not withstood the test of time. Currently, the ability of ultrasonography and CT to detect the bowel-wall thickening that goes with strangulation has made them more useful than plain films(Figure 9-5).

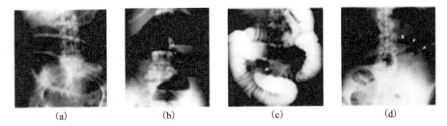

(a) Supine abdomen film shows obstruction with numerous loops of small bowel dilated; (b) Upright abdomen with small-bowel obstruction. Note different level of fluid in each loop, which differentiates it from small-bowel ileus; (c) Barium study shows site of obstruction caused by adhesion (arrow); (d) Upright abdomen film in advanced small-bowel obstruction with "string-of-beads" sign (arrows).

Figure 9-3　Mechanical small-bowel obstruction

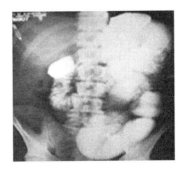

In this film, exposed after the patient had a barium meal, the jejunal loops are noted to be considerably dilated. The mucosal folds have not been obliterated even though there is distention; the appearance resembles that of stacked coins.

Figure 9-4　Adhesive band

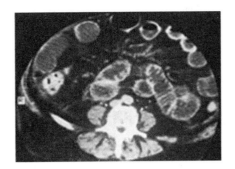

Intravenous contrast material fills the intramural portion of the markedly thickened small-bowel loops.

Figure 9-5　Computed tomogram of venous infarction of the small bowel

(3) Mechanical colon obstruction

1) Clinical and pathological manifestations: Colonic obstruction is usually caused by cancer . diverticulitis, Volvulus, hernia, and fecal impaction are other causes. The symptoms of obstipation and abdominal distention direct attention to the colon.

2) Imaging manifestations: In the presence of a competent ileocecal valve, colon obstruction is manifested by gaseous distention of the colon from the cecum to the site of obstruction(Figure 9-6). A varying amount of fluid is present but usually is not as prominent as in small-bowel obstruction. If the ileocecal valve is incompetent, the colonic gas may move into the small bowel and partially decompress the colon. The key observation is that there continues to be a disproportionate enlargement of the colon in relation to that of the small bowel. In sigmoid volvulus, two parallel, gas-distended colonic loops are seen rising out of the pelvis (Figure 9-7). In cecal volvulus, attention is usually directed to the left-upper quadrant, where the gas-distended cecum, which may mimic a gas-filled stomach, is observed (Figure 9-8). When plain films suggest colonic obstruction, the diagnosis should be confirmed by endoscopy or barium enema. Prompt decompression averts cecal perforation.

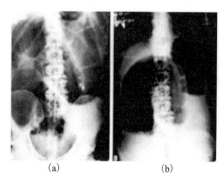

(a)   (b)

(a) There is marked distention of the proximal colon to the region of the splenic flexure. No appreciable amount of gas is present in the small bowel, indicating a competent ileocecal valve. The obstruction in this patient was in the sigmoid. The end of the gas column shown on a single film of this type does not necessarily indicate the site of obstruction; (b) Upright film of the patient shown in A.

Figure 9-6   Obstruction of the sigmoid colon

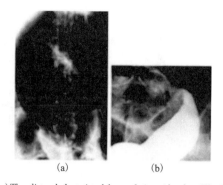

(a)   (b)

(a) The distended, twisted loop of sigmoid colon fills the entire abdomen giving an inverted U shape to the sigmoid colon; (b) Barium given rectally shows the "bird's beak" appearance at the site of the volvulus.

Figure 9-7   Sigmoid volvulus

(4) Strangulated obstruction

1) Clinical and pathological manifestations: Intestinal ischemia is a complication of bowel obstruction with high morbidity and mortality rates if left untreated, but clinical examination and radiographs lack sensitivity and accuracy to detect the early signs of it.

2) Imaging manifestations: CT is the imaging modality of choice for diagnosis of ischemia. The CT findings include bowel wall thickening with abnormal enhancement, increased attenuation of mesenteric fat (due to edema or engored mesenteric vessels) and intramural gas (Figur9-9). The bowel wall thickening, on average 8 mm, is circumferential segmental and caused by edema or hemorrhage. Compare to adjacent normal bowels, the enhancement is decreased in the involved bowel wall, but increased enhancement may be found in the hyperemic mucosa. Ascites can often be detected. If the bowel blockage is not removed, ischemia will progress in to necrosis, leading to mesenteric and even portal pneumatosis, and perforation. Identification of volvulus and closedloop obstruction is important since they present with high risk of bowel ischemia and require prompt surgery.

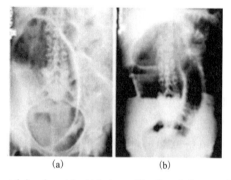

(a)   (b)

Recumbent (a) and upright (b) views. The distended cecum forms an oval-shaped radiolucency with the tip pointed upward and to the right. There is gas distention of the small intestine in the left-lateral portion of the abdomen. In B, note the gas-fluid level in the cecum and smaller levels in loops of small bowel. In the central abdomen, air-fluid levels are noted in the cecum and in the small bowel.

Figure 9-8   Volvulus of the cecum

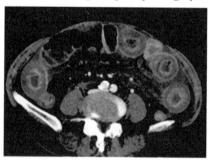

imageshows bowel wall thickening with abnormal enhancement, andincreased attenuation of mesenteric fat.

Figure 9-9   CT

（5）Paralytic （Adynamic）Ileus

1）Clinical and pathological manifestations: Laparotomy and other types of trauma may lead to impairment of intestinal motility. Hypothyroidism, drugs that inhibit intestinal motility, and hypokalemia also may cause an ileus pattern.

2）Imaging manifestations: Plain films usually show a proportionate distention of small bowel and colon（Figure 9-10）. Early in the process, the upright films show little fluid in the bowel. Occasionally, the paralytic process involves only the colon. The films then suggest colonic obstruction, but endoscopy or barium enema will eliminate this possibility. As with mechanical obstruction, colonic ileus may result in cecal perforation. Cecal diameters in the range of 12 cm or larger are reason for concern. Either cecostomy or colonoscopy can be used for decompression.

2. Acute abdominal trauma

1）Clinical and pathological manifestations: The mechanism of abdominal trauma can be penetrating or blunt types. In blunt force trauma, the most frequent affected organ is the spleen, followed by liver and kidney, while in penetrating injuries, it is the hollow

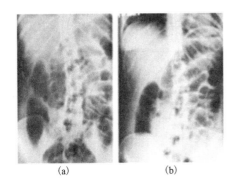

(a)　　　　(b)

Recumbent （a） and upright （b） projections show a considerable amount of gas in the small bowel and colon. Fluid levels are inconspicuous except in the cecum.

Figure 9-10　Adynamic ileus

visceral organs. Depending on the cause and manner of injuries, the spectrum and severity of splenic and liver involvement, as well as the associated complications, can be heterogeneous.

2）Imagingmanifestations: Contusions manifest as ill-defined hypodensity with decreased perfusion in the parenchyma on CT. When laceration of spleen or liver occur, linear shaped hypodense areas can be detected. Hematomas of the solid organs are frequently seen, showing oval-shaped, high-attenuation collections within the parenchyma （intraparenchymal hematomas）or beneath the capsular margin （subcapsular hematomas）. The use of IV contrast help identify pseudoaneurysm or contrast leak in the severely injuried patients. Contrast leak performs as a blob of contrast agent with an ill-defined edge, which retains the initial intensity in the late phase of contrast-enhanced CT. This pattern, indicating active bleeding, is commonly present with hemoperitoneum. Interventional embolization is desired for the patients to prevent haemorrhagic shock. Unlike contrast leak, accumulation of contrast agent in pseudoaneurysm follow a contrast-enhanced pattern of vessels.

（Yan Ronghua, Guo Zhuoxin, Wang Bin, Zhou Ziyi, Xiao Enhua, Liu Hui）

第十章

胃肠道

消化系统由长而弯曲的中空器官组成，从口腔到肛门，包括口腔、咽部、食管、胃、十二指肠、空肠、回肠和大肠。钡剂造影检查是常用的胃肠道检查手段之一，可显示其形态、大小、轮廓、蠕动及黏膜等情况；B超、CT、MRI检查还能进一步评估胃肠壁及腔外病变的情况。CT仿真内镜能与普通内镜检查一样显示肠腔内的病变，且其显示范围更广。

胃肠X线检查与普通的放射线检查不同：

(1)需要配备数字胃肠机或多功能X线检查(DR)。

(2)使用对比剂硫酸钡，它能充盈消化道不同部分并使消化道显影。

(3)检查前准备，即禁食、肠道清洁，检查常在清晨空腹下进行。

胃肠全程钡餐，即通过口服硫酸钡混悬液检查整个消化道，实际上，详细观察胃食管结合部、十二指肠及部分空回肠需依次显示并动态观察，而检查结肠，则最好选择钡灌肠检查。

第一节　检查方法

1.胸腹部透视

胸腹部透视是胃肠道造影吞钡前的检查步骤，以尽可能排除禁忌证。

2.造影检查

(1)钡餐：硫酸钡和水溶性碘剂是胃肠道常用的对比剂。单对比剂造影是传统的造影方法，稀释的钡混悬液扩张胃腔，同时使用加压的方法更好地显示病变。单对比钡灌肠需要使用低密度(浓度一般仅为15%～20%)的稳定钡混悬液，这因为钡灌肠是一种透视检查，充钡的结肠需要保持一定的透亮度。单对比硫酸钡混悬液进行钡灌肠时需照钡剂排空后的黏膜像。

目前，双重对比剂造影技术被广泛应用。双重分别指的是高密度的钡剂(阳性对比剂)和小苏打产生的气体(阴性对比剂)。胃肠道被气体充盈后，延展的黏膜表面黏附一层钡剂，即为双重对比相，它可以显示一些容易在单对比剂造影被漏诊的微小黏膜病变。

由于硫酸钡廉价、安全，大多胃肠道X线检查都使用硫酸钡作为对比剂。肠瘘、肠穿孔、肠梗阻、存在误吸风险或近期接受过胃肠道手术的患者，推荐用非离子型碘对比剂。

(2)血管造影：血管造影仅用于急性胃肠道出血的诊断和治疗，造影可明确出血的部位，并可进行选择性插管灌注血管加压素和栓塞控制出血。血管造影也可以评价门静脉高压指导外科治疗以及恶性肿瘤的血管供应和侵犯情况。

3.腹部CT和MRI

腹部CT和MRI是评估肠壁与壁外病灶及邻近器官的受压或侵犯情况的重要检查手段，有助于发现淋巴结受累及远处转移,肿瘤分期,最佳治疗方案的制定及治疗后监测和随访。

第二节 正常表现

1. X 线表现

(1)下咽部:上缘为会厌,与口咽相接,下缘至环状软骨水平并延续为颈段食管。站立正位片上,随着对比剂自口腔流向食管,下咽部中线两侧分别见充钡小囊,即会厌谷,由会厌与舌根部的间隙构成,其外下方可见另一对充钡的腔隙,称为梨状隐窝。鱼刺等异物容易存留在这些缝隙中。

(2)食管:食管是消化道的第一段。食管是一个肌性管道结构,起于第6颈椎水平环状软骨的下缘,下行至第11胸椎平面与胃贲门相接。食管长度25~30 cm,横行切断食管表现为扁平的管道,其组织结构层有:①黏膜,最内层,为被覆黏膜层,由上皮细胞(食管上段为具有抵抗力的复层鳞状细胞)、少量结缔组织和平滑肌组成;②膜下层:为柔软的结缔组织层,由血管、神经和淋巴组织组成;③肌层:内层是环形肌,外层是纵形肌;④外膜:可移动的外层筋膜组织,食管无浆膜层。

1)生理收缩性狭窄区:①环咽肌汇合处,在颈6平面后方由环咽肌所形成的切迹;②主动脉弓压迹;③左主支气管压迹;④横膈裂孔压迹。食管入口部为4个生理性压迹最窄的,故异物容易在此处停留。

2)蠕动:食管有3种可以区别的蠕动,即原发蠕动,由自主吞咽动作激发,贯穿食管全程;继发蠕动,由食物刺激及食管扩张引起,起始于主动脉弓水平,向下推行;第三收缩波,原发和继发蠕动都是推进性的,而第三收缩波则不是推进性的,表现为环形锯齿状,以患者卧位明显,可能为食管痉挛性收缩所致。

3)黏膜皱襞:当食管空虚时,可见2~3条纵行平行的黏膜皱襞,近贲门时聚拢。

4)食管胃结合部(胃食管前庭):食管是一个管状结构,但食管下端松弛时可表现为囊袋状,即前庭,管状区与囊袋状前庭的交界处称为食管胃前庭部(Wolf A 环),此环位于膈上;在此环以下,食管扩张表现为囊袋状(即膈壶腹)。在真正的胃食管结合部有另一个环(Schatzki B 环),即食管胃之间鳞状上皮的交界处。如果 B 环位于膈上说明存在膈疝。

(3)胃:胃呈"C"形,位于左侧腹腔。人为地将胃分成3部分:胃底,位于胃食管交界点水平线之上;胃体,位于胃底与角切迹之间的垂直部或水平部;胃窦,位于角切迹与幽门之间。

1)胃的形状和位置:与胃的张力和体型有关。矮胖体型者,胃的位置高而横,角切迹不明显,呈"牛角"型;中等体型者,胃呈"J"型,胃体几乎垂直,角切迹明显,幽门管与角切迹在同一水平,立位时,胃的最低点达髂嵴水平;瘦长体型者,胃呈"鱼钩"状,幽门管位于角切迹水平之上,立位时,胃的最低点位于髂嵴水平之下。当低张力胃出现在超重体型的个体时,有时出现类似消化性溃疡的症状。"瀑布"型胃:胃底成角后倒形成袋状,袋可深可浅,钡流自胃底倾泻而下类似瀑布。

2)胃黏膜:当胃空虚时,黏膜肌层收缩形成突向胃内的黏膜皱襞,当钡剂黏附黏膜面并进入黏膜沟时,在 X 线上表现为黑白相间的线状或曲线状结构,皱襞突入胃腔呈透明线状或带状影,延伸至胃的全长,皱襞的宽度不超过5 mm。必须注意,皱襞的形态不是一成不变的,因不同的生理状态而变化。由于双对比造影技术的发展,一种细小的黏膜结构或称之为微黏膜结构(胃小区)得以显示,表现为大量的卵圆形或尖角状透亮区,边缘为胃小沟,可见线状的钡剂黏附。

3)胃的蠕动:正常状态下,胃蠕动波起自胃体上部,胃大弯侧的波形较深,小弯侧较浅,透视下常可见2~3个连续的蠕动波。胃排空受食物的温度、种类和生理状态的影响,钡团在胃内停留的时间约1小时左右,如果所服钡剂的1/3量在胃内停留的时间超过6小时,则代表胃排空延迟。

(4)十二指肠:小肠的第一段呈"C"形,包绕胰头和胆总管,长约25 cm,分成球部、降段和水平段。球部是十二指肠的第一部分,在结构和功能上与胃窦基本一致,而其余部分则与小肠相似。在充盈状态下,球部呈三角形,轮廓光滑,幽门管开口于球基底部的中央。

(5)空回肠:真正意义的小肠由空回肠组成,它附着于后腹壁的肠系膜根部,使小肠可以自由地运动。小肠袢有两缘,固定缘,与肠系膜根部相连亦称系膜缘;游离缘,系膜缘的对侧,亦称对系膜缘。这一点对放射学家在认识某些疾病时非常重要，如淋巴瘤、种植性转移瘤、Crohn's 病易累及肠袢的系膜缘。空肠位于左上腹，而回肠位于右下腹及盆腔，回肠末端于右侧髂窝与盲肠汇合。

小肠黏膜表现为特征性的环形皱襞，当小肠非扩张状态时，环形及羽毛状皱襞同时存在，这种环形黏膜皱襞的数量及大小越接近回肠越减少，因此回肠的黏膜皱襞较平坦而非羽毛状，表现为带状。

小肠排空时间 7~9 小时，钡首到达盲肠的时间 2~6 小时。

(6)回盲部：回肠末端突入盲肠产生皱折，其功能类似括约肌，回肠浆膜不参与此结构的形成，此瓣膜功能为阻止盲肠内容物返流，X 线表现为"V"形充盈缺损。

(7)结肠：大肠长 1.5~1.7 m，位于腹腔周围，与小肠的区别点是结肠位于腹腔周围并有结肠袋，X 线上可将结肠区分为盲肠、升结肠、横结肠、降结肠、乙状结肠和直肠。结肠有两个曲，即肝曲和脾曲，两个曲均靠近后腹壁并有横结肠系膜附着，因此可自由运动，乙状结肠有更长的系膜附着，是易引起肠扭转的解剖基础。盲肠亦存在系膜而可以移动，亦是肠扭转发生的部位。当结肠充盈钡剂时，表现出特征性的结肠袋，近端结肠明显，至降结肠时肠袋变浅，直肠没有肠袋。结肠黏膜皱襞为横形，远段结肠皱襞与其长轴平行。

结肠的运动：有两种基本的不同形式的收缩：①局部收缩：使结肠产生折叠式的运动；②整体收缩。

2. CT 表现

(1)食管：食管是一个肌性管状结构，走行于胸主动脉右前方及脊柱前方，被覆一层脂肪组织。食管的密度与肌肉相似，厚度约 3 mm，管腔内可见气体(来源于吞咽的空气)。

(2)胃：胃底左后方是脾，右前方是肝左叶，胃体部位于更低的层面，与肝左叶、空肠、胰尾及脾关系密切，胃壁与十二指肠共同包绕胰头，其壁厚度正常在 2~5 mm，CT 显示其三层结构，由内到外分别为高密度的黏膜层，低密度的黏膜下层及高密度的肌层及浆膜层。

(3)十二指肠：十二指肠球部上接胃窦，向下走行(降部)并绕过胰头，水平向左(水平段)走行于腹主动脉前方及肠系膜上血管后方；肠壁厚度与小肠相近。

(4)小肠：肠壁厚约 3 mm，回肠末端可达 5 mm，空肠位于左上腹，回肠位于右下腹，增强扫描能较好地显示小肠系膜、腹膜、网膜等小肠肠腔外的结构。

(5)结肠：结肠内含有大量粪便，肠壁厚度大约 3~5 mm，轮廓光滑，边缘锐利。

3. MRI 表现

MRI 检查在胃肠道检查中应用越来越广泛，为了鉴别正常与异常表现，常需要使用对比剂，包括阴性对比剂(如硫酸钡、甘露醇等)和阳性对比剂(如顺超磁性氧化铁溶液、稀释的钆剂等)，引入方法包括口服法和灌肠。胃肠道壁的信号特点与肌肉类似。

第三节　基本病变

总体上讲，胃肠道是一个中空的肌性管道，在一个部位出现的病理改变在其他部位亦可出现，具有相同的 X 线表现，病变范围因部位而不同。

1. 溃疡性病变

溃疡性病变是胃肠道内壁的局限性缺损。溃疡的"火山口样"改变导致钡剂在缺损处积聚，而在 CT 或 MRI 上，它表现为凹陷性病变。胃肠造影时观察溃疡的方式有两种：正面观(正对溃疡面观察)和切线观(从侧面观察)。正面观，表现为圆形、边界清楚的钡剂聚集区；切线观，钡剂聚集区突出于胃轮廓线外(龛影)。溃疡周围常围绕一圈水肿带。肿瘤内亦可见溃疡，大多数是由溃疡恶变而来的，而恶性肿瘤伴发溃疡则较为罕见。良性、恶性溃疡鉴别详见表 10-1，图 10-1。

表1　良性、恶性溃疡鉴别

良性溃疡	恶性溃疡
突出于胃轮廓线之外	胃腔内溃疡
龛口周围的放射状黏膜皱襞	黏膜皱襞中断
溃疡圆形,轮廓清楚	溃疡周围黏膜不规则
溃疡周围组织水肿产生溃疡晕或袖口征	溃疡周围黏膜呈结节状
胃壁柔软,蠕动存在	胃壁僵硬

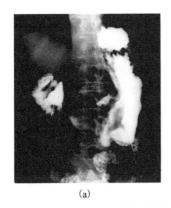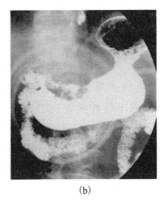

(a)　　　　　　　　　　　　(b)

(a)切线位投照显示胃小弯一处大的溃疡,突出于胃轮廓线之外,光滑、连续的黏膜皱襞放射状纠集至溃疡口部周围,提示良性病变。(b)恶性胃溃疡,切线位、加压投照,可观察到溃疡呈半月形,凸向胃腔内,溃疡周围黏膜皱襞中断、破坏。

图10-1　良性溃疡(a)和恶性溃疡(b)

2. 隆起性病变

隆起性病变指凸向腔内的病变。在钡剂检查时,因肿块占据空间而不能被钡剂充填称为充盈缺损,可由黏膜面、黏膜下或壁外病变引起。病变与正常肠管交界的形态有助于确定肿块位于腔内还是腔外。起源于黏膜面上的病变与肠管交界成锐角,而黏膜下病变则成钝角,腔外病变则成角更大。

(1)息肉:表现软组织密度的类圆形小结节。大部分是良性的增生性息肉,而腺瘤性息肉可具有恶变潜能,带蒂的息肉常为良性。息肉可发生在胃肠道任何部位,以大肠多见。

(2)肿块:肿块形态不规则,可伴或不伴有溃疡,可局限性地在胃肠壁内生长形成大息肉状或蕈伞状的外观,或环绕肠腔生长形成"餐巾环"样改变。病变部位的黏膜皱襞破坏或异常增粗。

(3)静脉曲张:另一种发生于胃和食管的隆起性病变。如食管静脉曲张,是门静脉阻塞引起的食管壁间的侧枝血管开放,最常见于肝硬化,钡造影时表现为正常黏膜皱襞扭曲成蚯蚓状,食管轮廓呈锯齿状。

3. 管腔狭窄

肠腔狭窄可由腔外生长的肿瘤压迫或肠壁自身生长的肿瘤引起,前者所致的肠腔狭窄轮廓光滑,而后者所致的肠腔狭窄情况与病变的性质和位置有关,良性病变引起的管腔狭窄常常轮廓光滑,管腔逐渐变细,黏膜结构完整。相对之下,不规则的管腔狭窄伴有胃肠壁僵直则提示恶性肿瘤。

4. 管腔扩张

中空脏器的扩张常由于远端梗阻,或神经、肌肉功能障碍所致。除机械性梗阻外,大多数肠管扩张是由于动力性肠梗阻所致,准确的机制尚不清楚,局限性肠扩张由局部刺激引起,因肠壁的自主神经丛受累所致;广泛性肠扩张由全身性疾病引起,最常见于外科手术后。肠道内在结构改变引起的扩张相对少见,在失弛缓症中,管壁的自主交感神经节细胞减少导致胃肠道不能弛缓而进行性扩张。

5. 憩室

胃肠道壁的囊袋状突出,分内压性(胃肠道壁局限性薄弱引起)和粘连性(胃肠道壁邻近的炎症粘连牵拉引起)两种,憩室壁通常具备胃肠道壁的各层结构。憩室可很小、多发,如结肠憩室;也可非常大,如食管憩室。钡餐造影切线位观察容易识别,表现为"烧瓶"样的突出物,其内见钡剂填充,边缘规整。憩室可能与溃疡龛影混淆,无肠壁痉挛且其内有黏膜结构有助于憩室的诊断。

第四节　常见疾病诊断

1. 慢性消化性溃疡

(1)临床与病理表现:正常情况下,胃肠道上皮细胞层具有防止腔内容物(如胃酸、消化酶、胆汁、和感染性物质)腐蚀的屏障。有些情况下,溃疡起源于肠壁间。黏膜缺血或炎症性肠病中炎症细胞在黏膜下层浸润是引起溃疡的主要原因。不管什么情况,胃肠黏膜表面一旦缺损,肠内容物对管壁的腐蚀将向各个方向延伸。如果邻近的上皮仍然正常,既使黏膜炎症和水肿,仍具有一定的抵抗力和完整性。

(2)影像表现:对比剂突出于管腔的轮廓线外是溃疡熟悉的 X 线表现(图10-2),胃肠道造影的早期应用就是为了寻找这种所谓的充钡龛影来诊断消化性溃疡。溃疡,即胃肠道表面形成的局限性缺损,当切线位投照时突出腔外或形成龛影,典型的溃疡起源于肠腔表面的溃烂。良性、恶性溃疡的鉴别主要基于其病理生理及其所致结构的变化,已在前面描述过。良性溃疡的诊断依据主要是溃疡周围的黏膜完整及黏膜皱襞可以直达龛口,典型的腺癌可见结节状、不规则的黏膜结构,表面可出现浅溃疡,溃疡边缘凹凸不平,浸润深部组织,而在巨大肿瘤较多见的是茶碟状的不规则溃疡深坑。

对于黏膜下间叶组织肿瘤,如平滑肌瘤或黏膜下转移瘤,溃疡形状多样,但是,由于上皮层不是首先受累,其溃疡口部常常锐利清楚,这也是胃肠造影中这类病灶呈现"牛眼征"和"靶征"的基础。

胃十二指肠消化性溃疡作为溃疡病变的基本征象,同样的概念也适合于其他胃肠道的溃疡性疾病。

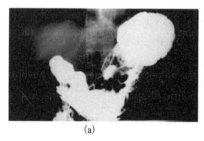 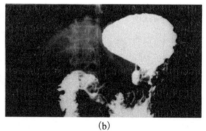

(a) (b)

双对比相(a)显示胃小弯侧充满钡剂的龛影,周围黏膜水肿,局部胃壁变形。切线位投照(b)清晰显示胃小弯溃疡,位于胃轮廓以外,黏膜皱襞放射状向溃疡口部纠集。

图10-2　胃小弯前壁胃溃疡

2. 平滑肌瘤

(1)临床与病理表现:平滑肌瘤是胃肠道最常见的良性肿瘤之一,起源于胃肠壁的平滑肌层,约80%的肿瘤生长于壁内并向腔内突出,约15%的平滑肌瘤向外生长,自浆膜层突向腹腔,5%左右的肿瘤向腔内外同时生长而呈哑铃状。小于 3 cm 直径的平滑肌瘤没有症状,当肿瘤增大后,因溃疡而出现消化道出血或因肿瘤引起的消化道输出路梗阻而出现恶心呕吐。根据影像学、内镜,甚至病理检查,常常难以鉴别平滑肌瘤与平滑肌肉瘤,两者的区分主要依据其生物学行为。

(2)影像表现:

1)X 线表现:大多数胃平滑肌瘤表现为不连续的黏膜下病变,在双对比剂造影出现肿块表面黏膜展平且相邻黏膜被推移，切线位观，肿瘤的边界与胃壁成直角或钝角；正面观，肿瘤的腔内面清晰、陡峭，边界清楚。肿瘤表面黏膜皱襞展平，正常胃小区存在。肌瘤可大可小，大于 2 cm 的肌瘤常出现溃疡，溃疡大小从 0.2~2 cm 不等，称为"牛眼征"或"靶征"。

2）CT 表现：胃平滑肌瘤表现为均匀软组织密度的规则肿块，其密度与骨骼肌类似，肿瘤常向胃腔内突出（图 10-3），为宽基的壁内肿瘤，偶尔肿瘤只向腔外生长。肌瘤可出现条纹状或丛状钙化，大多数钙化的肿瘤为良性胃肿瘤。尽管肿瘤表面存在溃疡，但肿瘤的边界仍光滑，且肿瘤与邻近器官间的脂肪间隙仍然存在。

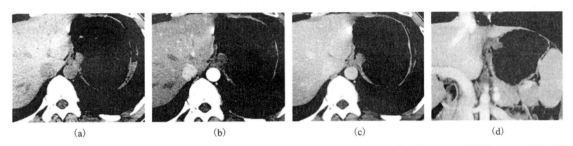

| (a) | (b) | (c) | (d) |

（a）CT 平扫显示胃底部密度均匀的肿块，凸向胃腔内生长，密度与骨骼肌类似。增强扫描动脉期（b）和静脉期（c），病灶轻度均匀强化；（d）增强扫描 CT 冠状位重建示病变与胃壁宽基底相连。

图 10-3　胃平滑肌瘤

3.肠结核

（1）临床与病理表现：肠道结核可以是原发，也可以是继发于身体其他部位的结核。85%~90% 的肠结核发生与回盲部，结核杆菌对淋巴组织的明显侵蚀性可以解析回盲部结核高发的现象。人类结核的病理表现与结核杆菌的毒力和宿主的免疫状态相关。早期，淋巴滤泡增大，继而因干酪坏死浸润肠壁，黏膜水肿和溃疡发生，并出现烧瓶状溃疡。由于结核肉芽肿形成而继发肠梗阻，最后因肠管明显狭窄而逐渐增加梗阻程度。所有的这些病理过程，代表病变既有破坏又有增生，且病程长。临床上，便秘，腹泻，腹痛，伴有肺结核高度提示肠结核的诊断。

（2）影像表现：

1）X 线表现：常表现为多种基本病变，然而，不同的患者表现不同。钡剂检查对肠结核的诊断有非常重要的价值，尽管没有病理诊断意义的 X 线征象，在结肠或小肠钡灌肠检查时，下述征象的出现提示肠结核。①跃征（Stirlin 征）：即病变肠段缺乏钡剂滞留，而其远近段肠管钡剂充盈良好，这是病变肠段痉挛、器质性挛缩或二者共同导致；②线征（图 10-4）：由于病变肠管器质性狭窄或激惹，在末端回肠出现的持续性的狭窄；③回盲部变形（图 10-4）：因为溃疡或结核结节增生使回盲部变形，X 线上，回盲部直角消失而变成钝角或趋向于与盲肠在一条线上，盲肠和（或）升结肠的肠袋变形或消失。盲肠常成角向下，当增生明显时，肠腔狭窄、缩短，受累肠管的轮廓可以光滑或呈不规则的"指印状"缺损，此时与肉芽肿性肠疾病或恶性病变常难以鉴别；④肠梗阻：通常见于小肠伴回肠袢中异常钡滞留；⑤黏膜变形或破坏：在病变区，由于水肿，黏膜皱襞不规则或增粗，肠蠕动紊乱。

2）CT 及 MRI 表现：通过腹部 CT 及 MRI 观察到的胃肠结核病变形式主要有两种：溃疡性病变与增殖性病变。回盲部肠壁增厚是最常见的 CT 表现。MRI 不仅能更敏感地发现受累肠段，而且能区分病变的性质。例如急性炎症引起的肠道病变通常在 T2 加权图像表现为高信号，可伴

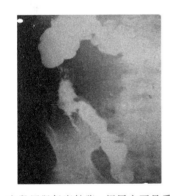

末段回肠轻度扩张，阑尾亦可见受累。升结肠和盲肠管腔呈线状狭窄（箭头），伴弥漫性溃疡。受累的肠管挛缩、变形，由于邻近的炎性组织增生和淋巴结肿大，使扩张的回肠末端与盲肠间距离加大，回盲部移位。

图 10-4　肠结核，盲肠和升结肠肠壁水肿，溃疡形成

有明显强化,而纤维增殖病变引起的肠壁增厚通常是 T2 低信号。在严重的病例中,肠壁环形增厚,邻近肠系膜粘连,可形成肿物样病变。CT 及 MRI 还能评估结核淋巴结病,以及腹腔、实质脏器及脊柱的受累情况,这些都是结核的常见表现。

4. 胃癌

(1)临床与病理表现:表浅的、可外科切除的胃癌常无临床症状,但一旦症状出现,往往已伴有肿瘤局灶浸润或转移。体重减轻和腹痛是最常见的首发症状,腹痛早期较为隐匿,表现为上腹部不适,如餐后饱胀感,后期可进展至剧烈而持续的疼痛,纳差和恶心症状亦较为常见。贲门部的病变常引起吞咽困难,当胃窦肿瘤导致胃腔狭窄时可引起呕吐症状。硬癌(即皮革胃)患者容易出现饱腹感。尽管只有 20% 的患者有黑便史,但对于胃肠道间叶组织肿瘤患者(如平滑肌瘤和平滑肌肉瘤),消化道大出血较常见。

早期胃癌无阳性体征,进展期胃癌患者可出现恶病质、肠梗阻、上腹部肿块、腹水、肝肿大或下肢水肿。伴有转移的胃癌患者可表现为锁骨上淋巴结(Virchow's 淋巴结)、腋窝前壁淋巴结或脐部(sister mary joseph's)淋巴结肿大,以及卵巢肿大(krukenberg's 瘤)。

(2)影像表现:

1)X 线表现:

①早期胃癌:早期胃癌指肿瘤局限于黏膜层或黏膜下层,不论有无淋巴结或远处转移。这个概念常提示疾病处于病程早期,病变较为局限,往往临床症状不明显。日本胃癌研究协会根据形态将早期胃癌分成 3 种主要类型。Ⅰ 型:息肉型,病变突出胃腔的高度大于 5 mm,影像学上表现为胃壁上小的隆起性病变。腺瘤样息肉可具有恶变潜能,因此任何大于 1 cm 的息肉,不论带蒂与否,应当作可疑早期胃癌处理。部分息肉型早期胃癌在穿透固有肌层前,肿瘤范围可能很大但没有临床症状。Ⅰ 型早期胃癌通常小于 2 cm,仅少数带蒂。Ⅱ 型:表浅型,可分为三种亚型,包括表浅隆起型(Ⅱa)、表浅平坦型(Ⅱb)及表浅凹陷型(Ⅱc)。表浅隆起型是指突出胃腔高度<5 mm 的早期胃癌。表浅凹陷型是指溃疡样的早期胃癌,而胃黏膜肌层未受侵。上述分型的胃癌在影像学上相应表现为扁平隆起、黏膜结节及表浅溃疡。Ⅱa 和Ⅱb 型常发生于胃窦部,而Ⅱc 型多发生于胃角。Ⅱ 型早期胃癌偶尔受累范围广泛,可累及胃的大部分。Ⅰ 型和Ⅱa 型在老年人多见。Ⅲ 型:溃疡型,病变穿透胃黏膜肌层达固有肌层,影像表现与胃溃疡相似,但其形态更不规则,周围纠集的黏膜皱襞局部可呈杵状、融合或中断改变,邻近黏膜可见结节形成。仔细分析上述影像表现常有助于与良性胃溃疡鉴别。

②进展期胃癌:进展期的胃癌是指肿瘤穿透固有肌层,常伴有邻近或远处转移。胃癌的形态分型最初由 Borrmann 提出,该分型可由放射、病理或内镜医师进行判断。该分型单纯基于大体病理表现将胃癌分为息肉型、溃疡型和浸润型。由于许多病变可同时具有上述多种形态,分型相互间常有重叠。Borrmann Ⅰ 型:息肉蕈伞型。Borrmann Ⅰ 型为巨大的息肉样或蕈伞状病变,呈不规则分叶状,直径大于或等于 3 cm,X 线表现:充盈相表现为大的、不规则状的充盈缺损;双重对比造影及加压相表现为边缘粗糙分叶状的不规则肿块影。在正面观,肿瘤基底部游离缘与邻近胃黏膜之间可见附钡白线影。巨大的肿块可占据胃腔大部分,但胃输出道梗阻并不常见。胃窦部息肉状肿块可经幽门管脱垂至十二指肠,表现为十二指肠球部肿块影。Borrmann Ⅱ 型:溃疡型。Borrmann Ⅱ 型,肿瘤呈"火山口"样,与邻近正常黏膜的分界锐利而呈现清晰的轮廓;溃疡直径常大于 3 cm,较小的溃疡在双重对比造影上难以与Ⅱc 型早期胃癌鉴别。病变早期可表现为糜烂或溃疡,随着疾病进展,正常的黏膜表面逐渐被病变取替。正面观上,恶性溃疡常不规则,偏心性生长,邻近见散在的肿瘤结节,溃疡口部常呈锯齿状、成角或裂隙状改变。黏膜皱襞往溃疡边缘集中,纠集的黏膜皱襞因肿瘤浸润而变得僵硬,或呈结节状、杵状及融合改变。在双重对比造影上,溃疡型胃癌的正面观可呈现"双环征",外环为肿瘤边缘,内环为溃疡边界;仰卧位加压相上,肿瘤内部的溃疡由钡剂填充。Borrmann Ⅲ 型:浸润溃疡型[图 10-5(a)]。Borrmann Ⅲ 型为浸润型和溃疡型的混合形态表现,但与溃疡型胃癌不同,该型胃癌的溃疡边缘缺乏清晰锐利的边界,另外,肿块外观往往比溃疡更明显。肿瘤在加压相表现为较大的不规则溃疡和溃疡周围的透亮缺损,在充盈相表现为充盈缺损影伴有局部胃壁僵硬,而且僵硬的范围超过溃疡本身,这是由肿瘤的弥漫性壁内浸润所致的。Borrmann Ⅳ 型:皮革胃。胃硬癌是

一种弥漫浸润性病变,伴随大量的纤维组织和结缔组织增生,导致胃壁增厚、胃腔缩小而类似皮革,称皮革胃。硬癌常累及胃的远侧部分,引起严重的狭窄。在进展期病例中,肿瘤可浸润全胃。胃窦部幽门前区比较局限的病变可导致胃窦缩短、成角,形成蜗牛胃。约40%病例仅见胃底或胃体部受侵而胃窦部正常,这样表现的胃癌在过去常被漏诊,双重对比造影在临床应用后,易被检出。

2)CT表现:除了胃癌发生的部位和形态,CT还能提供壁内浸润、腔外侵犯及远处转移等具有临床价值的信息,以帮助进行精确的术前评估并指导临床决策。国际抗癌协会参与制定的TNM分期标准是临床常用的胃癌分期系统。

T分期评估胃癌浸润的深度。在第八版TNM分期系统中,浸润黏膜层,黏膜下层,固有肌层,浆膜下层,浆膜层及邻近结构(由浅到深)的胃癌分别被归为T1a,T1b,T2,T3,T4a,T4b期。正常胃壁CT表现为三层结构,从内到外分别为:高密度的黏膜层,低密度的黏膜下层及高密度的肌-浆膜层。T1a期胃癌表现为黏膜增厚伴有强化,T1b期胃癌在此基础上还可见病变底部所处的低密度黏膜下层模糊、中断。由于固有肌层与浆膜层均表现为高密度且分界不明显,T2到T4a期胃癌在CT上鉴别可能较为困难。病灶邻近的浆膜层变得毛糙,或相邻腹腔脂肪间隙出现条索影,常提示肿瘤处于T4a期。CT发现病灶后,应进一步行胃镜下活检以明确其病理类型。

N分期评估受累淋巴结的数目。一般而言,短径>5~10 mm的淋巴结提示可疑淋巴结转移,但目前尚无统一标准。对于接受胃癌根治术的患者而言,淋巴结转移是肿瘤复发的独立危险因素之一。

M分期评估有无远处转移,如肝转移及腹膜转移。该分期在选择合适的临床治疗手段方面,尤其是对于筛选可能无法从胃切除术获益的患者,显得尤为重要。

CT是胃癌TNM分期的首选影像方法。高质量的多平面CT重建图有助于更好地显示胃壁的改变[图10-5(b)、(c)]。此外,CT分期的准确性还与肿瘤大小、强化方式及其组织学分型有关。对于存在CT禁忌证的患者,MRI是另一种替代性影像检查方法。MRI图像组织对比度高,这使得肿瘤侵犯显示更清晰。但是,扫描时间长、存在胃肠蠕动及呼吸运动相关伪影限制了MRI在临床实践中的广泛应用。

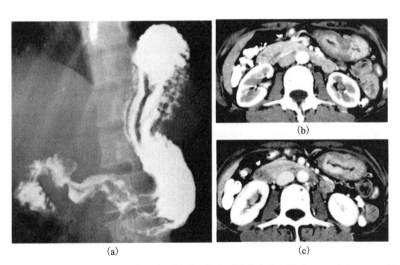

(a)胃窦部肿瘤浸润,管腔狭窄,管壁僵硬。箭头示肿块和溃疡形成。(b)和(c).CT图像显示胃壁增厚,黏膜明显强化,肿瘤边界不清。

图10-5 进展期胃癌(Borrmann Ⅲ型),浸润溃疡型

(颜荣华,郭焯欣,周广,邓志奇,丁竹远,肖恩华,刘辉)

Chapter 10

Gastrointestinal tract

The digestive system consists of long, curved hollow organs, from the mouth to the anus, including the mouth, pharynx, esophagus, stomach, duodenum, jejunum, ileum, and large intestine. Bariumradiography is one of the most common procedures performed to examine the changes of gastrointestinal tract in size, shape, contour, peristalsis and mucosa. B-mode ultrasound, CT and MRI examinations also contribute to the visibility of intramural and extrinsic abnormalities. Virtual endoscopy by CT can depict the endoluminal lesions as well as the conventional endoscopy does but in a wider field of view.

The X-ray examination of the gastrointestinal series differs in some aspects from ordinary radiographic procedures:

(1) It requires digital gastrointestinal machine or multi-functional DR;

(2) The use of contrast media, barium sulphate is essential to fill up various segment of the alimentary canal and renders the later roentgen visible;

(3) It requires preliminary preparation of the patient's G. I. tract fasting stomach on the day of examination and empty colon by cleansing enema for colon examination; the examinations are usually scheduled on the morning.

The term G. I. series, a complete study of the entire digestive tract after oral administration of Barium sulfate suspension. However, generally only the stomach with the gastro-esophageal junction, the duodenum and part of the jejunum are investigated in detail, complete examination of the esophagus and small bowel are usually performed only in cases with special pertinent problems and should be ordered separately. For examination of the colon, barium enema is the best choice.

Section 1 Method of examination

1. Thoracic and abdominal fluroscopy

The fluroscopy of the thoracic and abdomenis included as a preliminary part of barium meal studies. It is a scout film performed before swallowing barium to establish a baseline and to rule out potential contraindications of the examination.

2. Contrast examination

(1) Barium-meal study: Barium sulfate suspensions and iodinated water-soluble materials are the major categories of contrast agent used to examine the gastrointestinal tract. Single contrast study is a routine procedure. A diluted barium suspension is used to distend the lumen, at the same time, compression is applied to spread the barium over the mucosa in order bring out the lesion. The single-contrast barium enema requires a stable suspension

of low density, generally 15% to 20% w/v, since this is essentially a "see-through" examination and requires that the barium-filled colon be slightly radiolucent. Barium sulfate suspensions intended for the single-contrast barium enema must also produce a satisfactory postevacuation film.

Nowadays, double contrast study is widely adapted. Double contrast refers to high-density barium (positive contrast) and gas (negative contrast) produced by dry effervescent crystals. A double contrast view is obtained when the inner surface of mucosa is coated with a layer of barium and the lumen is fully distended with air. Examinations with double contrast are sensitive to visualize subtle mucosal irregularities which might be missed on single contrast studies.

Because of lower cost and greater safety, the majority of examinations are conducted using barium sulfate. In the setting offistula, perforation, obstruction, risk for aspiration or a history of recent gastrointestinal surgery, non-ionic iodine contrast is recommended.

(2)Angiograph: It is only used for diagnosis and therapeutic application in patients with acute gastro-intestinal hemorrhage where a bleeding site may be localized by selective angiography and thereby vasopressor agent is infused or embolic material is given to control the bleeding.

Besides, angiography is used to evaluate portal hypertension prior to shunt surgery and also usedto study the blood supply and vascular invasion in cases of malignancies.

3. Abdominal CT and MRI

Abdominal CT and MRI are essential imaging tools for the evaluation ofintramural and extraluminal lesions, as well as the compression or invasion to surrounding organs. CT and MRI can also help to detect lymph node involvement and distant metastasis, tumor staging, optimal therapies planning, and follow-up visit after treatment.

Section 2　Normal appearance

1. X-ray manifestations

(1)Laryngopharynx: It begins at epiglottis as the continuation of the oropharynx, extends inferiorly, and continues as the cervical esophagus at level of the cricoid cartilage. On the upright frontal view, following the contrast bolus from oropharynx down to the esophagus, one would see the barium filled sacs on both sides of the midline in pharynx, named epiglottic valleculaes, which are a pair of shallow spaces between the root of tongue and the epiglottis. Another pair of depressions with pooling of barium are the pyriform sinus, situated inferolateral to the epiglottic valleculaes. Ingested foreign bodies, especially fish bones, are commonly found in these spaces.

(2)Esophagus: The oesophagus is the first part of the digestive tract proper. The oesophagus is a tubular structure extending from the pharynx at the inferior border of the cricoid cartilage (approximately at the level of the 6th. Cervicle vertebra)to the cardiac orifice of the stomach (at the level ofthe 11th. thoracic vertebra). Its length varies among 25~30 cm. In cross section, it appears as a flattened tube. Basic tissue layers of the gut arethe followings: 1)Mucosa. Innermost, moist lining membrane. Epithelium (abrasion resistant stratified squamous in the upper oesophagus, simple beyond)plus a minor amount of connective tissue and smooth muscle. 2)Submucosa. Soft connective tissue layer, blood vessels, nerves, lymphatics. 3)Muscularis externa. Typical circular inner layer and longitudinal outer layer of smooth muscle. 4)Adventitia. Flexible outer fascial layer. Esophagus has no serosal layer.

1)Physiologic contractile stricture: There are 4 definite constrictionsin the normal esophagus: ① At the cricopharyngeal junction, indented by the posterior cricopharyngeal at the level of the C_6. ②At the level of the aortic arch; ③At the indentation of the left bronchus; ④At the level where the esophagus passes through the diaphragm. The lumen at the site of the upper constrictions is smaller than the fourth, so foreign bodies usually stay at one of the upper constrictions.

2) Motility of the esophagus: 3 types of peristaltic movements are recognizable. Primary peristalsis is usually initiated by the voluntary act of swallowing, which passes down the whole length of the esophagus. Secondary peristaltic wave, stimulated by distention, usually begins at the level of the remaining bulus. Anything not removed from the esophagus by the primary wave is cleared by a secondary stipping wave. And Tertiary wave gives a corkscrew appearance probably due to esophageal spasm, which isnon-propulsive while both primary and secondary waves are propulsive. These peristalsis is obviouswith patient lying down to avoid the gravity effect.

3) Plica mucosa: When the esophagus is empty, the mucosal coat of the lumen is thrown into 2-3 longitudinal folds and is usually defined with barium as paralleled lines throughout the esophagus, which gather above the cardia.

4) Esophagogastric junction: The esophagus for the most part is a tubular structure, except its lower end, which may form a sac when relaxed, the vestibule. The junction of the tubular area and vestibular portion is described as tubule-vestibular junction(ring A of Wolf), This junction is situated normally above the diaphragm. There is another ring around theesophagogastric junction (ring B of Schatzki). The B ring is the actual squamocolumnar junction between the esophagus and the stomach. If ring B is seen above the diaphragm, a hernia is present.

(3) Stomach: C shaped, left-sided abdominal cavity. The stomach is arbitrarily divided into 3 portions: the fundus, whichlies above the horizontal plane through the junction of the esophagus and the stomach; the body, which lies almost vertically or horizontally between the fundus and the incisura angularis; The antral portion is the part lies between the incisura angularis and the pylorus.

1) The shape and position of the stomach: They vary and depend upon the gastric tone and body built. In a short and stocky individual, the stomach is usually high in position and lies transversely, steerhorn in shape, and the incisura anglaris is not discernable. In a medium-sized individual, the stomach is J-shaped and the body of stomach tends to be vertical, the incisura is easily identified. The pylorus and the incisura are at the same level, the lowest portion of the stomach in the erect position tends to be at the level of the iliac crest. In a thin individual, the stomach is 'fish-hook' shaped, the pylorus lies above the level of the incisura angularis, the lowest portion lies below the level of the iliac crest in erect. When the hypotonic stomach occurs in an over-weighted individual, it is usually symptomatic, sometimes, suggestive of an ulcer syndrome. Cascade stomach: The fundus portion of the stomach becomes angulated backward and dowmward forming a pocket and separated from the stomach by a ridge. The pocket may be shallow or deep, and the barium mixture cascades into the body of the stomach from this pocket when patient is bending forward.

2) Mucosal pattern of the stomach: When the stomach is empty, the muscular layer contracts and throw the mucosa into folds (Rugae)which protrude into the interior of the stomach. When the barium mixture spreads over the mucosa and is getting in between the folds, they appear as white linear or curvilinear lines radiologically, and the rugae stand out as lucent lines or band-shaped shadows. In general, the width of the fold is no more than 5 mm. Since the advent of double contrast technique, a fine relief mucosal pattern also known as micromucosal pattern (called gastric aerea) is demonstrated. Radiologically, they present as a number of small, radiolucent areas in oval or polygonal shape, <1 cm in diameter diameter, with linear barium coating in the surrounding shallow gastric sulcus.

3) Gastric motility: In normal condition, the peristaltic waves in the stomach begin high up on the body. The waves become deeper as they spread along the greater curvature than that of the lesser curvature. Successive waves follow and usually 2-3 such peristaltic waves are visible underfluoroscopy. Gastric emptying depends upon many

factors such as temperature of the food, type of the meal, and physiological status of the patient. The main bulk of the barium meal should leave the stomach in an hour or more. Retention of barium suspension over 1/3 of the original amount in the stomach over =6 hours should be considered abnormal.

(4)Duodenum: First part of small intestine. Duodenum is C-shaped, 25 cm in length, curves around head of pancreas and it is the entry of common bile duct. This curve is subdivided into duodenal bulb, descending, horizontal and ascending portions.

Duodenal bulb, the first portion of duodenum is integrated both structurely and functionally with antrum of stomach, the reminder of duodenum resembles that of small intestine. In the filled state, the bulb is triangular in shape with smooth margin and the walls are slightly convex. The pylorus opens at the middle of the duodenal bulb base.

(5)Jejunum and Ilium: The small bowel proper, consisting of jejunum and ilium, is attached to the posterior abdominal wall by mesentery, the root of which extends obliquely from left upper quadrant to the right lower quadrant, and renders the small bowel freely movable. Any small bowel loop has two borders, a fixed border, facing the root of the mesentery is called mesenteric border, whereas the free border facing wasy the root is called antimesenteric border. This is of importance to radiologist because certain diseases, such as lymphoma, seeded metastasis and Crohn's disease tend to involve the mesenteric side of the loop. The jejunum usually lies in the left half of the abdomen while the ilium lies in the lower region and deep in the pelvis, with the terminal ilium arising out of the pelvis to meet the caecum.

The mucosal pattern of the small intestine gives a characteristic circular folds (plicae circularis). The combination of the plicae circularis and the villi feathery appearance when is viewed radiologically in the absence of distention. There is gradual deminition of the number and size of the plicae circularis toward the ilium, so the mucosal pattern of ilium is smoother and less feathery, giving a ribbon like appearance.

The evacuation time of small intestine is between 7-9 hours after ingestion of the barium meal. The head of barium column may reach caecum in 2-6 hours.

(6)Iliocaecal Junction: The terminal ilium projects into the caecum at its termination, producing folds that function as a sphinctor. The serosa of the ilium does not participate in this protrusion to prevent envagination of terminal ilium. This valve functions to prevent reflux from the caecum. Roentgenologically, it produces a v-shaped filing defect.

(7)Colon: The large intestine id approximately 5-51/2 feet in length and is situated peripherally in the abdomen. Distinguished from the small intestine by its peripheral location and by having haustrations. The colon has several radiologically identifiable segments caecum, ascending colon, transverse, descending, sigmoid colon and rectum. There are two flexures: hepatic and splenic flexures. Both flexures are posteriorly located while the transverse colon is anterior and is attached by mesentery—the transverse mesocolon. Thus it is freely retroperitoneal. The sigmoid colon is also attached by mesentery and may be very long, subjecting to volvulus (twisting). The caecum, in certain individual may have a mesentery, being mobile, so volvulus may also happen.

The colon when filled with barium mixture, it gives a characteristic appearance haustrations. They are prominent in proximal part of the colon and becomes indistinct toward the descending colon. No haustration seen in rectum.

The mucosal pattern of the colon often runs transversely but in its distal portion, it becomes parallel with the long axis.

The motility of the colon: There are basically two different forms of contraction: 1)Local contraction, gives the large bowel an "accordion" like appearance; 2)The extensive contraction.

2. CT manifestations

(1)Esophagus：Esophagus is a muscular tube that runs right and anterior to the thoracic aorta, and in front of the spine. The tube covered by a layer of adipose tissue, have a density close to the muscle with a wall thickness of about 3 mm and trapped gas (swallowed air)in the lumen.

(2)Stomach：Gastric fundus is situated right behind to the spleen and on the right front of the left hepatic lobe. The gastric body can be identified at a lower level, which has close relationship in anatomical location with the left hepatic lobe, jejunum, pancreatic tail and spleen. It surrounds the head of pancreas along with the duodenum. The gastric wall normally have a thickness of 2-5 mm and three layers can be detected on CT, from the inside out, including high-attenuated mucosa, low-attenuated submucosa and high-attenuated musculoserosal layers.

(3)Duodenum：As a continuation of the gastric antrum, the duodenum begins with the duodenal bulb, extend downwards (the descending part)which cupping the head of pancreas, then extend horizontally to the left (the transverse part)in front of the aorta and behind the superior mesenteric vessels. Its wall thickness is comparable to that of the small intestine.

(4)Small intestine：The wall thickness of small intestine is about 3 mm, while in terminal ileum it can be up to 5 mm. Jejunum is typically presented in the left upper quadrant, and the ileum, the distal portion of the small bowel, is predominantly located in the right lower abdomen. After contrast-enhancement, detailed evaluation can be performed on extraluminal structures such as mesentery, peritoneum and omentum.

(5)Colon：Colon contains a large amount of faeces. The wall is about 3~5 mm thickness with smooth contour and sharp edge on CT.

3. MRI manifestations

MRI is increasingly used in gastrointestinal examination. To distinguish normal from abnormal conditions, contrast agents are normally required, including negative contrast agents (barium sulfate, mannitol, etc.)and positive contrast agents (paramagnetic iron oxide solution, diluted gadolinium agent, etc.), which can be swallowed or administered by enema. The signal characteristic of gastrointestinal and esophageal wall on MRI is similar to that of the muscles.

Section 3　Basic pathologic changes

The gastro-intestinal tract can be considered, in general term, as a hollow, muscular tube. Pathologic alterations seen in one segment may be seen in any other segment and will manifest a similar radiographic appearance, regardless of the site. The incidences of those lesions, of course will vary from location to location.

1. Ulceration：Ulceration is a localized disruption and erosion in the inner surface of the gastro-intestinal tract. The "ulcer crater" results in a collection of barium being outside the normal lumen and it manifests as a depressed lesion on CT or MR. Radiographically, there are two ways a crater may be seen：on face(looking directly facing the ulcer" or in profile(looking from the side). Enface, a typical ulcer crater will be a distinct round, circumscribed unchanging collection of barium; on profile, this unchanging collection of barium will project outside the confine of the stomach(Niche). Quite often the ulcer is surrounded by an edematous ulcer collar. Ulceration may also occur within a tumor mass. One should remember that there are rare malignant ulcer but there are ulcerating malignancy. The differentiation of benign and malignant ulcers is shown in Table 10-1 and Figure 10-1.

Table 10-1 Radiological differential features between a benign gastric ulcer and ulcerating malignancy

Benign gastric ulcer	Ulcerating malignancy
Penetration beyond lumen	Intraluminal crater
Mucosal folds radiate to crater edge	Amputation of mucosal folds
Round, sharply circumscribed crater	Irregularity of surrounding mucosa
Edematous tissue surrounding	Nodularity of surrounding Mucosaan ulcer produces ulcer moundor collar.
Pliable, presence of peristalsis	Rigidity of wall

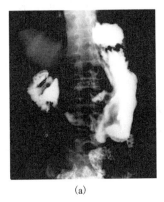 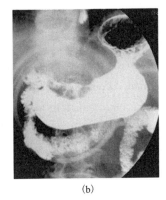

(a)   (b)

(a)Tangential, profile view of a large lesser curve ulcer projecting beyond the gastric margin. Smooth, tapering folds are seen extending to the edge of the ulcer crater, indicating its benign nature; (b) Malignant gastric ulcer, when viewed in profile and with compression, have a semicircular (meniscoid) appearance. The inner margin of the ulcer of the mass is convex toward the lumen. The folds leading to a malignant ulcer are irregular and blunted.

Figure 10-1 Benign(a)versus malignant(b)gastric ulcer

2. Protruding lesions

It refers to elevated lesions protruding in to the lumen. The space occupying mass produce filling defect on the barium. These may be true mucosal, submucosal or extrinsic. The abruptness of the junction of the lesion with normal bowel can help to localize the processes as either intrinsic or extrinsic. A mucosal lesion makes an acute angle with surrounding bowel while in a submucosal lesion the angle is less acute. A shallow extrinsic lesion smoothly indents the wall making a very obtuse angle.

(1)Polyps: It presents as a small round nodule with soft tissue density. The majority of polyps are known to be benign hyperplastic but an adenomatous polyp may have malignant potential. A poly attached by a narrow stalk is more likely to be benign. Polyp can occur anywhere along the length of the G. I. tract but more common in large bowel.

(2)Mass lesion: An irregular shaped mass, with or without ulceration, may grows in one space on the gastro-intestinal lining forming a large polypoid or fungating lesion, or encircles the bowel lumen resulting in a classical "napking ring" appearance. The normal mucosal folds are either destroyed or replaced by abnormal distended pattern.

(3)There is another type of producing lesion occurring in the stomach and esophagus. Varices in esophagus for instance, are collateral venous channels within the wall that open up when blood flow from the bowel to the liver via portal veins is impeded, most commonly due to cirrhosis of the liver. On the barium, they show as worm-like

309

filling defects that distort the normal mucosal folds and cause scalloping contour.

3. Stricture

Narrowing of the gut lumen may be due to compression by an extrinsic mass or a space occupying lesion that arises within the wall of the gut itself. In the former case, the narrowing usually has smooth margins, whereas in the latter case, it depends on the nature and location of the lesions. Smooth margin, tapering lumen, and intact mucosa are commonly seen in stricture caused by a benign lesion. Comparatively, irregular stricture with stiffness wall may indicate malignancy.

4. Dilatation

Dilatation of a hollow viscus is usually the result of distal obstruction or malfunction of the nerves and muscles in the intestines. Excluding mechanical obstruction, the most common cause of dilatation is probably adynamic ileus. The precise mechanism is often unclear. Localized ileus can result from local irritation, apparently when it involves the autonomic nerve plexi in the bowel wall. Generalized ileus is seen in systemic diseases and most commonly in the postoperative period. Dilatation caused by intrinsic structural changes in the bowel is relatively uncommon. In achalasia, decreased ganglion cells in the autonomic nerve plexi result in atony and progressive dilatation. Diverticulum: A benign outpouching of the gastro-intestinal tract at the point of weakness in the wall (pulsion type) or when the wall becomes adherent to an adjacent inflammatory process(traction type). Diverticulum generally contain all layers of the bowel wall. They may be relatively small, as in the colon, or quite large as in esophagus. There may be multiple diverticulosis as in the colon. It is readily recognizable on profile view of a barium meal, appearing as a flask-like protrusion with well-marginated barium collection. A diverticulum might be confused with an "ulcer crater", but the lack of spasm and the presence of mucosa within the deverticulum should suggest the diagnosis.

Section 4　Diagnosis of common diseases

1. Chronic peptic ulcer

(1)Clinical and pathological manifestations: The gastrointestinal epithelium is a resistant barrier to erosive luminal contents, such as gastric acid, digestive enzymes, bile, and infectious agents. In some cases, the ulcerating process begins within the wall. Mucosal ischemia or inflammatory cell aggregates in the lamina propria in inflammatory bowel disease may be the primary cause. In any case, once the surface is breached, the erosion extends in all directions. If the surrounding epithelium is otherwise normal, it remains relatively resistant and intact even though inflamed and edematous.

(2)Imaging manifestations:

A protrusion of contrast medium beyond the expected lumen of an organ is a familiar pattern (Figure 10-2). Indeed, an early application of gastrointestinal contrast was the search for the so-called barium-filled niche to diagnose peptic ulcers. An ulcer, being a hole in the luminal surface, protrudes or forms a niche when the surface is projected in profile. Ulceration is classically considered to arise from intraluminal insult. The classic signs distinguishing benign peptic ulcers from ulceration in malignancy are based on the pathophysiology and resulting configuration just described above. They depend mainly on the intact surrounding epithelium extending to the very edge of a benign crater. Adenocarcinoma typically produces a nodular, irregular epithelium. An ulcer in this surface has irregular edges that tend to be eroded along with the underlying tissue without much undermining. Erosion into an extensive tumor mass produces an irregular, saucer-shaped hole rather than a flat bottom.

Ulceration into a submucosal mesenchymal tumor such as a leiomyoma or a submucosal metastasis produces a variably shaped crater, but because the epithelium is not primarily involved its edge is often sharply defined. This is the basis for terms of GI series such asbull's-eye, target, and buttercupto describe these lesions.

Peptic ulceration in the stomach and duodenum has been used as the prototype here, but the same concepts apply anywhere in the gut.

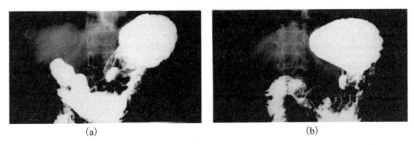

(a)   (b)

The double-contrast view (a)shows one fold running circumferentially around the barium-filled niche and some deformity of the lesser curve. Tangential, profile view (b) revealed a lesser curve ulcerclearly projecting beyond the gastric marginwith the folds radiating toward it.

Figure 10-2　Gastric ulcer on anterior aspect of lesser curve

2. Leiomyoma

(1) Clinical and pathological manifestations: Leiomyomas are one of the most common benign gastric neoplasms and GI stromal tumors. They arise from the smooth muscle layer of the gastric wall, and about 80% are endogastric lesions that remain intramural but grow toward the lumen. Another 15% of leiomyomas are exogastric tumors that remain subserosal but grow outward from the stomach toward the peritoneal cavity. The remaining 5% of tumors have both endogastric and exogastric components producing a dumbbell shape. Leiomyomas usually are asymptomatic when less than 3 cm in size. When larger, these tumors present with GI hemorrhage as a result of ulceration or nausea and vomiting secondary to mass effect or intermittent gastric outlet obstruction. It often is difficult to differentiate leiomyomas from leiomyosarcomas on the basis of radiologic, endoscopic, or even histopathologic criteria. Their classification ultimately depends on the biologic behavior of the lesion.

(2)Imaging manifestations:

1)X-ray findings: Most gastric leiomyomas appear as discrete submucosal lesions that have a smooth surface etched in white on double-contrast barium studies. When viewed in profile, the borders of these tumors form either right angles or slightly obtuse angles with the adjacent gastric wall. En face, the intraluminal surface of these tumors has distinct, abrupt, well-defined borders. The overlying mucosa usually is intact so that a normal areae gastricae pattern often is seen over these lesions. Leiomyomas vary greatly in size, and tumors larger than 2 cm in diameter often contain ulceration that is manifested radiologically by a central barium collection 0.2 to 2 cm in size, the so-called bull's-eye or target lesion.

2)CT findings: On CT, gastric leiomyomas present as smooth masses of uniform soft-tissue attenuation with a density similar to skeletal muscle. These masses usually project into the gastric lumen (Figure 10-3)with a broad mural attachment but occasionally may appear primarily exogastric in location. Leiomyomas may contain irregular streaks or clumps of mottled calcification and are the most commonly calcified benign gastric tumors. Although surface ulceration may be present, the outer borders of the leiomyoma are smooth, with preservation of the fat plane between the tumor and adjacent organs.

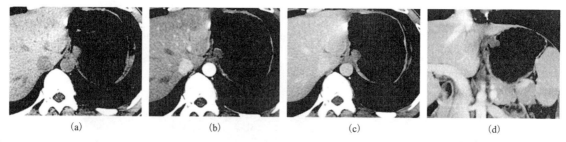

(a)   (b)   (c)   (d)

(a) Noncontrast CT scan shows a uniform density, endophyticmass with a density similar to skeletal muscle. Contrast-enhanced images show slight enhancement in arterial and venous phases(b and c); (d) Contrast-enhanced CT coronal image shows the lesion projecting into the gastric lumen with a broad mural.

Figure 10-3　Gastric leiomyoma

3. Tuberculosis of Intestine

(1) Clinical and pathological manifestations: Tuberculosis of intestinal tract may develop primarily within the intestine, or it may occur secondarily to a primary focus elsewhere in the body. Approximately 85 to 90 percent of the lesions are located in the ileocecal region. The apparent affinity of the tubercle bacillus for lymphoid tissue accounts for the occurrence in this region. Pathological picture in human tuberculosis is apparently related to the relationship between the virulence of the organism and the degree of immunity of the host.

In the early stage, enlargement of the lymph follicles occur. This may be followed by infiltration of the bowel wall, the overlying mucosa becomes swollen, ulceration develops due to caseous necrosis, and a ragged ulcer is formed. This destructive process may be associated with the formation of tuberculous granulomas. Eventually, the lumen of the bowel becomes markedly narrowed with gradual increasing obstruction. All these pathologic features represent either the destruction or the hyperplasia, and develop as a longstanding process (may last for a long time). Clinically, anorexia, diarrhea, and abdominal pain in a patient with pulmonary tuberculosis are strongly suggestive of intestinal tuberculosis.

(2) Imaging manifestations:

1) X-ray findings: Radiologically, it usually shows a mixture of various basic changes. However, any of them may be the predominant finding in different patients.

Barium examination has proved to be the greatest aid to the detection of this disorder. Although there are no pathognomonic roentgenologic signs, the presence of following features in the colon or small bowel barium enemas are strongly suggestive of this disease. ①Stirlin sign: There is a lack of barium retention in a diseased segment of ileum and caecum but with a column of barium remains on either side of the affected area. This phenomenon may result from spasm, organic contracture or a combination of both. ②String sign (Figure 10-4): A radiological sign shows persistent narrow stream of barium in distal portion of the small bowel due to increased irritability or organic stenosis. ③Distorted ileocecal region(Figure 10-4): The iliocecal valve may show a tendency to gap because of ulceration or granulation that progresses to fibrosis and results in retraction of the valve lips. This is represented radiographically by a broad-based triangular

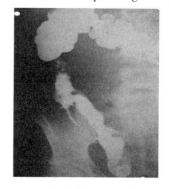

There is mucosal edema and ulceration of the ascending colon. The terminal ileum is edematous and slightly dilated, and the appendix also is infected. There is string-like narrowing (arrow) of the ascending colon and cecum with diffuse ulceration. Fistulous tracts extend from the contracted deformed cecum with adjacent inflammatory soft tissue mass and lymphadenopathy displacing the dilated, edematous distal ileum away from the cecum.

Figure 10-4　Tuberculosis of the cecum and ascending colon

appearance of the teminal ileum either the base toward the cecum. Loss of haustration in the cecum and ╱ or ascending colon is invariably present. The cecum is frequently conical with its apex pointing downward. When hyperplasia predominates the narrowing of lumen and shortening are more significant. The contour of the affectd bowel may present either smooth or irregular"finger-print" defects, and cannot be differentiated from those of other granulomatous diseases or from malignant lesios. ④Intestinal Obstruction: It is usually seen in the small bowel with abnormal retention of barium in the ileal loops. ⑤Distorted or destroyed mucosal folds: In the diseased area, the irregularity and prominence of the folds due to edema and disturbed motility often occur.

2)CT and MRI findings: On abdominal CT and MRI, there are two main forms of tuberculosis lesions found in the gastrointestinal tract: an ulcerative process and a hyperplastic reaction. Mural thickening involving the ileocecal region is the most common CT finding. Apart from being more sensitive to detect the affected bowel, T2-weighted imaging may also enable to characterize the cause of lesions. Bowel with active inflammation for instance, is of high signal intensity on T2WI and probably with remarkable enhancement, while wall thickening caused by fibrostenotic process may be T2 hypointense. In advanced diseases, concentric wall thickening together with adherence of adjacent mesentery may form a mass appearance. CT and MRI also offer the unique opportunity to evaluate the tuberulous lymphadenopathy and involvement of the peritoneum, solid viscera and spine, all of which are common manifestations of TB.

4. Gastric carcinomas

(1)Clinical and pathological manifestations: Gastric carcinomas typically produce no specific symptoms when they are superficial and surgically curable. Unfortunately, the disease often is locally advanced or metastatic at the time of clinical presentation. Weight loss and abdominal pain are the most frequent initial symptoms. The abdominal pain begins insidiously as upper abdominal discomfort that ranges in intensity from a vague sense of postprandial fullness to a severe, steady pain. Anorexia and nausea are often quite common. Dysphagia may be the main symptom associated with lesions of the cardia, and vomiting may occur if the tumor narrows the antrum. Other patients with scirrhous carcinomas (e. g. , linitis plastica)may have early satiety develop. Although melena occurs in 20% of patients, massive hemorrhage more commonly is seen with GI stromal tumors such as leiomyoma and leiomyosarcoma.

Early gastric cancer (EGC)has no physical findings. Patients with advanced gastric cancer may present with cachexia, small bowel obstruction, epigastric mass, ascites, hepatomegaly, or lower extremity edema. Metastases may also manifest as an enlarged supraclavicular lymph node (Virchow's node), large left anterior axillary or umbilical (Sister Mary Joseph's)lymph nodes, an enlarged ovary (Krukenberg's tumor)。

(2)Imaging manifestations:

1)X-ray findings:

①Early Gastric Cancer: Early gastric cancer is defined as carcinoma limited to the mucosa and submucosa regardless of the presence or absence of lymph node involvement and distant metastasis. This term clinically suggests a lesion that is early, confined, and asymptomatic. The Japanese Research Society for Gastric Cancer has divided EGC lesions into three morphologic types. Type I EGCs are polypoid lesions that protrude more than 5 mm into the lumen. Radiographically, they appear as small elevated lesions in the stomach. Adenomatous polyps can undergo malignant degeneration, so that any sessile or pedunculated gastric polyps greater than 1 cm in size should be viewed with suspicion for EGC. Some polypoid EGCs may be quite large and symptomatic without penetrating the muscularis propria. Type I tumors generally are smaller than 2 cm and only rarely pedunculated. Type II EGCs are also superficial lesions with elevated (IIa), flat (IIb), or depressed components (IIc). Superficial elevated lesions (IIa)lesions protrude less than 5 mm into the lumen. Superficial depressed lesions are ulcerations that do not penetrate the muscularis propria. These tumors present radiologically as plaquelike elevations, mucosal nodularity, and/or shallow areas of ulceration. Type IIa and IIb lesions usually involve the antrum; type IIc lesions more often involve the angulus. Type II lesions occasionally can be quite extensive, involving a large portion of the surface area of the stomach. Type I and IIa lesions are seen most frequently in the elderly population. Type III EGCs are excavated lesions that penetrate the muscularis mucosa but not the muscularis propria. They resemble gastric ulcers but with irregular ulcer craters, clubbing, fusion or amputation of radiating folds, and nodularity of the adjacent mucosa. Meticulous analysis of the radiographic findings of these lesions usually permits differentiation from benign gastric ulcers. If there is any doubt about the radiologic findings, then endoscopy with biopsy should be performed.

②Advanced Gastric Cancer: Advanced gastric cancer denotes tumor that has penetrated the muscularis propria and typically is associated with distant or contiguous disease. This tumor is identified by the radiologist, pathologist, and endoscopist in patterns that wereoriginally described by Borrmann. The classification is based solely on gross appearances: polypoid, ulcerated, infiltrating. There is considerable overlap in this classification because many lesions have mixed morphologic features. Borrmann Type 1: Polypoid-Fungating. These are large polypoid or fungating lesions that have irregular lobulation and measure 3 cm or greater in greatest diameter. Radiographically, these tumors produce large, irregular filling defects in the barium pool and cast an irregular tumor shadow with coarse lobulation on double-contrast and compression radiographs. On the nondependent surface of the stomach, these lesions, when viewed en face, are etched in white by a thin layer of barium trapped between the edge of the mass and the adjacent mucosa. Bulky lesions may significantly encroach on the lumen, but gastric outlet obstruction is uncommon. Polypoid antral tumors can prolapse through the pylorus into the duodenum and present as a mass at the base of the duodenal bulb. Borrmann Type 2: Ulcerated. These tumors have discrete, sharply defined borders so that the ulcer crater is clearly delineated from normal surrounding mucosa. These lesions typically exceed 3 cm in greatest diameter. When smaller, they may be difficult to differentiate from type IIc EGC on double-contrast barium studies. The primary site may appear as an erosion or ulceration, which, with progressive disease, replaces the mucosal surface. En face, these malignant ulcers are characterized by an irregular ulcer crater that is eccentrically located in a rind of neoplastic tissue. Discrete tumor nodules may be present in the adjacent mucosa, and these ulcers may also have scalloped, angular, or stellate borders. If there are radiating folds converging to the edge of the ulcer, they typically are blunted, nodular, clubbed, or fused as a result of tumor infiltration. On double-contrast barium studies, ulcerated carcinomas on the nondependent wall may be etched in white, producing a double ring shadow with the outer ring delineating the edge of the tumor and the inner ring indicating the edge of the ulcer. On prone compression views, the ulcer crater within the tumor mass fills with barium. Borrmann Type 3: Infiltrative-ulcerated(Figure 10-5a). These lesions have a mixed morphology with both infiltrative and ulcerated components. The ulceration does not have discrete borders however. The mass usually is more prominent than the ulcer. Compression images show a large irregular crater and a surrounding radiolucent defect. Barium pool images show a filling defect and stiffening of the gastric wall. Because there is diffuse mural infiltration, stiffening of the gastric wall extends beyond the cancer ulcer crater. Borrmann Type 4: Linitis Plastica. Scirrhous tumors of the stomach are diffusely infiltrating lesions that are associated with marked proliferation of fibrotic tissue and desmoplasia. This results in a grossly thickened stomach, with a shrunken lumen that has been likened to a leather bottle. The distal half of the stomach is most commonly involved and is severely narrowed. In advanced cases, the entire stomach is infiltrated by tumor. More localized tumors may be confined to the prepyloric antrum and appear as short, anular lesions with shelflike proximal borders. Nearly 40% of these patients have localized lesions in the gastric fundus or body with antral sparing. This fact was not appreciated until double-contrast barium techniques afforded adequate distention of the proximal stomach.

2) CT findings: Aside from tumor locations and morphologies, CT provide valuable information concerning

local tumor spread, lymph node involvement and distant metastasis. Accurate preoperative staging based on these factors guides treatment strategies. The tumor-node-metastasis (TNM) stages by the International Union against Cancer (UICC) is the major stage classification systems for gastric cancer.

T-staging of gastric cancer assess tumor invasion depth. In the 8th edition of TNM staging, tumor penetrating mucosa, submucosa, muscularis propria, subserosa, serosa and adjacent structures are classified as T1a, T1b, T2, T3, T4a, T4b gastric cancer, respectively. In general, the gastric wall is detected from the inside out as three layers on CT: high-attenuated mucosa, low-attenuated submucosa and high-attenuated musculoserosal layers. T1a shows mucosal thickening with enhancement on CT. A disruption of a low-attenuated layer at the lesion bottom, corresponding to submucosa, is additionally demonstrated in T1b. The invisible boundary between muscularis propria and serosa on CT make the differentiation of T2 to T4a difficult. However, the blurred serosal contour or strandlike densities extending into the perigastric fat indicate T4a. If a lesion is detected on CT, then endoscopy with biopsy should be performed to confirm the histopathologic findings.

N-staging assess the number of involved lymph nodes. Although there is no conclusive criteria on imaging, lymph nodes with a short-axis diameter of > 5 to 10 mm are commonly supposed to be pathologic. For patients undergoing curative resection for gastric cancer, lymph node metastases are an independent risk factor for recurrence.

M-staging evaluate the presence of distant metastases, such as liver metastases and peritoneal metastases. This staging is crucial for choosing appropriate treatment modalities, especially for selecting patients who might not benefit from gastrectomy.

CT is a primary imaging modality for TNM staging in patients with gastric cancer. High-quality multiplanar reformation (MPR) of CT improve the visualization of changes in the gastric wall layer structures (Figure 10-5b, c). The accuracy of TNM staging by CT also depends on tumor sizes, enhancement patterns, and the histologic subtypes. MRI is an alternative staging modality when CT is contraindicated for patients with gastric cancer. High soft-tissue contrast of MR imaging permits a better depiction of tumor invasion. Nevertheless, long acquisition times and artifacts related to peristaltic motion and respiration limit its wide application in clinical practice.

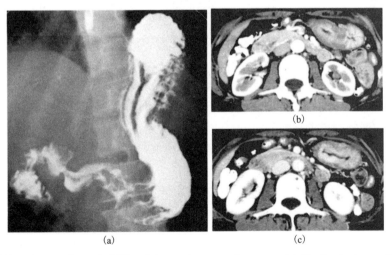

(a)   (b)

                                       (c)

(a) There is narrowing and rigidity of the gastric antrum due to mural infiltration by tumor. Note theinfiltration and ulcerations (arrows). (b) and (c). CT scans show the mural thickeningand strengthening. The edge of the tumor is ill-defined.

Figure 10-5 Advanced gastric cancer (Borrmann type 3): infiltrated, ulcerated

(Yan Ronghua, Guo Zhuoxin, Zhou Guang, Deng Zhiqi, Ding Zhuyuan, Xiao Enhua, Liu Hui)

第十一章

肝脏

第一节 检查方法

1. X 线检查

检查方法为 X 线平片与造影检查，X 线平片除观察肝脏内有无异常密度增高（钙化）或密度减低（如胆道积气）以外，其内部结构都不能显示。其次腹部 X 线平片可以观察肝上缘（即膈缘）有无异常隆凸；肝下缘（肠气衬托下）位置有无异常，若要观察其活动度则须透视。显示肝脏的轮廓与大小，以及肝血管的分布与走行、肝窦的显示等，则需要选择造影检查。X 线平片和透视只能大致了解肝的大小、轮廓、积气和钙化，诊断价值有限。

造影检查选择性腹腔动脉-肝动脉造影：肝血管造影是诊断肝脏肿块病变和门静脉高压症的重要方法。包括肝动脉的动脉期、毛细血管期及门静脉期（因同时有脾动脉显影），如果导管尖端插入肝总动脉又称之为超选择动脉造影。原发性或转移性肝癌及肝血管瘤，主要由肝动脉供血，肝动脉造影可显示肿瘤的血管结构，从而作出定位和定性诊断。肝动脉造影能显示肝内动脉分支。门静脉造影使门静脉及其属支显影，了解其解剖形态及血液动力学的改变、协助选择手术方式以及观察疗效等。门静脉造影方法很多，主要有3 种：脾门静脉造影，脐门静脉造影，经皮肝穿门静脉造影。

2. CT 检查

CT 是目前肝脏疾病最常用的检查方法之一。因其密度分辨率高，整体观较好，对肝脏占位性病变的定位、定性有重要价值。CT 检查方法：取仰卧位，先作平扫，后作增强扫描，以便更好地明确病变、病变性质并了解血管的情况。增强扫描依扫描的时间，可分为动脉期，门静脉期，门静脉晚期或肝实质期。

CT 表现：肝脏实质正常 CT 值 55~65 Hu，比脾脏高约 10Hu。肝脏肿瘤密度通常比正常实质低，但有时两者相差不大，因此有 10%~15% 的肿块 CT 平扫不能发现。CT 增强对肝脏占位性病变较敏感，较为常用的检查方法是双期扫描：动脉期和门静脉期。对主要由肝动脉供血的病变诊断价值较高，在动脉期上病变密度高于或等于肝实质密度，在门静脉期上病变密度低于肝实质密度。

3. MRI 检查

MRI 具有很高的软组织分辨率，能多角度、多序列成像，对肝脏病变的诊断和鉴别诊断有重有价值。肝脏检查一般包括 T1WI 和 T2WI。T1WI 上解剖关系较清楚，T2WI 对病变检出率更高。增强检查（包括 Gd-DTPA 动态对比增强和肝脏特异性 MRI 对比剂增强）能提供病变的血供情况。造影剂能缩短质子的弛豫时间，T1 和 T2 时间均缩短，T1 缩短更明显一些。增强扫描依扫描的时间，可分为动脉期，门静脉期，门静脉晚期或肝实质期。

第二节　正常表现

1.肝脏的位置

肝脏是上腹部最大实质性器官，位于在上中腹部、上方紧贴右膈下外缘紧靠腹壁、内侧与食管、右肾及肾上腺、胃、十二指肠、胰腺等器官，下方与结肠紧邻。正常肝脏呈楔形，右叶厚而大，向左逐渐变小变薄。超声检查可从任意方位显示肝脏形态；CT、MRI 则自横断、冠状、矢状位上显示肝脏形态。肝脏边缘光滑、棱角锐利。

2.肝脏的大小

肝脏的大小超声可以直接测量肝脏径线来评价肝脏大小。正常肝右叶前后径为 8~10 cm，最大斜径为 10~14 cm；左叶厚度不超过 6 cm，长度不超过 9 cm。多层螺旋 CT 及 MRI 检查，定量检测肝脏体积，但较费时，通常方法是测量肝叶最大径线并计算其间比例，以对各叶大小进行评价，正常肝右/左叶前后径比值约为 1.2-1.9，肝右/尾叶横径比例约为 2-3。

3.肝叶、肝段划分

肝脏分为左叶、右叶和尾叶。为了适应外科学需要，超声、CT、MRI 检查均可根据肝内血管分布特点把肝脏划分为若肝段。Couinaud 法通常以左、中、右肝静脉作为纵向划分标志、以门静脉左、右支主干作为横向划分标志，如此将肝脏划分为八个肝段，即尾叶为 Ⅰ 段，左外上段为 Ⅱ 段、左外下段为 Ⅲ 段、左内段为 Ⅳ 段，右前下段为 Ⅴ 段，右后下段为 Ⅵ 段，右后上段为 Ⅶ 段，右前上段为 Ⅷ 段（图 11-1）。

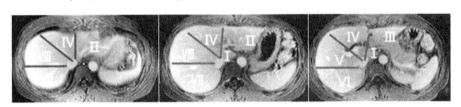

图 11-1　横断面压脂 T1WI 图像显示的 Couinaud 的肝脏 8 段

4.肝实质

（1）超声表现：正常肝实质表现为均匀一致的弥漫细小点状中等回声（图 11-2）。

（2）CT 表现：平扫、正常肝实质呈均匀软组织密度，比脾密度高，CT 值约为 55-75HU，其中的血管可表现圆形或管状低密度影［图 11-3(a)］；CT 多期增强检查可反映肝实质的供血特点、即动脉期强化并不明显，门静脉期强化达高峰，平衡期强化减弱［图 11-3(b)~(d)］。

（3）MRI 表现：正常肝实质信号均匀，T1WI 上呈中等信号，高于脾的信号，T2WI 上呈较低信号，明显低于脾的信号（图 11-4）；多期增强 TWI 上，肝实质强化表现与 CT 相同。

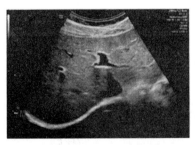

正常肝实质表现为均匀一致的弥漫细小点状中等回声，门静脉、肝静脉及其分支清楚显示，血管壁回声较强，血管腔无回声。

图 11-2　超声检查

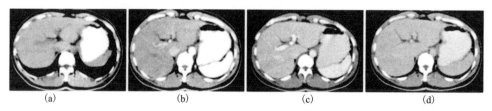

(a)横断面 CT 平扫；(b)横断面增强 CT 动脉；(c)横断面增强 CT 门静脉期；(d)横断面增强 CT 平衡期。

图 11-3　正常肝脏 CT 平扫及增强图像

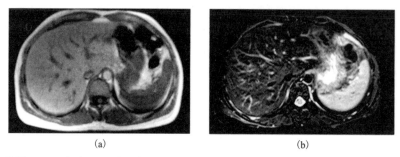

(a)横断面 T1WI 序列显示正常肝实质呈中等信号，高于脾脏信号；(b)横断面抑脂 T2WI 序列显示正常肝脏实质信号明显低于脾脏。

图 11-4　肝实质 CT 检查

5.肝血管

肝动脉和门静脉由肝门进入肝内继续分成各肝叶、段血管；肝静脉分支最后汇合形成左、中、右肝静脉，并于第二肝门进入下腔静脉。①DSA 检查，可以显示肝动脉、门静脉及其分支，在肝内呈树枝状分布，走行自然、边缘光滑；②超声检查，可清楚显示门静脉、肝静脉及其分支，血管壁回声较强，血管腔无回声（图 11-2）；③CT 检查，平扫时肝静脉和门静脉分支通常在表现为肝实质内条形或圆形低密度影，肝动脉分支则不能显示；多期增强检查，动脉期可显示肝动脉及其分支、表现为散在分布的线状、点状高密度影；门静脉期可见门静脉及其左右分支明显强化；平衡期左、中、右肝静脉发生强化；CTA 可从多方位显示血管的全貌；④MRI 检查，较大的门静脉、肝静脉及下腔静脉由于流空效应，于 SE 序列 T1WI、T2WI 上都表现无信号的管状结构，但肝内较小的血管则因流动相关增强效应而于 T2WI 上呈高信号的管状结构。MRA 可从不同方位更好地显示门静脉和肝静脉。

第三节　基本病变

1.X 线表现

肝脏体积明显增大时 X 线平片可见右膈顶升高，肝下角下移，肝内钙化性病灶可显示为高密度影。但肝区 X 线片价值有限，目前已少用。异常的血管造影表现有：①肝动脉增粗或变细；②血管受压移位；③异常新生血管；也称为肿瘤血管或病理血管，为粗细不均，走行紊乱的新生血管，是恶性肿瘤的重要征象；④血管浸润：血管壁的狭窄、闭塞、走行僵硬；⑤肿瘤染色：病灶内对比剂廓清延迟，毛细血管或静脉期呈密度增高影；⑥充盈缺损：病变区无血供，静脉期为无对比剂染色的空白区，常见于无血供的囊性病变或肿瘤的液化坏死；⑦静脉早显：即动脉期见到门静脉或肝静脉显影，多为肿瘤破坏血管造成动静脉短路所致；⑧门静脉充盈缺损：由癌栓所引起的充盈缺损，具有新生肿瘤血管供血，癌栓内也可见线状、片状强化影像。

2. CT 表现

(1)肝脏大小形态的异常：肝脏增大表现为肝缘边钝，肝叶形态饱满；萎缩则相反，肝硬化可见肝体积缩小，并肝结构的重建；肝轮廓凹凸不平呈结节状；肝各叶大小比例失常，常是尾叶与左叶较大而右叶较小；肝门和肝裂增宽。脾增大是诊断肝硬化的重要根据，其外缘前后径超过 5 个单元(一个肋骨或肋间隙称为一个肋单元)。

(2)肝脏边缘与轮廓异常：肝硬化再生结节或占位性病变可使肝脏轮廓凹凸不平，肝缘角变钝，失去正常的棱角而变圆，边缘呈锯齿状或波浪状改变。

(3)肝的弥漫性病变：为一组弥漫性肝细胞变性、坏死的疾病，可引起肝脏大小、形态、密度改变，如肝硬化、脂肪肝、血色病和肝豆状核变性等。CT 可见全肝或某一肝叶、肝段密度减低、增高或呈混杂密度。

(4)肝的局灶性病变：常见为肝囊肿、脓肿、寄生虫和各种肿瘤等病变。平扫多数表现为单发或多发的圆形、类圆形或不规则形肿块。增强后囊肿或乏血供病变表现为不强化或轻度强化。脓肿脓腔不强化，脓肿壁呈环形增强，轮廓光滑整齐，厚度均匀。海绵状血管瘤动脉期表现为边缘结节状强化，静脉期及延迟扫描可见增强的范围逐渐向中心扩展，最后整个血管瘤被造影剂"填满"。肝癌大部分在动脉期表现为明显的不均匀性强化，门静脉期强化程度迅速减低，低于周围正常强化的肝组织。

(5)肝血管异常：肝内血管可发生血管解剖学上的变异和病理性异常。CTA 具有类似 DSA 的诊断效果，能很好地显示肝脏血管的解剖变异，显示肿瘤的供血动脉。肿瘤对血管的侵犯，表现为血管边缘不规则及受压、移位；门静脉及肝静脉血栓或瘤栓显示为充盈缺损；动脉期出现门静脉或肝静脉显影则提示动静脉瘘。

3. MRI 表现

肝脏病变所致其轮廓、大小及形态改变的意义与 CT 相似；MRI 依据肝脏病变信号强化分为五个等级：①等信号：病变与肝实质信号相同；②极低信号：信号与肝内留空血管信号相同；③稍低信号：信号介于肝实质与留空血管信号；④稍高信号：信号介于脂肪与肝实质之间；⑤极高信号：信号与脂肪相同。肝脏实性肿瘤，多数具有细胞内水分增多的特征，在 T1WI 上显示为稍低信号，在 T2WI 上则为稍高信号；在 T1WI 上若病灶内见高信号，则提示出血或含脂肪成分；增强扫描后不同病变强化特点及方式与 CT 相似。

第四节 常见疾病诊断

1. 原发性肝细胞癌

(1)临床及病理表现：原发性肝细胞癌，通常称为肝癌，是肝脏最常见的原发性恶性肿瘤。男性患者多于女性。肝癌的病因复杂，已知与肝硬化、乙型肝炎病毒感染、和致癌物摄入有关。HCC 分为巨块型、结节型、弥漫型和小癌型。肝癌早期常无症状，中晚期常出现肝区痛、右上腹肿块、消瘦，甚者可出现发热、黄疸。血清 AFP 常增高。

(2)影像学表现：

1)CT 表现：平扫表现为低密度病灶或等密度灶，肿瘤边界可有包膜，可见一圈低密度带[图 11-5(a)、(b)]。多数肿瘤密度均匀，较大肿瘤因钙化、出血、坏死和囊变而致密度不均匀。动态 CT 增强表现：动脉期：绝大多数呈明显强化[图 11-6(a)、(b)]；实质期：绝大多数病灶密度迅速降低，低于周围正常强化的肝组织；门静脉和肝静脉受侵犯表现为血管增粗，密度不均，增强后可见腔内充盈缺损影(图 11-7)。许多肝硬化患者有门静脉血栓形成，许多肝癌患者有癌栓形成。这两个常见的表现可同时发生，区分血栓和癌栓非常重要。首先门静脉内如果是癌栓，它就会强化，动脉期最好显示；其次，如果门静脉内是癌栓，它常会导致血管直径的增加，有时癌栓内可能会出现新生血管。

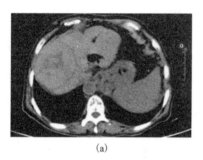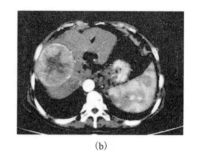

(a)　　　　　　　　　　　　　　　　　(b)

（a）肝癌 CT 平扫示肝 S7，8 稍低或等密度灶，肿瘤边界可有包膜，呈低密度环形影－"晕环征"；（b）肝癌 CT 动态增强扫描，动脉期见病灶明显强化。

图 11-5　肝癌

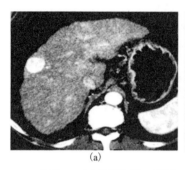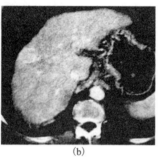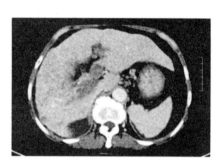

(a)　　　　　　　　　(b)

（a）肝癌 CT 动态增强扫描，动脉期肝 S8 病灶明显强化；（b）门脉期，病灶密度减低。

图 11-6　肝癌

在门静脉期 CT 上，门静脉主干和分支内可见低密度充盈缺损。

图 11-7　肝癌并门静脉癌栓

2）MRI 表现：原发性肝癌在 T1WI 上肝癌常呈低信号或等信号，在 T2WI 上常呈高信号。肿瘤边缘包膜和中心瘢痕在 T1WI 上常呈低信号，癌瘤信号常因出血、坏死、瘢痕而不均匀。注射造影剂后肝癌信号明显增强，可低于或高于正常肝的信号，境界更为清楚，其中低信号区（出血、坏死、瘢痕）则无强化。若有门静脉内瘤栓，可于低信号的门静脉中出现高信号块影［图 11-8（a）~（b）、图 11-9（a）~（b）、图 11-10（a）~（b）］。

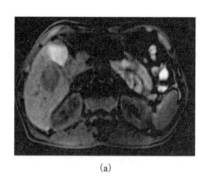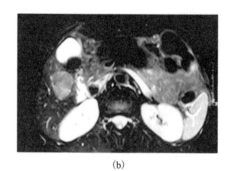

(a)　　　　　　　　　　　　　　　　　(b)

（a）SE T1WI 肝 S5 病灶呈低等混杂信号，可见部分低信号包膜；（b）肝癌，SE T2WI 病灶呈不均匀高信号，边界清楚。

图 11-8　肝癌

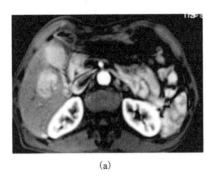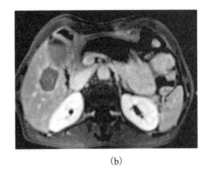

(a)   (b)

（a）在 T1WI 增强动脉晚期(约 35 秒)肝 S5 病灶与肝脏的其余部分相比，明显强化；（b）肝癌，
在 Gd-DTPA 门静脉期，与肝的其余部分相比，肝癌的包膜(箭头)表现延迟强化，然而肿块表
现迅速廓清，呈低信号。

图 11-9　肝癌

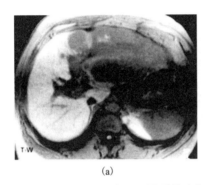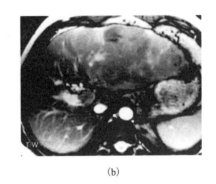

(a)   (b)

（a）SE T1WI，肝左叶肝癌，显示门静脉及右主支增粗；（b）肝癌伴癌栓，SE T2WI，门静脉流
空信号消失伴信号增高(箭头)。

图 11-10　肝癌伴癌栓

3）DSA 表现：肝癌主要由肝动脉供血，在造影中可见到动脉门静脉
瘘，门静脉受侵常见，肝静脉受侵少见（图 11-11）。

2.肝海绵状血管瘤

（1）临床及病理表现：肝海绵状血管瘤是肝脏最常见的良性肿瘤。
病灶通常为单发较小(直径 2 cm)，多发者(2 个以上)者占 50%。有时血
管瘤可以很大。血管瘤一般无包膜，切面呈囊状或筛状空隙，犹如海绵。
肝血管瘤常无任何临床症状，常为影像学检查时偶然发现，只有少数大
的血管瘤因压迫肝组织或邻近脏器，产生上腹部不适或腹痛。

（2）影像学表现：

1）CT 表现：平扫为球形或类圆形低密度区［图 11-12(a)］，但是在
肝硬化中表现为等或高密度。较大的血管瘤，其中心部分呈更低密度

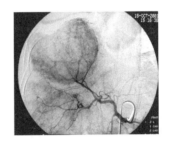

肝右叶巨大肝癌动脉期 DSA 显示肿
瘤血管不规则，染色；外周动脉呈弧
形压迫伴移位。

图 11-11　肝癌 DSA 检查

区，代表疤痕组织、血栓形成或陈旧性出血灶，钙化很少见。增强为动脉期扫描典型和常见表现为早期病
灶边缘强化［图 11-12(b)］，呈结节状高密度，代表瘤中的"血窦"，其密度与主动脉的密度相近，明显高于
正常肝；小血管瘤可立即完全强化。延时扫描可见增强的范围逐渐向中心扩展，且增强程度则逐渐减低，
最后整个血管瘤被造影剂"填满"，即整个血管瘤与肝的密度相等［图 11-12(b)、(c)］。强化不均匀，大血
管瘤可夹杂广泛的病灶内纤维化，显示瘤灶周边结节状强化，中心出现无强化区。小血管瘤强化类型也不
同，动脉期呈均匀强化。

2）MRI表现：血管瘤在T1WI上表现为均匀低信号区，T2WI上为高信号。较大的血管瘤则在其中心结构不均匀且T1WI信号更低，乃由于其中的血管和纤维化所致。T2WI对鉴别诊断很重要，血管瘤的T2WI信号很高，在重T2WI多回波上更明显，即所谓"亮灯"征［图11-13（a）~（c）］。血管瘤的表现不典型较少见，如不均匀性、快速强化、钙化、血栓形成、出血伴液液平面以及纤维化。

3）DSA表现：动脉期表现为病灶边缘出现点状或结节状强化，之后毛细血管强化，静脉期血管染色弥散，周边有环状强化。供血动脉无增宽，不出现动静脉分流（图11-14）。

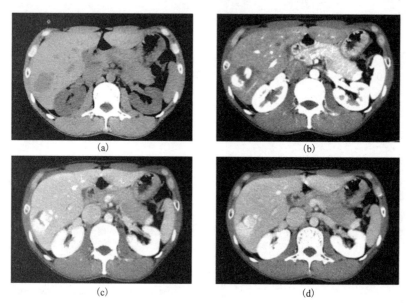

（a）CT平扫显示肝S6近包膜下低密度灶；（b）CT增强扫描，动脉期病灶周边结节、环形强化；（c）门脉期，病灶强化范围扩大，自周围向中央呈向心性填充方式强化；（d）延迟期，病灶几乎完全强化，与正常肝实质密度一致。

图11-12　肝血管瘤

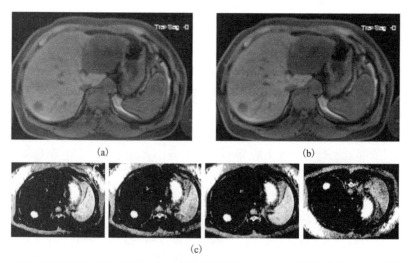

（a）T1WI脂肪抑制上肝S2及S7病灶呈圆形低信号灶；（b）T2WI脂肪抑制，病灶呈高信号；（c）T2WI多回波，随回波时间的延长，病灶信号无衰减，呈"亮灯征"。

图11-13　肝血管瘤MRI

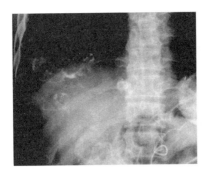

经腹主动脉造影，肝脏膈顶区见斑片状血管湖，主要分布在外周部分，无肿瘤血管。

图 11-14 肝血管瘤常规血管造影

3. 肝转移性肿瘤

（1）临床及病理表现：肝转移瘤比肝原发恶性肿瘤更常见。包括骨骼在内的全身任何部位的恶性肿瘤都可转移至肝脏。转移瘤主要由肝动脉供血。

（2）影像学表现：

1）CT 表现：平扫表现为大小不等的多发圆形低密度灶。增强扫描：大多数病灶呈边缘强化，中心低密度，延时扫描病灶无延时强化［图 11-15（a）、（b）］。血供丰富病例，动脉期整个病灶均匀或不均匀强化，门静脉期和延迟期病灶密度降低，呈等密度而不可见。

2）MRI 表现：多数转移瘤 T1WI 呈低信号，T2WI 呈高信号，瘤内有坏死、囊变、出血、钙化等改变时，则病灶内信号不均匀［图 11-16（a）、（b）］。

3）DSA 表现：转移瘤多数为少血供，呈低密度。少数富血供转移瘤可见肿瘤染色。因其敏感性、特异性低，又具有创性，现少用，但是可用来进行外科手术评价和经肝动脉进行化疗栓塞术。

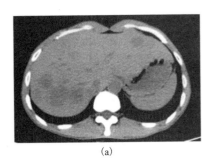
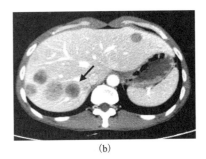

(a)   (b)

（a）CT 平扫肝内可见多发类圆形低密度灶，其内可见更低密度区；（b）CT 增强扫描，病灶周边轻度强化，中心更低密度区无强化，肝右叶病灶呈"牛眼征"（箭头）。

图 11-15 肝转移癌

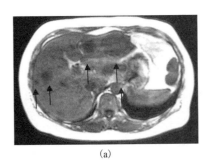
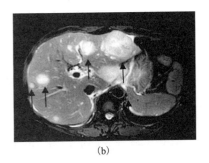

(a)   (b)

（a）SE T1WI，肝内多发类圆形低信号灶（箭头）；（b）SE T2WI，病灶呈高信号（箭头）。

图 11-16 肝转移癌 MRI

4. 肝囊肿

(1)临床及病理表现：真正的肝囊肿系肝内异常胆道囊状扩张，系肝内胆道发育不全且不与正常胆道连接。囊肿从数毫米到 10 cm 以上不等，可单发或多发。通常无临床症状，巨大囊肿可压迫肝脏和邻近器官，产生上腹部不适或腹痛等。

(2)影像学表现：

1)CT 表现：典型 CT 表现为边界光滑锐利的圆形或卵圆形低密度区，呈水样密度，CT 值 0~10 Hu。单发或多发，增强扫描囊肿无强化，可与血管瘤和转移瘤鉴别(图 11-17)。

2)MRI 表现：T1 加权呈低信号，T2 加权呈高信号，信号均匀，信号强度类似于脑脊液，注射 Gd-DTPA 增强扫描不强化，可与血管瘤鉴别[图 11-18(a)、(b)]。囊肿内出血是单纯性肝囊肿少见的并发症，表现为不均匀性高信号，当混合血液产物时在 T1 和 T2 加权图像上均可见有液液平面。此外，T1 信号升高也见于含有蛋白物质成分。对于这两种情况，在评估增强时使用减影图像法必不可少的。

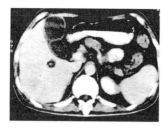

CT 增强示肝 S5 圆形水样无强化的低密度灶，边缘清楚光滑。

图 11-17　肝囊肿

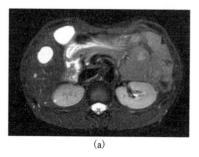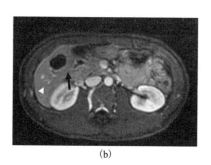

(a)　　　　　　　　　　　　(b)

(a)囊肿 MRIT2 加权像上在肝脏 S5 见一个圆形的水样高信号病灶(黑色箭头)，同时 S6 可见一小稍高信号的海绵状血管瘤(白色箭头)；(b)肝囊肿 MRI 增强 T1 增强扫描显示囊肿(黑色箭头)无强化，边缘光滑，但小血管瘤(白色箭头)可见有明显强化。

图 11-18　肝囊肿

5. 肝脓肿

(1)临床及病理表现：肝脓肿是由于阿米巴原虫和细菌感染而引起，一般病理过程为炎症导致阿米巴性肝炎或细菌性肝炎，病变部分坏死液化，后脓肿形成。脓肿可单发或多发，多见于肝右叶。病变发展可穿破膈而波及胸膜和肺，引起胸膜炎和肺脓肿。临床表现为高热、肝肿大、肝区疼痛。

(2)影像学表现：

1)X 线表现：透视和 X 线平片，偶可见肝区积气和出现气液平面，其余征象均缺乏特异性，诊断价值有限。

2)CT 表现：平扫显示为境界清楚的圆形低密度区。增强扫描脓腔不强化，脓肿壁呈环形增强，轮廓光滑整齐，厚度均匀。若腔内有气体和(或)液面则可确诊[图 11-19(a)、(b)]。

3)MRI 表现：肝脓肿在 MRI 上呈液体病变的信号特征。T1WI 上呈圆形、境界清楚的低信号区，其周围有一圈稍低信号晕围绕。T2WI 呈明显高信号，周边的环状壁亦稍呈低信号。注射 Gd-DTPA 增强扫描后这一圈晕呈高信号环。若腔内有气体和(或)液面则可确诊[图 11-20(a)~(d)]。DWI 序列显示脓肿腔内高信号，周围高信号，ADC 上脓肿腔内低信号，周围高信号。

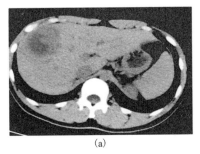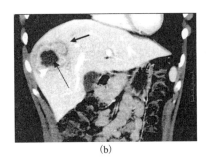

(a)　(b)

(a)CT平扫，肝S8见不均匀类圆形低密度灶，边缘模糊；(b)CT增强扫描：可见"环征"，外环低密度灶为水肿区(黑色箭头)，内环明显强化为脓肿壁(白色箭头)，中央坏死区域无增强(黑长箭头)。

图11-19　肝脓肿

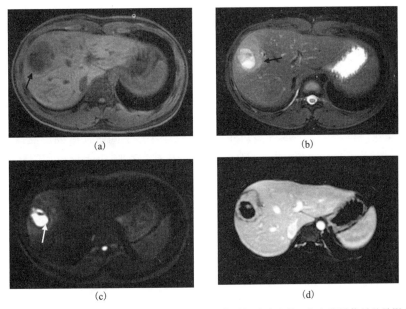

(a)　(b)

(c)　(d)

(a)在T1加权成像MRI上，肝脏S8可见一圆形低信号的脓腔病灶，伴有稍低信号的晕影(箭头)；(b)在T2加权成像上，脓腔呈高信号，内层低信号为脓肿壁，外层略高信号为水肿带(箭头)；(c)在DWI序列上，脓腔灶的坏死区域显示扩散受限，呈高信号，这是脓肿的特征性表现；(d)肝脓肿肝脓肿强化方式与CT类似。

图11-20　肝脓肿

6.脂肪肝

(1)临床及病理表现：脂肪肝(又叫肝脏脂肪变性)系过量脂肪尤其是甘油三酯在肝细胞内过度沉积所致。饮酒、肥胖症、酒精中毒性肝病或高脂肪、高胆固醇饮食等均可引起脂肪浸润。临床上，多无症状，重者伴肝功能损害，肝区不适、胀痛，或出现与病因有关的相关症状。

(2)影像学表现：

1)CT表现：平扫示肝脏普遍性或局限性的密度减低，而其内的血管走行没有变化。肝实质密度改变：CT诊断脂肪肝的标准一般参照脾脏，正常人平扫，肝CT值高于脾脏，肝脏CT值低于脾脏即可诊断为脂肪肝。正常肝实质密度高于血管，平扫血管影呈负影，肝静脉、门静脉分支清晰可辨。脂肪肝实质密度普遍下降，与肝内血管密度接近，使肝内血管影变得模糊或不能显示，严重脂肪肝时，肝脏密度低于肝内血管内血液密度，血管影可呈高密度。增强扫描，脂肪肝增强后仍保持相对低密度，仍低于脾脏，而肝内血管增强后特别清晰[图11-21(a)、(b)]。

尽管不能用脾脏信号来作为参照比较，MRI可见T1加权信号正常或稍高，局灶性者则T1加权上高于

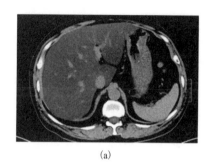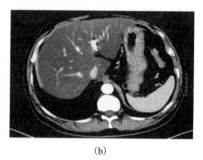

(a) (b)

(a)CT平扫：肝脏密度普遍降低，肝内血管密度相对增高；(b)CT增强扫描：肝实质轻度强化，肝内血管显示更清楚。

图 11-21 脂肪肝

正常肝组织，T2 加权和质子加权为稍高信号，脂肪抑制则显示病灶区低信号，肝内血管位置正常。脂肪抑制序列，如 STIR 序列上，信号不增高，细微变化难以鉴别时，需要同反相位来评估，同反相位上反相位信号减低。

7. 肝硬化

(1)临床及病理表现：肝硬化是以广泛结缔组织增生、坏死、瘢痕形成为特征的一类慢性肝病，肝细胞大量坏死，正常肝组织代偿性增生，形成许多再生结节，大小不一，同时伴肝内广泛纤维化，使肝小叶结构和血管结构紊乱。肝硬化患者肝癌的发病率增高。严重的并发症有肝功能衰竭和门脉高压导致食道静脉曲张破裂出血。肝硬化的病因甚多。

(2)影像学表现：

1)CT 表现：早期肝硬化 CT 表现可以为正常。进展期表现为肝体积缩小，并肝结构的重建。肝轮廓凹凸不平呈结节状，肝各叶大小比例失常，常是尾叶与左叶较大而右叶较小，肝门和肝裂增宽。脾增大是诊断肝硬化的重要根据，其外缘前后径超过 5 个单元，(一个肋骨或肋间隙称为一个肋单元)。病情进展者或伴有腹水。增强 CT 肝实质有不均匀强化[图 11-22(a)、(b)]。

2)MRI 表现：肝硬化对 T1 和 T2 弛豫时间的影响不明显。但是因为 Kupffer 细胞减少，用超磁氧化铁做造影剂时，吸收会减少。肝再生结节显示较好，T1WI 和 T2WI 呈低信号，超磁氧化铁造影时，肝再生结节因 Kupffer 细胞含量少，呈高信号[图 11-23(a)、(b)]。

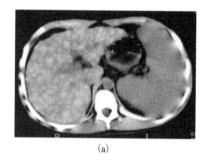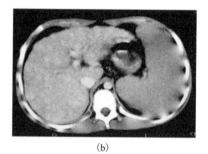

(a) (b)

(a)CT平扫，肝脏密度不均匀，可见略高密度结节，肝表面呈波浪状，脾大；(b)CT增强扫描，门脉期肝实质强化，平扫所见结节影部分已不甚明显。

图 11-22 肝硬化

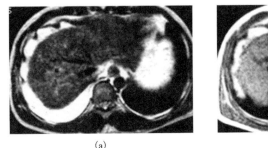
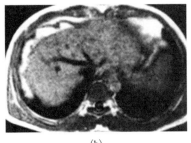

(a)　　　　　　　　　　　　　　(b)

(a)肝硬化 MRI SE T$_1$WI；(b)肝硬化 MRI SE T$_2$WI 肝右叶缩小，左叶大，脾大，肝内信号未见异常，肝右叶缩小，左叶大，脾大，肝内信号未见异常，右侧胸腔可见少量积液。

图 11-23　肝硬化

（袁友红，罗伟，李秀梅，蒋洪涛，毛志群，肖恩华，刘辉）

Chapter 11

Liver

Section 1　Method of examination

1. X-ray examination

Only an approximate estimate of liver contour and size, calcification and gas can be seen on the plain film appearances. It is useless in the diagnosis of liver diseases.

Hepaticangiography is useful to diagnosis thetumor of the liver. The blood supply of hepatocellular carcinoma comes mainly from the hepatic artery. Hepaticangiography can show the structure of the tumor, so can make the diagnosis of the location and the nature. Catheter-assisted angiography of the liver is performed via a catheter that is placed in either a selective or a superselective location. Celiac axis injection is inadequate for the detection of focal liver lesions. Selective or superselective injections with a slow infusion of iodinated contrast material and a prolonged filming sequence is the most accurate technique for detection of focal hepatic masses. Occasionally, oblique filming may be necessary.

2. CT examination

CT has become the mainstay for hepatocellular imaging because of its high spatial resolution and rapid acquisition times. The development of spiral CT scanning has had a significant impact on hepatic imaging. CT of the liver can be performed with or without contrast material. Scanning without the use of contrast material is the simplest but least informative method of performing CT of the liver.

Normal liver parenchyma has an attenuation of + 55 to + 65 HU. By comparison, the spleen measures 8 to 10 HU less than the liver. Hepatic tumors, unless well-differentiated primary neoplasms, do not contain glycogen; therefore, they are hypoattenuating relative to normal parenchyma. However, the difference in attenuation between parenchyma and tumor can be quite subtle on a noncontrasted study. This results in unenhanced CT being 10% to 15% less sensitive in detecting focal hepatic lesions than dynamic sequential enhanced CT.

Contrast-enhanced CT is a more sensitive examination for the detection of focal hepatic lesions. This permits two separate breath-held scans of the entire liver, one obtained during the arterial dominant phase and the other obtained during the portal venous dominant phase. This "dual-phase" examination is optimal for the evaluation of hypervascular lesions that may be isoattenuating to normal hepatic parenchyma on images acquired during the portal venous dominant phase of enhancement. Unlike the remainder of the liver, which receives the majority of its blood fromthe portal vein, these hypervascular lesions receive virtually their entire blood supply from the hepatic artery. Therefore, a dual-phase study with both hepatic arterial dominant and portal venous dominant phase images should be used in patients with known or suspected hypervascular tumors in whom determination of the extent of disease would affect therapy. The hepatic arterial dominant phase images maximize lesion detection, whereas the portal venous dominant phase images allow for evaluation of vascular structures and provide more optimal imaging of extrahepatic organs.

3. MRI examination

In general, both T1-and T2-weighted sequences are necessary for a complete examination of the liver. The T1-weighted images provide clear anatomic detail and high lesion detection. The T2-weighted images have greater lesion detection than T1-weighted images; although anatomy is less well defined. Numerous T2-weighted sequences also are available. Postcontrast T1-weighted images are a standard feature in many hepatic imaging protocols. These images are used to help with lesion characterization in those situations in which the unenhanced images are indeterminate. Gadopentetatedimeglumine (Gd-DTPA) is the most commonly used MR contrast agents. These agents shorten the relaxation times of protons in tissues in which the agent accumulates. Both T1 and T2 relaxation times are shortened, but the T1 relaxation times are shortened to a greater degree than the T2. Because of the short intravascular half-life of the gadolinium chelate, imaging of the liver after contrast administration requires rapid T1-weighted imaging, usually in the form of T1-weighted gradient-recalled echo sequences. Serial dynamic images are obtained during multiple phases of hepatic enhancement: precontrast, during the hepatic arterial dominant phase of enhancement from 20 to 40 seconds after initiation of the contrast bolus, during the portal venous dominant phase of enhancement at 50 to 100 seconds after the initiation of the contrast bolus, and during the equilibrium phase approximately 5 minutes after contrast injection. Lesions can be characterized as hypervascular or hypovascular and may demonstrate a characteristic pattern of enhancement.

Section 2 Normal appearances

1. The location and morphology of the liver

The liver is the largest substantial organ in the upper abdomen, which is close to the abdominal wall under the right diaphragm, and close to the right kidney and adrenal gland, stomach, duodenum, pancreas and other organs, and the lower part is close to the colon. The normal liver is wedge-shape, with the right lobe thickenedand large, while the left one gradually thinned. Ultrasound examination can show liver morphology from any direction; CT and MIRI show liver morphology from transverse, coronal and sagittal positions. The liver has smooth and sharp edges.

2. The size of the liver

Ultrasound can directly measure the diameter line of the liver to evaluate the size of the liver. The anterior and posterior diameter of the right lobe of normal liver was 8~10 cm, and the maximum oblique diameter was 10~14 cm. The thickness of the left lobe shall not exceed 6 cm and the length shall not exceed 9 cm. MSCT and MRI were used to quantitatively detect liver volume, but it was time-consuming. The usual method is to measure the maximum diameter line of the liver lobe and calculate the proportion between them to evaluate the size of each lobe. The ratio of the anterior and posterior diameter of the right/left lobe of normal liver is about 1.2-1.9, and the ratio of the transverse diameter of the right/tail lobe of liver is about 2-3.

3. Division of the liver lobes

The liver is divided into left lobe, right lobe and caudate lobe. In order to meet the needs of surgery, ultrasound, CT and MRI examinations can be divided into liver segments according to the characteristics of the distribution of blood vessels in the liver. According Couinaud method, the left, middle and right hepatic veins are used as the longitudinal division marks, and the left and right main branches of the portal vein are used as the transverse division marks. Thus, the liver is divided into eight liver segments, namely, the caudate lobe is segment I, the left outer upper segment is segment II, the left outer lower segment is segment III, the left inner segment is segment IV, the right anterior lower segment is segment V, the right posterior lower segment is VI, the right posterior upper segment is VII, and the right anterior upper segment is VIII (Figure 11-1).

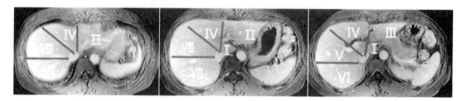

Figure 11-1   Fat suppression and cross section T1WI images showed 8 segments of Couinaud's liver

4. Liver parenchyma

On ultrasound examination, the normal liver parenchyma showed uniform diffuse fine speckled moderate echo (Figure. 11-2).

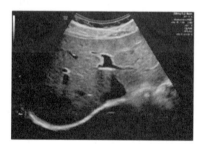

The portal vein, hepatic vein and its branches were clearly displayed, which the echo of vascular wall was strong, and there was no echo in the vascular cavity.

Figure 11-2   Ultrasound examination showed that the normal liver parenchyma showed uniform diffuse small dot-like moderate echo

The normal liver parenchyma showed uniform soft tissue density on plain CT scan, which was higher than that of the spleen. The CT value was about 55-75 HU, and the blood vessels showed round or tubular low-density shadows [Figure 11-3(a)]. CT multi-phase enhancement examination can reflect the blood supply characteristics of liver parenchyma, that is, the arterial phase enhancement is not obvious, the portal phase enhancement reaches the peak, and the equilibrium phase enhancement is weakened [Figure 11-3(b), (d)].

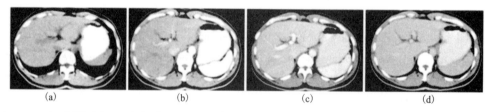

(a)   (b)   (c)   (d)

A cross-sectional CT plain scan(a); A cross-sectional enhanced CT artery(b); A cross-sectional enhanced CT portal vein phase(c); A cross-sectional enhanced CT balance phase(d).

Figure 11-3   Normal liver CT plain scan and enhanced images

MRI examination showed that the signal of the normal liver parenchyma was uniform. The signal on T1WI was medium, higher than that of the spleen, and the signal on T2WI was low, significantly lower than that of the spleen [Figure 11-4(a), (b)]. The enhancement of liver parenchyma was the same as that of CT in multistage enhanced T1WI

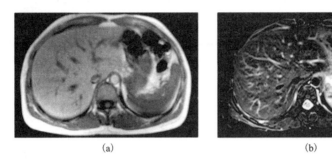

(a)　　　　　　　　　　　　(b)

The signal intensity of normal liver parenchyma was higher than that of spleen on cross-sectional T1WI(a), while that of normal liver parenchyma was lower than that of spleen on cross-sectional fat suppression T2WI(b).

Figure 11-4

5. Hepatic vessels

Hepatic artery and portal vein enter the liver through hepatic hilum and continue to be divided into each hepatic lobe and segmental vessel. The branches of the hepatic veins finally converge to form the left, middle, and right hepatic veins and enter the inferior vena cava at the second portal.

DSA examination can show the hepatic artery, portal vein and its branches, which are distributed in a dendritic manner in the liver, running naturally with smooth edges. Ultrasonography can clearly show portal vein, hepatic vein and its branches, strong echo in the vessel wall and no echo in the vessel cavity (Figure 11-2). In CT examination, hepatic vein and portal vein branches usually presented as bar or round low-density shadows in liver parenchyma during plain scan, while hepatic artery branches could not be shown. In the arterial phase, the hepatic artery and its branches were shown as scattered linear and dotted high-density shadows. At the stage of portal vein, the portal vein and its left and right branches were significantly enhanced; the left, middle and right hepatic veins were enhanced at the equilibrium phase. CTA can display the complete picture of blood vessels from multiple directions. MRI examination showed that the larger portal vein, hepatic vein and inferior vena cava showed no signal tubular structure on SE sequence T1WI and T2WI due to the effervescent cava effect, while the smaller blood vessels showed high signal tubular structure on T2WI due to the flow-related enhancement effect. MRA can better show portal vein and hepatic vein from different directions.

Section 3　Basic pathological changes

1. X-ray findings

When the liver volume increases significantly, the top of the right diaphragm can be seen on the plain film, and the inferior hepatic angle moves downward, and the intrahepatic calcified lesions can show high-density shadows. X-rays of liver area are of limited value and are rarely used now.

Abnormal angiographic findings include: Thinning or thickening of the hepatic artery; The pressure and displacement of the blood vessel; Abnormal new blood vessel; also called tumor blood vessel or pathological blood vessel, it is a new blood vessel with uneven thickness and disorder, which is malignant Important signs of tumor; Vascular infiltration: stenosis, occlusion, and stiffness of the blood vessel wall; Tumor staining: Contrast agent clearance in the lesion is delayed, and the capillary or venous phase shows increased density; Filling defect: no blood supply in the diseased area, no contrast in the venous phase, The blank area stained withreagent is common in cystic lesions without blood supply or tumor liquefaction necrosis; Venous early manifestation: that is, the portal vein or hepatic vein is visible in the arterial phase, which is mostly caused by the arteriovenous short circuit caused by the destruction of blood vessels by the tumor; Portal vein filling defect: filling defect caused by tumor thrombus, with new tumor blood vessels supplying blood, tumor thrombus Line-like and flake-like enhanced images can also be seen inside.

2. CT findings

(1) Liver size and shape. The enlargement of the liver is manifested by the blunt edge of the liver and the full shape of the liver lobe; the opposite is the case with atrophy. The liver cirrhosis shows the reduction of the liver volume and the reconstruction of the liver structure; the liver contour is uneven and nodular; the size of the liver lobes is abnormal, often the caudate lobe and the left lobe are larger and the right lobe is smaller; the hilum and fissure are widened. Enlargement of the spleen is an important basis for diagnosing liver cirrhosis. The anteroposterior diameter of the outer edge exceeds 5 units (a rib or intercostal space is called a rib unit).

(2) Liver edges and contours. Regenerative nodules or space-occupying lesions of liver cirrhosis can make the liver contour uneven, the liver edge angle becomes blunt, loses normal edges and corners and becomes rounded, and the edges are jagged or wavy.

(3) Diffuse liver disease. It is a group of diffuse liver cell degeneration and necrosis diseases, which can cause changes in liver size, shape, and density, such as liver cirrhosis, fatty liver, hemochromatosis, and hepatolenticular degeneration. CT showed that the density of the whole liver or a certain lobe or segment of the liver was decreased, increased, or showed mixed density.

(4) Focal lesions of the liver. Common diseases such as liver cysts, abscesses, parasites and various tumors. Most of the flat scans are single or multiple round, round or irregular lumps. After enhancement, cysts or poor blood supply lesions show no enhancement or mild enhancement. The abscess cavity is not strengthened, the wall of the abscess is enhanced in a circular shape, the outline is smooth and neat, and the thickness is uniform. The arterial phase of cavernous hemangioma is characterized by nodular enhancement on the edge, and the range of enhancement in the venous phase and delayed scanning gradually expands to the center, and finally the entire hemangioma is "filled up" with contrast agent. Most liver cancers show obvious uneven enhancement in the arterial phase, and the degree of enhancement in the portal vein phase decreases rapidly, which is lower than the normal enhancement of the surrounding liver tissue.

(5) Abnormal liver blood vessels. Vascular anatomy and pathological abnormalities can occur in blood vessels in the liver. CTA has a diagnostic effect similar to DSA, can well show the anatomical variation of liver blood vessels and show the blood supply arteries of the tumor. Tumor's invasion of blood vessels is manifested as irregular, compressed and displaced vascular edges; portal vein and hepatic vein thrombosis or tumor thrombus appear as filling defects; portal vein or hepatic vein visualization in the arterial phase indicates arteriovenous fistula.

3. MRI findings

The significance of the changes in contour, size and morphology caused by liver lesions is similar to that of CT; MRI is divided into five grades based on the signal enhancement of liver lesions: Iso-signal: the signal of the lesion is the same as the liver parenchyma; Very low signal: the signal and the liver Empty blood vessel signals are the same; Slightly low signal: the signal is between the liver parenchyma and the empty blood vessel signal; Slightly high signal: the signal is between the fat and liver parenchyma; extremely high signal: the signal is the same as the fat. Most of the solid tumors of the liver have the characteristics of increased intracellular water, which shows slightly low signal on T1WI and slightly high signal on T2WI; if there is a high signal in the lesion on T1WI, it indicates bleeding or contains fatty components; The enhancement features and methods of different lesions after enhanced scan are similar to CT.

Section 4　Diagnosis of common diseases

The purpose of the examinations of liver is to confirm the mass in the liver and to make sure its location and nature, and to differentiate the location in or out the liver, to know the blood vessel structure and its pathological changes, such as the reason of portal hypertension and side branch circulation.

1. Hepatocellular carcinoma (HCC)

(1) Clinical and pathological manifestations: Most common primary malignant tumor of the liver occurs predominantly in patients with underlying parenchymal liver disease. In general, men are affected more frequently than women. The main aetiological factors of HCC are cirrhosis, hepatitis B infection and carcinogens. HCC can be expansive (solitary, multifocal) or more rarely diffusely infiltrating. Patients present with abdominal pain and often have a palpable mass; jaundice, weight loss, and fever are often present. The serum alpha-fetoprotein is often elevated.

(2) Imaging manifestations:

1) CT findings: On precontrast CT, HCC may appear hypo-or iso-attenuation relative to the surrounding parenchyma. A tumor capsule may be visible in isoattenuating lesions as a thin peripheral hypoattenuating rim [Figure 11-5(a), (b)]. Most HCC appear homogeneous but inhomogeneous attenuation may be due to areas of calcification, necrosis or fatty metamorphosis. On dynamic contrast enhanced CT, HCC displays an early moderate to high degree of homogeneous enhancement on artery phase [Figure 11-6(a), (b)]. The contrast enhancement is transient and the lesion becomes iso-or hypoattenuating during the parenchymatous-venous phase [Figure 11-6 (b)]. Portal and hepatic vein invasion by HCC is observed as a filling defect within the contrast enhanced vascular lumen (Figure 11-7).

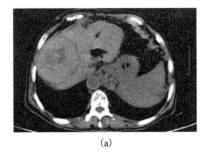
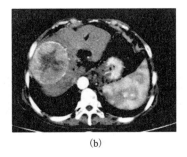

(a)　　　　　　　　　　　　　　(b)

(a) Precontrast CT appears isoattenuation lesioninsegments7 and 8, a tumor capsule may be visible as a thin peripheral hypoattenuating rim. (b) dynamic contrast enhanced CT displays a high degree of enhancement on artery phase.

Figure 11-5　HCC

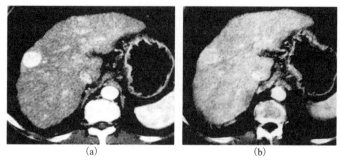

（a）dynamic contrast enhanced CT displays a high degree of enhancement in segments8 on artery phase；（b）the lesion attention becomes low during the venous phase.

Figure 11-6　HCC

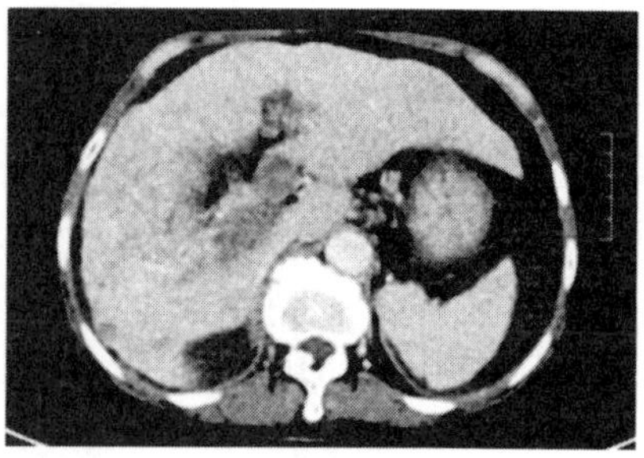

with portal vein cancerous emboli：it was found the filling defects within the trunk and branches of portal vein lumen on the portal venous phase CT.

Figure 11-7　HCC

2）MRI findings：

On T1-weighted images HCC is iso-or hypointensity. On T2-weighted images the majority of HCC are hyperintensity. The capsule, as well as the central scar, is usually markedly hypointensity on T1-weighted images. Frequently the signal intensity is inhomogeneous due to haemorrhagiaand scar and necrosis within the tumor. Dynamic contrast enhanced MRI with Gadolinium DTPA, which is able to detect more lesions than unenhanced MRI, shows an enhancement pattern similar to that observed on contrast enhanced dynamic CT［Figure 11-8（a），（b），Figure 11-9（a），（b），Figure 11-10（a），（b）］.

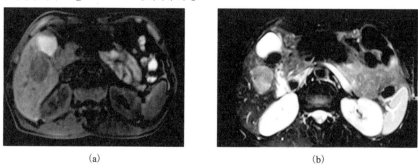

（a）The lesion（arrow）insegments5shows hypointensity on T1-weighted fat-saturated images；（b）The lesion（arrowa）in segments5is inhomogeneouslyhyperintensity on T2-weighted fat-saturated MRI.

Figure 11-8　HCC

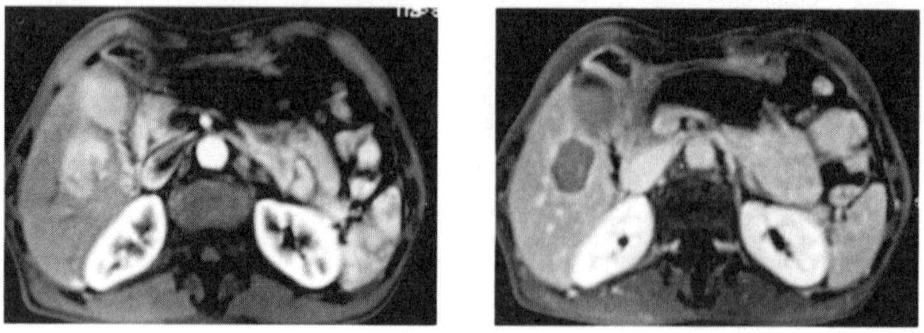

（a）The mass enhances obviously compared to the rest of the liver during late arterial phase.（~35 seconds）on T1-weighted image；（b）The capsule（arrow）of HCC shows delayed enhancement with Gd-DTPA on portal phase and the mass then washes out rapidly, becoming hypoattenuating in the portal venous phase, compared to the rest of the liver.

Figure 11-9　HCC

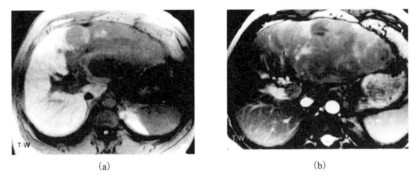

(a) with portal vein tumor thrombus (PVTT). The left lobe HCC shows the diameter of the main and right branches of portal vein increase on T1-weighted images; (b) with PVTT. Portal vein flow void signal disappeared with hyperintensity on T2-weighted images (arrow).

Figure 11-10　HCC

3) DSA findings: The blood supply of HCC comes mainly from the hepatic artery. Arterioportal blood shunting due to portal invasion is not uncommon. Portal vein invasion is frequently present whereas hepatic vein invasion occurs more rarely (Figure 11-11).

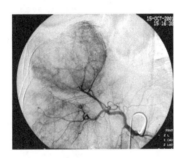

The massive HCC in the right lobe of liver shows irregular tumor vessels and staining on arterial phase DSA, while the peripheral artery shows compression with displacement.

Figure 11-11　DSA of HCC

2. Hepatic cavernous haemangioma

(1) Clinical and pathological manifestations: Cavernous haemangioma of liver are very common benign liver tumour of mesodermal origin. Cavernous haemangioma are usually small (2 cm diameter) and solitary. However, in 50% of cases they are multiple. Occasionally Cavernous Haemangioma may become very large. Cavernous haemangioma of the liver is composed of blood-filled fairly large or tortuous vascular cavities divided by thin, often incomplete, fibrous septa and lined by a single layer of flat endothelium. The lesions are usually asymptomatic but larger tumours may cause abdominal discomfort or pain.

(2) Imaging manifestations:

1) CT findings: On precontrast CT scans most cavernous haemangiomaappear as hypoattenuating relative to the adjacent liver parenchyma [Figure 11 - 12 (a)]. However, they may be iso-or even hyperattenuating in liver steatosis. The thrombosed, necrotic or fibrotic areas that are frequently present in larger lesions are lower in attenuation than the blood. Very rarely calcifications, particularly in large cavernous haemangioma are visible.

Mostcavernous haemangioma demonstrates a distinctive initial pattern of contrast enhancement during the arterial phase following intravenous bolus injection of contrast medium. This pattern is characterized by peripheral enhancement of one or more mural vascular nodular or globular structures which may partially encircle the tumour, the density is equal to the artery density[Figure 11-12(b)]. Later a progressive "fill-in" of the lesion from the periphery towards the centre seems to start from these peripheral vascular lakes[Figure 11-12(c), (d)]. At this stage the lesion may then become isoattenuating relative to the adjacent liver parenchyma. Huge cavernous haemangioma displays a more "atypical" contrast enhancement pattern consisting of mixed (central and peripheral) enhancement during the arterial phase and incomplete "fill-in" on the delayed scans. This pattern is explained by the presence of extensive areas of scar formation or of cystic cavities filled with fluid. A different pattern of enhancement is observed with some small haemangiomas. They may enhance homogeneously during the arterial phase and thus become completely hyperattenuating at that early phase. This is explained by the very small size of the vascular spaces in these small cavernous haemangioma.

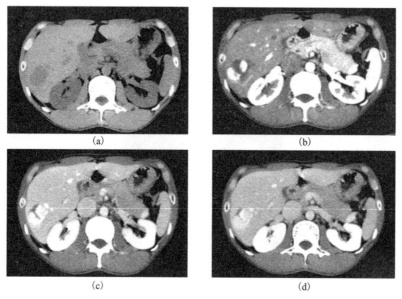

(a) The slightly hypodense lesion is founded near the subcapsular area in thesegment6of the liver on non-contrast CT scan; (b) Hepatic cavernous haemangioma, The lesion shows peripheral ring enhancement on arterial phase CT scan; (c) Hepatic cavernous haemangioma, The enhancement range of the lesion is enlarged with a centripetalfilling pattern on portal venous phase; (d) Hepaticcavernous haemangioma, The lesions is nearly complete enhanced on delayed phase and consistent with the density of normal liver parenchyma.

Figure 11-12　Hepatic cavernous haemangioma

2)MRI findings: On MRI, cavernous haemangiomaappear as well-defined lesions, with smooth borders and slightly lobulated shape. A low signal intensity on T1-weighted images and high signal intensity on T2-weighted imageswill be observed. The high signal intensity of cavernous haemangiomaon T2-weighted images are usually very homogeneous: the so called "light bulb" sign but in larger lesions it may be inhomogeneous due to the variable degree of fibrosis or haemorrhage within the lesion. Cavernous haemangiomaappear also higher in signal intensity than other hepatic neoplasms on T2-weighted images and this becomes particularly more evident on more heavily T2-weighted multiechoimages[Figure 11-13(a)~(c)]. Less frequently, hemangiomas may have atypical features such as heterogeneity, rapid enhancement, calcification, thrombosis, hemorrhage-and fluid-fluid levels, and fibrosis.

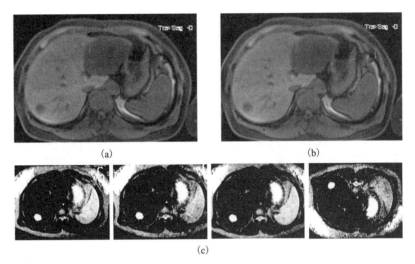

(a)　　　　　　　　　　　　　(b)

(c)

（a）There are two round hypointense lesions in segments 2and 7 of liver on T1-weighted fat-saturated image；（b）The lesions shows hyperintensity on T2-weighted fat-saturated image；（c）With the prolong of echo time and the lesion signal increase the hepatic hemangioma shows a "light bulb" sign on T2-weighted multiecho images.

Figure 11-13　Hepatic cavernous haemangioma

3）DSA findings：During the early arterial phase, punctate or nodular contrast accumulations in the peripheral sinusoids of the lesion are observed. During the late, capillary, and during the venous phase the staining becomes more diffuse while persistent ring shaped contrast puddlings are observed. The afferent artery does not have an increased calibre. There is usually no arterioportal shunting（Figure 11-14）.

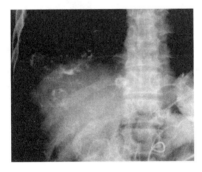

Patchy vascular lakes were found in the diaphragmatic apex of the liver by abdominal aortography and mainly distributed in the peripheral part without tumor blood vessels.

Figure 11-14　Hepatic cavernous haemangioma

3. Hepatic metastasis

（1）Clinical and pathological manifestations：Metastatic tumours in the liver are more common than primary malignant liver tumours. Liver metastases may arise from almost any malignant tumour in the body including bone. The vascular supply of most liver metastases is mainly of arterial origin.

（2）Imaging manifestations：

1）CT findings：Most metastatic liver lesions are focal with a round shape and sharply marginated border. Their size is extremely variable. On precontrast CT most liver metastases are visible as focal hypoattenuating areas relative to the adjacent liver parenchyma. On contrast CT some hypodense lesions may show rim enhancement, the central is hypodense. On delayed images no enhancement. Hypervascular metastases show early arterial enhancement but may become isoattenuating and thus invisible, during the portal venous or delayed phase of enhancement[Figure 11 -15(a), (b)].

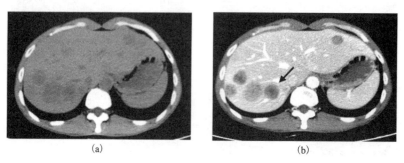

(a)   (b)

(a) Thereare multiple round mild hypointensity foci lesions in the liver on non-contrast CT scan and very low hypoattenuation areas could be seen in the central of lesion; (b) Hepatic metastasis. The lesions had slight ring enhancement on contrast-enhanced CT scan and no enhancement was found in the lower density area of the center. The lesion looks like "cow's eye sign" (arrow) in the right lobe of the liver.

Figure 11-15 Hepatic metastasis

2) MRI findings: Most hepatic metastases are hypointense on T1-weighted and hyperintense on T2-weighted images relative to the liver parenchyma. Metastases are often inhomogeneous in signal intensity due to haemorrhageand necrosisand calcification within the tumour[Figure 11-16(a), (b)].

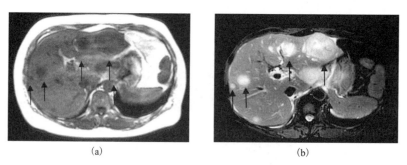

(a)   (b)

(a) There are multiple round hypointenselesions (arrow) in the liver on T1-weighted image MRI; (b) The lesions display hyperintense (arrow) on T2-weighted image fat-saturated MRI.

Figure 11-16 Hepatic metastasis

3) DSA findings: Most liver metastases is less vascular supply. Arteriography are visible as focal hypoattenuating areas. Hypervascular metastases show the tumour staining. Arteriography show is no longer used for the detection or characterization of liver metastases, but can be performed to display the arterial anatomy for planning surgical intervention or as part of transcatheter intra-arterial chemo-or embolotherapy.

4. Hepatic cyst

(1) Clinical and pathological manifestations: Cysts of liver are very common benign liver tumour Cysts from congenital origin arising from peripheral bile ducts. Their size is extremely variable, solitaryor multiple. They are frequent incidental findings on cross-sectional imaging studies of the liver. The lesions are usually asymptomatic but larger tumours may cause abdominal discomfort or pain.

（2）Imaging manifestations：

1）CT findings：On CT, small, circumscribed, round or oval homogeneously hypodense lesions with attenuation values between 0 and +10 HU are seen. Their size is extremely variable, solitaryor multiple. Following injection of contrast medium no enhancement of the cyst wall is seen. The administration of contrast medium will also help in the differential diagnosis with cavernous haemangioma and with metastasis(Figure 11-17).

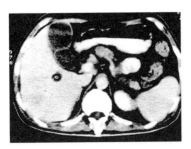

There is a water attenuation lesion in the right lobe of the liver with no enhancement and well-defined rim.

Figure 11-17　Hepatic cyst on CT

2）MRI findings：MRI features of simple hepatic cysts are well-defined homogeneous lesions with hypointense signal intensity on T1-weighted sequences and hyperintense signal intensity on T2-weighted sequences. Following Gadolinium injection cysts will show no enhancement, which can be helpful in the differential diagnosis with cavernous haemangioma[Figure 11-18(a), (b)].

In instances of intracystic hemorrhage, which is a rare complication in simple hepatic cysts, the signal intensity is high and heterogeneous, with a fluid-fluid level on both T1-and T2-weighted images when mixed-blood products are present. Also, elevated T1 signal can be seen in proteinaceous content. For both these circumstances, using imaging subtraction can be essential when assessing for the presence of enhancement.

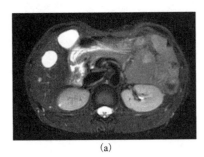 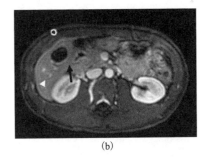

(a)　　　　　　　　　　　(b)

(a)There is a round watery hyperintensitylesion(black arrow)on T2-weighted fat-saturated image in the right lobe of the liver and a small cavernous haemangioma also is visible(white arrow); (b) Simple hepatic cyst onMRI. Thecyst(black arrow) appears no enhancement with smooth rim on contrast T1weighted fat-saturated image but the small hemangioma(white arrow)shows obvious enhancement.

Figure 11-18　Hepatic cyst on MRI

5. Hepatic abscess

（1）Clinical and pathological manifestations：Collection of pus that may be of pyogenic or nonpyogenic origin. Among the latter causes, amoebiasis are important.

（2）Imaging manifestations：

1）X-ray findings：Only a gas can be seen on the plain film appearances. It is useless in the diagnosis of hepatic abscess.

2)CT findings: The CT features of abscess on precontrast CT are round or ovoid area of varying size with inhomogeneous fluid attenuation. Following intravenous contrast medium an enhancing rim surrounding the lesion becomes apparent. In abscess gas bubbles or even a gas fluid level may be present[Figure 11-19(a), (b)].

3)MRI findings: MRI is equally able to detect and characterize liver abscess. The MRI appearance of abscess is characterized by liquid signal areas, that is can be seen round and a rim on T1 weighted image, a slightly low signal ring surrounding the lesion. T2 weighted image, the lesion is apparent high signal, a slightly low signal ring yet can be seen surrounding the lesion. Following intravenous contrast medium administration, an enhancing rim surrounding the lesion becomes apparent. The powerful diagnostic proof is to be seen the no signal gas in the abscess cavity(Fig 11-20a, b, c, d). It tends to have high signal within the abscess cavity and high signal at the periphery on DWI sequence but on ADC, it tends to have low signal within the abscess cavity and high signal at the periphery.

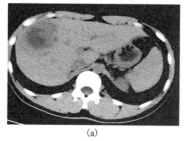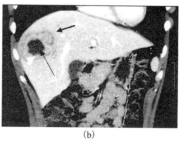

(a) (b)

(a)there is a round inhomogeneoushypo-attenuation lesion with fuzzy edge in the right lobe of the liver; (b)Hepatic abscess on enhanced CT scan. The "ring sign" can beseen, ahypo-attenuation shadow of the outer ringis the edema zone(black arrow), and the inner enhanced ring is the abscess wall (white arrow). There is no enhancement in the central necrotic area(long arrow).

Figure 11-19　Hepatic abscesson non-contrast CT

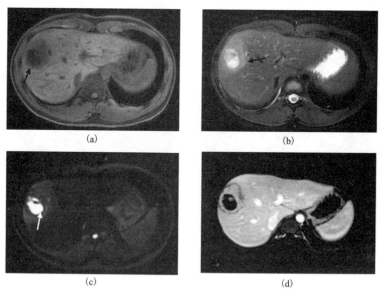

(a) (b)

(c) (d)

(a)there is a round hypointensitypurulent cavity lesion with a slightlyhypointensity signal halo (arrow)in the right lobe of the liver; (b)T2-weighted image MRI. The abscess cavity shows obvious hyperintensity with a mild hypointensity inner layer wall and the slightly hyperintensity outer layer wall represents edema zone (arrow); (c)Thenecrotic area in the pus cavity of lesion showes limited diffusion with a high signal on DWI sequence. It is the characteristic manifestation of abscess; (d)Hepatic abscess. The enhancement pattern of the abscess is similar to CT.

Figure 11-20　Hepatic abscesson T1-weighted image MRI

6. Fatty liver

(1) Clinical and pathological manifestations: Fatty liver (also called fatty metamorphosis of the liver and steatosis of the liver), is an excessive accumulation of triglycerides in the cytoplasma of the hepatocytes. Fatty liver infiltration is associated with a variety of conditions and diseases. Most common are excessive alcohol consumption, obesity, parenteral nutrition and steroids administration or excessive endogeneous production of steroids. Fatty infiltration of the liver usually will not cause any clinical symptomatology, although in some persons, vague upper quadrant pain may be reported. On clinical examination hepatomegaly may be noted and an elevation of enzymes such as transaminases alkaline phosphatases may be present.

(2) Imaging manifestations:

1) CT findings: Non-contrast CT will show generalized or focal reduction in attenuation of liver parenchyma with no distortion of underlying vessels. Whereas in normal individuals the attenuation value of the liver is slightly higher than that of the spleen, in fatty liver infiltration the attenuation values of both organs tend to be equal or the ratios may be reversed. Unenhanced portal and hepatic veins may have greater attenuation than surrounding parenchyma and so may'stand out' in a similar fashion to enhancing vessels in a normal liver. Comparison of hepatic attenuation with that of splenic parenchyma is useful[Figure 11-21(a), (b)].

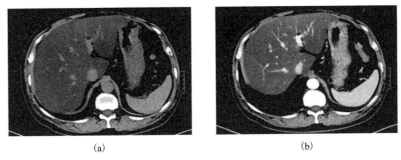

(a)　　　　　　　　　　　　　(b)

(a) Non-contrast CT, the attenuation of liver parenchyma is generally decreased. So the attenuation of intrahepatic vascular was relatively increased; (b) Contrast CT scan, the liver parenchyma was slightly enhancement and the intrahepatic vascular shadow was more clearly.

Figure 11-21　Fatty liver

2) MRI findings: Signal intensity of the liver on MR imaging will be skewed in the direction of fat and so will be increased on both T1-and T2-weighted spin-echo sequences, though the internal standard of the spleen will not be available, making subtle changes difficult to detect. Any increase in signal should not be present on fat-suppressed sequences such as STIR. It requires both in-and out-of-phase imaging and contrast to adequately assess. IP/OP: signal drop out on the out-of-phase sequence.

7. Hepatic cirrhosis

(1) Clinical and pathological manifestations: Hepatic cirrhosisis common chronic disease of the liver characterized by parenchymal necrosis, scarring and extensive fibrosis associated with parenchymal nodular regeneration leading to lobular and vascular disorganization. The main complications are liver failure and portal hypertension with intestinal bleeding from oesophageal varices. There is an increased incidence of hepatocellular carcinoma in patients with cirrhosis secondary to hepatitis. The aetiology of liver cirrhosis is multiple.

(2) Imagingmanifestation:

1) CT findings: During the early stage of liver cirrhosis the liver parenchyma may appear normal on CT. In the later stages there is overall loss of volume as well as volume redistribution. The increased nodularity of the liver

borders is well displayed on CT. The increase in the caudate lobe/right liver lobe ratio is a striking finding in liver cirrhosis and can usually be better evaluated on CT than on ultrasound. The widingportahepatisand liver fissure and enlargement of spleen can be seen. Ascitic fluid may be present. Following contrast enhancement an inhomogeneous degree of enhancement of the liver parenchyma is observed in the cirrhotic liver[Figure 11-22(a), (b)].

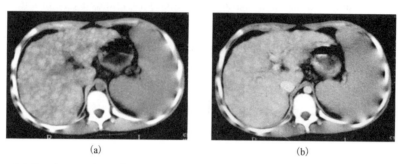

(a)   (b)

(a) Hepatic parenchyma shows inhomogeneous on non-contrast CT and hyper-attenuation nodule can be seen. The surface of liver is wavy and the spleen is large; (b) Hepatic cirrhosison contrast CT scan. The liver parenchyma was enhancementon portal phase and the nodular was not obvious to seen.

Figure 11-22   Hepatic cirrhosis

2) MRI findings: Cirrhosis does not significantly alter the T1 nor the T2 relaxations times but if supermagnetic iron oxide is administered as a contrast agent there is a reduced uptake because of the reduced number of Kupffer cells. Regenerative nodules are mostly hypointense on both the T1-weighted and T2-weighted images. If superparamagnetic iron oxide is administered these nodules may appear hyperintense relative to the liver parenchyma because they contain less Kupffer cells[Figure 11-23(a), (b)].

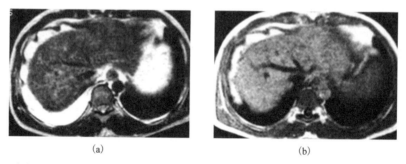

(a)   (b)

(a) Hepatic cirrhosison MRI SE T1WI; (b) Hepatic cirrhosison MRI SE T2WI The volume of the right lobe of the liver is reduced, the left lobe is relatively large, and the spleen is large. There is no abnormal signal in the liver. A small amount of effusion is found in the right pleural cavity.

Figure 11-23

(Yuan Youhong, JiangHongtao, Li Xiumei, Luo Wei, Mao Zhiqun, Xiao Enhua, Liu Hui)

第十二章

胆系

第一节 检查方法

1. X线检查

（1）普通 X 线检查：胆管系统普通 X 线检查主要为右上腹平片，其分辨力较低，只可显示一些含钙质成份较多的胆囊结石、胆囊壁钙化、钙胆汁和胆管积气等。有时胆囊扩大，在周围肠充气衬托下，可以显示胆囊轮廓。由于其诊断价值有限，随着近年超声、CT 等的广泛应用，胆管系统普通 X 线检查已基本被淘汰。

（2）造影检查

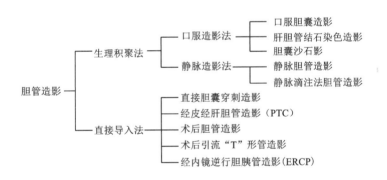

生理积聚法胆管造影以往应用较多，但是其图像质量较差、操作烦琐，而随着超声检查的普及与其图像质量的提高，特别是近年来 MRI 检查中 MRCP 的应用，生理积聚法胆管造影目前临床上也已很少应用。

直接导入法由于其可以进行后续的治疗，目前临床上仍较多采用，尤其是经皮经肝胆管造影（PTC）、经内镜逆行胆胰管造影（ERCP）与术后引流"T"形管造影。检查应在透视监视下进行，以保证安全，并使摄影满意。PTC 在非血管介入放射章节有专门介绍。

"T"形管造影指手术后经"T"形管注入对比剂作胆管造影，对观察胆管内残留结石或其他疾病，以及了解胆管与十二指肠的通畅情况，有较大帮助。

ERCP 指是将十二指肠纤维镜送至十二指肠降段，在透视监视下，经过十二指肠乳头插入导管注入对比剂，以显示胆管或胰管的方法，此方法对胆管系统结石、肿瘤的鉴别诊断（尤其中下段胆管）有重要价值，同时还可留置引流管达到治疗目的。

直接胆囊穿刺造影指不经剖腹而直接经皮胆囊穿刺注入对比剂（阳性碘剂、阴性气体或气体碘剂双重）使胆囊显影，同时可造影后留置引流管从而达到诊断与治疗目的，但由于穿刺成功率不高，且可造成胆瘘、腹膜炎等，现较少应用。

术中胆管造影指手术中直接经胆囊管、胆总管、胆囊、肝内胆管或十二指肠乳头注入对比剂使胆管显影。

2. 超声检查

检查前需禁食 8~12 小时,最好在清晨空腹时检查。一般采用仰卧位,必要时加用右前斜位、左侧卧位、坐位或站立位。右侧肋缘下斜切面与右肋间斜切面适合于观察胆囊与胆管。鉴别胆囊占位病变与结石应改变患者体位探查,如为结石则其影像随体位的改变而移动。B 型超声波检查是目前胆囊与胆管结石、炎症、肿瘤以及先天性胆管囊肿的诊断与鉴别诊断最常用的检查方法。

3. CT 检查

检查前禁食 8~12 小时,一般检查前口服 800~1000 mL 合适浓度的对比剂,如碘剂或水、脂肪等胃肠对比剂,这利于显示胃肠道而又不产生明显假影。CT 检查可分为平扫与增强,且多同时进行肝、胆、胰的CT 检查。常规扫描层厚、层距一般为 10 mm,重点部位可采取 2 mm 或 5 mm 的薄层扫描。

平扫可以显示含钙的结石与胆管梗阻的部位及部分胆囊、胆管肿块;增强扫描一般采用经静脉团注碘剂 80~100 mL 后扫描,增强扫描有助于更好地显示胆管形态与胆管周围的病变、区别血管与胆管,更好地显示胆囊形态及胆囊壁的病变。另外,CT 检查还可与口服与静脉胆管造影合并进行,更有利于胆管病变的显示。

4. MRI 检查

检查前禁食 8~12 小时,一般不需口服对比剂。胆管系统 MRI 检查多采用仰卧位,扫描序列有 SE、FSE、FSPGR 等,一般行横断位、冠状位、矢状位三方位 T1WI、T2WI 再加脂肪抑制扫描,必要时可加上MR 增强扫描与 MR 胰胆管造影(MRCP)。

MR 增强扫描指经静脉注入对比剂后扫描,根据注入的对比剂不同可分为两种:①常规 Gd-DTPA 动态增强,主要目的在于了解肿瘤的血液供应情况;②胆管特异性对比剂增强扫描,主要目的利用经胆管排泄的造影剂使胆囊与胆管呈明显高信号,但是这类增强扫描临床上尚未广泛采用。

MRCP 指采用长 TE 技术,获得重 T2 加权图像,同时合并脂肪抑制技术,使肝内外胆管、胆囊、胆囊管、胰管、胆总管等显示清楚(尤其是胆道扩张时),且与周围组织有明显的对比,产生类似于胆管造影的效果。主要用于分析胆管梗阻原因。

第二节 正常表现

1. X 线表现

PTC 或 ERCP 都能清楚地显示胆管。正常胆管显影密度均匀,边缘光滑。肝内胆管呈树枝状分布,走向自然,经逐级汇合后形成左、右肝管.再联合为肝总管:肝总管长 3~4 cm、内径 0.4~0.6 cm,向下续为胆总管,胆总管长 4~8 cm、内径 0.6~0.8 cm、末端与胰管汇合后共同开口于十二指肠乳头部。

2. 超声表现

横切面和纵切面上,胆囊呈圆形、类圆形或椭圆形,不超过 9 cm,前后径不超过 3 cm,壁厚 2~3 mm。胆囊腔表现为均匀无回声,胆囊后方回声增强,胆囊壁为边缘光滑高回声(图 12-1)。

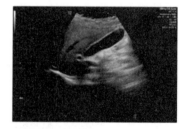

胆囊腔表现为均匀无回声,胆囊后方回声增强,胆囊壁为边缘光滑高回声。

图 12-1 正常胆囊超声检查

肝内胆管一般不能显示,高分辨超声可显示肝内胆管。其内径不超过 2 mm,肝外胆管位于门静脉前方,管壁薄而光滑。纵切面呈无回声长管状影、横切面呈小圆形无回声影。

3. CT 表现

平扫，胆囊通常位于肝门下方、肝右叶前内侧，横断层表现圆形或类圆形，直径 4~5 cm。胆囊腔表现均匀水样低密度，CT 值为 0-20 Hu，胆囊壁光滑锐利，厚度 2~3 mm，呈均匀薄壁软组织密度［图 12-2 (a)］。增强检查，胆囊腔内无强化，胆囊壁表现为细线样环状强化［图 12-2(b)］。

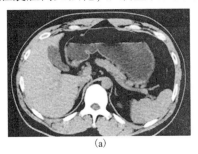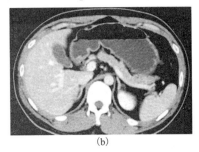

(a)　　　　　　　　　　　　　　(b)

(a) 正常胆囊 CT 平扫图像，胆囊腔呈均匀水样低密度，胆囊壁呈线样等密度，厚度约
2~3 mm，边缘光整；(b) 增强检查胆囊腔内无强化，胆囊壁表现为细线样环状强化。
平扫，正常肝内胆管不显示，肝外胆管尤其是胆总管通常可显示，特别是薄层扫描和
对比增强检查时，表现为小圆形或管状低密度影。

图 12-2　正常胆囊

4. MRI 表现

胆囊形状和大小与 CT 表现相同。胆囊腔内信号，T1WI 呈低信号，部分胆囊腔内 T1WI 信号不均，其腹侧为低信号，背侧为高信号，分别代表新鲜和浓缩胆汁［图 12-3(a)］，T2WI 呈高信号［图 12-3(b)］。

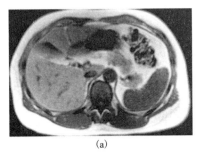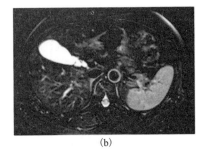

(a)　　　　　　　　　　　　　　(b)

(a) 胆囊腔内 T1WI 信号不均，其腹侧为低信号，背侧为高信号，分别代表新鲜和浓缩
胆汁；(b) 胆囊腔 T2WI 呈高信号。

图 12-3　正常胆囊

正常胆管内含有胆汁，普通 MRI 检查，肝内胆管多难以分辨，肝外胆管 T1WI 呈低信号，T2WI 呈高信号，表现为圆形或柱状影。

MRCP 正常肝内、外胆管表现为边缘光整的树枝状高信号；胆囊为类圆或卵圆形边缘光整的高信号（图 12-4）。

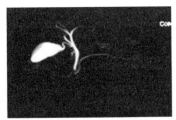

肝内外胆管结构呈边缘光整的树枝状高信号，
胆囊为类圆或卵圆形边缘光整的高信号。

图 12-4　MRCP 显示

第三节　基本病变

1. X 线表现

ERCP 及 PTC 为有创影像学检查，但均能很好的显示胆系的解剖结构。胆管异常主要表现为胆管扩张、狭窄、阻塞、管壁不规则和管腔内充盈缺损。一般情况下胆总管直径超过 1 cm 为胆总管扩张。

2. CT 表现

胆囊横断面直径超过 5 cm 时可考虑胆囊增大。胆囊壁增厚可为均匀性增厚，或不均匀、结节状增厚，增强扫描后增厚的胆囊壁可呈明显强化，见于炎症性和肿瘤性病变。肝总管和胆总管在 CT 横断面图像上表现为连续的管状低密度影，胆总管直径超过 1 cm 则考虑扩张。在扩张的胆管变细的层面，即为胆管狭窄段。胆系结石可分为高密度结石、等密度结石、低密度结石和环状结石，高密度结石在周围低密度胆汁的衬托下呈现特征性的靶征和新月征，等密度结石 CT 不易发现。胆囊肿瘤常表现为胆囊内软组织肿块，或胆囊壁增厚；胆总管肿瘤则可见胆总管壁增厚及局部软组织肿块。

3. MRI 表现

胆管内胆汁在 T2WI 上呈高信号，结石在高信号的胆汁衬托下呈低信号，容易显示；在 T1WI 多数结石与胆汁信号近似，呈低信号，部分结石信号可高于胆汁；在 MRCP 上，胆系结石亦呈低信号，若结石完全阻塞胆管，则 MRCP 可见扩张的胆管下端有杯口状或半月装低信号充盈缺损。胆管癌表现为胆管局限性狭窄，呈截断征象，多方位成像及增强扫描更有助于观察肿瘤的部位和范围；壶腹区占位病灶常引起胰胆管同时扩张，MRCP 上呈现双管征。

4. 胆道梗阻

根据扩张胆管范围、形态和梗阻端表现，有可能提示病变的性质：

（1）胆管大小、形态的改变：

1）肝内胆管：①中度—重度树藤状扩张，扩张胆管扭曲变形多见于恶性肿瘤梗阻；②轻度—中度树枝状、节段状、囊状呈比例扩张多见于良性病变梗阻。

2）肝外胆管：中度—重度扩张伴有肝内胆管，中度—重度树藤状扩张，多见于恶性肿瘤梗阻；②轻度—中度扩张伴有肝内胆管轻度—中度或无明显扩张，多见于良性病变梗阻。

3）胆囊：：①扩大，多见于胆囊颈、管或胆囊管与肝总管汇合良、恶性病变引起的梗阻；②缩小，多见于慢性胆囊炎；③口服胆囊造影不显影可见于胆囊病变、胆囊外的肝脏与胆道病变或胆囊缺如、患者原因及服药不正确等。

（2）扩张胆管密度、信号或回声的改变：

1）增高，CT 上高密度多提示含钙质高的结石；MRI 中 T1WI 明显高信号多见于含胆固醇或胆盐成分较多的结石，中等增高信号多见于结石或肿瘤；超声中的强回声多见于结石。

2）不改变，呈液性密度或信号，多见于近端良恶性梗阻所引起扩张的胆管。

3）降低或充盈缺损，CT 上胆管内低密度多见于含胆固醇等成分较多的结石，T2WI 或 MRCP 胆管内低信号可见于结石或肿瘤。

（3）梗阻部位：

1）肝内，扩张胆管局限于肝脏一侧，多提示病变位于肝内，常见原因：胆管癌、结石、炎症或肝癌等。

2）肝门部，扩张胆管累及全肝，多提示病变位于左、右肝管汇合部或周围，常见原因：胆管癌、肝总管结石、胆囊癌、肝癌及肝门淋巴结肿大等。

3）肝总管或胆总管，肝内胆管、肝总管扩张或伴有胆囊管、胆囊扩张，病变多位于胆总管或胰头部。常见原因：胆管癌、胰头癌、结石等，梗阻在胰腺以上多为胆管癌；梗阻在胰腺或以下三种均有可能，胆管癌与胰头癌胆道扩张明显，前者胆管壁不规则多见，后者胰头增大多见。

4)壶腹部，钩突内可见扩张胆管或呈现"双管征"（胆总管与胰管同时扩张），常见原因：结石或壶腹癌。

（4）梗阻部位形态：

1)截断征，扩张胆管在狭窄部位突然消失或呈锥状狭窄，狭窄移行段不超过 10 mm，多见于恶性肿瘤引起的梗阻。

2)移行性狭窄，扩张胆管在狭窄部位呈渐进性变窄、消失，狭窄移行段超过 20 mm，多见于良性病变引起的梗阻。

3)狭窄胆管、胆囊内缘光滑、柔软，多见于炎性病变；锯齿状、壁僵硬多见于恶性病变。

4)胆管病变范围较广，病变区胆管呈粗细相间的节段性分布，常见于原发性硬化性胆管炎。

5)结石致梗阻可见梗阻端呈倒杯口状表现。

第四节　常见疾病诊断

1. 先天性胆管囊肿

（1）临床及病理表现：先天性胆管囊肿又称为先天性胆管扩张症。1723 年 Vater 首先报道胆总管囊肿，1852 年 Douglas 总结了胆总管囊肿的临床特征，而 Caroli 则于 1958 年首先报道先天性肝内胆管囊肿。黄疸、腹痛、右上腹包块为三大主要的临床症状。肝内或外胆管囊状扩张且扩张囊状胆管不同程度与胆管分支或主干相通为其主要特点。最常用的检查方法为 USG，而诊断价值最高的方法为 MRCP。

Todani 根据囊肿部位与范围将胆管囊肿分为五型：

Ⅰ型：胆总管囊状或梭形扩张，最常见，占 80%～90%。

Ⅱ型：胆总管单发憩室，囊肿偏于一侧而胆总管正常，占 2%。

Ⅲ型：胆总管下端在十二指肠内囊状扩张并突入肠腔，占 1.4%～5%。

Ⅳ型：多发囊肿，肝内与肝外囊肿或多发肝外囊肿，占 19%。

Ⅴ型：单发或多发肝内胆管囊肿———Caroli 病。

Caroli 病又可分为两型：

Ⅰ型：肝内胆管囊状扩张；多伴胆管结石与胆管炎；无肝硬化与门脉高压。较多见。

Ⅱ型：肝内末端小胆管扩张而近端胆管无或轻度扩张；不伴胆管结石与胆管炎；多伴肝硬化与门脉高压。较少见。

（2）影像学表现：

1)X 线表现：X 线平片无特殊所见。PTC、ERCP 或直接穿刺囊腔注入对比剂，见肝内或肝外囊腔与胆道相通或直接显示囊状扩张的胆总管；在肝脏功能正常情况下，口服或静脉胆道造影则可显示对比剂进入囊腔，由此可确诊并可以根据囊腔所在位置分型。

2)USG：Ⅰ—Ⅳ型显示为胆总管部位或肝门区出现局限性扩张的无回声区，多呈椭圆形或梭形，可延伸至肝门或胰头部，壁薄，边界清晰。无回声区的近肝侧胆管一般无扩张，可显示与之相通，胆囊受压被推挤贴近腹前壁。

Caroli 病显示肝内沿胆管系统沿主要分支分布的多个圆形或梭形无回声区，边界回声增强且较清晰，在多方向观察可显示无回声区的狭窄处相互连通，或与肝内胆管的干支相连通。

3)CT 表现：Ⅰ型、Ⅱ型、Ⅳ型表现为肝门区液性密度占位病变，密度均匀，边缘薄而光滑；Ⅲ型表现为液性密度占位病变突入十二指肠腔。特点：①病变呈囊状或球状，外周一般不扩张；②静脉注射胆影普胺或口服胆管对比剂后 CT 扫描可见胆囊显影与对比剂通过肝管进入囊状病变；③囊肿较大时与肝、胰、肾、肾上腺囊肿表现可相似。

Caroli 病：近肝门区圆形或梭形的肝内胆管扩张，多不伴有末梢胆管扩张。Caroli 病的增强 CT 特征为"中心点征"，即在扩张的肝内胆管内强化点，代表门静脉。胆影葡胺静脉注射增强 CT 或口服胆道对比剂后 CT 扫描上见囊内增强，即可诊断 Caroli 病。

4）MRI 表现：病灶呈囊状、柱状或憩室状，由于病灶内含有胆汁，T1WI 上呈低信号；T2WI 呈高信号。有时，由于胆汁淤积，呈胆泥样改变，或者合并结石，T2WI 上可显示不均匀混杂信号或存在充盈缺损。

Ⅰ—Ⅳ型多表现为肝外胆管的囊状或梭状扩张，肝内胆管多不扩张或仅轻度扩张；Caroli 病多表现为肝内胆管的节段性扩张，且扩张的胆管沿胆管树分布而左右肝管与胆总管正常[图 12-5（a）、（b）]。

MRI 比较其他方法有明显的优势：①对囊性病灶敏感，尤其是 T*2WI 与 MRCP；②能从多方位观察病灶与胆管、肝实质以及临近器官的关系，其中，冠状面、矢状面 T2WI、MRCP 能较好显示囊肿与胆管树的解剖关系，尤其是 MRCP，能显示胆管树的全貌，借此能够准确地分型；③不需对比剂及其他损伤性操作，是先天性胆管囊肿诊断与分型的首选方法。

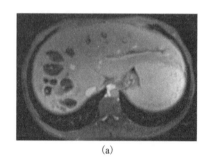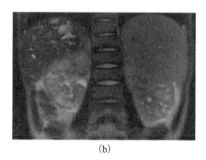

（a）　　　　　　　　　　　　　　　　　（b）

（a）T1WI 增强扫描显示扩张的肝内胆管围绕增强的门静脉，这称为"中心点"征（箭头）；
（b）在冠状位 T2WI 上，发现双肾内多发囊性病变，伴脾脏明显增大。

图 12-5　Caroli 病

（3）诊断与鉴别诊断：肝多发囊肿或多囊肝：表现为肝内散在分布的多发病灶，与胆管不相通，多囊肝可同时伴有其他脏器的多囊性病变。

2.胆囊炎

临床上按发病时间分为急性胆囊炎与慢性胆囊炎。

（1）急性胆囊炎：

1）临床及病理表现：急性胆囊炎多因结石梗阻、细菌感染、胰液反流等原因引起。主要临床表现为发热、右上腹痛及墨菲氏征阳性。病理表现主要为胆囊壁充血水肿、黏膜溃疡形成、胆囊扩大、囊壁增厚等，严重者可形成周围脓肿。首选检查方法为 USG。

2）影像学表现：

①X 线表现：有时 X 线平片可见增大的胆囊影，产气杆菌感染时胆囊区可见低密度的气体影像。一般不作造影检查。

②USG 表现：胆囊增大，常呈圆形或椭圆形，轮廓不光滑。胆囊壁弥漫性增厚，超过 3 mm，呈高回声带，其间为连续或间断的低回声带，即为"双边影"。胆囊内出现稀疏或密集的光点回声，后方无声影。胆囊内多见结石高回声伴后方声影。脂餐试验胆囊收缩功能差或丧失。

③CT 表现：胆囊壁增厚可超过 4 mm 以上，边缘模糊，周围水肿呈环状低密度影；胆囊扩大，横径大于 4.5 cm，内部可因积脓而密度增高；胆囊腔、壁或胆道系统内有时可见到低密度的气体影。增强 CT 见胆囊内侧黏膜层由于炎症引起的充血产生增强效应，呈致密细线条状阴影，其浆膜层由于水肿而形成一低密度带环绕胆囊全壁，这一征象较有价值。

④MRI 表现：很少做 MRI 检查，表现与 CT 基本一致。主要表现为胆囊壁增厚、胆囊扩大及周围积液，部分可见胆囊结石与周围脓肿。胆囊壁增厚是急性胆囊炎的主要影像表现，它的显示也是 MRI 相对于其他检查的主要优势所在，增厚胆囊壁较均匀，尤其内缘光滑，而浆膜可以不光滑，增强早期内层强化，延迟扫

描全层强化。

3）诊断与鉴别诊断：主要与引起胆囊壁增厚的疾病鉴别，包括肝硬化腹水致低蛋白血症、右心衰竭、肾脏疾病、糖尿病等，但后者一般无急性病史、胆囊多无扩大或胆囊结石等。

（2）慢性胆囊炎：

1）临床及病理表现：慢性胆囊炎可为急性胆囊炎的延续，也可为原发的慢性炎症，且常合并结石。临床表现较轻。病理表现主要为纤维组织增生与慢性炎症细胞浸润，引起囊壁增厚，肌肉组织萎缩，由此导致胆囊收缩功能减退。首选检查方法为USG。

2）影像学表现：

①X线表现：平片有时可显示胆囊影缩小，胆囊区可见钙化影。造影检查：生理积聚法造影胆囊不显影，在排除其他不显影的因素后，对慢性胆囊炎有诊断意义。

②USG表现：胆囊多缩小。胆囊壁增厚，回声增强，边缘粗糙。胆囊内见点状回声或沉积性光团，随体位改变而缓慢移动，常伴有胆囊结石高回声及后方声影，胆囊萎缩时胆囊内无回声区消失，仅在胆囊区见较高回声的弧形光带。脂餐试验胆囊收缩功能不良。

③CT表现：胆囊缩小，胆囊壁增厚，壁内可以有少量钙化影像、胆囊结石为慢性胆囊炎的主要表现，其中胆囊壁增厚为最重要、最常见的表现，瓷胆囊为最典型的表现。

④MRI表现：一般不需要MRI检查，其诊断价值也有限，其表现与CT相似，为胆囊壁增厚、胆囊结石与胆囊壁的钙化，但是对于胆囊壁的钙化MRI显示明显较CT差。

3）诊断与鉴别诊断：胆囊癌胆囊壁增厚非常明显且呈不规则增厚，以体部、颈部明显，如伴有胆囊周围肝实质侵犯或肝脏及淋巴结转移可以确诊。

3.胆系结石

（1）胆囊结石：

1）临床及病理表现：胆囊结石临床症状与结石所在大小、部位、有无梗阻及并发症等相关，程度从间歇期的右上腹不适到急性期的绞痛、呕吐、高热不等。胆结石成分为胆色素与胆固醇，有时可含有不同量的钙盐，由此可分为阳性结石（含钙成分较多，X线透过率降低）与阴性结石（含钙成分较少，X线透过率高）。首选检查方法为USG。

2）影像学表现：

①X线表现：10%~20%胆石是含钙的阳性结石，X线平片可以显示。这类结石大多在胆囊内，常多个堆积，从沙砾至蚕豆大，呈圆形、多边形或菱形，犹如一串葡萄或一堆石榴子，个别结石可以很大。80%~90%为阴性结石，X线平片不能发现，这时胆囊造影常显示为多数成堆充盈缺损，呈圆形或多面形，如石榴子样。有时结石过小或胆囊显影密度过高，卧位影常显示不清，需摄立位片或加压点片。

②USG表现：胆囊结石典型表现如下：胆囊内一个或多个强回声光团；回声光团可随患者体位的改变而移动；在强回声光团的后方有清晰的声影，声影是由于超声被结石反射和吸收，其能量高度衰减所致。另外，当结石填满胆囊时，又可称为填满型结石，这时胆囊无回声区消失，胆囊前半部呈弧形强光带，后方伴声影。当胆囊壁增厚时，则出现"囊壁-结石-声影"三合征（WES征）。泥沙型结石时，胆囊内可见后方伴声影的细小的高回声光点群。胆囊壁间结石则在胆囊壁内可见高回声光斑，后方伴彗星尾征或声影，体位改变时不移动。

③CT表现：由于含钙量不同而在胆囊区显示为单个或成堆的高密度、略高密度、等密度、低密度影，常呈环状或多层状，其位置多可随患者体位而改变。钙化性胆囊结石表现为高密度［图12-6（a）］，使其成为唯一能在CT扫描图像上清晰显示的类型，纯胆固醇结石在胆汁中呈低密度，而其他类型的胆囊结石与胆汁的密度相同，在CT上可能无法明确识别。

④MRI表现：胆囊结石在T1WI图像上信号多变，但在T2WI和MRCP图像上均呈无信号或低信号改变［图12-6（b）］，以T^*2WI上对比更为明显。研究表明，胆囊结石的信号与其内的脂质成分以及大分子蛋白均有密切关系。

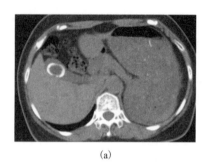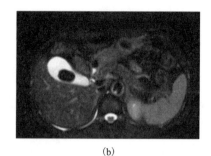

(a)   (b)

(a) 胆囊结石 CT：CT 平扫胆囊内见一圆形的高密度灶，称"环征"（箭头）；(b) 胆囊结石 T2WI：胆汁在 T2WI 呈高信号，胆汁勾勒出低信号的胆囊结石（箭头）。

图 12-6　胆囊结石

3）诊断与鉴别诊断

①钙化影：如肾内结核钙化、右肾结石及肾上腺钙化等表现形态不规则，且病灶多位于椎体后方而胆囊结石则位于椎体前方。

②阴性影像：如肠内气体、胆囊肿瘤等可以借助多方向检查、多体位观察等方法鉴别。

（2）胆管结石：

1）临床及病理表现：胆管结石按存在部位可分为可分为肝内胆管结石与肝外胆管结石；按发生部位可分为原发性胆管结石与继发性胆管结石（多继发于胆囊结石）。

肝内胆管结石临床表现不典型，间歇期可无症状，发作期表现为急性胆管炎，而间歇性发作为其临床特点。肝外胆管结石的典型表现为胆绞痛、黄疸、发热与寒战，即 Charoat 三联征。

胆管结石成分与胆囊结石基本相同，其中，肝内胆管结石以胆色素含钙结石较多见而继发性肝外胆管结石以胆固醇结石较多见，原发性肝外胆管结石以胆色素含钙结石较多见。首选检查方法为 USG。

2）影像学表现：

①X 线表现：X 线平片含钙阳性结石在胆道走行方向区域可见钙化影像。造影表现为单发、多发呈圆形、条状的充盈缺损，边缘光滑。

②USG 表现：胆管内见高回声团，呈圆形、斑点状、条束状，一般后方伴声影，同时多伴有结石部位以上的胆管扩张。当沿胆管、胆道走向出现双边样回声增强则提示胆管壁增厚。

③CT 表现：根据所含成分不同，可表现为胆道内高密度（含胆色素、钙质较多）、软组织密度、低密度（含胆固醇较多）、环状高低或高等密度（"靶征"）影像，多伴有远侧段胆管扩张[图 12-7（a）、（c）]。

④MRI 表现：信号特征与胆囊结石基本一致，表现为胆管内圆形或椭圆形无信号或低信号区[图 12-7（b）、（d）~（f）]，多伴有近侧胆道扩张、局部胆管壁的增厚等。

3）诊断与鉴别诊断：

胆管癌：USG 呈低或中等回声，后方无声影，病灶与管壁分界不清；CT 检查提示，胆管壁不规则增厚，病灶局限呈"截断征"等；MRI：MRCP 及 T*2WI 所显示胆道扩张与狭窄部位的恶性表现。术后吻合口狭窄与肝内胆管积气，可根据病史与临床症状鉴别。肝内钙化多不伴有胆管扩张。

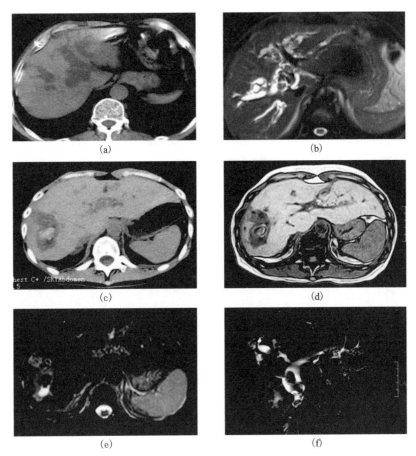

(a)CT平扫显示肝内胆管明显扩张；(b)同一患者T2WI上，肝内胆管内可见多发卵圆形充盈缺损，与胆管结石相符；(c)胆管结石CT：CT平扫，肝内胆管内可见多个高密度灶，与胆管内结石一致；(d)胆管结石MRI：T1WI上胆管结石可在同一患者表现为高信号或低信号灶；(e)胆管结石MRI：在T2WI上，扩张的肝内胆管内见多个充盈缺损信号；(f)胆管结石磁共振胰胆管造影(MRCP)肝内外胆管中见多个充盈缺损信号。MRCP是诊断胆管结石的金标准。

图12-7　胆管结石

4. 胆系恶性肿瘤

（1）胆囊癌：

1）临床及病理表现：胆囊癌为胆道系统最常见的恶性肿瘤，女性多见且多发于50岁以上。临床表现无特征，典型者可有右上腹痛、胆囊窝区包块，晚期可有黄疸。病理上以腺癌多见（85%），其次为鳞癌与类癌。约70%胆囊癌可以合并胆囊结石。

2）影像学表现：

①X线表现：X线平片诊断价值不大，造影检查价值也非常有限，目前已经很少采用，主要表现为病变侵犯胆总管、胆囊管引起的胆管狭窄、梗阻或肿块引起胆囊不显影、充盈缺损等。

②USG表现：一般根据胆囊癌形态改变可分为三型。腔内型(15%~23%)：从胆囊壁突入腔内的单发、多发乳头状肿块，可有较宽的不规则基底或草莓样，而蒂难以显示，胆囊腔存在，多为较早期表现；壁厚型(15%~22%)：胆囊壁呈现局限性或弥漫性不均匀增厚，内侧表面不平整，以胆囊颈部、体部明显；肿块型(41%~70%)：胆囊为软组织肿块占据，胆囊腔大部或完全消失，多为晚期表现。另外，还有作者将胆囊癌分有：阻塞型：肿瘤侵犯胆囊管造成阻塞，胆囊扩大，这一型肿块多较小；混合型：胆囊壁显示不规则增厚，同时具有腔内型与壁厚型的表现。声像图上，病灶呈低回声或不均匀回声，无声影，伴有结石时，可见高回声光团及声影，另外出现胆囊与胆管扩张、肝脏直接侵犯、肝脏或其他脏器转移、淋巴转移等表现。

③CT 表现：肿块分型与 USG 相同。肿块表现为软组织密度，胆囊癌一般为多血供病变增强有明显强化且延续时间长，这与肝细胞癌的"速升速降"特点有区别。当临近肝组织出现低密度区（带），则为直接侵袭肝的征象。同时有肝总管远侧肝内、外胆管的扩张和钙化等伴随影像，也可出现肝门部淋巴结增大、腹水、肝内转移灶等晚期肿瘤改变[图 12-8(a)、(b)]。

④MRI 表现：分型同上。胆囊癌病灶 T1WI 上多呈稍低或等信号；在 T2WI 图像上呈中等度的高信号；病灶强化较明显，且延续时间长，这与肝细胞癌的"速升速降"特点有区别。胆囊周围的脂肪层消失提示肝脏侵犯。

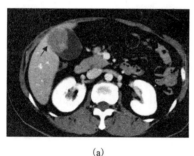 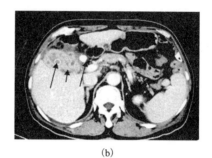

(a)   (b)

(a) 腔内型胆囊癌 CT：中度强化、胆囊腔内突起软组织肿块，胆囊与肝组织之间的间隙消失（箭头）；(b) 弥漫性胆囊癌 CT：胆囊壁弥漫性增厚（短箭头）伴不均匀强化，胆囊内可见多个结石（长箭头）。

图 12-8 胆囊癌

3）诊断与鉴别诊断：

①慢性胆囊炎：与厚壁型胆囊癌难以区别，但一般前者胆囊壁增厚程度较轻，且无周围侵犯或远处转移。

②胆囊良性肿块：如息肉、肉芽肿、腺瘤，一般良性肿块多在 1 cm 以内，不浸润胆囊壁且胆囊壁软而光滑，也无周围侵犯或远处转移，引起胆道梗阻或偶阻塞胆囊管导致胆囊扩大时程度也较轻。

（2）胆管癌：

1）临床及病理表现：多发生在较大胆管，8%~31%发生在肝内胆管；37%~50%在肝外胆管近段；4%~36%在肝外胆管远段。50~70 岁多。临床上以无痛性进行性黄疸或腹痛伴黄疸等为主要表现。病理上以腺癌多见，按形态可分为浸润型，最多见，易引起局限性狭窄而无明显肿块；肿块型（结节型），局部肿块较明显而胆道梗阻不明显；乳头状息肉样型，少见，为管腔内肿块。胆管癌生长缓慢，易引起到梗阻，多因合并症而死亡。

2）影像学表现：

①X 线表现：X 线平片无特殊意义。PTC 可显示肿瘤的部位与近端扩张的胆管及其形态，浸润型多产生局限性狭窄，肿块型与息肉样型多表现为充盈缺损。ERCP 主要从下端显示肿瘤的形态与侵袭范围，表现与 PTC 相似。ERCP 与 PTC 结合，定性诊断可达 90%以上。

②USG 表现：在扩张的胆管远端显示肿块图像，呈乳头状或不规则的低回声至稍高回声，其内回声分布不均匀，后方无声影。乳头状息肉样或肿块型表现由管壁突入扩张的胆管腔内，或充满胆管腔，与胆管壁无分界。浸润或结节浸润型表现为扩张的胆管远端突然狭窄或截断，但无明显肿块显示，梗阻部位管壁内缘不规则。间接征象为病变以上的胆管系统明显扩张；肝门部淋巴结肿大；肝弥漫性增大或肝内转移病灶。

③CT 表现：肿块表现同 USG。有人按肿块发生部位分为四型。周围型（也就是胆管细胞型肝癌）：起源于左右肝管以远的胆管，表现为肝实质内肿块，邻近伴有扩张胆管或钙化灶；肝门型：起源于左右肝管或肝总管近端 10 mm 以内，为"Y"形或不规则形肿块[图 12-9(a)、(b)]；肝外胆管型：起源于左右肝管汇合处 10 mm 以远至 Vater 壶腹，表现为条状或不规则肿块；壶腹型：病灶位于 Vater 壶腹或胰头下部，表现为不规则肿块。增强扫描早期强化不明显，可有延迟强化。此外，梗阻部位以上胆管呈中度—重度树藤状

扩张，梗阻部位呈现截断或突然狭窄表现，梗阻部位薄层扫描可显示管壁内缘不规则，壶腹癌可表现"双管征"，可伴有胆道结石、局部肝萎缩与其他脏器转移等。

④MRI表现：病灶形态与梗阻特征同USG、CT。在T1WI呈低或等信号；T2WI上呈稍高信号；DWI呈不均匀高信号，不均匀强化，有延时强化[图12-10(a)、(d)]。MRCP可以很好地显示胆管扩张的程度与范围以及梗阻的形态特点，同PTC和ERCP比较，作为一项无创伤的检查方法，已日益被临床所认识。

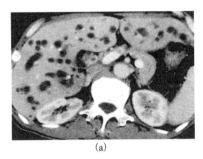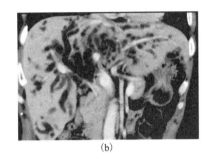

(a)　　　　　　　　　　　(b)

(a)胆总管上段管壁显著增厚伴管腔狭窄，CT扫描门静脉期增厚管壁显著强化；(b)冠状位CT可清晰显示肝门胆管癌累及的范围，诊断为Bismuth-Corlette I型肝门胆管癌。

图12-9　肝门胆管癌(Klatskin瘤)

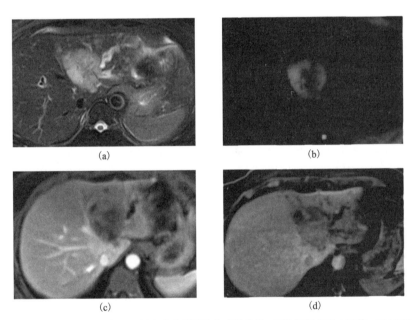

(a)T2WI上，左肝可见轻度不均匀高信号肿块伴瘤周病灶，可见扩张的肝内胆管；(b)DWI序列上外周高信号的"靶征"表现支持肝内胆管细胞癌；(c)肿块在静脉期上显示呈不均匀性中度强化；(d)左肝肿块表现为延迟强化，5分钟肝实质成像有均匀强化趋势。

图12-10　肝内胆管细胞癌

3)诊断与鉴别诊断：

主要与引起黄疸的其他慢性胆管梗阻疾病鉴别，常见的是胆管结石或结石引起的炎症，可从USG上结石的声影，PTC、ERCP、MRCP等显示胆管狭窄与扩张的程度与形态等方面鉴别。但是由于结石、炎症与胆管癌互为成因且长混合出现，有时鉴别有一定困难。

(袁友红，罗伟，李秀梅，蒋洪涛，毛志群，肖恩华，刘辉)

Chapter 12

Biliary system

Section 1   Method of examination

1. X-ray Examination

(1)Common X-ray: The plain film of the right upper quadrant abdomen is the major method of common X-ray examination of biliary system. But its ability of diagnosis anddifferential diagnosis is poor and it can only distinguish some calcium in content, for example, cholecystic calculus, calcification of cholecystic wall, calcium bile, gas in bile duct and so on. Sometimes, the outline of cholecyst can be distinguished, because enlarged cholecyst is set off by the gas around. Because its diagnostic value is limited and, in recent years, ultrasonography (US) and computed tomography (CT)have been applied widespreadly, the plain films are applied seldom in the diagnosis of the biliary systemic disease.

(2)Contrast examination: The contrast examination of biliary system concludes two methods: physiologically evacuating and directly introducing. Oral Cholecystography and intravenous cholecystocholangiography of physiologically evacuating are applied most frequently past, however, with US, CT, MRI, especially MRCP applied in the clinical more and more, physiologically evacuating contrast examinations of biliary system are chosen seldom or never today because of its poor image quality and complicated operation.

Because the directly introducing contrast examination of biliary system can not only diagnose the disease, but be used to treat as well, some of them, for instance, percutaneous transhepatic cholangiography(PTC), endoscopic retrograde cholangiopancreaticography (ERCP), "T" draining-tube-graphy post of the operation are performed frequently in the clinic. In order to enhance the safety of the operation and the quality of the image, directly introducing contrast examinations of biliary system are generally applied under supervision of the fluoroscopy. PTC will be introduced in the chapter of interventional radiology.

"T" draining-tube-graphy is a method of directly introducing contrast examination of biliary system, in which contrast medium is injected directly through "T" draining-tube that is fixed during operating of biliary system. It is able to observe if there are remaining calculi in the biliary tract and if it is unobstructed between bile duct and duodenum.

ERCP is a method that the operator, firstly, send duodenal fiber scope into the descending portion of duodenum, then introduce contrast medium into the bile duct and pancreatic duct through papilla of duodenum under supervising of the fluoroscopy and at last photograph. With contrast medium into the bile ducts and pancreatic duct through catheter, ERCP can display its dimension and form. It isn't only very important in the diagnosing and differential diagnosing between bile duct calculus and tumor, but also able to treat through fixing draining tube, especially to the middle and lower level bile duct.

Percutaneous cholecystography (PTC) can display dimension and interior cava form of cholecyst by way of injecting contrast medium, for example, iodine, gas or iodine and gas at the same time, through the catheter after the operator punctures into cholecyst percutaneously and directly under supervising of the fluoroscopy. Besides its diagnosic values, PTC also has all kinds of treating advantages by way of fixing draining pipe in the cholecyst. In recent years, PTC, however, has hardly been performed in the clinical because of its complications, for instance, the fistula of cholecyst or bile duct, peritonitis, and so on.

Contrast examination of biliary tract during operating displays biliary tract by way of directly injecting contrast medium into cystic duct, choledochus, cholecyst, intrahepatic bile duct or papilla of duodenum when abdomen is opening.

2. Ultrasonography(US)

The patients have to fast about 8 to 12 hour before US examination and it is the best time when their stomach is empty in the morning. Supine position is the generalposition of US examination and, when necessarily, the patient have to adopt right-anterior-inclined position, left-lateral position, sitting position or standing position. Right-inclined-cut images under rib or between ribs are suit to display and observe the cholecyst or the bile duct. In order to differentiate cholecystic tumor and calculus, the patient needs to change his position. The calculus in the cholecyst will change its position with the patient's position changing. Today, US is the most frequent method of diagnosis and differential diagnosis about the calculus, phlegmasia, neoplasm of cholecyst or bile duct and congenital biliary duct cyst.

3. Computed tomography(CT)

The patients have to fast about 8 to 12 hour before CT examination and take800 ~ 1000 mL, proper concentration contrast medium which is proper to display stomach and bowel but develop obvious artifact, for example, iodine medium, water, fat medium and so on. The CT examination of the biliary tract includes precontrast scan and postcontrast scan. Moreover, the liver, the biliary tract and pancreas are usually performed at the same time. The thickness and index of the routine CT scan of the biliary tract is 10 mm respectively and gracile layer scan, for example, whose thickness and index is 5 mm, 2 mm or less 2 mm respectively, may be performed in the focal position.

The precontrast scan can display the calculus contained calcium, the position of obstruction of biliary tract and some neoplasm of cholecyst and biliary tract. The postcontrast scan is usually the scan after bolus injecting intravenously iodine contrast medium about 80 ~ 100 mL and it is valuable to display the size and the form of the biliary tract and the lesion of the biliary tract round, to differentiate the biliary tract from vessel and to manifest better the size and the form of the cholecyst and the lesion of the cholecyst paries. In addition, It is beneficial to display the lesion of the biliary tract when the CT scan is performed along with oral cholecystography and intravenous cholecystocholangiography.

4. Magnetic resonance imaging(MRI)

The patients have to fast about 8 to 12 hour before MRI examination and, generally, do not need to take contrast medium. Supine position is the routine position of MRI examination indiagnosing the diseases of the biliary tract and the sequences of the MRI scan include spin echo(SE)、fast spin echo(FSE)、fast spoiled gradient recalled echo(FSPGR) and so on. MRI usually includes T1WI, T2WI and fat-suppression(FS) of axial, coronal and sagittal and, when necessarily, it may also plus postcontrast MRI and MR cholangiopancreatography (MRCP).

The postcontrast MRI is a method of MR scanning after contrast medium is bolus injected transvenously and includes two kinds according to different contrast medium：(1)The routine postcontrast MRI, in which Gd-DTPA is used the most frequently among all kinds of contrast medium and the main purpose of which is to comprehend the condition of blood providing. (2)Specific contrast MRI of the biliary tract, whose main purpose is to display better the cholecyst and the biliary tract because most of these contrasts evacuate through the biliary system. But it has not been applied extensively because of its cost and other reasons.

MRCP is a kind of technology that it gets T^*2WI through making use of the technology of longer TE and fat-suppression (FS). MRCP can not only display clearly intra-and extrahepatic bile duct, cholecyst, cystic duct, pancreatic duct, choledochus, but it can also develop high contrast between the biliary duct and tissue round. The diagnostic and differentially diagnostic value of MRCP is similar to the oral cholecystography and intravenous cholecystocholangiography. Today MRCP is used mainly to analyze the reasons of the obstruction of biliary tract.

Section 2　Normal appearances

1. X-ray findings

Both PTC and ERCP can clearly show the bile duct. Normal bile duct manifests density uniform, smooth edge. The common hepatic duct is 3~4 cm long and 0.4~0.6 cm in diameter. The common bile duct is 4~8 cm in length and 0.6~0.8 cm in inner diameter. The end ofthe common bile duct is opened at the papilla of duodenum.

2. Ultrasound findings

On the transverse and longitudinal sections of ultrasonography, the gallbladder is round, quasi round or oval. The length of the gallbladder is no more than 9 cm. The anteroposteriordiameter of the gallbladder is no more than 3 cm, its wall thickness is 2~3 mm. The cystic cavity was homogeneous and anechoic, and the echo behind the gallbladder is enhanced. The gallbladder wall is highly echogenic with smooth edges (Figure 12-1).

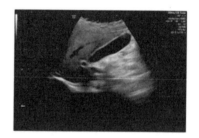

Figure 12-1　Normal gallbladder
Ultrasound examination shows that the gallbladder cavity was homogeneous and anechoic, the echo behind the gallbladder is enhanced, and the gallbladder wall is smooth and hyperechoic.

Intrahepatic bile duct can not be shown in general, but high resolution ultrasound can show the intrahepatic bile duct. Its inner diameter is not more than 2 mm, the extrahepatic bile duct is located in front of the portal vein, and its wall is thin and smooth. The longitudinal section showed no echo, while the transverse section showed small round without echo.

3. Computed tomography(CT) findings

The gallbladder is usually located below the hepatic hilum and medial to the right lobe of the liver, with round or quasi-round in transverse section, with a diameter of about 4~5 cm. The gallbladder cavity shows uniform water-like low density, and the CT value was about 0-20 HU. The gallbladder wall is smooth and sharp, with a thickness of about 2 ~ 3 mm, presenting uniform parenchyma soft tissue density [Figure 12 - 2(a)]. On enhanced examination, there is no enhancement in the gallbladder cavity, and the gallbladder wall show thin linear annular enhancement [Figure 12-2(b)].

On plain scan, the normal intrahepatic bile duct is not shown, but the extrahepatic bile duct, especially the common bile duct, can usually be shown, especially when thin layer scan and contrastive enhancement examination, showing small round or tubular low-density shadow.

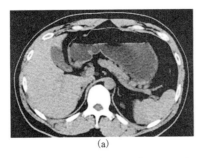
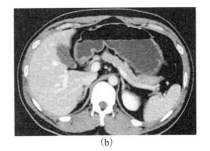

(a)　　　　　　　　　　　　　　　(b)

The gallbladder cavity shows uniform water low density, gallbladder wall shows linear isodensity, thickness is about 2~3 mm, and edge is smooth(a). There is no enhancement in the gallbladder cavity, and the gallbladder wall shows fine linear ring enhancement(b).

Figure 12-2　Normal gallbladder CT plain scan image and enhancement

4. Magnetic resonance imaging (MRI) findings

The shape and size of gallbladder examined by MRI are the same as that of CT. The signal intensity of gallbladderis homogeneous on T1WI and hyperintensity on T2WI. The signal intensity of some gallbladder is heterogeneous on T1WI, low signal on ventral side and high signal on back side, which respectively represent fresh and concentrated bile[Figure 12-3(a)]. T2WI has a high signal [Figure 12-3(b)].

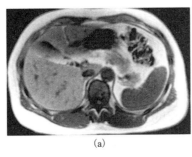
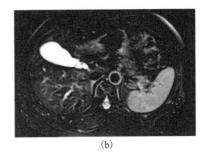

(a)　　　　　　　　　　　　　　　(b)

The signal of gallbladder cavity on T1WI is uneven. its ventral side is low signal, dorsal side is high signal, representing fresh and concentrated bile respectively(a). The signal of gallbladder cavity on T2WI is high signal(b).

Figure 12-3　Normal gallbladder on T1WI and T2WI

The normal bile duct contains bile, while the ordinary MRI examination and intrahepatic bile duct are difficult to distinguish. The extrahepatic bile duct presents low signal on T1WI and high signal on T2WI, showing round or columnar shadow.

MRCP illustrates that normal intrahepatic and external bile ducts show dendritic high signals with smooth edges. The gallbladder is a high signal with rounded or ovoid edges (Figure 12-4).

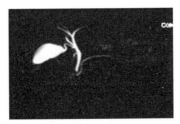

it shows that the structure of intrahepatic and extrahepatic bile ducts is dendritic high signal with smooth edge, and the gallbladder is round or oval high signal with smooth edge.

Figure 12-4　MRCP finding

357

Section 3   Basic pathologic changes

1. X-ray Examination findings

ERCP and PTC are invasive imaging examinations, but both can well show the anatomy of the biliary system. Bile duct abnormalities are mainly manifested as bile duct dilation, stenosis, obstruction, irregular wall and filling defect in the lumen. Under normal circumstances, the diameter of the common bile duct is more than 1 cm, which means the common bile duct is dilated.

2. Computedtomography(CT) findings

Gallbladder enlargement can be considered when the cross-sectional diameter of the gallbladder exceeds 5 cm. The thickening of the gallbladder wall can be uniform thickening, or uneven and nodular thickening. After enhanced scanning, the thickened gallbladder wall can be significantly enhanced, in view of the inflammatory and tumorous lesions. The common hepatic duct and the common bile duct appear as continuous tubular low-density shadows on the CT cross-sectional image. The common bile duct is considered to be dilated if the diameter of the common bile duct exceeds 1 cm. The narrowed segment of the bile duct is the narrowed section of the dilated bile duct. Gallstones can be divided into high-density stones, iso-density stones, low-density stones and ring stones. High-density stones show characteristic target signs and crescent signs against the surrounding low-density bile. Isodense stones are not easy to find on CT. Gallbladder tumors often appear as soft tissue masses in the gallbladder, or without thickening of the gallbladder wall. Common bile duct tumors can show thickening of the bile wall and local soft tissue masses.

3. Magneticresonance imaging(MRI) findings

The bile in the bile duct shows high signal on T2WI, and stonesare low signal under the background of high signal bile, which is easy to show. On T1WI, most stones are similar to bile signal, showing low signal, and some stones have higher signal than bile. On MRCP, Biliary stones also show low signal intensity. If the stones completely block the bile duct, MRCP shows a cup-shaped or semi-monthly low signal filling defect at the lower end of the expanded bile duct. Cholangiocarcinoma manifests as limited bile duct stricture, showing signs of truncation. Multi-directional imaging and enhanced scanning are more helpful to observe the location and extent of the tumor. Occupying lesions in the ampullary area often cause simultaneous dilation of the pancreaticobiliary ducts, and the MRCP presents a double duct sign.

4. Biliary obstruction

According to the extent, shape and performance of the obstructed end of the dilated bile duct, it may indicate the nature of the lesion:

(1) The size and the form change of biliary tract. Middle to high tree and vine shape dilatation of the intrahepatic bile ducts, which are wrenched and transformed, are mostly observed in the obstruction of malignant tumors, but low to middle proportional branch or bladder dilatation of the intrahepatic bile ducts are mostly shown in the obstruction of good lesions. Middle to high dilatation of the extrahepatic bile duct along with middle to high tree and vine dilatation of the intrahepatic bile ducts are mostly observed in the obstruction of malignant tumors, but low to middle proportional dilatation of the extrahepatic bile ducts along with not or low to middle proportional branch or bladder dilatation of the intrahepatic bile ducts are mostly shown in the obstruction of benign lesions. The amplification of the cholecyst is mostly observed in the obstruction of benign or malignant lesions originating from the neck of gallbladder, cystic duct or confluence of the neck of gallbladder and cystic duct. The diminution of the cholecyst is mainly shown in the chronic cholecystitis. No developing of oral cholecystography may be the lesion

from the cholecyst, the liver, the biliary tract or other reasons from the patient.

（2）The density, signal or echo changing of the dilatant biliary duct. Increasing of density is mainly observed in the calculus on CT, which contains more calcium, while highly increasing of signal is mainly observed in the calculus on T1WI of MRI, which contains more cholesterol and less biliary sal. On US, middle increasing of echo is mainly observed in the calculus or tumor while highly increasing of echo is mainly shown in the calculus, which often is accompanied with "sound shadow". No changing, whose density or signal is same as the fluid, are usually observed in the dilated bile duct because of the close bile duct benign or malignant. The local decreasing of the density or filling defect of CT is often shown in the calculus, which contains more cholesterol, and its of T2WI or MRCP is mainly seen in the calculus or tumor.

（3）The spot of the obstruction. When the dilatation of bile ducts limit in one side, the spot of the obstruction usually is in the liver, which shows the lesion of the same side liver, for example, cholangiocarcinoma, calculus of bile duct, phlegmonosis or hepatocarcinoma and so on. When the dilatation of bile ducts have come up to all of the liver, the spot of the obstruction usually is located at the porta hepatis and the reasons of the obstruction often are cholangiocarcinoma, calculus of the common hepatic duct, carcinoma of gallbladder, hepatocarcinoma or tumefaction of the portal lymph node and so on. When the dilatation of biliary ducts include cystic duct and cholecyst but intrahepatic bile ducts and common hepatic duct, the spot of the lesion usually is located at the choledochus or the head of the pancreas, which includes cholangiocarcinoma, carcinoma of the pancreas head, calculus of the biliary tract and so on. If the spot of the obstruction lies above the head of the pancreas, the lesion is mainly cholangiocarcinoma. If the spot of the obstruction lies at or under the head of the pancreas, cholangiocarcinoma, carcinoma of the pancreas head, calculus of the biliary tract all are possible, the high dilatation of which are usually cholangiocarcinoma whose dissepiment is mainly not smooth or carcinoma of the pancreas head whose characteristic often is the augmented head of the pancreas and the low dilatation of which is mostly the calculus of the choledochus. The obstruction reasons of the duodenal ampulla are calculus or carcinoma of ampulla, which shows the bile duct dilatation of the uncinate process of pancreas or the dilatation of the choledochus and pancreas duct at the same time, so called "bi-duct manifestation".

（4）Morphology of obstruction. Truncation sign, the dilated biliary tract suddenly disappears at the stenosis or becomes a cone-shaped stenosis, and the transitional segment of the stenosis does not exceed 10 mm, which is more common in obstruction caused by malignant tumors. Migrating stenosis, the dilated biliary tract gradually narrows and disappears at the stenosis site, and the migration section of the stenosis exceeds 20 mm, which is more common in obstruction caused by benign lesions. The narrow bile duct and the inner edge of the gallbladder are smooth and soft, which are more common in inflammatory lesions; serrated and stiff walls are more common in malignant lesions. The scope of biliary tract lesions is wide, and the bile ducts in the lesion area are distributed in thick and thin segments, which are common in primary sclerosing cholangitis. Obstruction caused by stones can be seen in the form of an inverted cup at the obstructed end.

Section 4　Diagnosis of common diseases

1. Congenital biliary duct cyst

（1）Clinical and pathological manifestations: The congenital biliary duct cyst has been called the congenital cholangiectasis once. Dr. Vater firstly reported choledochal cyst in 1723 and, in 1852, Dr. Douglas summarized the clinical characteristic of choledochal cyst and then, in 1958, Dr. Caroli, as the first man, reported congenital intrahepatic bile duct cyst. The icterus, abdominal ache and right upper quadrant mass of abdomen are three major clinical symptom of the congenital biliary duct cyst. Its main characteristic is that the cystic dilating of intra-and extrahepatic bile ducts communicate different-levelly with branch or major duct of the biliary tract. The most general method of imaging examination is US but the method of the most highly diagnostic value is MRCP.

Basing on the spot and the coverage of cysts, Dr. Todani classified the congenital biliary duct cyst into 5 types.

The type A is that the choledochus show cysticly or fusiformly dilated. It is 80－90 percent of all, most frequently. The type B is the choledochal cyst, which looks like simple diverticulum but the choledochus is normal. It is about 2 percent of all. The type C is that the choledochus of inferior extremity cysticly dilates, which enters the cava of the dodecadactylon, It is about 1.4－5 percent of all. The type D shows poly-cysts, which are intra-and extrahepatoic cysts. It is about 19 percent of all. The type E displays simple-or poly-cysts in the liver parenchyma, so called "Caroli disease".

The "Caroli disease" can also be classified into 2 types. The characteristics of the type A are cystic dilatation of intrahepatic bile duct, frequently accompanied with bile duct calculus and cholangitis and no cirrhosis and portal hypertension. The characteristics of the type B are cystic dilatation of distal end intrahepatic bile duct, accompanied seldom or never with bile duct calculus and cholangitis and frequent along with cirrhosis and portal hypertension.

(2) Imaging manifestations:

1) X-ray findings: The plain film has not special value in diagnosing the congenital biliary duct cyst. If PTC, ERCP or directly puncturing cholecystography shows communicating between cysts and intra-or extrahepatic bile ducts or directly displays the cysticly dilated choledochus, we can pathologically diagnose and also classify the congenital biliary duct cyst. Sometimes, we can also pathologically diagnose the congenital biliary duct cyst when the oral cholecystography or the intravenous cholecystocholangiography shows contrast medium of cyst from bile ducts.

2) Ultrasound findings: The A, B, C, and D type of the congenital biliary duct cyst manifest no echo area of the limited dilatation of the choledochus or porta hepatic bile duct. They do not show only ellipse or fusiform shape, but distinct border as well. They may also extend to the porta hepatis or the head of pancreas. The intra-or extrahepatic bile ducts beyond the cystic lesion often are not dilated but they may appear communicating with the cystic lesion. The cholecyst is usually pushed near the forearm of abdomen.

"Caroli" often manifest no echo area of multi-round or multi-fusiform around the main branch of the intrahepatic bilary duct. The lesions mostly appear high and clear echo of the border and it is communicated between cystic lesions or between the cystic lesions and the main branch of the intrahepatoic bile ducts.

3) Computed tomography(CT) findings: The A, B, C and D type of the congenital biliary duct cyst manifest impartial fluid density and the gracile, smooth, glossy border lesions of porta hepatis. The C type of the congenital biliary duct cyst appears fluid density lesion which extends into the duodenal lumen. The CT characteristic of the congenital biliary duct cyst are cystic or ball lesions and no bile duct dilating beyond lesions, the cholecyst developing and contrast medium in cystic lesions after intravenous cholecystocholangiography or oral cholecystography and manifestation similar to liver, pancreas, kidney or suprarenal gland cyst when the diameter of the cystic lesion is big.

"Caroli" mainly displays round or fusiform dilatation of intrahepatic bile duct near porta hepatis but no dilatation of end-brush bile duct. The characteristics of CT enhancement of "Caroli" is "central dot" sign, enhancing dots within the dilated intrahepatic bile ducts, representing portal radicles. Another way we can pathologically diagnose "Caroli" if the density of cystic cava is increased after intravenous cholecystocholangiography or oral cholecystography.

4) Magneticresonance imaging (MRI) findings: The lesions show cystic, column or diverticulum and thesignal

第四篇　腹部与盆腔

of theirs is low on T1WI and high on T2WI because of their cholestasis inside.

The A, B, C and D type of the congenital biliary duct cyst manifest the obviously cystic or fusiform dilatation of extrahepatic bile duct but no or light dilatation of intrahepatic bile duct. However, "Caroli" mainly shows partly or segmentally dilating of intrahepatic bile ducts, which distribute along with the branch of the bile duct, but no dilating of the right hepatic duct, the left hepatic duct, the common hepatic bile duct and the choledochus. The "central dot" sign is also seen on enhancement of MRI[Figure 12-5(a), (b)].

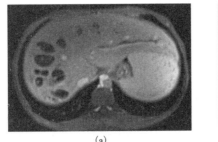
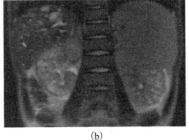

(a)　　　　　　　　　　　　　　　(b)

(a) The dilated intrahepatic bile duct surrounds the enhanced portal vein on contrast T1WI, which is called "central dot" sign(arrow); (b) Multiple cystic lesions were found in both kidneys with large spleen on Coronal T2WI.

Figure 12-5　Caroli disease

The transparent superiorities of the biliary tract MRI include: The sensitivity to the cystic lesions, especially on T*2WI and MRCP; The ability of observing relationship between the lesion and bile duct, liver parenchyma, organs close to the lesion and so on, for example, the coronal plane of T2WI, the sagittal plane of T2WI and MRCP, especially for MRCP, which can manifest the anatomic relationship between cyst and branch of biliary tract; Not needing to enhance and injuringly operate.

(3) Diagnosis and differential diagnosis

Intrahepatic multi-cysts and polycystic liver manifest idlely distributed cystic multi-lesions in the liver and their characteristic is no communicating between the lesion and bile ducts, associated with extrahepatic cystic mass.

2. Cholecystitis

The cholecystitis is classified into acute cholecystitis and chronic cholecystitis in the clinic.

(1) Acute cholecystitis

1) Clinical and pathological manifestations: The cause of the acute cholecystitis is mainly the obstruction of biliary tract calculus, the bacterial infection, the regurgitation of pancreatic juice and so on. The fever, right hypochondrial region and manifestation of the "Murphy's sign" are main clinical situation of the cholecystitis. The pathology mostly manifests hyperemia and edema of cholecystic wall, mucosal ulceration, amplification of cholecyst, thickening of cholecystic wall, abscess around and so on. The best method of examination is US.

2) Imaging manifestations:

①X-ray findings: Attimes, we can see the imaging of the dilated cholecyst because of cholecystitis or imaging of gas in the area of cholecyst because of the rod able to develop gas. The contrast medium examination is seldom or never used in diagnosing acute cholecystitis.

②Ultrasound findings: The gall bladder mostly enlarges and it usually appears round or oval-shap and unsmooth outline. The cholecystic wall manifests diffusely thickening, over 3 mm, and the high-low echo tape that there are continuous or intermittent low echo between high echo tapes. We can generally observe the high echo of calculus in the cholecyst, the post of which usually appear "sound shadow", if there are calculuses in the gall badder. Moreover, the ability of gallbadder contracting will descend or lose after eating fat.

③Computed tomography(CT) findings: The acute cholecystitis usually develops thickness more than 4 mm and clouding border of the gall bladder wall but manifestation of annular and low density because of its edema. The gall bladder, sometimes, amplificates, of which the diameter is more than 4.5 cm, and the density of the cholecystic cava often is high relative to water because of empyema of gallbladder. At times, we can observe manifestation of low density gas in the gallbladder cava, in its wall or in biliary tract. The mucous layer of the acute cholecystitis manifests enhancement by reason of phlegmonosis on the contrast CT, which appears strip or slight hyperattenuation, and a low density band formed in the serosa layer around the whole wall of gallbladder due to edema, which is very value in diagnosing the acute cholecystitis.

④Magnetic resonance imaging(MRI) findings: It is seldom used in diagnosing the acute cholecystitis and the MRI performance is in accordance with the CT basically. The acute cholecystitis mainly manifests thickened cholecystic wall, amplificated cholecystic cava and the fluid accumulating around the cholecyst but cholecystolithiasis or surrounding abscess in part. The cholecystic wall thickening is the major manifestation of acute cholecystitis and its ability of displaying also is main advantage of MRI relative to other methods in diagnosing acute cholecystitis. The characteristic of the thickened gall bladder wall usually are thickening impartial, intraborder smooth, serous membrane coarse and all of wall enhancement on delaying contrast MR scanning but intralayer's earlier enhancement.

3) Diagnosis and differential diagnosis: It is necessary for us to differentiate with other diseases, for example, hypoproteinemia by reason of the cirrhosis of liver, right heart failure, kidney's diseases, diabetes mellitus (DM) and so on. They generally haven't the history of acute disease, cholecyst enlargement or holecystolithiasis.

(2) Chronic Cholecystitis

1) Clinical and pathological manifestations: The chronic cholecystitis often comes from the acute cholecystitis but other original diseases and mostly mergers cholecystolithiasis. Its clinical performance is light and its major pathologies are the proliferating of fibrous tissue and chronic inflammatory cell infiltration so that they cause the cholecystic wall thickening, muscle atrophy and the hypofunction of gallbladder contraction. The best method of examination is US.

2) Imaging manifestations:

①X-ray findings: At times, we can see the decreased size cholecyst or the calcification in the cholecystic area. We can pathologically diagnose the chronic cholecystitis if no developing on oral cholecystography or intravenous cholecystocholangiography after eliminating other reasons.

②Ultrasound findings: We can usually observe the cholecyst contracting, its wall thickening and its echo reinforcing but its asper border. If there are cholecystolithiasises, we can observe its high echo, which areable to slowly move with posture changing, and "sound shadow". If the cholecyst has been atrophied, we can not observe fluid echo inside and only see the higher echo curve zone in the area of the cholecyst. Moreover, the contracting function of gallbladder usually decreases after eating fat.

③Computed tomography(CT) findings: We can usually observe manifestations of gallbladder atrophy, its wall thickening and, at times, a sprinkle of calcification in the gallbladder wall or cholecystolithiasis. Its wall thickening is the most important feature and frequent demonstration, the calcification of gallbladder wall is the most typical manifestation in diagnosing chronic holecystitis.

④Magnetic resonance imaging(MRI) findings: It is seldom used in diagnosing the chronic cholecystitis and the MRI performance is in accordance with the CT basically. The chronic cholecystitis mainly manifests cholecystic wall thickening, gallbladder atrophy with wall calcificating. But the ability of displaying the calcification of gallbladder wall is a great deal lower than the CT.

3)Diagnosis and differential diagnosis: The irregular thickening of cholecystic wall in carcinoma of gallbladder is more obvious than that of in chronic cholecystitis and that is mainly observed at thecervical and body of gallbladder. Basing on the irregular thickening of cholecystic wall accompanied with invasion of the liver parenchyma or liver parenchyma metastasis or lymph nodes metastasis, we can pathologically diagnose carcinoma of gallbladder.

3. Gall stone

(1)Cholecystolithiasis

1)Clinical and pathological manifestations: The clinical symptom of the cholecystolithiasis has something to do with its dimension, spot, obstruction or not and complication or not and so on. At times, there are not clinical symptoms or right upper quadrant malaise and, on the other hand, the symptoms of cholecystolithiasis also may be colicky pain, emesis, highly fever and so on when it is acute. The component of cholecystolithiasis includes bile pigments, cholesterol or, at times, calcium salt of different degree and cholecystolithiasis can be classified into two types. The cholecystolithiasis is called positive calculus when it contains more calcium and more X-ray is obstructed and it is called negative calculus when it contains less calcium and less X-ray is obstructed. The best method of examination is US.

2)Imaging manifestations:

①X-ray findings: 10-20 percent of cholecystolithiases are positive calculi and can be displayed by the plain film. Most of cholecystolithiases, which dimensions are about from sand to fava but part of the biggest, appear round, polygon, rhombus and stacked, which look like a string of vines. 80-90 percent of cholecystolithiasises are negative calculi and cann't be displayed by the plain film. Most of negative cholecystolithiases show filling defect of round or polygon on cholecystography.

②Ultrasound findings: The manifestations of typical cholecystolithiases include mass of one or more high echo, which can be moved with the posture changed, and clear "sound shadow" back of the high echo mass, which is emerged from highly attenuated echo energy by reason of refecting and absorpting of cholecystolithiases. Moreover, when the cholecyst is filled up with calculus, no echo area of the cholecyst will disappear and the front of cholecyst appear curve and high echo tape while there is "sound shadow" back of the cholecyst. When the cholecystolithiasis is accompanied with the thickening of the cholecystic wall, we can observe the manifestation which is made up of wall, calculus and "sound shadow". When the cholecystolithiasis is in its wall, we, at times, can observe more or less light spot of high echo, "sound shadow" and its characteristic of not moving with the patient's posture.

③ Computed tomography (CT) findings: The cholecystolithiasis may be displayed hyperattenuation, isoattenuation or hypoattenuation in the cholecyst with different level calcium on CT and they appear annular or multiplayer. Calcified gallbladder stones arehyperattenuating to bile, making them the only type to be clearly visualized on CT scan images[Figure 12-6(a)]. Pure cholesterol stones are hypoattenuating to bile, and other gallstones are isodense to bile and these may not be clearly identified on CT.

④Magnetic resonance imaging(MRI) findings: Gallbladder stones showed no signal or low signal on T2WI and MRCP images [Figure 12-6(b)], especially on T*2WI, although the signal of Gallbladder stones is variable. Many investigations have demonstrated that the signal of cholecystolithiasis is highly related to the content of its lipid and large molecular protein.

3) Diagnosis and differential diagnosis: Other positive lesions, for example, calcification of the kidney tubercle, adrenal calcification or calculus of the right kidney, mostly show irregular form and locate back of the vertebral body while cholecystolithiasis often lie in front of the vertebral bodyon lateral plain film. The neoplasms of the cholecyst have to refer to many examinations and its clinical manifestation.

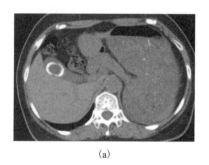
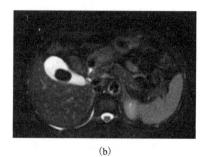

(a)   (b)

(a)Gallstones on CT. There is a round rim hyperattenuation lesion in the gallbladder(arrow) and means "rim sign"; (b)Gallstones on MRI T2WI. Gallstones shows low signal outlined by markedly hyperintense bile within the gallbladder hypointensity on T2WI(arrow).

Figure 12-6   Gallstones

(2)Bileduct calculus

1)Clinical and pathological manifestations: The calculus of bile duct is classified into two types: The calculus of intrahepatic bile duct and the calculus of extrahepatic bile duct based on the existing spot or the primary calculus and the following calculus based on the originating spot.

The clinical manifestation of the intrahepatic bile duct calculus isn't typical. Most havn't manifestation in intermittent period while most show manifestation of acute cholangitis in acute period and intermittent attacking is its clinical characteristic. The typical manifestation of the calculus of extrahepatic bile duct is biliary colic, icterus, fever and chill, so called "Charoat triad".

The component of the bile duct calculus is same as the cholecystic calculus. Most of the calculi of intrahepatic bile duct are calcium. Most of following calculi of extrahepatic bile duct are cholesterol calculus while most of primary calculus of extrahepatic bile duct are calculus of bile pigment. The best method of examination is US.

2)Imaging manifestations:

①X-ray findings: The positive calculus of calcium, at times, appears manifestation of calcification on the plain film which lie in the area of the biliary duct and filling defect of simple or multiple, round or strip and smooth border on contrast examination.

②Ultrasound findings: The calculus of bile duct shows round, blotch or strip high echo and"sound shadow" along with the bile duct while the bile ducts above of high echo are usually dilated.

③ Computed tomography (CT) findings: Routine contrast-enhanced CT is moderately sensitive to choledocholithiasis with a sensitivity of 65%~88%. The calculus of bile duct may be hyperattenuation (the calculus contains more bile pigment or calcium), isoattenuation or or hypoattenuation (the calculus contains more cholesterol)in the bile duct with different level calcium on CT and, at times, they also appear annular or multilayer high or low density, so called "Target". If the stone is outlined by thin shell of density it shows "rim sign". The bile ducts above of calculus are usually dilated [Figure 12-7(a), (c)].

④Magnetic resonance imaging (MRI) findings: MRCP haslargely replaced ERCP as the gold standard for diagnosis of choledocholithiasis, able to achieve similar sensitivity (90%~94%) and specificity (95%~99%), without ionizing radiation, intravenous contrast, or the complication rate inherent in ERCP.

Filling defects are seen within the biliary tree on thin cross-sectional T2 weighted imaging. Care should be taken not to use thick slabs for the diagnosis as volume averaging may obscure smaller stones. However, if the diagnosis has already been secured by ultrasound or CT, maybe there is no additional value of MRCP. The signal characteristic of the bile duct calculus is in accordance with the gall bladder calculus basically and it mostly shows round or oval shape low intensity or no signal lesion [Figure 12-7(b) ~ (f)]. The bile ducts above of calculus are usually dilated and most of the local bile duct walls are thickened.

3) Diagnosis and differential diagnosis

On US, cholangiocarcinoma manifests low or middle echo while there isn't "sound shadow" and there isn't clear delimitation between the wall of the bile duct and the lesion. On CT, cholangiocarcinoma demonstrates irregular thickening of the bile wall and the local interruption of the biliary tract. On MRCP or T*2WI, there are local bile duct constriction and bile duct dilatation of malignant tumor. The stoma constriction post of the operation or the gas of the intrahepatic bile duct usually can be differentiated from their history and clinical symptoms. Intrahepatic calcification is not accompanied by biliary dilatation.

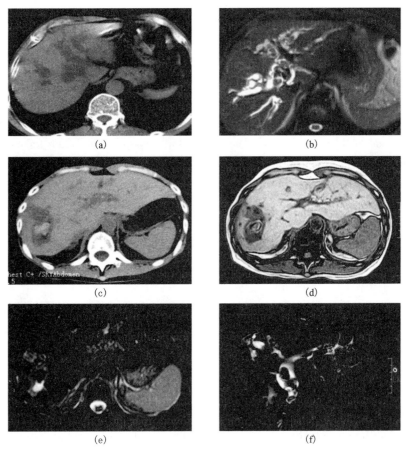

(a) The intrahepatic bile duct is dilated obviously on non-contrast CT; (b) Bile duct calculus. There are much ovoid filling defects seen within the intrahepatic bile duct on T2WI in the same patient and this is consistent with an intraductal calculus; (c) Bile duct calculus of CT. There are much hyper-attenuation lesion seen within the intrahepatic bile duct on non-contrast CT and is consistent with intraductal calculus; (d) Bile duct calculus of MRI. Bile duct calculus can appear high signal intensity or low signal intensity on T1WI images at same patient; (e) Bile duct calculus of MRI. Multiple filling defect signals are found in intrahepatic bile ducts with bile duct dilation on T2WI images; (f) Bile duct calculus MPCP. Multiple filling defect signals are found in intrahepatic and extrahepatic bile ducts. Magnetic resonance cholangiopancreatography (MRCP) has become the gold standard for the diagnosis of bile duct stones.

Figure 12-7 Bile duct calculus

4. Maligant tumor

（1）Gallbladder carcinoma

1）Clinical and pathological manifestations: The gallbladder carcinoma is the most general malignant tumor of the biliary system and are mainly reported in women over 50 years old. Most of them havn't charactistic clinical manifestation while part may show right hypochondrial region, mass of gallbladder fossa or icterus of lateperiod tumor and so on. 85 percent of gallbladder carcinomas are adenocarcinoma and others may be squamous carcinoma or carcinoid. 70 percent of gallbladder carcinomas are usually accompanied with cholecystolithiasis.

2）Imaging manifestations:

①X-ray findings: The value of the plain film is little indiagnosing gallbladder carcinoma and the diagnostic value of cholecystography is limited. The gallbladder could not be visualized in the oral cholecystography procedure or filling defect of the cholecyst. The invasion of hilar bile duct can lead to bile duct stricture with obstruction. In recent years, cholecystography procedure has been replaced step by step by US, CT, MRI.

②Ultrasound findings: Based on the form of gallbladder carcinoma, it is mostly classified into three types: The intracavum type, the pachy wall type and the mass type. The intracavum type (15% ~ 23%) comes from the cholecystic wall and appears simple or multiple nipple tumors. Most of them have irregular and broad basis and their cholecystic cava can still be observed while the pedicel of the tumor is shown seldom, which are mostly earlier period manifestation of gallbladder carcinoma. The pachy wall type (15% ~ 22%) shows limited or diffused asymmetrical thickening wall, of which the intraborder isn't irregular. Most of them originate from the neck or the body of the gall bladder. The mass type (41% ~ 70%) is most frequent and is mostly late period gallbladder carcinoma. The cholecystic cavum is partly or completely occupied by soft tumor. In addition to the above, there are obstruction type and mixed type in some literatures. The characteristic of the obstruction type is the obstruction of cystic duct because of the tumor's occupying or offending and the dilatation of cholecystic cavum, of which the tumors are frequently small. The mixed type has the characteristic of the intracavum type and the pachy wall type at the same time.

On US, most of gallbladder carcinomas manifest low or no echo while there are not "sound shadow". When it is accompanied with cholecystolithiasis, we can observe itshigh echo mass and "sound shadow". In addition, we can usually observe manifestations of dilatation of cholecyst or bile duct, direct invasion of the liver, metastasis of the liver or otherorgans, lymphatic metastasis and so on.

③Computed tomography(CT) findings: The classification of gallbladder carcinoma is same as the US. The gallbladdercarcinomas mostly manifest the density like soft tissue and mild enhancement[Figure 12-8（a）,（b）] while a little long duration unlike the characteristicic of hepatocarcinoma with "rapid wash in and wash out". At times, we can observe manifestations of dilatation of cholecyst or bile duct, direct encroaching of the liver, metastasis of the liver or otherorgans, lymphatic metastasis and so on. If we observe low density lesion in liver parenchyma around the tumor of gallbladder carcinoma, we can diagnose liver invaded from gallbladder carcinoma.

④Magnetic resonance imaging(MRI) findings: The classification of gallbladder carcinoma is same as the US. The signal ofgallbladder carcinoma is low or equal to soft tissue on T1WI and high on T2WI. Most of gallbladder carcinomas have obvious enhancement and long duration unlike the characteristic of hepatocarcinoma with "rapid wash in and wash out". We can diagnose liver parenchyma invasion by reason of gallbladder carcinomas with the fat signal around cholecyst disappearing.

3）Diagnosis and differential diagnosis: At times, it is difficult to differentiate the chronic cholecystitis from the pachy wall type of gallbladdercarcinoma. However, the thickening wall of chronic cholecystitis is lighter and equalizedlier than gallbladder carcinoma and chronic cholecystitis does not invade adjacent tissues and distant metastasis.

The characteristics of benignneoplasm, for example, polyp, granuloma, adenoma and so on, include that their diameter is, generally, no more than 10 mm, that their walls are soft and smooth and that there are not offending around and distant metastasis.

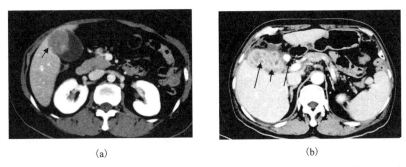

(a)　　　　　　　　　　　　(b)

(a) Intraluminal gallbladder carcinoma on CT. There is a round soft mass protruding into the gallbladder cavity with mild enhancement. And the space between gallbladder and liver tissue is disappeared(arrow); (b) Diffuse gallbladder carcinoma on CT. It is diffuse mural thickening of gallbladder(short arrow) with heterogeneous enhancement. Gallstones are present (long arrow).

Figure 12-8　Intraluminal gallbladder carcinoma

(2)Cholangiocarcinoma

1)Clinical and pathological manifestations: Most cholangiocarcinoma are located in big ducts, 8-31 percent of which lie in the intrahepatic ducts while 37-50 percent of which lie in close segment of the extrahepatic ducts and 4-36 percent of which lie in the choledochus or "Vater ampulla". The painless and advancing icterus or the icterus accompanied with abdominal pain are the major clinical manifestation of cholangiocarcinoma. Most of cholangiocarcinoma are adenocarcinoma. Based on the forms of cholangiocarcinoma, they can be classified into three types: The infiltrating type, the mass type and the intraductal type. The infiltrating type is the most commonly type and easily lead to local constriction when small tumor. The lesion of the mass type is obvious very much while the obstruction because of it is light relatively. The intraductal type is seldom and mainly appear the tumor of duct cavum. The characteristic of cholangiocarcinoma is slowly growing, easily obstructing bile duct and mainly die from its complication.

2)Imaging manifestations:

①X-ray findings: The plain film hasn't special value in diagnosing cholangiocarcinoma. PTC can display the spot of cholangiocarcinoma and the form of close segment dilatation of bile duct. The infiltrating type mostly appears locally constricted while the mass type and the nipple polypoid type mainly manifest filling defect. ERCP is able to demonstrate the spot and the coverage of the lesion with direction of the inferior-to-superior. Based on PTC and ERCP at the same time, 90 percent ofcholangiocarcinomacan be pathologily diagnosed.

②Ultrasound findings: The lump of the cholangiocarcinoma is located at the inferiority of the dilated bile duct and appears low or middle and mammillary or irregular echo. The echoes of cholangiocarcinoma most are not asymmetrical and, unlike bile duct calculus, there is not "sound shadow". The mass type and the nipple polypoid type mainly manifest local lump in the bile duct cava or the bile duct cava filled with tumor while there isn't delimitation between the bile duct wall and the lump. The infiltrating type or the mass-infiltrating type display the biliary tract unexpectedly constricted or interrupted and, at the same time, irregular intraborder of the obstructed spot but not having obvious lump. In addition to the above, there are other manifestations, for example, bile duct dilatation above the lump, lymph node tumefaction of porta hepatis, metastases of the liver or other organs.

③Computed tomography(CT) findings: CT manifestation of cholangiocarcinoma is same as that of the US. Based on the original spot of the cholangiocarcinoma, it is classified into four types: The circumference type, the porta hepatis type, the extrahepatic bile duct type and the ampulla type. The circumference type tumors, so called cholangioma or liver tumor of bile duct cell, originate from the bile duct wall beyond right or left hepatic duct. They manifest the lump in the hepatic parenchyma along with the dilatation of circumferential bile duct or, at times, the calcification in the lump. The porta hepatis type tumors originate from the wall of right hepatic duct, left hepatic duct or the 10 mm close segment of common hepatic duct and the lump appear "Y" or irregular[Figure 12-9(a), (b)]. The extrahepatic bile duct type tumors originate from the wall of the close segment common hepatic duct to "Vater ampulla" and the lumps appear strip or irregular. The "Vater ampulla" type tumors originate from the wall of "Vater ampulla" or the bottom of pancreas head and the lumps appear irregular.

Most of cholangiocarcinoma havn't high enhancement in early period of contrast scanning but they may have delayed enhancement.

In addition to the above, the bile ducts beyond the spot of the obstruction generally display tree and vine shape dilatation from middle to high and the obstruction spot appears to be interrupted or unexpectedly constricted. With the obstruction spot gracilely scanned, the intraborder often is irregular. The ampulla carcinomas usually display the manifestation of bi-duct. Moreover, biliary tract calculus, atrophying of local liver or metastases of other organs are usually observed in some cholangiocarcinoma.

④Magnetic resonance imaging (MRI) findings: MRI is the imaging modality of choice, as it can best visualize all three the tumor itself, the biliary ducts and the blood vessels, all of which are essential for determining resectability. Appearances on MR are similar to those described above for CT, except that MR is more sensitive to contrast enhancement and bile duct visualization. The form of the tumor and the characteristic of obstruction are same as the US or the CT. The signal of the cholangiocarcinoma is low or equal to that of hepatic parenchyma on T1WI while slightly high on T2WI. Compared with PTC and ERCP, MRCP is able to display the level and coverage of bile duct dilating and the characteristic of the obstruction. A peripherally hyperintense "target" appearance on DWI favors cholangiocarcinoma over hepatocellular carcinoma[Figure 12-10(a) ~ (d)].

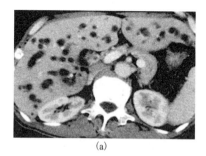
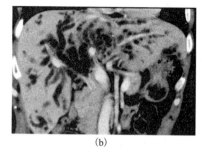

(a) (b)

(a)The wall of the upper segment of the common bile ductis significantly thickened with bile duct stenosis and was accompanied by significant enhancement in portal venous phase CT scan; (b)Hilar cholangiocarcinoma(Klatskin tumor). The extent of hilar cholangiocarcinomais clearly shown on coronal CT and it is diagnosed as hilar cholangiocarcinoma Bismuth-Corlette(BC) type I.

Figure 12-9   Hilar cholangiocarcinoma(Klatskin tumor)

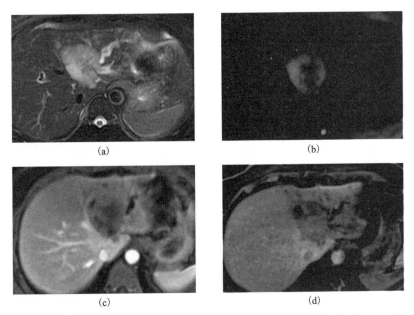

(a) Heterogeneous slightly high signal mass with peritumoral focus is found in the left liver and intrahepatic bile duct is dilatation on T2WI；（b）Intrahepatic cholangiocarcinoma. A peripherally hyperintense "target" appearance on DWI favors cholangiocarcinoma；（c） Intrahepatic cholangiocarcinoma. The tumor shows heterogeneous moderate enhancement in portal vein phase；（d）Intrahepatic cholangiocarcinoma. The left liver tumor shows delayed enhancement and tended to be homogeneous after 5 minutes at parenchymal phase imaging.

Figure 12-10   Intrahepaticcholangiocarcinoma

3）Diagnosisand differential diagnosis：The cholangiocarcinoma have to be differentiated with other chronic diseases, especially calculus of bile duct and chronic phlegmonosis by reason of bile duct calculus, that can lead to obstruction of biliary tract. When we diagnose the cholangiocarcinoma, it is very important for us to synthesize the history, the clinical situation, the spot, the dimension and blood supplying of the lesion by US, CT or MRI, the dilated or constricted characteristic of biliary tract by MRCP, PTC, ERCP or US.

（Yuan Youhong, Jiang Hongtao, Li Xiumei, Luo Wei, Mao Zhiqun, Xiao Enhua, Liu Hui）

第十三章

胰腺

第一节　检查方法

1. X 线检查

腹部 X 线平片在发现胰腺内的钙化方面具有一定的价值(图 13-1)；胃肠造影、低张十二指肠造影价值较低，主要根据胰腺周围器官位置、形态改变推断胰腺病变；ERCP 是显示胰腺导管的有价值的方法，可用于慢性胰腺炎、胰腺癌、壶腹癌的鉴别诊断；DSA 可用于胰腺富血管功能性胰腺神经内分泌肿瘤的诊断。

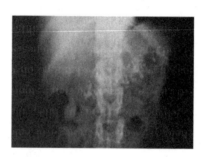

图 13-1　慢性胰腺炎患者腹部平片显示散在沙粒样钙化

2. CT 检查

CT 平扫与增强扫描是胰腺疾病常用的影像学方法，需空腹饮水，口服稀释阳性对比剂，常规先行平扫，多同时多期增强扫描，方法同肝脏。平扫能够显示胰腺与周围结构的关系及胰腺形态大小密度等改变，增强扫描有利于显示胆管、胰管、未造成外形改变的小病灶及与周围血管的关系。CTA 有利于准确判断胰周动脉、静脉的情况。

3. MRI 检查

MRI 是超声与 CT 检查的重要补充，常规行平扫 T1WI 与 T2WI，抑脂技术可更好的显示胰腺及病变，能够敏感的检出病变(小的胰岛素瘤)、清楚显示病变的细节及确定其组织成分(如肿瘤出血)，有利于胰腺疾病诊断与鉴别诊断。MRCP 是显示胰管的最佳检查方法，能够完整显示胰管及胆道，主要用于观察胰管及胆道的形态及通畅情况。

第二节　正常表现

1. 胰腺的位置、形态、大小

胰腺位于腹膜后肾前间隙内,前面隔网膜囊与胃相邻,后方有下腔静脉、门静脉和脾动静脉等重要结构,其胰头被十二指肠环抱,胰尾抵达脾门。胰腺形似弓状,凸面向前,平对第 1-2 腰椎,长 17~20 cm,宽 3~5 cm,厚 1.5~2.5 cm,正常胰管内径≤2 mm。正常胰腺形态多为蝌蚪型(胰头粗,体尾逐渐变细),其次为哑铃型(头、尾粗、体部较细)及腊肠型(头、体、尾粗细大致相等)。

2. 胰腺的分部

胰腺分为头、颈、体、尾 4 部分,各部之间无明显界限。一般胰尾位置高,胰头位置低。钩突是胰头下方向内延伸的楔形突出、其前方为肠系膜上动、静脉,外侧是十二指肠降段,下方为十二指肠水平段。

3. 胰腺实质

(1)X 线表现:ERCP 示正常胰管自胰头部向尾部斜行,管径逐渐变细,最大径不超过 5 mm,边缘光滑整齐,主胰管上有一些分支,有时还可显示位置高于主胰管的副胰管。

(2)超声表现:正常胰腺在其长轴切面上边缘整齐、胰头稍膨大,其下方向左后的突出部为钩突。超声还可显示胆总管胰内段,主胰管多数可见,为胰腺实质内的两条平行而光滑的中、高回声线即主胰管壁;正常胰管内径≤2 mm(图 13-2)。

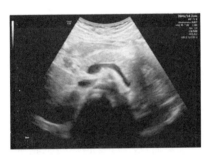

胰腺形似弓状,凸面向前,信号均匀,脾静脉
沿胰腺体尾部后缘走行,是识别胰腺的标志。

图 13-2　胰腺实质超声表现

(3)CT 表现:可清楚显示胰腺的轮廓、密度、形状和大小。正常胰腺边缘光滑或呈小分叶状;密度均匀,低于肝实质,年长者其内常因脂肪浸润而有散在小灶性脂肪密度,增强后密度均匀增高(图 13-3)。脾静脉沿胰腺体尾部后缘走行,是识别胰腺的标志。胰管位于胰腺实质内,可不显示或表现为细线状低密度影。

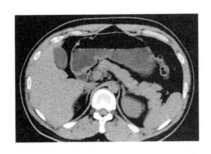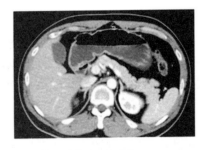

正常胰腺实质密度均匀,增强密度均匀增高,边缘呈小分叶状。

图 13-3　实质 CT 表现

（4）MRI 表现：腹膜后高信号脂肪组织有助于勾画出胰腺轮廓。在 T1WI 和 T2WI 上，胰腺为均匀较低信号结构，与肝实质信号相似，应用 T1WI 抑脂序列，胰腺呈相对高信号表现（图 13-4）；其背侧的脾静脉由于流空效应可呈无信号影，有助于勾画出胰腺的后缘，胰头位于十二指肠曲内，十二指肠内液体表现为 T2WI 高信号影。

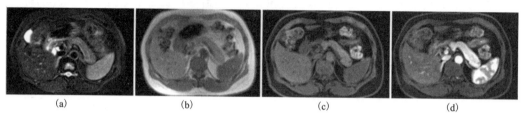

(a)横断面抑脂 T2WI 序列显示正常胰腺实质信号高于肝脏、低于脾脏；(b)横断面 T1WI 序列显示正常胰腺实质信号高于脾脏；(c)横断面抑脂 T1WI 序列，胰腺呈相对高信号表现；d 横断面抑脂 T1WI 序列增强动脉期胰腺明显均匀强化。

图 13-4　胰腺 MRI 表现

第三节　基本病变

1. X 线表现

X 线平片可发现胰腺区钙化及胰管结石；ERCP 的异常表现有胰管阻塞、狭窄，边缘不规则，腔内充盈缺损，胰管走行异常，分支僵硬、短缺及排列不整齐，也可粗细不均匀呈串珠状或囊状扩张。ERCP 对诊断慢性胰腺炎、胰头癌和壶腹癌有一定帮助。

2. CT 表现

（1）胰腺大小和外形异常：胰腺弥漫性增大多为急性胰腺炎表现；胰腺肿瘤则常表现为胰腺局部增大；胰头癌往往还伴有胰腺体尾部萎缩；胰腺萎缩及脂肪浸润则胰腺轮廓呈羽毛状改变。

（2）主胰管的异常：扩张的胰管在 CT 上多表现为胰腺中央带状低密度影，增强扫描后显示更为清晰；慢性胰腺炎可致胰管串珠状或囊状扩张。

（3）胰腺密度异常：胰腺炎由于胰腺组织的液化坏死则表现为胰腺实质密度不均匀；胰腺肿瘤多为乏血供肿瘤，增强扫描后往往强化低于正常胰腺实质而表现为低密度肿块，肿瘤中央的液化坏死则表现为更低密度影；功能性胰岛细胞瘤在增强扫描后明显强化，非功能性胰岛细胞瘤则往往与胰腺密度相近而有较明显强化。

（4）胰腺边缘及周围异常：炎症渗出及肿瘤浸润常常使胰腺周围脂肪间隙密度增高，胰腺边界模糊不清；渗出较多时胰腺周围可见条片状低密度积液；肾前筋膜增厚则是胰腺炎周围组织异常的常见征象。

3. MRI 表现

胰腺大小、形态异常的意义与 CT 相似。不同病变 MRI 有其不同的信号变化：胰腺癌在 T1WI 上常表现为低或等信号，在 T2WI 上主要为高信号，肿瘤内出现出血、液化坏死而呈混杂高信号；胰岛细胞瘤的信号较为均匀，尤其是功能性者。胰腺囊性病变在 T1WI 上为低信号，在 T2WI 上为高信号，囊腺瘤常为多房性，其内可见软组织信号分隔及壁结节影。急性胰腺炎由于充血、水肿及胰液外渗，胰腺实质在 T1WI 上信号减低，在 T2WI 上信号增高。慢性胰腺炎 T2WI 上可呈混杂信号，胰腺或胰管内钙化或结石为无信号影；胰管扩张，MRCP 显示为条带状或串珠状高信号影。

第四节　常见疾病诊断

1. 急性胰腺炎

（1）临床与病理表现：急性胰腺炎是胰蛋白酶原溢出被激活成胰蛋白酶引发胰腺及周围组织自身消化的一种急性炎症。发病前多有酗酒、暴饮暴食或胆道疾病史，临床上表现为突发上腹痛并可出现休克，疼痛向腰背部放射，伴有恶心、呕吐、发热和血胰酶增高等为特点。病变程度轻重不等，轻者以胰腺水肿为主，临床多见，病情常呈自限性，预后良好，又称为轻症急性胰腺炎或急性水肿型胰腺炎，占80%~90%；少数重者的胰腺出血坏死，常继发感染、腹膜炎和休克等，病死率高，称为重症急性胰腺炎或出血坏死型胰腺炎。

（2）影像学表现：

1）X线表现：X线平片主要表现为上腹部肠曲扩张，或表现肺底炎性表现或胸腔积液等。

2）CT表现：对于了解病变的程度与范围很有帮助，在提供腹部及腹膜后综合信息方面具有优势。急性水肿型胰腺炎平扫表现为胰腺体积明显肿大，多为弥漫性增大；由于胰腺水肿，胰腺实质密度减低；炎性渗出，胰腺边缘模糊，与周围分界不清，肾周筋膜增厚；增强扫描胰腺均匀强化。急性出血性坏死性胰腺炎除胰腺增大更加明显外，还可出现胰腺内坏死的更低密度区或出血的高密度灶，同时炎性渗出更明显，可见胰腺周围积液或腹水，液体可进入小网膜、肾周、结肠旁沟及胸腔内，并发症一般为假性囊肿，多由于积液没能够完全吸收造成；增强扫描水肿区可强化，坏死区无强化［图13-5（a）、（b）］。

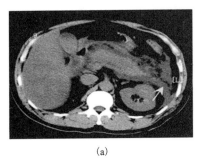 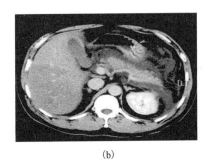

(a)　　　　　　　　　　　　(b)

平扫（a）及增强（b）示胰腺体积普遍性增大，边缘不清，胰周脂肪间隙模糊，可见低密度渗出性改变，左侧肾前筋膜明显增厚。

图13-5　急性胰腺炎

3）MRI表现：由于炎性细胞浸润、水肿、出血坏死等改变，胰腺体积增大，形状不规则，边缘模糊不清，T1WI表现为低信号，T2WI表现为高信号，注射Gd-DTPA增强扫描后灌注正常的胰腺组织出现强化，坏死组织区不强化。坏死性胰腺炎出血区T1WI、T2WI可表现为高信号，胰周积液及炎症表现为相应改变，假性囊肿表现为长T1长T2信号，其他同CT（图13-6）。

（3）诊断与鉴别诊断：急性胰腺炎常有明确病史、体征及化验检查结果，结合影像学表现，诊断较易，但影像学表现有助于确定病变病理情况、腹膜后表现及有无并发症。

2. 慢性胰腺炎

（1）临床与病理表现：多由急性胰腺炎反复发作而形成，多造成胰腺广泛纤维化，质地变硬呈结节状，腺泡及胰岛均有不同程度的萎缩消失，胰管与间质可有钙化和结石形成。临床上常有上腹痛，且反复出现，可合并糖尿病或胆道疾病等。

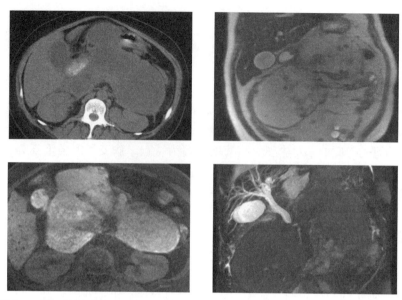

轴位 CT 平扫示整个胰腺区巨大不均质低密度包块,与周围脂肪界限不清,冠状位 T2WI 示大片液体高信号内斑片状低信号影,轴位抑脂 T1WI 示病灶内部明显高信号,厚层 MRCP 可见肝内外胆管扩张,胆总管远端梗阻。

图 13-6 急性胰腺炎 MRI 表现

(2)影像学表现:

1)X 线表现:X 线平片可于胰腺走形区发现致密、多发的小结石及钙化;ERCP 对慢性胰腺炎比较敏感,多表现为多发性狭窄、扩张并存,串珠样或管状。

2)CT 表现:对胰腺实质的显示更为准确,对钙化的显示更为敏感。阳性表现:胰腺大小可正常、缩小或增大;胰管可呈管状、串珠状扩张,部分伴有胆总管扩张;出现胰管结石或沿胰管分布的胰腺实质性钙化,为特征性表现;胰内或胰外假囊肿形成;肾周筋膜增厚等(图 13-7)。

3)MRI 表现:胰腺大小形态改变同 CT,由于胰腺纤维化,T1WI 脂肪抑制像和 T2WI 可表现为低信号,增强后无强化或强化不明显,合并假性囊肿时表现为长 T1 长 T2 信号,钙化表现为长 T1 短 T2 信号。

(3)诊断与鉴别诊断:慢性胰腺炎,特别是导致胰头局限性增大时,与胰腺癌难以鉴别,一般慢性胰腺炎胰头增大以纤维化为主,T1WI 和 T2WI 均为低信号,强化特征与体尾一致,但胰腺癌增强扫描动脉期为低密度或低信号,慢性胰腺炎伴钙化、假性囊肿多见,胰腺癌更易引起胰腺邻近血管侵犯或包埋,同时也可出现转移。

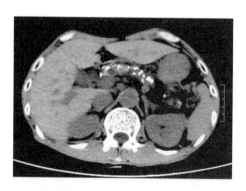

CT 平扫显示胰腺体积缩小,胰头体尾散在分布斑点片状钙化。

图 13-7 慢性胰腺炎 CT 表现

3.胰腺内分泌肿瘤

(1)临床与病理表现：胰腺内分泌肿瘤最常见的为胰岛细胞瘤，占胰腺肿瘤的1%~2%，常好发于在30~60岁，无明显的性别倾向。多为孤立病变，1%~2%与多发性内分泌肿瘤Ⅰ型(MEN-I)有关，其特征为甲状旁腺、垂体和胰腺三联征，临床症状和体征与其细胞类型和生物活性有关。这些肿瘤可根据其是否分泌足够的活性化合物而大致分为综合征(胰岛素瘤、胃泌素瘤、胰高血糖素瘤、血管活性肠肽、生长抑素瘤)或非综合征性肿瘤。

(2)影像学表现：

1)X线表现：平片不能诊断胰腺神经内分泌肿瘤。

2)CT表现：胰腺内分泌肿瘤多为富血供性，边界清楚，可出现钙化或囊性改变；较小肿瘤密度均匀、边界清楚、血供丰富，较大肿瘤密度可能不均匀，包含囊性或坏死区；胰腺内分泌肿瘤在早期动脉期(25~35 s)出现峰值增强，但在动脉晚期对比不明显，易漏诊(图13-8)。

3)MRI表现：检出敏感性与CT相似。相对于胰腺实质，胰腺内分泌肿瘤在T1WI上呈低信号，在T2WI上表现为高信号，注射Gd-DTPA增强扫描后相对胰腺实质表现为高强化或富血供。

(3)诊断与鉴别诊断：主要与原发内分泌疾病的鉴别，要靠影像检查，如果影像学检查发现有胰腺肿瘤的存在，加上有激素水平的改变，可诊断胰腺内分泌肿瘤。

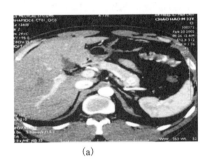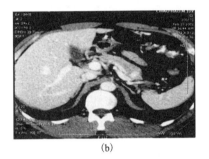

(a) (b)

(a)为动脉期，(b)为静脉期，胰尾处小肿物动脉期强化明显，门静脉期仍有强化，但不如动脉期明显。

图13-8 胰岛素瘤

4.胰腺癌

(1)临床与病理表现：胰腺癌为胰腺最常见的恶性肿瘤，占95%，为胰腺导管细胞癌，60%~70%发生在胰腺头部，其次为体、尾部或全胰癌，好发于40岁以上男性，发病率随年龄增大增加，早期无症状，晚期可出现持续性腹痛、进行性黄疸与体重减轻三大症状，侵犯周围结构是出现相应症状。胰腺癌预后较差，5年生存率仅约5%。

(2)影像学表现：

1)X线表现：X线平片价值不大；胃肠道钡餐造影可显示中晚期病变，主要表现为癌症对邻近胃、十二指肠的压迫或侵犯；ERCP表现取决于肿瘤与胰管的关系，可表现为主胰管受压移位或局限性不规则狭窄至完全截断，远端胰管扩张；PTC胆总管下端梗阻，形态呈圆钝、平滑或小结节状影，充盈扩张的胆总管可有移位性改变。

2)CT表现：胰头体尾癌具有相应部位胰腺肿块，平扫多为低密度影，少量为等或高密度；肿瘤较大可显示局部隆起，较小时外形可正常，全胰腺癌表现为整个胰腺或大部分成低密度影；肝内胆管、胆总管、胰管不同程度扩张；增强扫描，动脉期表现为均匀、不均匀低密度灶，边缘不规则环状强化，静脉期为低密度，但与正常胰腺密度差较动脉期减小(图13-9)；侵犯胰周血管及远处脏器、淋巴结转移。

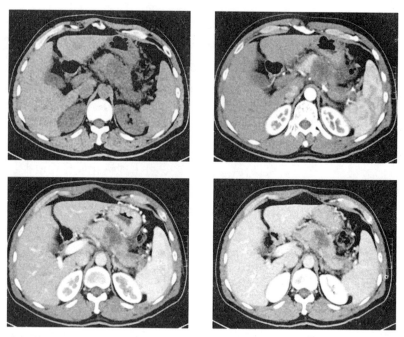

平扫与增强三期扫描显示胰体部肿块、局部隆起，平扫稍低密度，增强扫描强化不明显，呈低密度区。

图 13-9　胰腺癌 CT 表现

3）MRI 表现：主要表现为肿块，轮廓不规则，与正常胰腺分界不清；T1WI 多为低信号，T2WI 可表现为不均匀高信号；强化特征、侵犯转移表现与 CT 相似，MRI 增强扫描实质期 T1WI 脂肪抑制像有利于淋巴结转移的显示。

（3）诊断与鉴别诊断：中晚期胰腺癌诊断较为容易，胰腺癌主要与慢性胰腺炎鉴别，炎性病变胰管多呈串珠状扩张，可见胰腺萎缩及钙化，肾周筋膜增厚，无淋巴结转移。

（袁友红，罗伟，李秀梅，蒋洪涛，毛志群，肖恩华，刘辉）

Chapter 13

Pancreas

Section 1 Method of examination

1. X-ray examination

Abdominal plain film has certain value in finding pancreas calcification (Figure 13 − 1). The value of gastroenterography and hypotonic duodenography is relatively low in the diagnosis of pancreatic disease, which mainly infers pancreatic lesions according to the location and morphological changes of organs around the pancreas; ERCP is a valuable method to display pancreatic duct, which can be used for the differential diagnosis of chronic pancreatitis, pancreatic cancer and ampullary cancer; DSA can be used for the diagnosis of pancreatic neuroendocrine tumor with rich vascular.

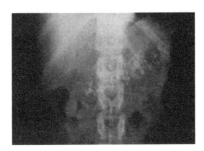

Figure 13−1　Abdominal plain film of chronic pancreatitis shows scattered sandy calcification

2. CT examination

CT plain scan and enhanced scan are the common imaging methods of pancreatic diseases, which usually need fasting drinking water, oral diluted positive contrast agent. The method of plain scan and multi-phase dynamic enhanced scan is the same as that of liver scan. Plain scan can show the relationship between the pancreas and its surrounding structures, and the changes of the shape, size and density of the pancreas. Enhanced scan is helpful to show the bile duct, pancreatic duct, small lesions without pancreas appearance changes and its relationship with the surrounding vessels. CTA is helpful to judge the condition of peripancreatic artery and vein.

3. MRI examination

MRI is an important examination method besides ultrasound and CT in pancreatic diseases. MRI plain scan T1WI and T2WI, especially fat suppression technology, can sensitively detect lesions (such as small insulinoma), clearly show the details of lesions and determine their tissue components (such as tumor bleeding), which is conducive to the diagnosis and differential diagnosis of pancreatic diseases. MRCP is the best method to display the pancreatic duct. It can display the pancreatic duct and biliary tract completely and it is mainly used to observe the shape and patency of the pancreatic duct and biliary tract.

Section 2　Normal appearances

1. The position, shape and size of the pancreas

The pancreas locates in the retroperitoneal space between the anterior renal space, adjacent to the anterior omentum sac of the stomach, and behind the inferior vena cava, portal vein and splenic artery and vein. The head of the pancreas is surrounded by the duodenum, and the tail of the pancreas reaches the hilum of the spleen. The pancreas is arched, convex forward, flat to the 1st~2nd lumbar vertebrae, 17~20 cm long, 3~5 cm wide, 1.5~2.5 cm thick, and the normal pancreatic duct diameter ≤2 mm. The normal shape of pancreas is mostly tadpole type (pancreas head thick, body tail gradually thin), followed by dumbbell type (head, tail thick, body thin) and sausage type (head, body, tail roughly equal thickness).

2. The parts of the pancreas

The pancreas is divided into four parts: head, neck, body and tail, with no distinct boundaries between the parts. The position of pancreatic tail is high while the head is low in general. The uncinate process is a wedge-shaped protrusion extending inwards in the inferior direction of the head of the pancreas. In front of the uncinate process are the superior arteries and veins of the mesentery, and the lateral part is the descending part of the duodenum, and the lower part is the horizontal part of the duodenum.

3. Pancreatic parenchyma

(1) X-ray findings: X-ray examination of ERCP show that the normal pancreatic duct is inclined from the head of the pancreas to the tail, the diameter gradually thinned, the maximum diameter is no more than 5 mm, the edge is smooth and neat, there are some branches on the main pancreatic duct, and sometimes the position of the accessory pancreatic duct is higher than the main pancreatic duct.

(2) Ultrasound findings: Ultrasound examination of normal pancreas in the long axial section of the upper edge of neat, slightly enlarged pancreatic head, its downward direction after the left protrusion is uncinate process. Ultrasonography can also show the internal segment of the common bile duct. The main pancreatic duct is mostly visible, and there are two parallel and smooth middle and hyperechoic lines in the pancreatic parenchyma. Normal pancreatic duct diameter ≤2 mm (Figure 13-2).

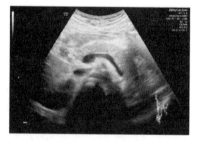

The shape of pancreas is like an arch The convex surface is forward.
The signal is uniform. The splenic vein runs along the posterior edge
of the body and tail of pancreas. It's a marker of the pancreas.

Figure 13-2　ultrasound findings of normal pancreas

（3）CT findings：CT examination can clearly show the pancreatic contour, density, shape and size. Normal pancreas margin is smooth or small lobulated. The density was uniform, lower than that of liver parenchyma, and the elderly often had scattered focal fat density due to fat infiltration, and the density increased uniformly after enhancement （Figure 13-3）. The splenic vein runs along the posterior margin of the pancreatic body, which is a marker for identification of the pancreas. The pancreatic duct is located in the pancreatic parenchyma and may not appear or appear as a linear low-density shadow.

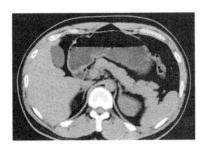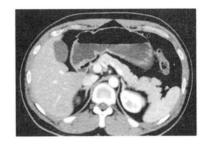

The density of normal pancreatic parenchyma was uniform. The enhancement density was increased evenly, and the edge was lobulated.

Figure 13-3　Plain CT scan of cross section clearly showed pancreas

（4）MRI findings：MRI examination of high signal adipose tissue in retroperitoneum helps to outline the pancreas. On T1WI and T2WI, the pancreas showed a homogeneous and low signal structure, similar to that of the liver parenchyma. T1WI lipid suppression sequence showed a relatively high signal performance in the pancreas （Figure 13-4）. The dorsal splenic vein may show no signal shadow due to the flow-empty effect, which helps to delineate the posterior edge of the pancreas. The head of the pancreas is located in the curvature of the duodenum, and the fluid in the duodenum presents high signal shadow of T2WI.

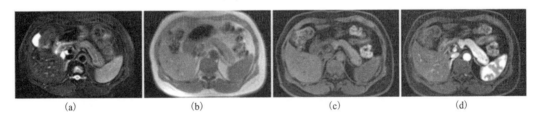

(a)　　　　　　　　(b)　　　　　　　　(c)　　　　　　　　(d)

Cross-sectional fat suppression T2WI sequence shows that the signal of normal pancreatic parenchyma is higher than that of liver and lower than that of spleen（a）; Cross-sectional T1WI sequence shows that the signal of normal pancreatic parenchyma is higher than that of spleen（b）; Cross-sectional fat suppression T1WI sequence shows relatively high signal of pancreas（c）; Cross-sectional fat suppression enhanced T1WI sequence shows the pancreas is obvious homogeneous enhancement in arterial phase.

Figure 13-4　MRI findings of normal pancreas

Section 3　Basic pathological changes

1. X-ray findings

Plain film can find calcification and pancreatic duct stones in the pancreatic area. Abnormal manifestations of ERCP include pancreatic duct obstruction, stenosis, irregular edges, filling defects in the cavity, abnormal pancreatic duct movement, stiffness, shortage and irregular arrangement of branches, or irregularities Uniformly beaded or cyst-like expansion. ERCP is helpful in the diagnosis of chronic pancreatitis, pancreatic head cancer and ampullary cancer.

2. CT findings

The size and shape of the pancreas are abnormal: Diffuse enlargement of the pancreas is mostly manifested by acute pancreatitis. Pancreatic tumors often manifest as local enlargement of the pancreas. Cancer of the head of the pancreas is often accompanied by atrophy of the body and tail of the pancreas. Pancreatic atrophy and fat infiltration show the outline of the pancreas is feathering changes. Abnormality of the main pancreatic duct: The dilated pancreatic duct usually appears as a low-density band in the center of the pancreas on CT, which is more clear after enhanced scanning; chronic pancreatitis can cause beaded or cystic dilatation of the pancreatic duct. Abnormal pancreatic density: Pancreatitis is manifested by uneven density of pancreatic parenchyma due to the liquefaction and necrosis of pancreatic tissue; pancreatic tumors are mostly tumors with poor blood supply. After enhanced scanning, the enhancement of the pancreatic parenchyma is often lower than normal and appears as a low-density mass. The liquefaction necrosis is manifested as infarct density; functional islet cell tumors are significantly enhanced after enhanced scanning, and non-functional islet cell tumors tend to be similar to the pancreas with more obvious enhancement. Abnormal edges and surroundings of the pancreas: Inflammatory exudation and tumor infiltration often increase the density of the fat space around the pancreas, and the pancreas borders are blurred; when there is more exudation, there are patches of low-density fluid around the pancreas; the prerenal fascia is thickened It is a common sign of abnormal tissues surrounding pancreatitis.

3. MRI findings

The significance of abnormal pancreas size and shape is similar to that of CT. MRI of different lesions has different signal changes: pancreatic cancer often shows low or equal signal on T1WI, and mainly high signal on T2WI. Hemorrhage, liquefaction and necrosis in the tumor are mixed with high signal; the signal of islet cell tumor is more uniform, especially functional ones. Pancreatic cystic lesions have signals on T1WI and high signals on T2WI. Cystic adenomas are often multilocular with soft tissue signal separation and mural nodules. In acute pancreatitis, due to hyperemia, edema, and extravasation of pancreatic juice, the signal of the pancreatic parenchyma decreases on T1WI, and the signal increases on T2WI. Chronic pancreatitis may show mixed signals on T2WI, with calcification or stones in the pancreas or pancreatic duct as no signal shadow; pancreatic duct dilation, MRCP shows a band-like or beaded high signal shadow.

Section 4 Diagnosis of common diseases

1. Acute pancreatitis

(1) Clinical and pathological manifestations: Acute pancreatitis is an acute inflammation in which trypsinogen spillover is activated and trypsin causes the pancreas and surrounding tissues to digest themselves. Most of the patients had a history of alcoholism, overeating or biliary tract diseases before the onset. The clinical manifestations were sudden upper abdominal pain and shock. The pain radiated to the waist and back, accompanied by nausea, vomiting, fever and elevated serum trypsin.

The severity of the disease is different. The mild is mainly pancreatic edema, which is common clinically. The condition is often self-limiting and the prognosis is good. It is also known as mild acute pancreatitis or acute edematous pancreatitis, accounting for $80\% \sim 90\%$. In a few severe cases, pancreatic hemorrhage and necrosis are often secondary to infection, peritonitis and shock, with high mortality, which is called severe acute pancreatitis or hemorrhagic necrotizing pancreatitis.

(2) Imaging manifestations:

1) X-ray findings: Plain film mainly showed distention of upper abdominal flexure, or inflammatory expression

of lung bottom or pleural effusion.

2）Computed tomography（CT）findings：It is helpful to understand the extent and scope of the lesions，and has advantages in providing comprehensive information of abdomen and retroperitoneum. The plain scan of acute edematous pancreatitis showed that the volume of pancreas was obviously enlarged，mostly diffuse enlargement. Due to pancreatic edema，the density of pancreatic parenchyma was reduced. Inflammatory exudation，the edge of pancreas was blurred，the boundary with the surrounding was unclear，and the perirenal fascia was thickened. Enhanced scan showed that the pancreas was uniformly enhanced（Figure 13-5）.

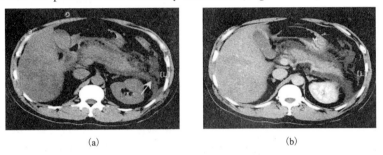

(a)   (b)

Plain scan（a）and enhanced scan（b）showed that the volume of pancreas was generally enlarged，the edge was unclear，the fat space around pancreas was blurred，low-density exudative changes were visible，and the left anterior renal fascia was significantly thickened（a↑）.

Fig. 13-5　CT findings In acute pancreatitis

3）Magnetic resonance imaging findings：Due to inflammatory cell infiltration，edema，hemorrhage and necrosis，the volume of pancreas increased，the shape was irregular，and the edge was blurred. On T1WI，the signal intensity of pancreas was low，and on T2WI，the signal intensity was high. After GD-DTPA enhancement，the normal perfusion pancreatic tissue was enhanced，and the necrotic tissue was not enhanced. The hemorrhage area of necrotizing pancreatitis showed high signal on T1WI and T2WI，peripancreatic effusion and inflammation showed corresponding changes，pseudocyst showed long T1 and long T2 signal，others were the same as CT（Figure 13-6）.

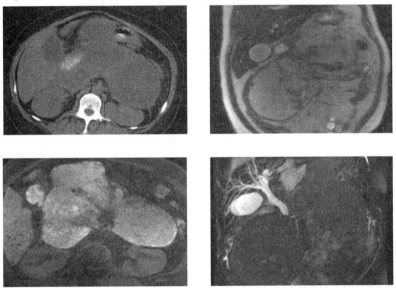

Axial CT plain scan showed a huge heterogeneous low-density mass in the whole pancreatic region，with unclear boundary with surrounding fat. Coronal T2WI showed a large area of liquid high signal and patchy low signal shadow. Axial fat suppression T1WI showed obvious high signal inside the lesion. Thick layer MRCP showed dilatation of intrahepatic and extrahepatic bile ducts and distal obstruction of common bile duct.

Figure 13-6　CT and MRI findings in acute pancreatitis

（3）Diagnosis and differential diagnosis: Acute pancreatitis often has a clear history, signs and laboratory examination, combined with imaging findings, diagnosis, but imaging findings are helpful to determine the disease, retroperitoneal manifestations and complications.

2. Chronic pancreatitis

（1）Clinical and pathological manifestations: Most of chronic pancreatitis are caused by recurrent acute pancreatitis, resulting in extensive fibrosis of the pancreas, hardening and nodular texture, atrophy and disappearance of acini and islets in varying degrees, calcification and stone formation in pancreatic duct and stroma. Clinical often have epigastric pain, repeated, can be combined with diabetes or biliary diseases.

（2）Imaging manifestations

1）X-ray findings: On plain film, dense and multiple small stones and calcifications could be found in the pancreatic transitional zone. ERCP is more sensitive to chronic pancreatitis, which is characterized by multiple stenosis, dilatation, beaded or tubular.

2）Computed tomography（CT）findings: The display of pancreatic parenchyma is more accurate and the display of calcification is more sensitive. Most of positive manifestations are found: the size of the pancreas can be normal, reduced or increased; the pancreatic duct can be tubular, beaded expansion, some with common bile duct expansion; pancreatic duct stones or pancreatic solid calcification distributed along the pancreatic duct are characteristic manifestations; intrapancreatic or extrapancreatic pseudocyst formation; perirenal fascia thickening, etc. (Figure 13-7).

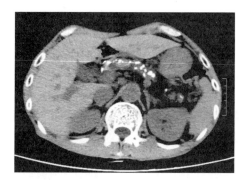

Plain CT scan showed that the volume of pancreas was reduced, and there were scattered patchy calcifications in the head, body and tail of pancreas.

Figure 13-7   CT findings in chronic pancreatitis

3）Magnetic resonance imaging findings: The size and shape of pancreas were similar to CT findings. Due to pancreatic fibrosis, fat suppression on T1WI and T2WI can show low signal, no enhancement or no obvious enhancement after enhancement. When combined with pseudocyst, it shows long T1 and long T2 signal, and calcification shows long T1 and short T2 signal.

（3）Diagnosis and differential diagnosis: It is difficult to differentiate chronic pancreatitis from pancreatic cancer, especially when it leads to localized enlargement of the pancreatic head. In general, the enlargement of the pancreatic head of chronic pancreatitis is mainly caused by fibrosis, which manifests low signal on T1WI and T2WI, and the enhancement features are consistent with the body and tail. However, the arterial phase of enhanced scan of pancreatic cancer is low density or low signal. Chronic pancreatitis with calcification and pseudocyst are common, and pancreatic cancer is more likely to cause blood loss of the adjacent pancreas, tube invasion or embedding, and metastasis.

3. Pancreatic endocrine tumor

(1) Clinical and pathological manifestations: Pancreatic endocrine tumor is usually called "islet cell tumor", which accounts for 1% ~ 2% of pancreatic tumors. It usually occurs in 30−60 years old, and has no obvious gender tendency. Most of them are solitary lesions. 1% ~ 2% of them are related to multiple endocrine tumor type I (MEN-I), which is characterized by the triad of parathyroid, pituitary and pancreas. These tumors can be divided into syndromic (insulinoma, gastrinoma, glucagonoma, VIPoma somatostatin) or nonsyndromic tumors according to whether they secrete enough active compounds.

(2) Imaging manifestations

1) X-ray findings: Plain film cannot diagnose pancreatic neuroendocrine tumor.

2) Computed tomography (CT) findings: Pancreatic endocrine tumors are mostly hypervascular, with clear boundary and sometimes calcification or cystic changes may occur. Smaller tumors have uniform density, clear boundary and abundant blood supply, while larger tumors may have uneven density, including cystic or necrotic changes. Pancreatic endocrine tumors show peak enhancement in the early arterial phase (25 ~ 35 s), but the contrast is not obvious in the late arterial phase, which is easy to be missed (Figure 13−8).

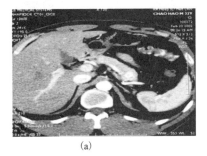 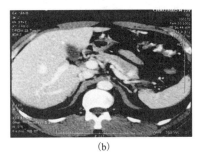

(a)　　　　　　　　　　　　　(b)

A-arterial phase and B-venous phase. The small mass at the tail of pancreas has obvious enhancement in arterial phase, and there is still enhancement in portal venous phase, but not as obvious as that in arterial phase.

Figure 13−8　CT findings of insulinoma

3) Magnetic resonance imaging: The sensitivity of MR is similar to that of CT. Compared with pancreatic parenchyma, pancreatic endocrine tumors showed low signal on T1 and high signal on T2. After GD-DTPA enhancement, pancreatic endocrine tumors showed high enhancement or rich blood supply.

(3) Diagnosis and differential diagnosis: It mainly depends on imaging examination to differentiate from primary endocrine diseases. If imaging examination finds the existence of pancreatic tumor and changes of hormone level, it can differentiate from primary endocrine diseases.

4. Pancreatic cancer

(1) Clinical and pathological manifestations: Pancreatic cancer is the most common malignant tumor of the pancreas, accounting for 95%. It is pancreatic ductal carcinoma. 60% ~ 70% occurs in the head of pancreas, followed by body, tail or whole pancreatic cancer. It occurs in men over 40 years old. The incidence rate increases with age. There is no symptom in the early stage. There are three major symptoms of persistent abdominal pain, progressive jaundice and weight loss. The prognosis of pancreatic cancer is poor. The 5−year survival rate is only about 5%.

(2) Imaging manifestations

1) X-ray findings: Plain film is of little value and gastrointestinal barium meal examination can show middle

and advanced lesions, mainly manifested as compression or invasion of adjacent gastroduodenum by cancer. ERCP performance depends on the relationship between tumor and pancreatic duct, which can show compression and displacement of main pancreatic duct or local irregular stenosis to complete amputation, distal pancreatic duct dilatation and PTC common bile duct obstruction, with round, smooth or small nodular shadow The dilated common bile duct may be displaced.

2) Computed tomography (CT) findings: The tumors in the head, body or tail of the pancreas have corresponding pancreatic masses. Most of them are low-density on plain scan, and a few are equal or high-density. When the tumor is large, it can show local uplift, and when it is small, it can be normal in appearance. The whole pancreas cancer showed low-density shadow of the whole pancreas or most of the pancreas. The intrahepatic bile duct, common bile duct and pancreatic duct of pancreatic cancer were dilated in varying degrees. On contrast-enhanced scan, the arterial phase showed homogeneous and uneven low-density lesions with irregular ring enhancement at the edge, the venous phase was low density but the density difference between the lesion and normal pancreas was smaller than that in arterial phase (Figure 13-9). Pancreatic cancer may invade peripancreatic blood vessels, distant organs and lymph nodes.

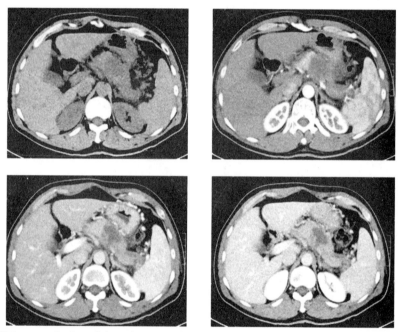

Plain scan and enhanced three-phase scan showed pancreatic body mass, local uplift, plain scan slightly low density, enhanced scan was not obvious, low density area.

Figure 13-9　CT findings of pancreatic cancer

3) Magnetic resonance imaging findings: The main manifestations on MRI were mass, irregular contour and unclear boundary with normal pancreas. Most of them manifested low signal on T1WI and uneven high signal on T2WI. Enhancement features and characteristics of infringement transfer were similar to CT. Fat suppression on T1WI in solid phase of MRI enhanced scan was conducive to the display of lymph node metastasis.

(3) Diagnosis and differential diagnosis: The diagnosis of advanced pancreatic cancer is relatively easy, and pancreatic cancer is mainly differentiated from chronic pancreatitis. In inflammatory lesions, pancreatic duct showed Beaded dilation, pancreatic atrophy and calcification, perirenal fascia thickening, and no lymph node metastasis.

(Yuan Youhong, Jiang Hongtao, Li Xiumei, Luo Wei, Mao Zhiqun, Xiao Enhua, Liu Hui)

第十四章

脾脏

第一节　检查方法

1. X线检查

正常情况下，脾脏的轮廓可以通过脾周脂肪的衬托在X线平片上予以显示，脾脏外伤和出血能使脾脏影肿大并使其边缘变模糊。但是，超过58%的腹部平片不能清楚地显示脾脏轮廓。胃泡向中央移位是脾脏肿大的间接征象，但正侧位照片是更准确和有意义的技术。

2. CT检查

CT检查，特别是螺旋CT检查在大部分的患者中可以选择性地用于脾脏的检查。在可能的情况下应进行静脉下注射对比剂的增强CT检查。怀疑脾脏钙化时可用CT平扫检查。在平扫和增强CT上脾脏的CT值比肝脏低，为5~10 Hu。

3. MRI检查

脾脏的T1像比肝脏的长，而脾脏的T2像比肝脏的短。所以在T1加权像脾脏信号比肝脏低，在T2加权像脾脏信号比肝脏高。在无静脉对比增强的图像上脾实质的信号强度是均匀的，但由于血管的波动和呼吸的运动使脾脏的信号变得不均匀。团注磁共振对比剂Gd-DTPA扫描后60秒，脾脏动脉期相表现为不规则曲线样(拱形样)细微强化(图14-1)，这种状态很快达到平衡变成均匀强化。这种斑片状不均匀强化在CT增强早期也可能显示出来。

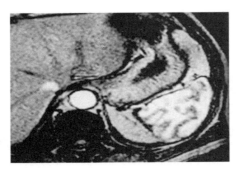

注射Gd-DTPA增强扫描动脉期显示弧形假影。

图14-1　正常脾脏MRI

器官特异性和组织特异性对比剂使得MRI对脾脏病理改变的分析很有价值，顺磁性物质氧化铁被在脾脏中红细胞产生的巨噬细胞和在肝脏内的 Kupffer 细胞所吞噬,这样使得正常脾脏和肝脏的信号降低,而无网状内皮系统的异常组织保持正常信号甚至为高信号,所以 MRI 造影检查对脾脏具有很大的意义。

第二节　正常表现

1. 脾脏位置、形态、大小

脾是人体最大的淋巴器官,具有储血、造血、清除衰老红细胞和进行免疫应答的功能。脾位于左季肋部。脾厚径:以脾膈面弧度做切线,该线至脾门距离即为脾厚径,正常不超过 4.5 cm;脾长径:为脾内上缘至外下缘的距离,正常范围为 8~12 cm;脾静脉内径:脾门处脾静脉内径小于 0.8 cm。

2. 脾脏分部

脾可分为膈、脏两面,前后两端和上下两缘。膈面光滑隆凸,对向膈。脏面凹陷,中央有脾门,是血管、神经、淋巴管出入之处。在脏面,脾与胃底、左肾、左肾上腺、胰尾和结肠脾曲相毗邻。

3. 脾实质

(1)超声表现:正常脾形态与切面方向有关,可呈半月形或类似三角形,外侧缘为弧形,内侧边缘凹陷;脾门有脾动、静脉出入,为无回声平行管状结构;包膜呈光滑的细带状回声,脾实质呈均匀中等回声,略低于肝实质回声。CDFI 显示脾静脉及其分支呈蓝色血流,脾门处脾动脉呈红色血流(图 14-2)。

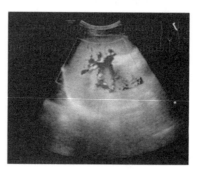

正常脾实质呈均匀中等回声,形态呈半月形或类似三角形,外侧缘为弧形,内侧边缘凹陷;脾门有脾动、静脉出入,为无回声平行管状结构;包膜呈光滑的细带状回声。CDFI 显示脾静脉及其分支呈蓝色血流,脾门处脾动脉呈红色血流。

图 14-2　脾脏超声表现

(2)CT 表现:平扫,脾形态近似于新月形或为内缘凹陷的半圆形,密度均匀并略低于肝脏;脾内侧缘常有切迹,其中可见大血管出入的脾门。增强扫描,动脉期脾呈不均匀明显强化而呈花斑状;静脉期和实质期脾的密度逐渐达到均匀(图 13-3)。正常脾外缘通常少于 5 个肋单位(肋单位为同层 CT 上一个肋骨或一个肋间隙的长度)。

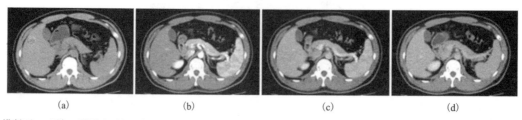

(a)　　　　　　　(b)　　　　　　　(c)　　　　　　　(d)

(a)横断面 CT 平扫,脾形态近似于新月形或为内缘凹陷的半圆形,密度均匀并略低于肝脏,脾内侧缘常有切迹,其中可见大血管出入的脾门;(b)增强扫描,动脉期脾呈不均匀明显强化而呈花斑状;(c)静脉期和(d)实质期脾的密度逐渐达到均匀。

图 14-3　脾脏 CT 表现

（3）MRI 表现：脾在横断层上表现与 CT 类似，冠状位显示脾的大小、形态及其与邻近器官的关系要优于 CT 横断层。脾信号均匀，由于脾内血窦丰富，故 T1 及 T2 弛豫时间比肝、胰长（图 13-4）。脾门血管呈流空信号。增强扫描影像表现同 CT。

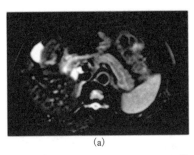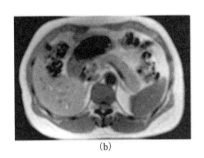

（a）横断面抑脂 T2WI 序列显示正常脾脏信号高于肝脏、胰腺信号；（b）横断面 T1WI 序列显示脾脏信号低于肝脏、胰腺信号。

图 14-4　脾脏 MR 表现

第三节　基本病变

1. CT 表现

（1）脾脏大小异常：CT 横断面图像脾脏外侧缘对应的肋单元超过 5 个应考虑脾脏增大，该指标反映脾脏前后径大小；脾脏下缘低于正常肝脏下缘时应考虑脾脏增大，该指标反映脾脏上下径。

引起脾肿大的病因很多：①炎症性：伤寒、败血症、结核、疟疾等；②淤血性：门静脉高压、心脏病等；③增殖性：溶血性贫血、真红细胞增多症；④肿瘤性：恶性淋巴瘤、白血病、转移瘤等；⑤寄生虫性：血吸虫病等；⑥胶原病性：红斑狼疮、类风湿、淀粉样变性等。最常见的原因是白血病、网织细胞增多症、疟疾。

（2）脾脏密度异常：脾脏密度高于肝脏密度常提示脂肪肝存在。脾脏原发或继发性肿瘤多表现为局限性低密度病灶。脾脏钙化在 CT 上表现为高密度，可能原因有结核、梗死、包虫病、脓肿和静脉石。部分患者有活动性结核，许多患者有肺内结核性病灶和胸膜肥厚。结核的钙化灶为多发不规则圆形影，较小且散在分布于脾脏内。有些报道认为不透 X 线的钙化灶由于钙质含量高表现为边界清楚且较小。脾梗死 CT 典型表现为脾内三角形低密度影，基底位于脾的外缘，尖端指向脾门，边缘可清晰或略模糊。

2. MRI 表现

脾脏占位性病灶多呈局限性异常信号，由于正常脾在 T2WI 上为高信号，因此容易掩盖肿瘤性病变，增强扫描有助于识别病灶及病变的性质。脾囊肿在 T1WI 上呈低信号，在 T2WI 上为高信号，境界清楚。

第四节　常见疾病诊断

1. 正常变异和先天异常

正常变异和先天异常包括先天性异常、副脾、游走性脾、无脾、多脾、脾性腺融合、肾后脾等。

（1）副脾：

1）临床与病理表现：副脾是正常脾组织的先天性结节，在胚胎发生过程中，融合失败可导致一个或多个结节分离；副脾很常见，腹部 CT 检查中发生率约 16%，尸检中高达 30%；可以是单发或多发，直径通常不超过 4 cm，最常见于脾门。

2)影像学表现：

①X 线表现：X 线平片对于副脾无诊断价值。

②CT 表现：副脾常表现为圆形或无蒂结节，密度和增强特征与脾脏相似[图 14-5(a)、(b)]；如果在脾门处发现肿块，其增强方式与邻近脾脏不同，应考虑其他诊断。

③MRI 表现：副脾应与肿大淋巴结区分开来，因为在不同的脉冲图像上，副脾的信号强度和增强程度与脾一致。副脾的信号强度通常与脾脏的信号强度相同，助于其诊断。

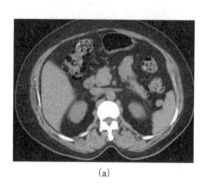
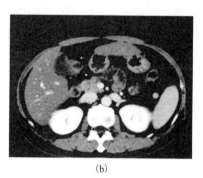

(a)　　　　　　　　　　　　(b)

(a)脾下缘内侧见大小约 1 cm 的软组织密度灶，平扫密度与脾组织类似；(b)同一患者静脉期 CT 显示病灶与脾组织同步均匀强化。

图 14-5　副脾 CT 表现

(2)多脾综合征

1)临床与病理表现：多个脾块，脾的数目可为 2~6 个。也被称为左侧异构，是一种异位综合征，其中多个脾脏为先天性左侧异构的一部分，常伴其他腹部器官位置和心血管的异常，女性更常见，其临床表现与相关的病理学有关。

2)影像学表现：

①X 线表现：X 线平片对多脾综合征的诊断无价值。

②CT 表现：特点是多个脾脏而无母脾，其密度与正常脾相同，强化方式类似。多脾发生在患者左侧，也可能位于双侧，最常见的相关特征是下腔静脉中断伴奇静脉或半奇静脉的延续(图 14-6)。

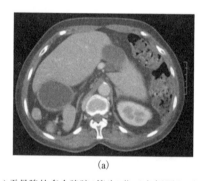
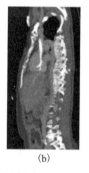

(a)　　　　　　　　　　　　(b)

(a)无母脾的多个脾脏(箭头)位于右侧膈肌下，下腔静脉阻断，同时显示内脏反位；(b)多脾综合征。同一患者 MIP 显示下腔静脉阻断，通过奇静脉延续至上腔静脉。

图 14-6　多脾综合征 CT 表现

③MRI 表现：信号特征与正常脾组织类似，表现为 T1 低信号，T2 高信号，增强后表现与 CT 类似。

(3)游走脾：脾位于正常位置以外的腹腔内其他部位，CT 与 MRI 可清楚显示异位脾的位置与形态，其密度或信号与强化表现与正常位置脾相同。

2.脾外伤

（1）临床与病理表现：脾脏是钝性创伤后最常损伤的内脏器官，可发生在钝性或穿透性损伤后，或继发于医疗性损伤（即医源性），患者可能表现为左上腹部、左胸痛、左肩部疼痛（膈肌刺激）和低血压或休克症状。脾损伤包括裂伤、血肿（包膜下或实质内）、活动性出血、假性动脉瘤或动静脉瘘、脾梗死。

（2）影像学表现：

1）X线表现：X线平片不能直接发现脾创伤，但可能发现相关的损伤，如肋骨骨折、胸腔积液。

2）CT表现：CT是评价脾创伤的首选方法。由于动脉期脾脏呈不均匀性强化（斑马或迷幻脾脏）可误诊脾脏撕裂/挫伤，因此脾脏实质损伤应在门静脉期进行评估。裂伤表现为线性或条状低密度灶（图14-7）。包膜下血肿可表现为导致脾脏周围液性低密度灶并导致脾结构扭变形。活动出血表现为高密度（80~95Hu）物质，这是由于对比剂外渗，延迟期病灶体积增大。假性动脉瘤和动静脉瘘在初始扫描时与活动性出血相似，但在延迟期和血池成像时病灶不增大。

3）MRI表现：脾外伤的影像表现MRI与CT类似，但由于MRI成像时间慢，较少用于脾外伤检查。

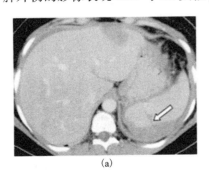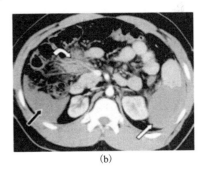

(a)　　　　　　　　　　　　(b)

（a）线状低密度灶（箭头）延续至脾包膜周围，伴包膜下血肿。注意血肿导致的脾脏实质变形特点，这一特征有助于与脾脏周围腹膜出血的鉴别。肝左外侧叶可见挫伤；（b）脾撕裂。脾脏的后半部份无强化，被高密度的"哨兵凝块"（白色直箭头）包围。注意肠系膜血肿（白色曲线箭头）和右侧结肠旁沟的腹腔积血（黑色箭头）。

图14-7　脾撕裂CT表现

3.脾血管瘤

（1）临床与病理表现：又称脾静脉畸形、脾海绵状畸形或脾慢流静脉畸形，多见于30~50岁的成年人，多数无症状，偶然发现。脾脏血管瘤由非肿瘤性、无包膜、大小不等的血管组成，包括毛细血管和海绵状血管，含有缓慢流动的血液。

（2）影像学表现：

1）X线表现：平片通常无法诊断脾血管瘤，有时可发现脾的增大或钙化。

2）CT表现：平扫显示低密度肿块，增强后显示向心性充盈（从周围向内填充），较大的病灶填充更慢，也可能填充不完全和不均匀。

3）MRI表现：大多数血管瘤的信号特征与肝血管瘤相似，与正常脾实质比较，T1WI表现为等信号至低信号，T2WI表现为高信号，增强表现为早期结节性向心性增强和延迟期均匀强化，而较小的病灶可在增强后即刻表现为均匀增强和延迟期仍然强化。

4.脾梗死

（1）临床与病理表现：脾梗死可由多种过程产生，包括供血动脉、脾本身或静脉引流。可表现为左上象限疼痛，可有发烧和畏寒等症状，部分人甚至可表现为弥漫性腹痛，约40%脾梗死患者无症状；形态学上典型的梗死是受累脾组织的呈锥体楔形改变，其顶端指向脾门，底部位于脾周包膜。

（2）影像学表现：

1）CT表现：CT通常是首选的影像学检查，最好在门静脉期进行，以避免在动脉期出现的不均匀性强化。影像学特征可因梗死的分期而异：超急性期，CT 可能显示混杂增强的区域，代表出血性梗死的区域；脾梗死典型表现为周围楔形低强化区、多发性梗死表现为低密度非强化灶，间隔正常强化的脾组织（图 14-8）；慢性期，梗死可能完全消失，但常可见梗死后纤维化收缩导致的体积逐渐缩小伴周围正常脾脏肥大，如果梗死液化，可能留下中心为液性密度的囊性病变。

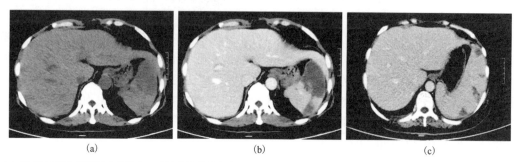

(a)CT 平扫见脾实质密度不均匀，可见片状稍低密度区；(b)静脉期 CT 显示病灶呈楔形改变，尖端指向脾门，无强化；(c)脾多发梗死。门静脉期 CT 显示脾外周多发楔形无强化的低密度灶，提示脾梗死。

图 14-8　脾梗死 CT 表现

2)MRI 表现：脾梗死的敏感性和影像表现与 CT 类似，陈旧性脾梗死，在轴位 T2 上表现为低信号瘢痕伴包膜回缩（图 14-9），但 MRI 较少用于脾的急性梗死。

5. 脾淋巴瘤

（1）临床与病理表现：也称为淋巴瘤脾脏受累，是脾脏最常见的恶性肿瘤，多为继发性的，原发性和继发性脾淋巴瘤均可引起左上腹部疼痛，常出现发热、盗汗和体重减轻等症状。

（2）影像学表现：

1)CT 表现：常见脾肿大，平扫可见脾脏内部单发或多发稍低密度灶，边界不清或清楚，增强扫描呈轻度不规则强化，与正常脾实质分界清楚，可伴有腹膜后淋巴结肿大，也可表现出累及其他器官和系统的征象（图 14-10）。

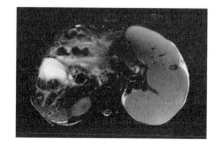

肝硬化、脾大患者，脾陈旧性梗死在轴位 T2 上表现为低信号瘢痕伴包膜回缩。

图 14-9　脾陈旧性梗死 MRI 表现

2)MRI 表现：可仅表现为脾脏弥漫性增大，也可表现为单个或多个大小不等的圆形肿块，边界不清，T1WI、T2WI 均表现为不均匀混杂信号，增强扫描轻度强化，信号较正常脾脏低，典型可呈"地图"分布，可伴有腹膜后淋巴结肿大。

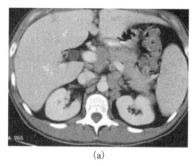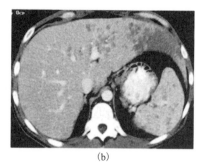

(a)非霍奇金淋巴瘤表现以腹膜后和腹腔淋巴结病变，由于明显的淋巴结受累，脾脏肿大，强烈提示该病；(b)尽管肝脏和脾脏无明显肿大，但两个器官都存在低密度灶。化疗后几个月，病灶消失。

图 14-10　脾淋巴 CT 表现

（袁友红，罗伟，李秀梅，蒋洪涛，毛志群，肖恩华，刘辉）

Chapter 14

Spleen

Section 1　Method of examination

1. X-ray examination

Splenic injury or hemorrhage can enlarge the splenic shadow and blur its borders, normally outlined by perisplenic fat on plain radiographs. However, the splenic outline is invisible in up to 58% of plain abdominal radiographs. Medial deviation of the stomach bubble is an indirect sign of splenic enlargement, but cross-sectional techniques are more accurate and definitive.

2. CT examination

CT, especially with helical scanning, is the imaging study of choice for evaluation of the spleen in most cases. CT should be performed with intravenous contrast enhancement, when possible. Unenhanced CT should also be performed if calcifications are suspected. The spleen tends to have slightly lower CT numbers than the liver on both unenhanced and enhanced CT by approximately 5 to 10 HU.

3. MRI examination

T1 of spleen is longer than that of liver, and splenic T2 is shorter. Therefore, the spleen is hypointense to liver on T1-weighted images and hyperintense on T2-weighted images. On images obtained without intravenous contrast, the parenchymal splenic signal intensity is homogeneous, but the spleen often appears heterogeneous because of artifacts from vascular pulsation and respiratory motion. Up to 60 seconds after bolus administration of a gadolinium chelate, arterial phase images of the spleen show curvilinear (" arciform ") differential enhancement (Figure 14-1). This pattern quickly equilibrates to uniform enhancement. A similar pattern of striped heterogeneous enhancement may be seen on early-phase enhanced CT.

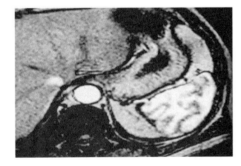

Arterial-phase, gadolinium-enhanced MR with arciform artifact.

Figure 14-1　Normal spleen

Organ-specific or tissue-specific contrast agents may make magnetic resonance imaging (MRI) more useful for splenic pathology. Particulate superparamagnetic iron oxides are phagocytosed by red pulp macrophages in the spleen and Kupffer cells in the liver resulting in signal loss in the normal splenic and hepatic tissue. Abnormal tissue without reticuloendothelial uptake retains normal but higher signal, and thus has greater conspicuity.

Section 2　Normal appearances

1. The position, shape and size of the spleen

The spleen is the largest lymphoid organs in the human body, which has the functions of blood storage, hematopoiesis, clearance of senescent red blood cells and immune response. The spleen is located in the left seasonal rib cage. The thickness diameter of the spleen: take the radian of the diaphragmatic surface of the spleen as the tangent, and the distance from the line to the spleen gate is the thickness diameter of the spleen, normally no more than 4.5 cm. The length diameter of the spleen: the distance from the upper edge of the spleen to the lower edge of the spleen, and the normal range is 8~12 cm. The internal diameter of splenic vein: the internal diameter of splenic vein at the hilum is less than 0.8 cm.

2. The parts of the spleen

The spleen can be divided into two parts: diaphragmatic and visceral surfaces, anterior and posterior ends and upper and lower margins. The diaphragmatic surface is smooth and convex opposite to diaphragm. The visceral surface is sunken with splenic hilum in the center which is the entrance and exit of blood vessels, nerves and lymphatic vessels. On the visceral surface, the spleen is adjacent to the fundus of stomach, left kidney, left adrenal gland, tail of pancreas and splenic flexure of colon.

3. Splenic parenchyma

The normal shape of the spleen in ultrasound examination is related to the direction of section, which can be in the shape of a half-moon or similar triangle, with an arc at the outer edge and a depression at the inner edge. There are splenic arteries and veins in and out of the card door, which is anechoic parallel tubular structure. The capsule showed smooth and fine band echo, and the spleen parenchyma showed uniform and medium echo, slightly lower than that of liver parenchyma. CDFI shows blue blood flow in the splenic vein and its branches, and red blood flow in the splenic artery at the hilum (Figure 14-2). On CT scan, the shape of the spleen was similar to that of a crescent or a semicircle with a concave inner edge, and the density was uniform and slightly lower than that of the liver. The medial margin of the spleen often has a notch, with the splenic hilum opening and closing with large vessels. In arterial phase, the spleen showed inhomogeneous enhancement and floriferous pattern. The density of the spleen gradually reached homogeneous in the venous and parenchymal phases [Figure 14-3(a) ~ (d)]. The outer margin of the normal spleen is usually less than 5 costal units (the costal units are the length

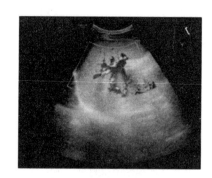

The normal splenic parenchyma was homogeneous and moderately echoic in shape of meniscus or similar triangle, with arc-shaped outer edge and concave inner edge. The splenic artery and vein were in and out of the portal, which was an anechoic parallel tubular structure. The capsule was smooth and thin-band-like echo. CDFI showed blue blood flow in splenic vein and its branches, and red blood flow in splenic artery at splenic hilum.

Figure 14-2　Ultrasonic findings of spleen

of one rib or intercostal space on the same CT scan). MRI examination of the spleen on the transverse section is similar to CT, coronal position shows that the size, shape and the relationship between the spleen and the adjacent organs is better than CT transverse section. The spleen signals are uniform, and T1 and T2 relaxation time is longer than liver and pancreas due to abundant blood sinuses in the spleen [Figure 14-4(a), (b)]. The vessels in the splenic hilum show emptysignal. The enhancment scan was the same as CT.

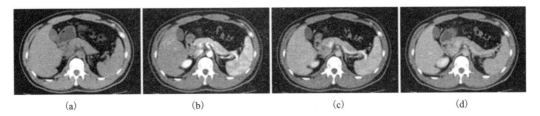

Cross-sectional CT plain scan showed that the shape of spleen was similar to crescent shape or semicircle with concave inner edge, and the density was uniform and slightly lower than that of liver There were often incisions on the medial edge of spleen, in which the splenic hilum with large blood vessels could be seen (a). The spleen showed uneven enhancement and flower spots in arterial phase(b). The venous phase(c) and the parenchymal phase(d), the density of spleen gradually reached uniformity.

Figure 14-3   CT findings of spleen

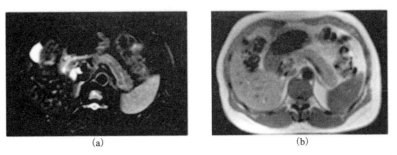

The cross-sectional fat suppression T2WI sequence showed that the signal of normal spleen was higher than that of liver and pancreas(a). The cross-sectional T1WI sequence showed that the signal of spleen was lower than that of liver and pancreas(b).

Figure 14-4   MRI findings of spleen

Section 3   Basic pathological changes

1. CT findings

(1) Spleen size: There are more than 5 rib units corresponding to the lateral edge of the spleen in the CT cross-sectional image. The enlargement of the spleen should be considered. This index reflects the size of the anterior and posterior diameter of the spleen; when the lower edge of the spleen is lower than the lower edge of the normal liver, the enlargement of the spleen should be considered. This indicator reflects the upper and lower diameter of the spleen. There are many causes of splenomegaly: 1) Inflammatory: typhoid fever, sepsis, tuberculosis, malaria, etc. 2) Congestive: portal hypertension, heart disease, etc. 3) Proliferative: hemolytic anemia, polycythemia vera. 4) Neoplastic: malignant Lymphoma, leukemia, metastasis, etc. 5) Parasitic: schistosomiasis, etc. 6) Collagen disease: lupus erythematosus, rheumatoid, amyloidosis, etc. The most common causes are leukemia, reticulocytosis, and malaria.

(2) Spleen density: Spleen density higher than liver density often indicates the presence of fatty liver. Primary or secondary tumors of the spleen are mostly localized low-density lesions. Splenic calcification is high-density on CT. The possible causes are tuberculosis, infarction, hydatid disease, abscess and phlebolith. Some patients have active tuberculosis, and many patients have tuberculous scars and pleural hypertrophy in the lungs. The calcifications of tuberculosis are multiple irregular round shadows, small and scattered in the spleen. Some reports believe that X-ray opaque calcification foci are clear and small due to high calcium content. CT of splenic infarction

typically presents a triangular low-density shadow in the spleen, the base is located at the outer edge of the spleen, the tip points to the splenic hilum, and the edge can be clear or slightly blurred.

2. MRI findings

Splenic space-occupying lesions often show localized abnormal signals. Since the normal spleen is high signal on T2WI, it is easy to cover up the tumorous lesions. Enhanced scanning helps to identify the lesions and the nature of the lesions. The splenic cyst showed low signal on T1WI and high signal on T2WI with a clear boundary.

Section 4 Diagnosis of common diseases

1. Normal variation and congenital anomaly

They include congenital abnormality, accessory spleen, migratory spleen, asplenia, polysplenia, splenic gland fusion, Retrorenal spleen and so on.

(1)Accessory spleen

1)Clinical and pathological manifestations: Accessory spleen is a congenital nodule of normal spleen tissue. During embryogenesis, failure of fusion may lead to separation of one or more nodules. It is very common and the incidence of accessory spleen is about 16% in abdominal CT examination, while as high as 30% in autopsy. Accessory spleen can be single or multiple, the diameter is usually not more than 4 cm, the most common in the splenic hilum.

2)Imaging manifestations

①X-ray findings: Plain film has no diagnostic value for accessory spleen.

②CT findings: The accessory spleen usually presents as round or sessile nodules with similar density and enhancement features as the spleen [Figure 14-5(a), (b)]. If a mass is found in the splenic hilum, its enhancement mode is different from that of the adjacent spleen, other diagnosis should be considered.

③MRI findings: The accessory spleen should be distinguished from the enlarged lymph nodes, because on different pulse images, the signal intensity and enhancement degree of accessory spleen are consistent with that of spleen. The signal intensity of accessory spleen is usually the same as that of spleen, which is helpful for its diagnosis.

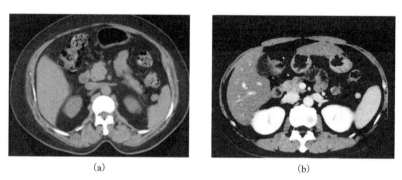

(a)   (b)

(a)CT showed a soft tissue density of about 1 cm on the medial side of the lower edge of the spleen, and the density on plain scan was similar to that of the spleen; (b)In the venous phase of the same patient, CT showed that the lesion and spleen were enhanced simultaneously and evenly.

Figure 14-5 CT findings of accessory spleen

（2）Polysplenia syndrome

1）Clinical and pathological manifestations：Multiple spleen masses, the number of spleens can be 2-6, also known as left isomerism. Polysplenia syndrome is an ectopic syndrome, in which multiple spleens are part of congenital left isomerism. It often accompanied by other abdominal organ location and cardiovascular abnormalities, more common in women, and its clinical manifestations are related to the relevant pathology.

2）Imaging manifestations

①X-ray findings：Plain film has no value in the diagnosis of polysplenia syndrome.

②CT findings：Polysplenic syndrome is characterized by multiple spleens without maternal spleen. Its density is the same as that of normal spleen, and its enhancement mode is similar. Polysplenia may occur on the left side or on both sides of the patient. The most common related feature is interruption of the inferior vena cava with the continuation of the azygos vein or hemiazygos vein［Figure 14-6(a), (b)］.

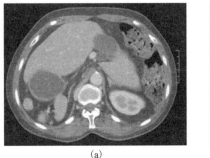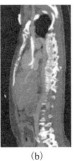

(a)　　　　　　　　(b)

（a）Cross sectional CT showed that multiple spleens without maternal spleen（arrow）were located under the right diaphragm, inferior vena cava was blocked, and visceral inversion was also shown；（b）MIP reconstruction of CT scan in the same patient showed that the inferior vena cava was blocked and extended to the superior vena cava through the azygos vein.

Figure 14-6　CT findings of polysplenic syndrome

③MRI findings：The signal characteristics of MR were similar to those of normal splenic tissue, showing low signal on T1 and high signal on T2, and similar to those of CT.

（3）Migratory spleen

The spleen is located in other parts of the abdominal cavity other than the normal position. CT and MRI can clearly show the position and morphology of the ectopic spleen, and its density or signal and enhancement are the same as the normal spleen. 2. Splenic trauma

（1）Clinical and pathological manifestations：Spleen is the most common internal organ damaged after blunt trauma. It can occur after blunt or penetrating trauma, or secondary to medical injury（iatrogenic）. Patients with splenic trauma may present with left upper abdomen, left chest pain, left shoulder pain（diaphragmatic stimulation）and hypotension or shock. Splenic trauma includes laceration, hematoma（subcapsular or parenchymal）, active hemorrhage, pseudoaneurysm or arteriovenous

fistula, and splenic infarction.

（2）Imaging manifestations

①X-ray findings：Plain film cannot directly detect splenic trauma, but may find related injuries, such as rib fracture, pleural effusion.

②CT findings：CT is the first choice to evaluate splenic trauma. Since the inhomogeneous enhancement of the spleen in arterial phase (zebra or hallucinogenic spleen)can be misdiagnosed as splenic laceration / contusion, the splenic parenchymal injury should be evaluated in portal venous phase. Splenic laceration showed linear or strip low-density focus [Figure 14-7(a), (b)]and splenic subcapsular hematoma may lead to liquid low-density foci around the spleen and torsion deformation of splenic structure. Splenic active bleeding is characterized by high density (80-95 Hu)substance, which is due to the extravasation of contrast medium and the increase of lesion volume in the delayed phase. Splenic pseudoaneurysms and arteriovenous fistulas were similar to active bleeding on initial scan, but did not increase in delayed phase and blood pool imaging.

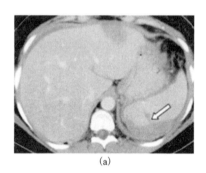 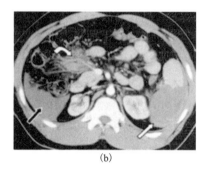

(a)   (b)

(a) On plain CT scan, the linear hypodense focus (arrow) extended to the splenic capsule with subcapsular hematoma. Attention should be paid to the deformation of splenic parenchyma caused by hematoma, which is helpful to differentiate from perisplenic peritoneal hemorrhage. Contusion can be seen in the left lateral lobe of the liver; (b) On enhanced CT scan, the latter part of the spleen showed no enhancement and was surrounded by high-density "sentinel clot" (white arrow). Note the mesenteric hematoma (white curvilinear arrow)and hemoperitoneum in the right paracolonic sulcus (black arrow).

Figure 14-7 CT findings of splenic laceration

③MRI findings: The imaging manifestations of splenic trauma on MRI are similar to those on CT, but due to the slow imaging time of MRI, it is seldom used in the examination of splenic trauma.

3. Splenic hemangioma

(1) Clinical and pathological manifestations: Splenic hemangioma, also known as splenic venous malformation, splenic cavernous malformation or splenic slow flow venous malformation, is more common in adults aged 30 to 50 years old. Most of them are asymptomatic and occasionally found. Splenic hemangioma is composed of non-neoplastic non encapsulated blood vessels of different sizes, including capillaries and cavernous vessels, with slow flowing blood.

(2)Imaging manifestations

1)X-ray findings: Splenic hemangioma cannot be diagnosed by plain film, sometimes splenic enlargement or calcification can be found.

2)CT findings: Plain scan showed low density mass, while enhanced showed centripetal filling (filling from the surrounding to the inside)and most of larger lesions filled more slowly, which may also be incomplete and uneven filling.

3)MRI findings: MR signal characteristics of most hemangiomas are similar to those of hepatic hemangiomas. Compared with normal splenic parenchyma, splenic hemangioma showed isointensity to hypointensity on T1WI and hyperintensity on T2WI. The enhanced scan of splenic hemangioma showed early nodular centripetal enhancement and delayed homogeneous enhancement and small splenic hemangiomas showed homogeneous enhancement and delayed enhancement.

4. Splenic infarction

(1) Clinical and pathological manifestations: Splenic infarction can be caused by a variety of reasons, including feeding artery, spleen itself or venous drainage. Patients with splenic infarction can appear left upper quadrant pain, accompanied by fever and chills and other symptoms and some people can even show diffuse abdominal pain, about 40% of patients with splenic infarction asymptomatic. Morphologically, the typical splenic infarction showed a pyramidal wedge-shaped change, with the top pointing to the splenic hilum and the bottom at the perisplenic capsule.

(2) Imaging manifestations

1) CT findings: CT is usually the preferred imaging examination of splenic infarction and imaging features may vary with the stage of infarction. In the hyperacute phase of splenic infarction, CT may show areas of mixed density, which represents the area of hemorrhagic infarction. The typical manifestations of splenic infarction are peripheral wedge-shaped non enhancement area and multiple infarction are low-density non enhancement foci with normal enhancement intervals [Figure 14-8(a) ~ (c)]. In the chronic phase, splenic infarction may be normal, but it is often seen that the volume gradually shrinks due to fibrosis contraction after infarction with normal splenic hypertrophy around. If the infarction liquefies, cystic lesions with liquid density in the center may be left.

2) MRI findings: The sensitivity and imaging findings of splenic infarction are similar to those of CT. T2W showed low signal scar with capsule retraction (Figure 14-9). But MRI is rarely used in acute splenic infarction.

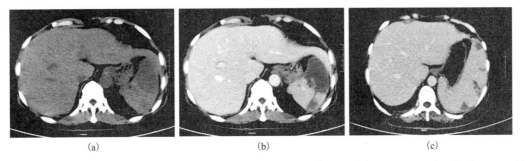

(a) (b) (c)

(a) Plain CT scan showed that the density of splenic parenchyma was not uniform, and there were some low density areas; (b) Enhanced CT scan in venous phase showed wedge-shaped lesions with tip pointing to splenic hilum without enhancement; (c) CT in portal vein phase showed multiple wedge-shaped low-density lesions without enhancement around the spleen.

Figure 14-8　CT findings of splenic infarction

5. Splenic lymphoma

(1) Clinical and pathological manifestations: Splenic lymphoma is the most common malignant tumor of the spleen and it is mostly secondary. Primary and secondary splenic lymphoma can cause pain in the left upper abdomen and patients often have symptoms of fever, night sweats, weight loss and so on.

(2) Imaging manifestations

1) CT findings: Splenomegaly is common in patients with splenic lymphoma. On plain CT scan, splenic lymphoma showed single or multiple slightly low-density foci with unclear or clear boundary. On enhanced CT scan, splenic lymphoma showed mild irregular enhancement with clear boundary with normal splenic parenchyma. It

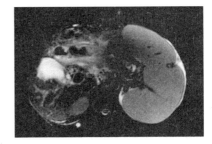

MRI axial T2 showed low signal scar with capsule retraction.

Figure 14-9　MRI findings of old splenic infarction

may be accompanied by retroperitoneal lymph node enlargement, and may also show signs of involvement of other organs and systems [Figure 14-10(a), (b)]

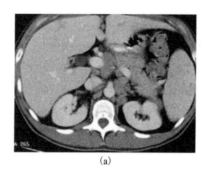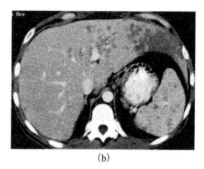

(a)   (b)

(a) CT findings of non Hodgkin's lymphoma are retroperitoneal and abdominal lymph node lesions. Splenomegaly and obvious lymph node involvement strongly suggest the disease; (b) Although the same case of liver and spleen no obvious swelling, but there are low-density lesions in both organs. A few months after chemotherapy, the lesion disappeared.

Figure 14-10   CT findings of splenic lymphoma

2) MRI findings: Splenic lymphoma can only show diffuse enlargement of the spleen, but also can show single or multiple round masses of different sizes with unclear boundary. Them showed heterogeneous mixed signal on T1WI and T2WI and slightly enhanced on contrast-enhanced scan, which lower signal than normal spleen and typical "map" distribution. Splenic lymphoma may be accompanied by retroperitoneal lymphadenopathy.

(Yuan Youhong, Jiang Hongtao, Li Xiumei, Luo Wei, Mao Zhiqun, Xiao Enhua, Liu Hui)

第十五章

泌尿系统

泌尿系统包括肾、输尿管、膀胱和尿道，X线诊断，主要是运用腹部X线平片和泌尿系造影检查，CT优于常规X线检查，而MRI在评估病变内部结构及恶性肿瘤的转移、复发等方面优于CT。

第一节　检查方法

1. X线检查

(1)腹部X线平片(KUB)：是泌尿系统的常规检查方法，可观察肾脏的大小、形态和位置，了解泌尿道有无阳性结石和(或)钙化，并做各种泌尿系造影前的参考片。

(2)排泄性尿路造影：又称静脉肾盂造影(IVP)，是将有机碘液注入静脉内，经肾排泄，几乎全部经肾小球滤过排入肾盏、肾盂，并从肾盂流经输尿管至膀胱。本法简单易行，危险性小，不但可观察整个泌尿系统的解剖结构，还可了解肾脏的排泄功能，是临床上最常用的一种泌尿系统X线检查方法。

(3)逆行性尿路造影：包括逆行肾盂造影和逆行膀胱造影。前者是在膀胱镜指导下，将导管插入输尿管内并逆行注入对比剂而使肾盏、肾盂、输尿管和膀胱充盈显影，本法适应于静脉法不显影或显影不良及不适于做排泄性尿路造影者。逆行膀胱造影是将导尿管经尿道插入膀胱，然后注入对比剂而使膀胱充盈显影的方法。

(4)主要包括腹主动脉造影与选择性肾动脉造影，通常采用Seldinger技术经皮股动脉穿刺插管，在影像监视下将导管送入腹主动脉，并将导管顶端置于肾动脉开口上方(腹主动脉造影时)或置于一侧肾动脉内(选择性肾动脉造影时)，快速注入对比剂并连续摄片。血管造影主要用于检查肾血管病变，特别是肾动脉狭窄与闭塞，确定其部位和范围并行介入治疗，也可发现肾动脉瘤和肾动脉畸形等。

2. CT检查

(1)平扫检查：肾与输尿管CT检查无需特殊准备，膀胱CT检查需在膀胱充盈尿液状态下进行。常规取仰卧位采用横断层面扫描(轴位CT)，层厚和层距10 mm，病灶较小时局部可加薄层扫描。肾脏扫描范围自肾上腺区开始至肾下极下缘，如需同时观察输尿管，则继续向下扫描至输尿管膀胱入口处，盆腔(膀胱)扫描范围自耻骨联合下缘开始向上连续逐层扫描至髂骨嵴高度，或由上至下连续扫描。

(2)增强检查：常规增强扫描方法是向静脉内一次快速注射水溶性有机碘对比剂如60%泛影葡胺或相同碘含量的非离子型对比剂60~100 mL，注射完毕对比剂后立即按普通扫描的方法进行扫描，必要时可进行动态增强扫描，肾脏双期或多期扫描，以发现小的病灶。

(3)CT血管成像(CTA)：在静脉内快速注入含碘对比剂，在肾动脉期进行图像采集，并对容积数据进行三维重组，可获得类似X线肾动脉造影所得图像(图15-1)。

(4)CT尿路成像(CTU)：其原理与CTA类似，是在肾脏排泄期进行图像采集，并对肾盂、肾盏、输尿管、膀胱容积数据进行三维重组,可获得类似 IVP 检查所得图像。

3. MRI 检查

(1)平扫检查:肾与输尿管常规 MRI 检查以横断面(轴位)扫描为主,必要时再辅以冠状位或/(和)矢状位扫描,应用 T1WI 并脂肪抑制技术有助于对肾解剖结构的分辨及含脂肪性病变的诊断。

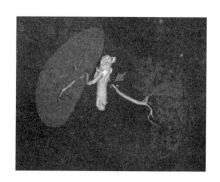

(2)增强检查:方法是向静脉内快速注入顺磁性对比剂 Gd-DTPA 后,即行 T1WI 扫描,可进一步确定病变的存在,判断病变的起源,提供病变的内部结构、边缘状况及血液供应等信息。

左肾动脉开口处狭窄(箭头所示)。

图 15-1　肾动脉 CTA

(3)MR 尿路成像(MRU):MRU 主要用于肾盂输尿管梗阻性病变的诊断,不用对比剂即能显示扩张的肾盏、肾盂和输尿管,类似常规 X 线尿路造影图像,适于碘过敏患者,IVP 重度积水或不显影者应用。

(4)MRI 血管成像(MRA):MRA 通常作为肾动脉及其较大分支病变的筛查方法,诊断准确性尚不如 CTA 检查。

第二节　正常表现

1. X 线表现

(1)肾:腹部 X 线平片可显示肾的轮廓、大小和位置。正常肾影呈蚕豆形,位于脊柱两侧,外缘为凸面,内缘凹陷为肾门。成人肾影长 12~13 cm,宽 5~6 cm,通常位于胸(T_{12})-腰(T_3)水平之间,右肾比左肾低 1~2 cm。由仰卧位改为立位,肾影可下降 1~5 cm,侧位双侧肾影与脊柱重迭。尿路造影(图 15-2)可观察肾盂、肾盏的形态。正常肾盂形态变异较大,多呈喇叭状,少数呈分支状或壶腹状,边缘光滑整齐。肾盏分肾大盏和肾小盏,肾大盏呈长管状,顶端或尖部与数个肾小盏相连,基底部与肾盂相连;肾小盏呈短管状,末端稍膨大,其顶端由于肾乳头的直接突入而呈杯口状凹陷。正常肾盂轮廓清晰,大小肾盏边缘均光滑整齐。

(2)输尿管:在腹部平片上正常输尿管不能显示。尿路造影片上输尿管为细长条状致密影,全长 25~30 cm,上端与肾盂相延续,沿脊柱的两侧向前下行,入盆腔后,先向后下外行,继而转向前内,斜行进入膀胱。输尿管正常有三个生理狭窄区,即与肾盂相连处、跨越真骨盆边缘处及输尿管膀胱连接处。正常输尿管轮廓清晰,充盈均匀,可有折曲。

(3)膀胱:正常膀胱呈软组织密度影,由于与周围组织结构之间缺乏自然对比,平片难以显示。造影片可显示膀胱内腔,其大小和形态取决于充盈程度及与周围器官的关系。膀胱正常容量为 300~500 mL,充盈较满的膀胱呈椭圆形,横置于耻骨联合上方,边缘光整,密度均匀。如充盈未满或处于收缩状态,其粗大的黏膜皱壁可使边缘不整齐而呈锯齿状。此外,在膀胱底两侧输尿管开口之间有时可见一横形透明带,为输尿管嵴,勿误为病变。

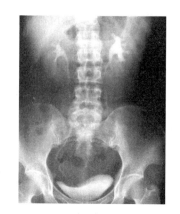

图 15-2　正常排泄性尿路造影

2. 肾血管造影表现

腹主动脉造影与选择性肾动脉造影检查可显示三个期相,即肾动脉期、肾实质期和肾静脉期。肾动脉期可清晰地显示肾动脉主干及分支,正常由粗变细,分布均匀,边缘光滑,无扩张、狭窄、中断和过度迂曲等表现;肾实质期,整个肾实质弥漫性显影,可清楚显示肾的轮廓、大小和形态;肾静脉期,肾静脉显影但不很清晰。

3. CT 表现

（1）肾：平扫，在横断层面上，肾位于脊柱两侧，表现为圆形或椭圆形软组织密度影，边缘光滑锐利。在肾的中部层面见肾门内凹，有肾动脉、静脉和输尿管进出。肾实质密度均匀，CT 值为 30~50Hu，一般不能分辨皮、髓质。增强检查，肾强化表现取决于对比剂用量、注射速度及扫描时间。常规剂量团注法增强检查早期（注药后约 1 分钟内），肾血管和皮质明显强化，而髓质仍维持较低密度，此时皮、髓质可清晰分辨；注药后约 2 分钟，髓质明显强化，程度类似或超过肾皮质，皮、髓质分界不再清晰，此时肾盂肾盏也开始强化；注药 5~10 分钟后，肾实质强化程度减低，肾盂肾盏则呈高密度。

（2）输尿管：平扫，自肾盂向下连续层面追踪，多可见正常输尿管腹段，呈点状软组织密度影，位于腰大肌前缘处。盆段输尿管一般难以识别。增强检查，注药 5~10 分钟后延迟扫描，输尿管因管腔内充盈对比剂而呈点状致密影，连续追踪可观察输尿管全程。

（3）膀胱：平扫检查，膀胱大小和形态与充盈程度有关，一般呈圆形或椭圆形，膀胱腔内尿液呈均一水样低密度。在周围低密度脂肪组织及腔内尿液的对比下，膀胱壁显示为厚度一致的薄壁软组织结构，内外缘均光整。增强检查，注入对比剂后早期膀胱壁即强化；30~60 分钟后延迟扫描，膀胱腔呈均匀高密度。如对比剂与尿液混合不均，则出现液—液平面。

4. MRI 表现

（1）肾：常规 SE 序列检查，在 T1WI 像上，肾皮质呈中等强度信号，肾髓质低于皮质信号。T2WI 像上，整个肾实质均呈较高信号，皮髓质难以分辨。富含脂肪的肾窦在 T1WI 和 T2WI 上分别呈高信号和中等信号。肾动脉和肾静脉由于流空效应而呈无信号带状影。注射 Gd-DTPA 后增强检查，肾脏强化程度和形式类似 CT 增强检查。

（2）输尿管：在 T1WI 或 T2WI 横断面检查时，自肾盂连续向下追踪可识别部分腹段输尿管，呈点状低信号影。

（3）膀胱：膀胱内尿液呈均匀长 T1 低信号和长 T2 高信号；膀胱壁的信号强度在 T1WI 和 T2WI 像上分别高于和低于腔内尿液信号。

（4）磁共振尿路成像（MRU）：正常含尿液的肾盂、肾盏、输尿管和膀胱皆呈高信号，类似正常 X 线排泄性尿路造影图像。

第三节　基本病变

1. 腹部 X 线平片表现

（1）肾、输尿管和膀胱区高密度影：多为泌尿道阳性结石所致。肾盂、肾盏结石可有不同形态；输尿管结石位于其走行区内，易见于三个生理狭窄处；膀胱结石常呈椭圆形，横置于耻骨联合上方。肾区内高密度钙化影也可见于肾结核、肾癌或肾囊肿等。

（2）肾轮廓改变：肾影增大或部分增大并局部外突，主要见于肾盂积水、肾肿瘤或肾囊肿；肾边缘分叶状或波浪状改变可见于胎儿性分叶肾和慢性肾盂肾炎；肾周脓肿和血肿可使肾轮廓消失。

2. 尿路造影表现

（1）肾盂、肾盏受压变形移位：多为肾内肿物所致，如肾囊肿、肾肿瘤、血肿和脓肿等。

（2）肾盂、肾盏破坏：可因肿瘤或结核等引起，表现为肾盂、肾盏边缘不规则，呈虫蚀状或鼠咬状乃至正常结构完全消失。

（3）肾盂、肾盏、输尿管和膀胱内充盈缺损：表现为病变区内无对比剂充填，为突入腔内病变或腔内病变所致，如肿瘤、结石、血肿和气泡等。

（4）肾盂、肾盏、输尿管和膀胱扩张积水：可单侧或双侧，多为梗阻所致，原因有肿瘤、结石、血块、炎性狭窄或外在性压迫等。

3.肾血管造影表现

(1)肾动脉狭窄:因病因不同,狭窄的部位、程度、形态和范围也各不相同,主要见于大动脉炎、动脉粥样硬化等。

(2)其他有肾动脉瘤,肾动静脉畸形和肾动脉栓塞等。

4.CT 表现

(1)肾:肾实质异常主要是各种密度不同的肿块,水样密度囊性肿块见于各种肾囊肿,无强化;低密度、软组织密度或混杂密度肿块多为各种类型良、恶性肾肿瘤,可有不同程度和形式的强化;高密度肿块常为外伤后血肿。肾盂、肾盏常见异常是高密度结石、梗阻所致扩大积水以及肿瘤所致软组织密度肿块。肾周异常主要包括肾周脂肪密度增高、筋膜增厚或(和)积液(积血),多为炎症、外伤所致,也可见于肿瘤的周围侵犯。

(2)输尿管:主要异常表现是梗阻造成的扩张积水,显示为输尿管明显增粗,呈水样低密度,于梗阻端层面有可能发现高密度结石影或软组织密度肿块,后者常为输尿管肿瘤。

(3)膀胱:主要异常是膀胱肿块和膀胱壁增厚。与膀胱壁相连的腔内肿块既可为膀胱肿瘤,也可为血块或结石,除密度差异外,结石与血块的位置通常随体位发生改变,可资鉴别。膀胱壁弥漫性增厚多为各种类型炎症或慢性梗阻所致,局限性增厚见于膀胱肿瘤,也可为膀胱周围炎症或肿瘤累及膀胱。

5.MRI 表现

肾、输尿管和膀胱病变依组织成分和病变性质而有不同的信号特征:富含水份的病变如肾囊肿或扩张的肾盂、肾盏和输尿管,均呈长 T1 低信号和长 T2 高信号;T1WI 和 T2WI 上呈混杂信号的肾实质肿块,形态不规则,增强检查呈不均一强化,为肾癌常见特征;MRU 检查,扩张的肾盏、肾盂和输尿管皆呈明显高信号;膀胱 MRI 异常形态改变类似 CT 检查所见。

第四节　比较影像学

泌尿系统疾病的影像学检查方法较多。常规 X 线检查包括 X 线平片、尿路造影和血管造影,CT 和 MRI 检查也已广泛应用于临床。要选择适宜的检查方法,充分发挥它们各自的优势,就必须对泌尿系统各种不同检查方法的适用症、应用价值和限度有一个全面的了解,除了考虑患者的安全、舒适和费用外,主要取决于临床申请的要求,即要达到准确诊断的目的,又要获得较高的性价比。

虽然 CT 和 MRI 在泌尿系统的应用已越来越普及,但某些常规 X 线检查方法如腹部平片和尿路造影等对病变的发现乃至定性诊断仍有重要的价值,且具有简便、经济的特点,目前在泌尿系统影像诊断中应用仍然非常广泛。对于常规 X 线检查难以发现的病变或虽有异常发现但难以作出确切诊断的病变,则需 CT 或 MRI 检查以进一步明确诊断。

各种影像检查方法的临床应用:

1.腹部 X 线平片

腹部 X 线平片虽可显示肾脏的轮廓、大小和位置,但不能显示输尿管,膀胱也只是偶尔可见且不很清楚,其在泌尿系统中的最大应用价值是诊断阳性结石和评价病理性的钙化。常规 X 线平片对阳性的肾结石和膀胱结石一般能作出准确诊断,结合尿路造影检查对输尿管阳性结石也可作出正确诊断,但对泌尿道阴性结石则无能为力。此外,当右肾区显示有高密度结石影时,常需摄侧位 X 线平片,以鉴别右肾结石与胆囊结石或淋巴结钙化。

2.尿路造影

在泌尿系统疾病的诊断中仍然具有重要价值,几乎适应于泌尿道所有方面——肾、输尿管和膀胱疾病的诊断,如结石、结核、肿瘤、畸形和积水等。能证实尿路结石的部位,了解有无阴性结石,了解肾盂、肾盏和输尿管扩张积水的情况。特别是在肾结核的早期阶段，即可显示肾实质的病变和肾盂、肾盏的改变，其价值优于 CT 和 MRI，因此临床疑为泌尿道结核(肾、输尿管和膀胱)的患者应首选尿路造影。对于肾盂内肿瘤，尤其是早期较小肿瘤的确定，尿路造影是最佳检查方法；对于肾实质内的肿瘤也能提供肾盂、肾盏受压、移位和变形等占位病变的间接征象，对膀胱、输尿管肿瘤也有一定的诊断价值；尿路造影亦是诊断异位肾、游走肾、肾盂输尿管重复畸形等先天异常的有效和首选的检查方法。

3. 肾血管造影(包括 DSA)

肾血管造影是诊断肾血管病变如肾动脉狭窄、闭塞、肾动脉瘤的金标准，其价值优于 CTA 和 MRA，还可用于观察肾肿瘤的血供情况及行化疗和(或)栓塞等介入性治疗。

4. CT

当前，CT 检查在泌尿系统疾病的诊断中已越来越显示它的重要性。CT 可直接评估肾脏的形态和功能，还可了解腹膜后软组织的情况(包括淋巴结、肾上腺、主动脉、下腔静脉等)；在盆腔 CT 可评估膀胱及周围软组织和淋巴结。对多数泌尿系统疾病，如肿瘤、结石、炎症、外伤和先天性畸形等，CT 都具有很大的诊断价值，不但能作出准确诊断，且能确定病变范围，从而有助于临床治疗。目前公认 CT 是泌尿系统肿块性病变(如肾实质内肿瘤、膀胱癌等)的最有效的检查方法，既能提供定性诊断的信息，还可对恶性肿瘤进行分期。因此，通过其他影像检查方法发现的可疑肿块性病变尤其是肾肿块都应进行 CT 检查(平扫+增强)。

CT 血管造影(CTA)是近年来发展的一项新的技术，肾血管 CTA 并三维重建可显示副肾动脉、主动脉后肾静脉等异常以及象肾动脉狭窄、闭塞和动脉瘤等病变，其检查的诊断价值目前仍在研究之中。

5. MRI

在泌尿系统疾病诊断中的应用已日趋广泛，极佳的软组织分辨力使其能很好的评估肿块性病变，对确定病变的组织成份和内部结构均有较高的价值，对于泌尿系统的恶性肿瘤如肾癌、膀胱癌等能较为准确地显示肿瘤侵犯的深度、范围、邻近器官有无受累、有无瘤栓及远处转移，还可确定肿瘤有无复发，其价值优于 CT 检查。由于 MRI 对钙化病变不敏感，因而很少用于泌尿系统结石的检查。

MRU 是近年来 MR 成像技术的临床发展，其在泌尿系统疾病特别是梗阻性病变中的诊断价值较大，是 IVP 的一种准确、安全、无创的替代方法，其临床应用目前仍在不断探索中。

影像分析和诊断原则：

影像诊断是主要的临床诊断方法之一，在观察和分析泌尿系统常规 X 线检查影像时，首先应注意照片质量是否满足诊断要求。例如，检查位置是否准确，摄影条件是否恰当，造影期相是否全面等，否则将直接影响病变的分析和诊断。例如临床怀疑泌尿道结石时，若胃肠道内有较多内容物和气体，则可干扰结石的观察，影响诊断的准确性。在观察和分析泌尿系统 CT 和 MRI 影像时，应注意检查范围是否充分，扫描方式、位置是否准确及检查序列是否全面等。

熟悉泌尿系统 X 线、CT 和 MRI 的正常影像学表现和基本病变的影像学表现是进行影像学诊断的基础；全面细致的图像观察，发现并确认异常病变，认真分析病变的特点，再密切结合临床资料和其他有关的检查结果进行综合分析判断，是作出正确影像学诊断的关键。例如临床怀疑肾输尿管结核的患者，若尿路造影显示肾盂、肾盏边缘不规则和(或)肾实质内有一团对比剂集聚灶，且输尿管出现不规则狭窄和扩张呈串珠状改变，结合临床症状(如尿频、尿痛、血尿等)和实验室检查尿中查出结核杆菌，即可确立诊断。

在观察和分析泌尿道异常影像学表现时，应注意观察病变的部位、大小、形态、密度和边缘特点，单侧还是双侧，单发还是多发，实质性或是囊性，及与邻近组织和器官的关系，注意找出一个或几个有主要意义的影像学表现，从而提出初步的影像学诊断。多数泌尿系统病变需通过几种检查方法综合分析，才能作出准确地诊断，特别是对肿瘤性病变应综合分析和评估 CT 或 MRI 平扫与增强后的特征，并注意检查期相，才能确定病变的位置、范围和性质并作出正确地诊断。例如，尿路造影显示肾盂肾盏受压、移位但无破坏，常提示肾实质内占位病变，进一步行 CT 检查，如显示肾实质内圆形均一水样低密度灶且增强检查病灶无强化,则可诊断为肾囊肿,若肾实质内肿块病变呈中等或略低密度或密度不均匀,增强检查病灶有明显不均一强化,则多可诊断为肾癌。

第五节 常见疾病诊断

1. 泌尿系结石

结石是泌尿系统的常见病,主要原发于肾和膀胱,输尿管和尿道结石多由上泌尿道下移而来。结石的成份不同,X 线检查时形状、密度也不同,多数结石含有钙盐,密度较高,能在 X 线平片上显示称为阳性结石,少数结石如尿酸盐类结石,含钙少,X 线平片不能显示称为阴性结石。应该指出,有相当高比例的阴性结石可由 CT 或 USG 发现。

(1)肾结石:

1)临床与病理表现:肾结石可单发或多发,单侧或双侧(约 10%),一般位于肾盂或肾盏内,病理改变主要是梗阻、积水和感染。典型临床表现为腰痛和血尿,如合并感染,则可伴有尿频、尿急、尿痛等。

2)影像学表现:腹部平片检查,表现为肾区内圆形、卵圆形、鹿角形或不定形高密度影(图 15-3),密度可均匀一致,也可不均或有分层。侧位片观察,肾结石多与脊柱重叠。尿路造影主要用于检查阴性结石,表现为肾盂、肾盏内充盈缺损,也可确定可疑影是否在肾内,还能了解患肾的功能。CT 平扫能确认肾盂和肾盏内高密度结石的存在。

(2)输尿管结石:

1)临床与病理表现:输尿管结石常由肾结石下移而来,易停留在三个生理狭窄处,结石引起梗阻可造成梗阻以上尿路不同程度扩张积水。典型表现为下腹部疼痛并可向会阴部放射,同时伴有血尿。

2)影像学表现:X 线平片和 CT 平扫都表现为输尿管走行区内米粒大或黄豆大的高密度影(图 15-4)。尿路造影可确定致密影是否位于输尿管内,并能显示阴性结石。排泄性尿路造影和 CT 还可显示结石上方的输尿管和肾盂、肾盏的扩张积水。MRU 亦可显示结石所致的输尿管扩张积水。

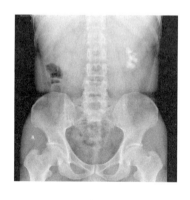

图 15-3 腹平片示左肾区多发点状高密度影

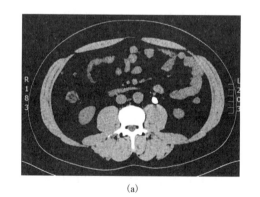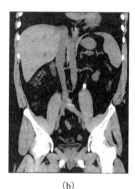

(a) (b)

横断位及冠状位 CT 示左侧输尿管上段内可见点状高密度影。

图 15-4 输尿管结石 CT 表现

(3)膀胱结石:

1)临床与病理表现:膀胱结石有原发和继发两种,前者形成于膀胱,后者由肾结石经输尿管下降而成。典型表现为排尿疼痛,尿流中断,尿频、尿急和血尿等。

2)影像学表现:主要行 X 线平片检查,表现为耻骨联合上方圆形或椭圆形致密影,大小可不一,边缘可光滑或毛糙,密度可均匀、不均或分层,结石可随体位而改变位置为其特点。膀胱造影可进一步确定结石并可发现阴性结石。CT 和 MRI 一般不作为膀胱结石的常规检查方法。

2. 泌尿系统感染

(1)泌尿系统结核：

1)临床与病理表现：泌尿系结核多继发于肺结核，主要侵犯肾，然后蔓延至输尿管及膀胱。肾结核初期为皮质感染，其后蔓延至髓质，于肾乳头形成干酪样溃疡，继而造成肾盏和肾盂破坏。如病变进一步向下蔓延则引起输尿管壁增厚、僵直和管腔狭窄甚至闭塞。膀胱结核初期膀胱黏膜充血、水肿，形成不规则溃疡和(或)肉芽肿，晚期则膀胱壁增厚并发生挛缩。肾结核干酪化病灶可发生钙化，甚至全肾钙化称为肾自截。泌尿系结核的主要临床表现为尿频、尿痛、脓尿和血尿，可伴有消瘦，乏力和低热等全身症状。

2)影像学表现：

①X 线表现：腹部 X 线平片常无异常发现，有时可见肾区有云絮状或环状钙化影，甚至全肾钙化。尿路造影检查，早期肾小盏边缘不整如虫蚀状，溃疡空洞与肾盏相通时，可见肾实质内团块状造影剂与受累肾盏相连，受累肾盏可变形狭窄。病变进展导致肾盂、肾盏广泛破坏或形成肾盂积脓时，排泄性尿路造影常不显影。逆行尿路造影可见肾盂肾盏扩大形成一不规则的空腔。输尿管结核可使输尿管边缘不整，管腔出现不规则狭窄与扩张呈串珠状，晚期导致输尿管僵硬、短缩甚至闭塞。膀胱结核早期可无明显改变或仅见边缘略不规则，晚期膀胱挛缩，体积变小，膀胱造影呈典型小膀胱，有时可见"输尿管反流"征象。

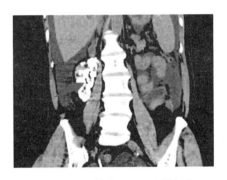

图 15-5　冠状位 CT 示右肾钙化

②CT 表现：在肾结核早期，CT 检查可显示肾实质内低密度灶，边缘不整。病变进展显示肾盏、肾盂扩张，呈不规则多房变形，CT 值接近水的密度。晚期肾可萎缩变形，肾皮质变薄。CT 亦可见多发点状或不规则高密度钙化影，甚至全肾钙化(图 15-5)。输尿管结核表现为输尿管管壁增厚，管腔不规则狭窄和扩张。膀胱结核表现为膀胱壁增厚，边缘不规则和容积变小。

③MRI 表现：类似 CT 所见，MRU 表现犹如尿路造影所见。

(2)肾脓肿：

1)临床与病理表现：多由血源性感染所致，也可由于尿路逆行感染而引发。临床主要表现为发热，肾区胀痛，实验室检查尿中有细菌生长。

2)影像学表现：

①CT 表现：早期 CT 主要表现为肾实质内低密度影，边界模糊，脓肿成熟期可见类圆形低密度灶，增强扫描病灶周围(脓肿壁)可见环形强化，部分脓肿内可见气体影。

②MRI 表现：以成熟期肾脓肿为例，平扫时病灶多呈 T1WI 低信号，T2WI 高信号，增强 T1WI 检查，病变周边可见环形强化(图 15-6)。

3. 泌尿系统肿瘤

(1)肾癌：

1)临床与病理表现：肾癌是最常见的肾恶性肿瘤，病理上起源于肾小管上皮细胞，多位于肾上下极，呈不规则实质性肿块，内可有出血、坏死和囊变，晚期可发生肾周组织的直接侵犯、淋巴转移和血行转移。典型临床表现是无痛性血尿和腹部肿块。

2)影像学表现：

①X 线表现：可见肾影增大，呈分叶状或局部突出，偶可见肿瘤钙化。尿路造影由于肿瘤压迫或侵蚀肾盏可见肾盏伸长、变形、狭窄乃至闭塞，边缘不整或出现充盈缺损；肿瘤范围较大而波及多个肾盏，可使

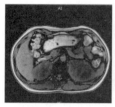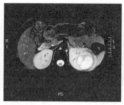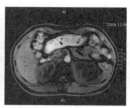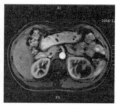

左肾内可见长 T1 长 T2 信号影，增强扫描呈轻度环形强化。

图 15-6 肾腔肿 MRI 表现

各肾盏聚集或分离；肿瘤压迫或侵蚀肾盂可造成肾盂受压、变形、破坏或出现充盈缺损。肾动脉造影，肾癌表现为网状和不规则杂乱血管影伴有造影剂池状充盈，相邻血管发生分离移位。

②CT 表现：目前，CT 是肾癌最有效的检查方法，平扫表现为肾实质内类圆形或不规则肿块，较大者可突向肾外，肿块密度低于或类似邻近肾实质，可均一，也可不均一，内可有不规则低密度区，少数可有点状或不规则钙化。增强检查，早期肿瘤多有明显不均一强化，其后由于周围肾实质强化而呈相对低密度(图 15-7)。CT 也可显示肾癌与肾包膜及周围组织的关系。

③MRI 表现：类似 CT 所见，常呈混杂信号肿块，T2WI 上病变周边常见低信号带，代表肿瘤的假性包膜。Gd-DTPA 增强肿块呈不均一强化。MRI 亦可确定肾静脉和下腔静脉内有无瘤栓及其范围。

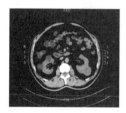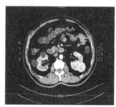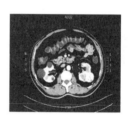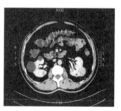

横断位 CT 示，左肾肿块密度不均匀，伴有不规则的低密度区域，对比增强后，肾透明细胞癌表现为"快进快出"。

图 15-7 肾癌 CT 表现

3)鉴别诊断：

①肾血管平滑肌脂肪瘤：瘤内脂肪密度或信号的存在是其特征。但乏脂肪的肾血管平滑肌脂肪瘤与肾透明细胞癌在 CT 表现相似，通常肾透明细胞癌更容易瘤内出血坏死而密度不均，增强后多表现为"快进快出"；而肾血管平滑肌脂肪瘤增强后主要表现为瘤内血管性结构强化，其他结构不强化。

②肾盂癌：肾盂癌主体位于肾盂，而肾癌位于肾实质内；肾癌的强化程度常高于肾盂癌。需要注意的是，晚期肾癌累及肾盂后与肾盂癌影像学很难区分，需要进一步病理诊断。

(2)肾盂癌：

1)临床与病理表现：肾盂癌病理上多为移行细胞癌，常呈乳头状生长，又称乳头状癌。肿瘤发生于肾盂或肾盏，可向输尿管和膀胱种植。临床表现主要为无痛性全程血尿。

2)影像学表现：

①X 线表现：腹部平片检查多无异常发现，尿路造影可见肾盂、肾盏内有固定不变的充盈缺损，形态不规则，肾盂和肾盏可伴有不同程度的扩大。如肿瘤侵犯肾实质可致肾盏变形移位，如肿瘤移植到输尿管可造成小的充盈缺损和不完全梗阻。因肿瘤血管少，肾动脉造影意义不大。

②CT 表现：为肾窦区肿块，CT 值高于尿液而低于肾实质，增强扫描轻中度均匀或不均匀强化，排泄期强化减退，肾窦脂肪受压、变薄或消失(图 15-8)。

③MRI 表现：类似 CT，在 T1WI 上肿块信号强度高于尿液，而在 T2WI 上则低于尿液。

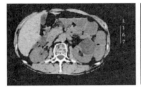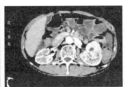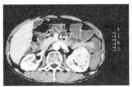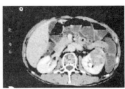

横断位 CT 表现为左肾窦内肿块,其 CT 值高于尿液,低于肾实质,增强扫描轻中度不均匀强化,排泄期强化减退,肾窦内的脂肪显示被压缩。

图 15-8 肾盂癌 CT 表现

(3)膀胱癌:

1)临床与病理表现:多数膀胱癌为来自上皮组织并呈乳头状生长的乳头状癌,可单发或多发,好发于膀胱三角区及两侧壁。肿瘤自膀胱壁突向腔内,并可侵犯肌层,进而延伸至周围组织和器官。部分肿瘤呈浸润性生长而造成膀胱壁局限性增厚。临床主要症状是无痛性肉眼血尿,可伴尿频、尿急、尿痛和排尿困难。

2)影像学表现:

①X 线表现:膀胱造影表现为自膀胱壁突向腔内的结节状或菜花状充盈缺损,大小不等,基底部常较宽,侵犯肌层时致局部膀胱壁僵硬和形态固定。

②CT 表现:CT 扫描显示为自膀胱壁向腔内突入的软组织密度肿块,局部膀胱壁不规则增厚。增强早期肿块多为均一强化[图 15-9(a)、(b)],延迟扫描,由于膀胱腔内充盈对比剂,肿块则表现为低密度充盈缺损。

③MRI 表现:类似 CT。CT 和 MRI 还可发现邻近组织和器官的侵犯及淋巴结的转移。

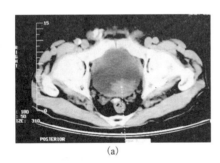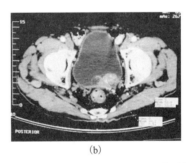

(a) (b)

(a)CT 平扫,肿瘤自膀胱左后壁突向腔内,呈软组织密度肿块,表面不规则;(b)CT 增强早期,肿块强化,形态不规则。

图 15-9 膀胱癌 CT 表现

(4)肾血管平滑肌脂肪瘤:

1)临床与病理表现:血管平滑肌脂肪瘤是肾脏较为常见的良性肿瘤,为一种无包膜的错构瘤性的肿块,由血管、平滑肌和脂肪组织构成。肿瘤一般为孤立性,大小不等,可自数毫米直至 20 cm,少数(约 20%)可合并有结节性硬化。临床上肿瘤生长缓慢,可无症状或因并发出血而产生腹痛。

2)影像学表现:

①X 线表现:平片和尿路造影,肿块较大时可致肾轮廓改变,肾盂、肾盏受压、移位和变形。肾动脉造影可显示丰富迂曲的肿瘤性血管。

②CT 表现:CT 典型表现为肾实质内边界清楚的混杂密度肿块,肿块内有明确的脂肪成份,增强扫描肿块内脂肪性低密度区无强化,而软组织密度区(代表血管和平滑肌组织)则普遍性增强。

③MRI 表现:类似 CT 所见,在 T1WI 和 T2WI 上均呈混杂信号肿块,内有脂肪性高信号或中等信号灶,

应用 T1WI 并脂肪抑制技术, 脂肪灶信号明显下降。

4.肾脏囊性病变

(1)单纯性肾囊肿:

1)临床与病理表现:单纯性肾囊肿极为常见,为一种薄壁充满液体的囊肿,可单发或多发,多发生在皮质,呈圆形或类圆形,大小不等。临床上一般无症状,但较大囊肿可表现有腹部不适或触及腹部肿块。

2)影像学表现:

①X 线表现:较大囊肿平片可见肾轮廓改变,偶见囊肿壁弧线状钙化。尿路造影可见肾盂、肾盏受压、移位和变形,但无破坏。

②CT 和 MRI 表现:为边缘清晰锐利的圆形或椭圆形水样密度或信号强度灶。增强检查病变无强化(图15-10)。

(2)多囊肾:

1)临床与病理表现:多囊肾系遗传性病变,以成人型多见,一个重要特点为双肾布满多发大小不等的囊肿,囊内含有水样液体,常合并有多囊肝。临床上通常在中年后发病,表现为腹部肿块、高血压和血尿,晚期可发生肾衰竭。

2)影像学表现:

①X 线表现:平片可见双肾影增大,轮廓呈分叶状。尿路造影可见双侧肾盂、肾盏受压、变形、移位、拉长和分离,呈"蜘蛛足"样改变。

②CT 和 MRI 表现:CT 和 MRI 检查可发现双肾布满多发、大小不等圆形或卵圆形水样密度或信号病变,增强扫描病变无增强,部分囊内可有急性出血性密度和信号,肾体积增大变形,边缘呈分叶状(图15-11),常可同时发现多囊肝。

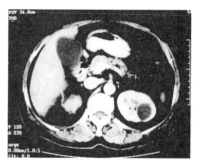

CT 增强,左肾外部圆形水样低密度灶,边缘清晰锐利,病变无强化。

图 15-10　左肾单纯性囊肿 CT 表现

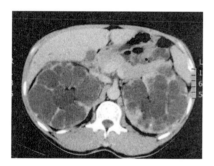

CT 示双侧肾脏多发大小不等的圆形或椭圆形肿块病变,呈水样密度,未见明显强化。

图 15-11　多囊肾 CT 表现

3)鉴别诊断:

主要与多发单纯性肾囊肿相鉴别。典型多囊肾表现为双侧肾轮廓增大,肾盂、肾盏可扭曲,常合并多囊肝;后者表现为多个无强化的囊性灶,但肾脏增大不明显,且无阳性家族史。

5.泌尿系统先天异常

(1)临床与病理表现:泌尿系统的胚胎发育过程较为复杂,包括肾曲管和集合系统的连接,肾轴的旋转及肾自盆腔上升至腰部等,因而泌尿系统的先天异常较为常见且种类繁多,包括数目、结构和位置异常以及其他异常。临床上可无症状或因并发症而出现梗阻、感染等表现。

(2)影像学表现:

1)肾盂、输尿管重复畸形(双肾盂、双输尿管):即一侧或双侧肾各分上、下两部分,分别有一套肾盂和输尿管,重复输尿管可相互汇合,也可分别汇入膀胱,尿路造影可清楚显示这种畸形。CT 和 MRI 尤其是增强检查可进一步确定诊断(图15-12)。

2)异位肾：系胎儿期肾的上升过程发生异常所致，异位肾大多位于盆腔内，少数可居膈下、髂窝甚至胸腔内。平片可显示异位侧肾区无肾影，尿路造影、CT和MRI增强均能发现肾位置异常。

3)孤立肾：系一侧肾未发育(单侧肾缺如)。平片见一侧肾影缺如，对侧肾影相对增大。尿路造影辅以CT和MRI检查能明确诊断。腹主动脉造影可见缺如侧无肾动脉。

4)马蹄肾：两肾的一极且多为下极相互融合形如马蹄称为马蹄肾。尿路造影可显示肾位置较低，肾旋转不良，两肾下极相互融合，而上极远离脊柱，肾盂、肾盏常有扩大。CT和MRI均可显示两肾下极的肾实质于脊柱前方相连(图15-13)。

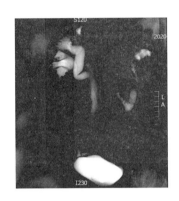

图15-12　MRU示右肾双肾盂畸形

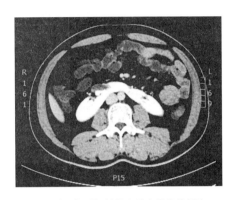

CT显示双肾下极的肾实质在脊柱前相连。

图15-13　马蹄肾CT表现

6.泌尿系统外伤

(1)肾外伤：

1)临床与病理表现：依据出血部位以及损伤程度可分为肾包膜下血肿、肾周血肿、肾挫伤及肾撕裂伤。临床主要表现为患侧腰部疼痛、血尿，严重者可出现休克。

2)影像学表现：肾包膜下血肿主要表现为患侧肾包膜下新月形高密度影；而肾周血肿范围一般较广，但局限于肾筋膜囊内，表现为肾周围高密度影。肾挫伤依据出血量、尿液溢出量及残存肾实质水肿程度，可表现为肾实质内高密度、混杂密度或低密度影，但肾包膜及肾实质连续。肾撕裂伤表现为肾实质连续性中断，其内间隔以高密度的血液及低密度的尿液(图15-14)。

上述均为急性肾外伤后影像学表现，随着时间推移，血肿可慢慢吸收、液化而呈低密度。

MRI：血肿的形态学表现与CT检查相似，但其T1WI和T2WI上的信号强度随血肿期龄而异。

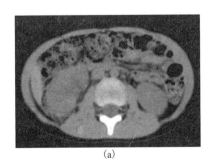
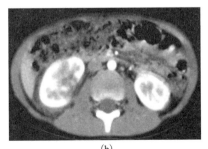

(a)　　　　　　　　　　(b)

CT显示右肾下极肾皮质不连续，肾周可见片状稍高密度影。

图15-14　肾挫伤CT表现

7. 肾梗死

(1)临床与病理表现：急性肾梗死是指肾动脉主干及分支血栓形成或栓塞，导致动脉管腔狭窄或闭塞，造成肾或局部肾组织坏死，从而影响肾功能的一种疾病。急性肾梗死临床表现缺乏特异性，大多数患者有"三联症"：持续的腰腹疼痛、血清乳酸脱氢酶升高及蛋白尿。

(2)影像学表现：急性肾脏梗死 CT 直接征象表现为：①肾脏楔形或扇形低密度无强化或延迟期轻度强化影，与周围正常组织界限清楚，尖端指向肾门，底部位于肾脏表面；②广泛性梗死表现为肾脏大范围无强化区、甚至全肾无强化，其内可见部分索条影，增强各期肾盂内均无造影剂填充。

急性肾脏梗死 CT 间接征象表现为：①肾周脂肪间隙密度增高，呈斑片状磨玻璃样密度影；②肾周间隙积液，积液分布不均匀；③肾周筋膜增厚。

肾动脉造影为金标准，但其为有创检查，CTA 目前已取代肾动脉造影，用于观察急性肾梗死时肾动脉病变，对于肾动脉闭塞、充盈缺损以及肾动脉瘤有很好的显示效果。

MRI 不需要注射对比剂即能显示肾脏梗死灶，但因检查时间长，常不用于急诊患者。

（陈翔宇，柴甜，李亚，刘梅桃，肖恩华，刘辉）

Chapter 15

Urinary system

The urinary system consists of the kidneys, ureters, bladder and urethra. X-ray diagnosis mainly makes use of the plain film of abdomen and the urinary contrast examination. Computed tomography (CT) is preferable to conventional X-ray examination, whereas MRI has an advantage over CT in evaluating the internal structure of the lesion and metastasis and recurrence of malignant tumor.

Section 1   Method of examination

1. X-ray examination

(1) Plain film of the abdomen (KUB): The plain film, the routine examination of the urinary system, is performed to observe the size, shape and position of the kidneys, and obtain an evidence of positive calculi or calcification in the region of the urinary tract, and also provide a preliminary view before performing all kinds of contrast examinations.

(2) Excretory urography: Excretory urography is also known as intravenous pyelography (IVP). Iodine medium is administered intravenously and excreted by kidneys. All of them is almost filtrated through glomerulus into the renal calyces and pelvis, and flow from renal pelvis to bladder via ureters. This test, readily performed and with less danger, not only may shows the anatomical structures of the entire urinary tract, but is able to evaluate the excretory function of the kidneys. Therefore, it is clinically the most common used X-ray examinal modality of urinary system.

(3) Retrograde urography: Retrograde urography includes retrograde pyelography and retrograde cystography. The former is that a catheter is introduced via a cystoscope into the ureter and the contrast medium is injected retrogradely, thus making the renal calyces, pelvis, ureters and bladder demonstrating. This technique is preferred for patients for whom IVP is impractical or is adequately not visible and IVP is not fit at all. Retrograde cystography involves the insertion of a catheter via the urethra into the bladder, followed by injection of the contrast medium, thus making the bladder showing.

(4) Renal angiography: Renal angiography mainly includes abdominal aorta angiography and selective renal arteriography. Usually using seldinger technique, a fine catheter is inserted percutaneously into the femoral artery and advanced under fluoroscopic guidance into the abdominal aorta. The tip of the catheter is placed at the upper of origin of the renal artery (abdominal aorta angiography) or into renal artery of one side (selective renal arteriography). After rapidly injecting the contrast medium, a series of sequence X-ray films are taken. Main purpose of the angiography is to examine the lesions of renal vessel, particularly the narrowing and occlusion of renal artery, and determine the position and range of the lesions and perform interventional therapy, and also detect renal aneurysm and renal artery malformation etc.

2. CT examination

(1) Plain scan: No special preparation is needed for CT scan of the kidneys and ureters, but CT examination of the bladder requires the patient with a urine-distented bladder. The patient is placed in supine position on the examination table. Scanning is conventionally performed in body cross-section (axial CT), with 10 mm slice thickness and slice interval. Local thin slice scan is suggested for the smaller focuses. The range of renal CT scan is from adrenal region to inferior margin of lower pole of kidney. If needing to visualize the ureters simultaneously, the scanning is continuously performed downwards up to the level of ureterovesical junction. The pelvic cavity (the bladder) CT scan is performed upwards at consecutive levels from inferior margin of pubic symphysis to height of iliac crest, or is continuously performed from superior to inferior.

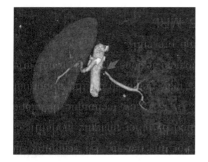

Left renal artery orifice stenosis (Indicated by the arrows).

Figure 15-1   CTA

(2) Contrast scan: The method of conventional contrast scan is that approximate 60 ~ 100 mL of the water soluble organic iodide contrast media or the non-ionic contrast media of the same dosage iodine are rapidly given intravenously, and a series of tomograms are immediately taken as plain scan after the injection. When necessary, dynamic contrast scan, renal double phases or multi-phases scan may be performed to detect the small focuses.

(3) CT angiography(CTA): Injecting iodine contrast agent rapidly in the vein, then collecting images at the renal artery stage, and recombining the volume data in three dimensions (Figure 15-1), Images similar to X-ray renal arteriography can be obtained.

(4) CT urography(CTU): The principle of CTU is similar to that of the CTA. Image collection was carried out during the renal excretory stage, and three-dimensional recombination of renal pelvis and renal calyces, ureters and bladder volume data, then can obtain images similar to those obtained by IVP examination.

3. MRI examination

(1) Plain scan: Routine MRI scanning of the kidneys and ureters is mainly performed in cross-sectional (axial) plane. When necessary, coronal and (or) sagittal scanning may also be added. Using T1-weighted images (T1WI) with a fat inhibition technique will help to identify anatomical structure of the kidneys and diagnose the lesions containing fat.

(2) Contrast scan: After paramagnetic contrast medium Gd-DTPA is rapidly injected intravenously, T_1WI scanning is immediately performed. Obtaining images can help further to determine presence and source of the lesions, provide the information of the lesions about internal structure, marginal state and blood supply and so on.

(3) MR urography (MRU): MRU is mainly used to diagnose the obstructive lesions of renal pelvis and ureters. Without contrast, it can demonstrate the dilatational calyces, pelvis and ureters. MRU image is similar to that of routine X-ray urography, therefore, it is suitable for patients who is high sensitive to iodine or have severe hydrops or is complete non-visualization to IVP.

(4) MRI angiography (MRA): MRA is often used as a screening method for renal artery and its larger branches, and its diagnostic accuracy is not as good as CTA.

Section 2　Normal appearances

1. X-rays findings

(1) The kidney: Plain film of the abdomen can show the renal contour, size and position. Normal shadows of the kidneys are bean-shaped, situated in the flank of the vertebral column. Each adult kidney is about 12 to 13 cm long, 5 to 6 cm wide, and has convex lateral margins and concave medial margins called renal hila. The kidneys are usually located between 12 thoracic vertebra to 3 lumbar vertebra, and right kidney is slightly 1 to 2 cm lower than the left. The kidneys in an upright position are 1 to 5 cm lower than those in a supine position. Bilateral shadows of the kidneys overlap the vertebral column in a lateral view.

Urography (Figure 15-2) can visualize the shape of the renal calyces and pelvis. Normally, the renal pelvis, with a great number of variations in shape, are mostly like "loudspeaker" with smooth margins, a small number like "bifurcation-like" or "bellied-like". The renal calyces are comprised of major calyces and minor calyces. The former is of long-tube shape, and connects with a few minor calyces at its apices or tips, and also links up renal pelvis at the bases; the minor calyces are like short-tube with slight expansive ending, and their tops appear "cupping-like" invagination due to the renal papillae directly projecting toward the calyx beneath it. The normal renal pelvis should be clearly outlined, and the margins of major and minor calyces should be fine and sharp.

(2) The ureter: The ureters can not be normally shown on plain film of the abdomen. On the urography film, the ureters appear as the compact shadows of narrow, long-tube shape, and are about 25 to 30 cm long. The ureters are continuous with the renal pelvis at superior end, traveling downward and forward along the flank of the vertebral column into the pelvic cavity, firstly running backward and inferolaterally in the pelvic cavity, then turning towards anteromedially and finally entering the bladder wall obliquely. The normal ureters have three sites of natural narrowing-the ureteropelvic junction, the bony pelvic brim and the ureterovesical junction, and are should be outlined clearly, filled uniformly and flexible.

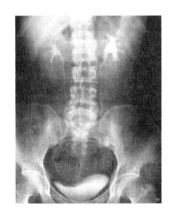

Figure 15-2　Normal excretory urography.

(3) The bladder: The normal bladder presents with the shadow of a soft-tissue density and can be rarely seen on the plain film duo to lacking the natural contrast in comparision with surrounding tissues and structures. The urography film may show the internal lumen of the bladder. Its size and shape depend on the amount of contrast medium filled and relationship to the peripheral organs. Normal capacity of the bladder is 300 to 500 ml. When filled well, the bladder is elliptic and lies transversally above the pubic symphysis, with smooth edge and uniform density. If the bladder is not well filled or is being in contracted state, the thick mucosal fold may make its edge irregular like "sawtooth". In addition, sometimes a transversal hyaline band can be seen between the bilateral ureteric orifices opening the base of the bladder, called ureteral crest, no misdiagnosed pathology.

2. Renal angiographical findings

Abdominal aorta angiography and selective renal arteriography may show three phases of the vessels filling: arterial, nephrographic and venous. In the arterial phase, the trunk of renal artery and its branches can be clearly visualized, and are normally from thick to thin, distributed uniformly, with smooth margins, without the findings such as dilatation, stenosis, discontinuance and excessive tortuosity etc. In the nephrographic phase, the contrast media are spread all over the renal parenchyma, so that the renal contour, size and shape can be clearly demonstrated. In the venous phase, the shadows of renal veins can be seen but not be clear.

3. CT findings

（1）The kidney: Plain scanning. On the cross-sectional slice, the kidneys lie in the flank of the vertebral column and appear as the shadow of circular or elliptical soft-tissue density with smooth and sharp margins. In the middle levels of the kidney, we can see the concave renal hila through which the renal arteries, renal veins and ureters pass. The density of the renal parenchyma is uniform, with a CT number 30 to 50 Hu. Generally, the cortex and the medulla can not be distinguished. Contrast scanning. The findings of renal enhancement depend on the amount of contrast medium, speed of injection and scanning time. If contrast scanning is administered by bolus IV injection with the conventional dosage, in the early stage (in about 1 min after injection), the renal vessels and the cortex are enhanced obviously, whereas the medulla still maintain the lower density. At this moment, the cortex can be clearly distinguished from the medulla; About 2 min after injection, the medulla is enhanced obviously, and the degree of enhancement is similar to the cortex or in excess of it. The corticomedullary boundary is no longer clear. Meanwhile, the renal pelvis and calyces also begin to become intensified; In 5 to 10 min after injection, the degree of enhancement of the renal parenchyma is diminished, whereas the renal pelvis and calyces become maximally enhanced.

（2）The ureter: Plain scanning. If CT scanning is continuously performed from the renal pelvis downwards, the abdominal portion of normal ureters can be often shown with the dot shadows of the soft-tissue density situated in anterior margin of the psoas major. Generally, it is difficult to identify the pelvic portion of the ureters. Contrast scanning. If denay contrast scanning is performed in 5 to 10 min after the injection, the ureters appear as the dot compact shadows duo to intraureteral contrast medium collecting. The entire course of ureters can be visualized by a series of consecutive levels scanning.

（3）The bladder: Plain scanning. The size and shape of the bladder are related to the degree of urine filling. It is generally circular or elliptical. Urine in the bladder is presented with uniform water low-density. Under contrasting with surrounding low-density fat tissues and urine in the bladder, the wall of the bladder appears as the soft-tissue structure of thin wall with uniform thickness and smooth, regular margin (internal and external). Contrast scanning. The wall of the bladder is immediately enhanced in the early stage after the contrast medium is injected. With the delay scanning after 30 to 60 min, the lumen of the bladder presents with even high density, or fluid-fluid level when the contrast medium and urine are blended unevenly.

4. MRI findings

（1）The kidney: MRI of the kidneys is performed with conventional SE sequences. In T1-weighted images (T1WI), the renal cortex appears the middle signal, whereas the signal of the renal medulla is lower than that of the renal cortex. In T2-weighted images (T2WI), the entire renal parenchyma is demonstrated with the higher signal, and renal cortex and medulla can not be readily distinguished from each other. Renal sinus with abundant fat separately appear high signal on T_1WI and middle signal on T2WI. Because of the flow void effects, the renal arteries and renal veins are demonstrated with the band shadows without signal. By Gd-DTPA contrast examination, the degree and pattern of the renal enhancement are similar to CT contrast scan.

（2）The ureter: When T1WI or T2WI cross sectional scanning is continuously performed from the renal pelvis downwards, abdominal segments of the ureters, with dot low signal shadows, may be partially identified.

（3）The bladder: Urine in the bladder presents with uniform low signal of long T1 and high signal of long T2. Signal degree of the wall of the bladder is higher on T1WI and lower on T2WI than that of urine in the bladder.

（4）Magnetic resonance urography (MRU) The normal renal calyces, renal pelvis, ureters and bladder containing urine present with high signal, similar to image of normal X-ray excretory urography.

Section 3　Basic pathologic changes

1. Findings of abdominal plain film

(1) The high density calcification shadows at the areas of the kidneys, ureters and bladder: They result commonly from the positive calculi of the urinary tract. The stones of the renal pelvis and calyces may have the different shapes, The ureteral stones are situated in the their courses and often seen at the point of three physiological narrowing; The bladder stones commonly appear as ellipse and lie transversally above the pubic symphysis. The high density calcification shadows within the renal areas can be also visualized in the other diseases, such as renal tuberculosis, carcinoma of kidney or renal cyst etc.

(2) The change of renal contour: The hydronephrosis, renal tumor or renal cyst may demonstrate the renal enlargement or partial enlargement followed by local protrusion; A renal lobulated or wave edge may be seen in fetal lobulated kidney and chronic pyelonephritis; The perinephric abscess and hematoma may make the renal contour disappear.

2. Findings of urography

(1) Compression, distortion and displacement of the renal pelvis and calyces: Resulting commonly from the mass within kidney such as renal cyst, tumor, hematoma and abscess.

(2) Destruction of the renal pelvis and calyces: This may be caused by the tumor or tuberculosis etc, and appears as irregular edges of the renal pelvis and calyces similar to "moth-eaten" or "rat-bite" and even perfect disappear of the normal structure.

(3) Filling defect within the renal pelvis, calyces, ureters and bladder: presenting without contrast medium filled at the area of the lesion. That results from the lesion projecting into cavity or the intrinsic lesion, such as tumor, calculi, blood clot and gas etc.

(4) Dilatation and hydrops of the renal pelvis, calyces, ureters and bladder: Unilateral or bilateral, they result most commonly from the obstruction caused by tumor, calculi, blood clot, inflammatory narrow or extrinsic compression etc.

3. Findings of renal angiography

(1) Stenosis of renal artery: The position, degree, shape and range of the stenosis depend on different causes for the disease. The main causes include takayasu arteritis and atherosclerosis etc.

(2) The other findings: including aneurysm of renal artery, renal arteriovenous malformation and embolism of renal artery etc.

4. CT findings

(1) The kidney: Abnormalities of the renal parenchyma are mainly all kinds of different density masses. All types of renal cyst appear often as the cystic mass of water density without enhancement; The masses of low density, soft-tissue density or ununiform density are usually the findings of all types of benign and malignant renal tumors, followed probably by the varying degrees and patterns of enhancement. Post-traumatic hematoma is often shown with the high density mass. Common abnormal findings of the renal pelvis and calyces include the high density calculi, the dilatation and hydrops caused by obstruction, and the soft-tissue density mass caused by the tumor. The perinephric abnormalities mainly include the perinephric fat density heighten and the thickening or (and) hydrops (hematocele) of fascia, which are mostly caused by the inflammation and trauma, and may be also caused by peripheric invasion of the tumor.

(2) The ureter: The main abnormal findings are the dilatation and hydrops caused by the obstruction,

appearing as ureteral obvious enlargement with water low density. In the level of obstructive point, it is possible to detect the calculus shadow of high density or the soft-tissue density mass which may most commonly be ureteral tumor.

(3) The bladder: The main abnormalities include the mass of the bladder and the thickness of bladder wall. The mass connected with the bladder wall within the lumen is either the bladder tumor or the blood clot or the calculus. Except for density difference, the position of the calculus and blood clot usually changes with the posture, that can help identification. The diffuse thickness of the bladder wall results commonly from various inflammation or chronic obstruction, whereas the localized thickness may be caused by the bladder tumor, as well as the involvement of bladder by the peripheric inflammation or tumor

5. MRI findings

By MRI, the lesions of the kidneys, ureters and bladder may have different signal characteristics according to different composition and property of the nidus: The lesion containing mainly water, such as renal cyst or dialated renal pelvis, renal calyces and ureters, appears as long T1 low signal and long T_2 high signal; Carcinoma of kidney is commonly characterized as the solid mass of mingled signal with irregular shape on the T1WI and T2WI, and nonuniform enhancement on MRI contrast scanning; The dialated renal pelvis, renal calyces and ureters are demonstrated with obvious high signal by MRU; Abnormal MRI findings of the bladder are similar to CT examination.

Section 4　Basic comparative imaging

There are many kinds of imaginal methods for the diseases of urinary system. The conventional X-ray examinations include the abdominal plain film, urography and angiography. CT and MRI scanning have been vastly used in clinic. To select a appropriate modality and give full play to the respective advantages, one needs a thorough understanding of the indications, utilized value and limitation about all different kinds of imaginal methods of the urinary system. The selection of methods depends mainly on the clinical question asked in addition to considerations of patient safety, patient comfort, and cost, not only achieving the purpose of accurate diagnosis but acquiring a higher ratio of diagnosis to price as well.

The utility of CT and MRI in urinary system are popularized more and more, but some conventional X-ray examinational methods, such as abdominal plain film and urography etc, have still the significant value to the detection and the qualitative diagnosis of the pathological lesions, and have the simple, convenient and economical characteristics. At present, they are still utilized very vastly in the imaging diagnoses of urinary system. In order to further determine diagnosis, the CT and MRI are required for the lesions which is difficultly found by conventional X-ray examinations, and so are for the lesions which may be found with abnormality but can not be accurately diagnosed by them

The clinical application of all kinds of imaging examinations:

1. Plain film of the abdomen

In the plain film, the contour, size and position of the kidneys may be shown, but the ureters can not be shown, the bladder can be also seen only occasionally and is not clear. Its greatest utility in the urinary system is to diagnose the positive calculi and to evaluate the pathological calcifications. The conventional X-ray plain film can generally make a accurate diagnosis to the positive renal stone and bladder stone, and can also make a correct diagnosis to the positive ureteral stone if combining with the urography, whereas it is helpless to evaluate the negative stones of urinary tract. In addition, when the right renal region appears the hyperdense calculus shadow, a lateral plain film is often required to differentiate the right renal stone and the cholecystolithiasis or the calcification of lymph nodes

2. Urography

The urography, still having important value, is nearly suitable for the diseases of all aspects of urinary tract kidneys, ureters and bladder, such as calculus, tuberculosis, tumor, malformation, hydrops and so on. It can confirm the position of urinary calculi, and understand the presence of negative calculi, and understand the situation of dilatation and hydrops of renal pelvis, calyces and ureters as well. Particularly in the early stage of renal tuberculosis, urography may demonstrate the lesions of renal parenchyma and the changes of renal pelvis, calyces, and have an advantage over CT and MRI, so it should be firstly considered for the patient who is clinically suspected of the tuberculosis of urinary tract. Urography is the best modality for the definition of intrapelvic tumor, particularly the earlier and smaller tumor; For the intraparenchymal tumor, it can also provide the indirect signs of occupying lesion, such as compression, displacement and distortion of renal pelvis and calyces; Urography is also of certain diagnostic value to the tumor of ureter and bladder; as well it is a efficient and firstly considered method of congenital abnormality such as ectopic kidney, wandering kidney and duplication of renal pelvis and ureters etc.

3. Renal angiography (including DSA)

Renal angiography is a gold standard of diagnosis of renal vascular disease such as stenosis, occlusion and aneurysm of renal artery and has an advantage over CTA and MRA. It can be also utilized to observe the blood supply of renal tumor and perform interventional therapy such as chemotherapy and (or)embolism etc.

4. CT

At present, CT have played a more and more important role in the diagnosis of diseases of urinary system. CT may directly assess the morphology and function of the kidneys, and also understand the appearance of the retroperitoneal soft tissues (lymph nodes, adrenals, aorta, inferior vena cave). In the pelvic cavity, CT can evaluate the bladder, as well as surrounding soft tissues and lymph nodes. CT is of very great diagnostic value for a vast majority of the diseases of urinary system, such as tumor, calculi, inflammation, trauma, congenital malformation and so on. CT can not only make an accurate diagnosis but also determine the range of the lesion, thus helping clinical therapy. Currently, CT has been recognized to be the most efficient examination of the mass lesion of urinary system, as it can not only provide qualitative diagnostic information but stage malignant tumor as well. For this reason, CT scanning should be performed to evaluate suspected mass lesion, particularly renal mass identified by other imaging modalities.

CTA is a new technique developed in recent years. Renal vessels CTA with three-dimensional reconstructed images may demonstrate the abnormalities such as accessory renal arteries and retroaortic renal veins, and the pathological lesions such as renal artery stenosis, occlusions and aneurysms etc. Its diagnostic value is still in research presently.

5. MRI

The use of MRI in the diagnosis of urinary diseases is becoming widespread day and day. The outstanding soft-tissue resolution offered by MRI makes it well suited for evaluating the mass lesions, and it is very valuable to defining the histological component and internal structure of the lesion. For malignant tumors of urinary system such as renal carcinoma and bladder cancer etc, MRI may accurately show the depth and range of tumor invasion, the circumstances of surrounding organs involved, the presence of tumor embolus and distal metastases, and may also determine whether there is recurrence of malignant tumors, thus having the value over CT. As MRI is not sensitive to calcification, it is rarely utilized to examine the calculi of urinary system.

MRU is another clinical development of MR imaging technique in recent years. It is of very great diagnostic value to the urinary diseases, particularly the obstructive lesions, and is a accurate, safe and noninjurious substitutive method for IVP. Its clinical application is still presently in continuous exploration.

Analytic and diagnostic principle of images:

The imaging diagnosis is one of methods of the important clinical diagnoses. In observing and analyzing the images of urinary system offered by conventional X-ray examination, one should firstly notice whether the film quality can satisfy the requirements of diagnosis or not, for example, whether examinal position is accurate, whether imaging condition is appropriate, whether contrasting phase is perfect and so on, otherwise these will directly affect the analysis and diagnosis of the lesions. For example, when suspecting the calculi of urinary tract clinically, if there are a great number of contents and gases in the gastrointestinal tract, they will may disturb the observation of calculi and affect the accuracy of diagnosis.

In observing and analyzing the images of urinary system offered by CT and MRI, one should notice whether the range of examination is full and whether scanning pattern, position and sequence are perfect.

It is the basis of imaging diagnosis to know normal and elementary pathological imaging findings of X-ray, CT and MRI. It is the key of correct imaging diagnosis toanalyze and assess comprehensively by observing carefully the images, finding and determining abnormal lesion, analyzing seriously the characteristics of lesion, and combining closely with clinical material and other related examination. For example, for patient suspected with renal and ureteral tuberculosis clinically, if the urography present with the irregularity of renal pelvic and calyceal margins, and (or)the collecting focus of bolus contrast medium in the parenchyma, and irregular stricture and dilatation of the ureter like "a string of beads", the diagnosis of tuberculosis may be established by combining with clinical symptoms (frequent micturition, pain in urination, hematuria etc) and experimental examination (with tubercle bacillus in urine).

In observing and analyzing the abnormal imaging findings of urinary tract, one should notice to observe the lesions about their position, size, shape, density and marginal feature, and unilateral or bilateral, single or multiple, solid or cystic, and relationship to adjacent tissues and organs, trying to find out one or a few significant imaginal findings, thereby putting forward a preliminary imaging diagnosis. For the most of urinary diseases, only by comprehensively analyzing a few imaginal methods can you make the accurate diagnosis. Particularly for tumor lesion, only by comprehensively analyzing and assessing the features of plain scan and contrast scan in CT or MRI, and noticing the phase of scanning, can you determine the position, range and quality of the lesion and make a correct diagnosis. For example, the compression, displacement but no destruction of renal pelvis and calyces shown by urography often indicate the occupying lesion in parenchyma. By performing further CT examination, if CT demonstrates the circular, uniform water hypodense lesion in parenchyma and the lesion is not enhanced in contrast scanning, it may be diagnosed as renal cyst; if the mass lesion in parenchyma is of middle or slightly low or ununiform density and has obvious ununiform enhancement in contrast scanning, the diagnosis of renal carcinoma may be usually established.

Section 5　Diagnosis of common disease

1. Stones of the urinary tract

The urinary calculi, which are the common disease of urinary system, originate primarily in the kidney and the bladder. Ureteric and urethral calculi are mostly from migrating down of the upper urinary tract stones. In the X-ray examination, the shape and density of the stones depend on their component. The majority of calculi, which can be visualized duo to containing calcium and having higher density on the X-ray plain film, are known as the positive stone (radiopaque). A small number of calculi such as uric acid stones, which are not visible on the X-ray plain film duo to only containing quiet less calcium, are known as the negative (radiolucent) stone. It should be indicated that a quiet high proportional negative stones may be detected by CT or USG.

(1) Renal calculi

1) Clinical and pathological manifestations: Renal stones, single or multiple, unilaterally or bilaterally (about 10%), are usually located in the renal pelvis and calyces. The pathologic changes of renal stones are mainly obstruction, hydrops and infection. Typical clinical manifestations are lumbodynia and hematuria, and may be accompanied by frequent micturition, urgency of urination and pain in urination if concurring urinary infection.

2) Imaging manifestations:

Plain abdominal film may show the high density shadows of circular, elliptical, staghorn or indeterminate shape in the renal region(Figure 15-3). The density of stones is either uniform or ununiform or storeyed. On the lateral view, renal stones generally overlap the spinal column; Urography, used mainly as the examination of negative stones, may demonstrate the filling defect within the renal pelvis and calyces, and can determine whether the suspicious shadow is within the kidney, and can also understand the function of the ill kidney; CT plain scanning may confirm the presence of high density calculus in the renal pelvis and calyces.

(2) Ureteric calculi

1) Clinical and pathological manifestations: Ureteric stone is commonly from the renal stone which migrates down via the ureter and is easily stagnated at three physiological narrowing points. The obstruction resulting from stone can lead to varying degrees of dialatation and hydrops of the urinary tract above the obstructed point. The patient presents typically with the lower abdominal pain that may radiate to the perineum and is simultaneously accompanied by hematuria.

2. Imaging manifestations

Both X-ray plain film and CT plain scanning can show the high density shadow of grain or soybean size along the course of the ureter[Figure 15-4(a), (b)]; Urography may define whether the compact shadow is within the ureter and may demonstrate the presence of negative calculus. Excretory urography and CT scanning can also show the dilatation and hydrops of the renal pelvis, calyces and ureters above the stone, as it is on MRU.

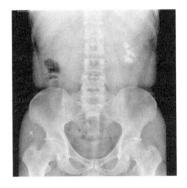 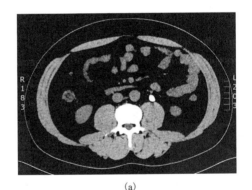 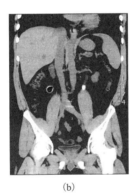

(a)　　　　　　　　(b)

Punctate high-density shadows can be seen in the upper part of the left ureter.

Figure 15-3　X-ray shows that multiple dot-like high-density shadows can be seen in the left kidney area.

Figure 15-4　Ureteric calculi

(3) Bladder stones

1) Clinical and pathological manifestations: There are two types of the bladder stones, primary and secondary.

The former form in the bladder, whereas secondary stones are from the renal stones which pass from the renal pelvis to bladder via ureters. The typical manifestations are urodynia, interruption of urine flow, frequent micturition, urgency of urination and hematuria etc.

2) Imaging manifestations: X-ray plain film, being chief modality, may show circular or elliptical compact shadow above the pubic symphysis probably with different size, smooth or crude margin, uniform or ununiform or storeyed density. The stone is characterized by that it can alter position with the change of posture; Cystography can further define the stone and may detect the negative stone; CT and MRI are generally not utilized as routine modality of examination for the bladder stone.

3. Urinary system infection

(1) Tuberculosis of the urinary system

1) Clinical and pathological manifestations: Urinary tuberculosis (TB) is generally considered to be secondary to pulmonary tuberculosis, which invades mainly into the kidneys and then extends to the ureters and bladder. Renal tuberculosis is initially infected in the cortex, and then spreads to the medulla and forms caseous ulcer at the renal papilla, and afterwards leads to the destruction of the renal pelvis and calyces. With progressive development, the lesion may extend downwards and cause the thickening and rigidity of the ureteral wall, and in turn result in the stricture, even occlusion of the ureteral lumen. The pathological changes of bladder tuberculosis include the hyperemia and edema of the bladder mucosa, the formation of irregular ulcer and(or) granuloma in the early stage, and thickening of the bladder wall and formation of a contracted bladder in the later period. The caseous lesion of renal tuberculosis can produce calcification, and even result in calcification of entire kidney called autonephretomy.

The chief clinical manifestations of urinary tuberculosis are frequent micturition, pain in urination, pyuria and hematuria, and may accompany general symptoms such as emaciation, hypodynamia and low fever etc.

2) Imaging manifestations:

① X-ray findings: The plain film of the abdomen has often not abnormal finding, and sometimes could demonstrate the cloudy or ringlike calcified shadows in the renal region, even entire renal calcification. In the early stage of disease, the urography may show the irregularity of minor calyceal margins described as "moth-eaten". When the ulcerocavernous lesion is connected with the renal calyces, the bolus contrast medium in the parenchyma can be seen to link with the involved calyces which may be of the deformation and stricture. With advancement of the disease, when resulting in the vast destruction of the renal pelvis and calyces or forming pyonephrosis, the excretory urography is often no visible. The retrograde urography may demonstrate the dilated renal pelvis and calyces forming a irregular cavity. Ureteral tuberculosis may make the ureteral edges irregular, appearing irregular stricture and dilatation like "a string of beads", and finally leading to the ureteral rigidity, shortening, even occlusion in the later stage. Tuberculosis of the bladder may has not obvious changes or only has irregular edge seen in the early stage, but appears as a contracted bladder and has volumn reduced in the later stage. Cystography presents with a typical small bladder, and sometimes may demonstrate "vesicoureteral reflux sign".

② CT findings: In the early stage of renal TB, CT scanning may show the low density lesion within the parenchyma with irregular margins. In progressive disease, the renal pelvis and calyces are demonstrate with dilatation and present with irregular multilocular deformation having CT number approximate to water. In the later stage, the kidney may appear the atrophy and distortion, and the renal cortex become thin. CT can also show multiple dot or irregular high density calcified shadows, even entire renal calcification (Figure 15-5). Ureteral TB may present with the thickening of ureteral wall, irregular stricture and dilatation of ureteral lumen. Bladder TB may appear as the thickening of bladder wall, the irregulation of bladder margin and the reduction of bladder volumn.

③ MRI findings: Finding of MRI is similar to that of CT, whereas finding of MRU is nearly the same as urography.

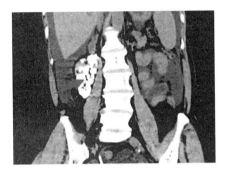

Figure 15-5　CT can show entire renal calcification

(2) Renal abscess

1) Clinical and pathological manifestations: It is mostly caused by blood borne infection, and can also be caused by retrograde urinary tract infection. The main clinical manifestations were fever, renal distension and pain, and laboratory examination shows that bacterial growth can be found in urine.

2) Imaging manifestations:

① CT findings: Early CT mainly shows low-density shadow in renal parenchyma with fuzzy boundary. In mature stage of abscess, circular low-density lesions could be seen. Circular enhancement could be seen around the lesions (abscess wall) and gas shadow could be seen in some abscesses.

② MRI findings: Taking mature renal abscess as an example, the lesions showed low signal on T1WI and high signal on T2WI. On enhanced T1WI, circular enhancement could be seen around the lesions (Figure 15-6).

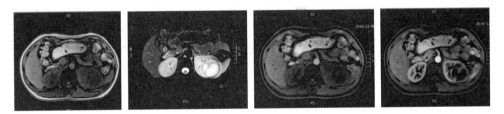

Long T1 and long T2 signal shadows can be seen in the left kidney, and the enhanced scan shows a slight ring enhancement.

Figure 15-6　MRI of renal abscess

3. Tumors of the urinary system

(1) Renal carcinoma

1) Clinical and pathological manifestations: Renal carcinoma, the commonest malignant neoplasm of the kidney, originates pathologically from the renal tubular epithelial cell, and is often located in upper and lower pole of the kidney, and presents with irregular solid mass probably followed by hemorrhage, necrosis and cystic degeneration. In the end-stage, renal carcinoma may occur direct invasion of the perinephric tissues, metastases of lymph nodes and blood stream. Typical clinical manifestations are the painless hematuria and the mass of the abdomen.

2) Imaging manifestations:

① X-ray findings: Abdominal plain film may show the enlargement of renal shadow appearing as the "lobulated-like" or local protrusion, occasionally the calcification of the neoplasm. Urography will show the extension, distortion, stenosis, even occlusion of the renal calyces because of the compression or invasion of the carcinoma, irregularity of the calyceal outline and filling defects within the calyces. If the tumor is large and involves many calyces, the aggregation and separation of the renal calyces may be shown. The compression and invasion of the carcinoma on renal pelvis may result in the compressed, distortion and destruction of the renal pelvis, or occurrence of filling defect. On renal angiographical film, renal carcinoma appears as the reticular and irregular vessels images followed by "pudding filling" of the contrast medium within the kidney. The neighbouring vessels occur separation and displacement.

②CT findings: Currently, CT is the most efficient examination of renal carcinoma. CT plain scanning presents with the elliptical or irregular mass within renal parenchyma. The larger mass may project out of the renal outline. The density of the mass is lower than that of neighbouring parenchyma or similar to it, uniform or ununiform, probably accompanied by the areas of irregular low density, and the dot or irregular calcification in a small number of cases. By contrast scanning, the tumor usually has obvious uneven enhancement in the early stage, and then presents a relative low density duo to enhancement of the neighbouring renal parenchyma (Figure 15-7). CT can also show the relationship between renal carcinoma and perinephrium and perinephric tissues.

③MRI findings: Similar to CT, present commonly with a mingled signal mass. The low signal band is often seen in the periphery of mass lesion on T_2WI, representing the pseudocapsule of the tumor. In Gd-DTPA contrast scan, the mass is shown with a ununiform enhancement. MRI can also help to determine presence of the tumor embolus and its range within renal veins and inferior vena cava.

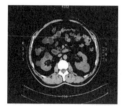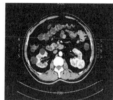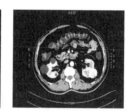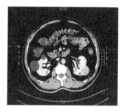

ununiform mass, accompanied by the areas of irregular low density, after contrast enhancement, renal clear cell carcinoma is more like to be manifested as "fast in and fast out".

Figure 15-7　CT findings of left renal carcinoma

3) Differential diagnosis

①Renal angiomyolipoma is characterized by the presence of fat density or signal in the tumor. However, the CT findings of renal angiomyolipoma with adipose deficiency and renal clear cell carcinoma are similar. Usually, renal clear cell carcinoma is more prone to hemorrhage and necrosis, and the density is heterogeneous. After contrast enhancement, renal clear cell carcinoma is more like to be manifested as "fast in and fast out", while renal angiomyolipoma mainly shows the enhancement of vascular structure in the tumor, and other structures are not enhanced.

②Carcinoma of the renal pelvis is mainly located in the renal pelvis, while the renal carcinoma is located in the renal parenchyma. It should be noted that it is difficult to distinguish advanced renal carcinoma from renal pelvic carcinoma in imaging, and further pathological diagnosis is needed.

(2)Renal pelvic carcinoma

1) Clinical and pathological manifestations: Renal pelvic carcinoma, also known as papillary carcinoma, is mostly transitional carcinoma pathologically and often grows like papillary. The tumor forms in the renal pelvis and calyces, and may have implantation into the ureter and the bladder. Clinical manifestation is mainly painless

hematuria involving entire urine.

2）Imaging manifestations：

① X-ray findings：Plain film of the abdomen is generally normal. Urography may show persistent irregular filling defect within the renal pelvis and calyces which can be followed by varying degrees of enlargement. Tumor invasion into the renal parenchyma may cause the distortion and displacement of the renal calyces. Tumor implantation into the ureter may result in intraureteric small filling defect and incomplete obstruction of the ureter. Renal angiography is of little usefulness, as the tumor is typically avascular.

② CT findings：CT scanning appears as the mass in the renal sinus that its CT number is higher than that of the urine and lower than that of the renal parenchyma. In contrast-enhanced scan, mild to moderate homogeneous or heterogeneous enhancement, and decreased enhancement in excretory phase (Figure 15-8). The fat within renal sinus appears to be compressed, thinned or disappeared.

③ MRI findings：Similar to those of CT. Signal intensity of the mass is higher than that of the urine on T1WI, but lower than it on T2WI

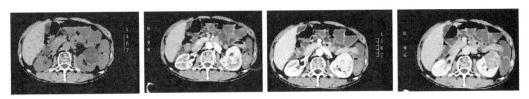

Left renal pelvic carcinoma CT contrast scanning appears as the mass in the renal sinus that its CT number is higher than that of the urine and lower than that of the renal parenchyma, In contrast-enhanced scan, mild to moderate heterogeneous enhancement, and decreased enhancement in excretory phase. The fat in the renal sinuses is compressed and thinned.

Figure 15-8　CT findings of pelvic carcinoma

（3）Carcinoma of bladder

1）Clinical and pathological manifestations：The vast majority of bladder cancer, single or multiple, is the papillary carcinoma arising from the epithelium and growing like papillary, and occur most commonly in the trigonal region and both lateral wall of the bladder. The tumor grows up from the bladder wall projecting into the lumen, and may also invade the bladder muscle, and may further spread to peripheric tissues and organs. Some of the tumors may lead to the regional thickening of the bladder wall duo to infiltrative growth of the tumor. The chief symptom of bladder carcinoma is painless gross hematuria, probably followed by frequent micturition, urgency of urination, pain in urination and dysuria.

2）Imaging manifestations：

① X-ray findings：Cystography presents with the nodular or cauliflower-like filling defect projecting from the bladder wall into the lumen, varying in size, commonly with broad base. The tumor invading deep muscle may result in the rigidity and a fixed shape of regional bladder wall.

② CT findings：CT scanning shows a soft-tissue density mass projecting from the bladder wall into the lumen and the irregular thickening of regional bladder wall. In an early stage of contrast scan, the mass usually occurs uniform enhancement [Figure 15-9(a), (b)]. However, in the delay contrast scan, the mass appears as a low density filling defect duo to the filling of contrast medium in the bladder.

③ MRI findings：Similar to CT. CT and MRI are also able to detect the invasion of perivesical tissues and organs, and metastases of lymph nodes.

（4）Renal angioleiomyolipoma

1）Clinical and pathological manifestations：Angioleiomyolipoma is a common benign tumor of the kidney.

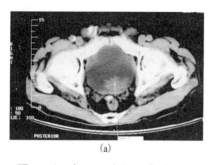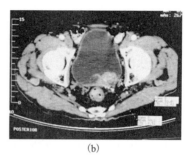

(a)   (b)

CT scanning shows a soft-tissue density mass projecting from the bladder wall into the lumen and the irregular thickening of regional bladder wall, the mass usually occurs uniform enhancement(A: precontrast; B: In an early stage of contrast scan).

Figure 15-9   CT findings of bladder cancer

Being a benign renal hamartoma mass without capsule, it is histologically composed of angiomatous, smooth-muscle and adipose elements. The tumor is usually solitary, variably sized from a few mm to 20 cm. A small number of patients (about 20%) may concur tuberous sclerosis. Clinically, the tumor tends to grow slowly, and probably presents without symptoms, or occurs abdominal pain duo to concurring hemorrhage.

2) Imaging manifestations:

① X-ray findings: On the plain film and urography, the larger mass may result in the renal outline changed, and compression, displacement and distortion of the renal pelvis and calyces. Renal arteriography may show the abundant tortuous tumor vessels.

② CT findings: Typical presentation of CT is a sharply demarcated mingled density mass in the renal parenchyma with clear and definite fat element. On contrast scanning, the areas of fat low density within mass are not enhanced, whereas the areas of soft-tissue density, representing vessels and smooth-muscle tissue, are vastly enhanced.

③ MRI findings: Similar to that of CT. Both T1WI and T2WI show the mingled signal mass with high or middle signal fat focuses within the tumor. By using T1WI with a fat inhibition technique, the signal intensity of fat focuses is obviously reduced.

4. Cystic lesions of the kidney

(1) Simple renal cyst

1) Clinical and pathological manifestations: Simple renal cyst, extremely common, is a cystic lesion having a thin outer wall and being full of fluids. This disease is commonly located in the cortex, single or multiple, circular or elliptic, varying in size. Generally, there are not any clinical symptoms, but the larger cyst may manifest with uncomfortable feeling of the abdomen or palpating abdominal mass.

2) Imaging manifestations:

① X-ray findings: Plain abdominal film may show distortion of the renal outline in the larger renal cyst, and occasionally arcline calcification of the cystic wall. On urography film, the renal pelvis and calyces may be compressed, displaced and distorted, but no destroyed.

② CT and MRI findings: CT and MRI show a sharply demarcated circular or elliptic mass lesion with water density or signal intensity that does not enhance with contrast scanning (Figure 15-10).

(2) Polycystic renal disease

1) Clinical and pathological manifestations: Polycystic kidney is an inherited disease and the most common in

adult. An important feature of this disease is the presence of bilateral, multiple, variably sized cysts containing water-like fluids in it, often concurring polycystic liver disease. Clinically, symptomatic presentation is usually after the mid-ages, manifesting with abdominal mass, hypertension and hematuria, or occurring renal failure in the end-stage.

2）Imaging manifestations:

① X-ray findings: Plain abdominal film may show enlargement of bilateral renal outline appearing as "lobulated". Urography may display compression, distortion, displacement, extension and separation of bilateral renal pelvis and calyces, presenting a change as "arachnodactyly-like".

② Ct and MRI findings: CT and MRI may detect bilateral distributed, multiple, variably sized, circular or elliptic mass lesions with water density or signal intensity that do not enhance with contrast scanning. Acute hemorrhagic density or signal can be seen in some of the cysts. Renal volumn presents with enlargement and disformation, and the renal marginal outline presents as "lobulated-like" （Figure 15-11）. Polycystic liver is often found simultaneously.

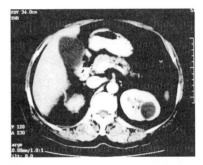

a sharply demarcated circular mass lesion with water density that does not enhance with contrast scanning.

Figure 15-10　CT findings of simple left renal cyst

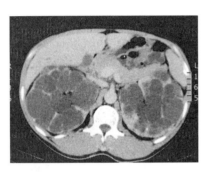

CT shows bilateral distributed, multiple variably sized, circular or elliptic mass lesions with water density or signal intensity that do not enhance with contrast scanning.

Figure 15-11　CT findings of polycystic kidney

3）Differential diagnosis

It is mainly differentiated from multiple simple renal cysts. Typical polycystic kidney is characterized by bilateral renal contour enlargement, renal pelvis and calices can be distorted, often accompanied by polycystic liver；The latter shows multiple cystic lesions without enhancement, but the renal enlargement is not obvious, and there is no positive family history.

5. Congenital abnormalities of the urinary system

（1）Clinical and pathological manifestations: The embryonic development of urinary system is a very complex course including the junction of renal convoluted tubules and renal collecting system, the rotation in the renal axis and ascending of the kidneys from pelvic cavity to lumbar part etc. Therefore, congenital abnormalities of urinary system are very common and exist a number of types including the abnormalities of number, structure, position and the others. Clinically, the patient is of no any symptoms, or appears manifestations of the complication about obstruction and infection etc.

（2）Imaging manifestations:

1）Duplication of renal pelvis and ureters （double pelvis and double ureters）

Namely, unilateral or bilateral kidney is divided into upper and lower two parts which have separately a set of the renal pelvis and ureter. Double ureters either converge each other or drain separately into the bladder. Urography may clearly demonstrate this malformation. CT and MRI, particularly contrast scanning, may further determine the diagnosis (Figure 15-12).

2) Ectopic kidney

Ectopic kidney results from the abnormality of ascending course of the kidney in the fetal stage and is mostly located in the pelvic cavity. A small number of ectopic kidney may be located in subdiaphragmatic region, iliac fossa, even thoracic cavity. Plain film can not show the shadow of normal kidney in renal region of ectopic side. All of urography, CT and MRI contrast scanning can detect the abnormality of renal position.

3) Solitary kidney

That is, one of two kidneys has been not developed (absence of unilateral kidney). Plain film can not show renal shadow of absent side, whereas the contralateral renal shadow is relatively hypertrophied. Urography, with CT and MRI examination, can confirm the diagnosis. Abdominal aorta angiography can confirm that there is not renal artery in the absent side.

4) Horseshoe kidney

That one pole (mostly the lower pole) of two kidneys is joined each other, like horseshoe, is known as horseshoe kidney. Urography may show the low-lying and malrotated kidneys. The lower poles of two kidneys are mixed together, whereas the upper poles are distal to vertebral column. The renal pelves and calyces are commonly shown with enlargement. Both CT and MRI may confirm that the renal parenchymas of two renal lower poles are merged in front of vertebral column (Figure 15-13).

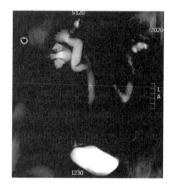

Figure 15-12 MRU shows double renal pelvis on the right side

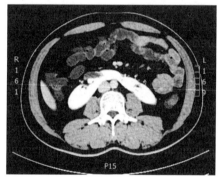

CT confirms that the renal parenchymas of two renal lower poles are merged in front of vertebral column.

Figure 15-13   CT findings of horseshoe kidney

6. Urinary system trauma

(1) Renal contusion

1) Clinical and pathological manifestations: According to the location of hemorrhage and the degree of injury, it can be divided into subcapsular hematoma, perirenal hematoma, renal contusion and renal laceration. The main clinical manifestations were lumbago and hematuria on the affected side. Shock may occur in severe cases.

2) Imaging manifestations:

Renal subcapsular hematoma mainly showed crescent shaped high-density shadow under the renal capsule on the affected side, while the perirenal hematoma generally had a wide range, but was limited to the renal fascial sac, showing high-density shadow around the kidney. According to the amount of bleeding, urine overflow and the degree of residual renal parenchyma edema, renal contusion can be manifested as high density, mixed density or low density shadow in renal parenchyma, but the renal capsule and renal parenchyma are continuous. Renal laceration showed continuous interruption of renal parenchyma with high density of blood and low density of urine (Figure 15-14a, b).

All of the above are imaging findings after acute renal contusion. With the time passed by, the hematoma can be slowly absorbed, liquefied and presented low density.

MRI: The morphology of hematoma was similar to that of CT, but the signal intensity on T1WI and T2WI varied with the age of hematoma.

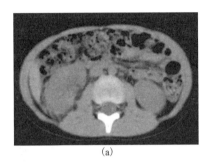 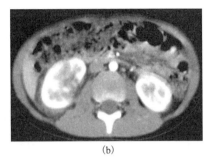

(a)   (b)

The renal cortex of the lower pole of the right kidney is discontinuous, and a patchy slightly higher density shadow can be seen around the kidney.

Figure 15-14　Renal contusion CT

7. Renal infarction

(1) Clinical and pathological manifestations: Acute renal infarction refers to the thrombosis and embolism of the main renal artery and branches, leading to stenosis or occlusion of the arterial lumen, resulting in renal or local renal tissue necrosis, thereby affecting renal function. The clinical manifestations of acute renal infarction are lack of specificity, and most patients have a "triad": persistent abdominal pain, elevated serum lactate dehydrogenase, and proteinuria.

(2) Imaging manifestations:

CT direct signs of acute renal infarction are as follows: 1) The kidney is cuneate or fan-shaped with low density without enhancement or mild enhancement in the delayed phase, clearly demarcated from surrounding normal tissue, with the tip pointing to the hilum and the bottom on the surface of the kidney. 2) The manifestation of extensive infarction is that there is no renal enhancement in a large area, or even in the whole kidney. There are some cable shadows in the renal pelvis, and no contrast agent filling in the renal pelvis at all stages of enhancement.

CT indirect signs of acute renal infarction are as follows: 1) The density of perirenal fat space increased, showing patchy ground glass like density shadow. 2) Perirenal space has effusion, and the distribution of effusion is not uniform. 3) Perirenal fascia thickened.

Renal arteriography is the gold standard, but it is an invasive examination. Now, CTA has replaced renal arteriography in the observation of renal artery lesions in acute renal infarction, and has a good effect on renal artery occlusion, filling defect and renal aneurysm.

MRI can show renal infarction without injection of contrast agent, but it is often not used in emergency patients due to the long examination time.

(Chen Xiangyu, Chai Tian, Li Ya, Liu Meitao, Xiao Enhua, Liu Hui)

第十六章

肾上腺

第一节　检查方法

1. CT 检查

（1）平扫：无需特殊准备，宜选用快速、高分辨率 CT 机。常规取仰卧位横断层面扫描，采用 4~5 mm 薄层并靶扫描技术，扫描范围自膈顶开始扫描至肾门平面。

（2）增强：常规方法是用非离子型碘对比剂 60~100 mL 快速静脉注射后立即扫描。多数肾上腺病变尤其是肿块性病变需行 CT 增强检查。

2. MRI 检查

（1）平扫：肾上腺 MRI 检查宜使用中、高场强 MR 成像系统。常规行 SE 序列横断面扫描，扫描层厚为 3~5 mm，必要时再辅以冠状位或矢状位扫描。应用 T1WI 或 T2WI 并脂肪抑制技术有助于含脂肪性病变的诊断，应用梯度回波序列的同相位和反相位成像技术，可帮助确定在细胞水平同时含水与脂质的病变，有利于肾上腺腺瘤的鉴别诊断。

（2）增强：方法是向静脉内快速注入顺磁性对比剂 Gd-DTPA 后即行 T1WI 并脂肪抑制技术检查，多数肾上腺肿块性病变需行 MRI 增强扫描。

第二节　正常表现

1. CT 表现

肾上腺位于两肾上极上方，与肾同包于肾筋膜囊内。平扫检查，在周围低密度脂肪组织对比下，正常肾上腺能够清晰显示，为软组织密度影，边缘光滑，无外突结节，CT 值为 30~50 Hu。其形态因人而异，在 CT 不同层面上也各有不同，右侧肾上腺常呈斜线形、倒"V"形或倒"Y"形，左侧者多为倒"V"形、箭头形或三角形。通常用侧支厚度和面积来估计肾上腺大小，正常侧支厚度小于 10 mm，面积小于 150 mm^2。增强检查：正常肾上腺呈均一强化，一般不能分辨皮、髓质。

2. MRI 表现

平扫检查，在横断层面上，正常肾上腺的表现与 CT 类似，其信号强度因检查序列而异，常规 T1WI 和 T2WI 影像上，信号强度类似正常肝实质，且明显低于周围脂肪信号；T1WI 或 T2WI 并脂肪抑制技术，信号强度明显高于周围被抑制的脂肪组织，呈相对高信号。注射 Gd-DTPA 增强检查，正常肾上腺发生强化。

第三节　基本病变

1. CT 表现

常见异常表现为肾上腺肿块,其大小、形态和密度与其组织类型相关。水样密度类圆形肿块见于含液的肾上腺囊肿,也可见于脂类丰富的肾上腺腺瘤;均一软组织密度肿块并有不同程度均一强化,常见于肾上腺腺瘤、嗜铬细胞瘤或转移瘤;密度不均且内有脂肪性低密度灶的肿块是肾上腺髓脂瘤的特征表现;较大软组织密度肿块伴有坏死、囊变所致的低密度灶,并呈不均一强化,可见于嗜铬细胞瘤、肾上腺皮质癌或神经母细胞瘤等。

双侧肾上腺弥漫性增大,而密度和形态仍维持正常,为肾上腺增生表现。双侧肾上腺变小代表肾上腺萎缩,常见于垂体功能低下或特发性肾上腺萎缩,也可见于 Cushing 腺瘤。

2. MRI 表现

主要异常表现为肾上腺肿块,其大小、形态、信号强度及增强表现与病变组织类型有关。长 T1 和长 T2 且无强化的类圆形肿块多为肾上腺囊肿;T1WI 和 T2WI 上均与肝实质信号类似的类圆形肿块,可见于肾上腺腺瘤和肾上腺转移瘤,前者在梯度回波反相位像上信号强度明显下降,具有特征;不均质肿块,内含可为脂肪抑制技术所抑制的高信号灶,是肾上腺髓脂瘤的特征表现;较大类圆形或分叶状肿块,信号不均,内有水样或出血信号灶,并呈不均一强化,可见于嗜铬细胞瘤、肾上腺皮质癌或神经母细胞瘤。

3. 比较影像学

对于肾上腺疾病的影像学检查,常规 X 线检查如腹部 X 线平片、尿路造影、腹膜后充气造影等基本上无价值,除 X 线平片可显示肾上腺病变的异常钙化外(多为其他原因行 X 线平片检查时意外发现),这些常规方法已极少使用或已废弃,而目前公认 CT 是肾上腺疾病最有效的和首选的检查方法,MRI 多作为 CT 检查之后的补充手段。

CT 检查肾上腺病变的优点是:解剖关系明确,密度分辨力高,易于发现小至几毫米的病变,可确定病变的侧别、数目、大小和范围,且肾上腺病变的 CT 表现可能反映出病变的一些组织特征,因此有助于确定病变的性质。在观察和分析肾上腺病变的 CT 影像时,应熟悉正常肾上腺及其相邻解剖结构的 CT 表现,了解肾上腺病变的分类和基本病变的 CT 表现,在此基础上,注意观察肾上腺病变的大小、形态、密度及增强后的表现等。根据不同类型病变的 CT 表现,再密切结合临床症状、体征和实验室检查资料,多数肾上腺病变都能够作出准确诊断,因此临床上疑为肾上腺的病变均应行 CT 检查。

应当指出,CT 检查肾上腺病变也有一定的限度。对肾上腺区较大肿块,有时难以判断肿块的起源;也并非所有肾上腺疾病 CT 检查均有异常发现,如约有 50% 肾上腺皮质增生,虽有功能异常,但肾上腺形态和大小可无明显变化,在 CT 上可表现正常;此外,CT 对肾上腺的某些非功能性肿瘤与肾上腺转移瘤难以鉴别,诊断在很大程度上依赖于临床资料。

对于肾上腺疾病的检查,MRI 常作为 CT 检查的补充手段,其优点是:可多方位、多参数、多序列成像;易于确定肾上腺区较大肿块的起源;组织分辨力高,能较为准确地显示肿块并反映病变的组织特征,从而有利于病变的定性诊断;利用梯度回波正、反相位检查,能较为可靠地鉴别富含脂类的肾上腺腺瘤与不含脂类的肾上腺转移瘤。在肾上腺病变的 MRI 影像观察和分析中,应注意肿块的数目、大小、侧别、形态和不同序列的信号强度及增强表现,以确定肿块的起源,推断肿块的可能性质,结合临床表现和实验室检查结果,大多数肾上腺肿块可作出明确诊断。MRI 的不足是不易发现肾上腺小肿块（<1 cm）,也不能可靠地显示肾上腺增生和肾上腺萎缩。

第四节　常见疾病诊断

肾上腺组织结构复杂,能产生多种激素,肾上腺的病变依其对肾上腺功能的影响与否分为三种类型,即肾上腺功能亢进性病变，肾上腺功能低下性病变和肾上腺非功能性病变。

1. 肾上腺功能亢进性病变

（1）Cushing 综合征：

1）临床与病理表现：Cushing 综合征依病因可分为垂体性、异位性和肾上腺性。垂体性和异位性占全部 Cushing 综合征的 70%～85%，是由于垂体肿瘤、增生或异位肿瘤分泌过多促肾上腺皮质激素（ACTH），导致双侧肾上腺增生，腺体弥漫性增大；肾上腺性 Cushing 综合征占 15%～30%，是因肾上腺腺瘤（Cushing 腺瘤）或皮质癌自主分泌皮质醇所致，由于血中皮质醇增高，从而反馈性抑制垂体 ACTH 的分泌，造成非肿瘤部位肾上腺萎缩。

临床上 Cushing 综合征最常发生在中年女性，典型表现为向心性肥胖、满月脸、皮肤紫纹、痤疮、骨质疏松、高血压和月经不规则等。

2）影像学表现：

①肾上腺增生：目前，对于肾上腺增生主要依靠 CT 和 MRI 做出形态上的诊断，表现为双侧肾上腺弥漫性增大，侧支增粗、变长，但肾上腺的形态和密度保持不变，明显增大时，边缘可有一些小的结节。应该指出，有些肾上腺增生虽有功能异常，但形态和大小可无明显变化，与正常肾上腺不能区分。

②Cushing 腺瘤：CT 表现为单侧肾上腺圆形或卵圆形肿块，边缘光滑，密度低而不均匀，增强检查，肿块呈轻至中度强化，同侧肾上腺非病变处和对侧肾上腺萎缩。MRI 检查，肿块信号强度类似或略高于肝实质，因腺瘤细胞内富含脂质，故在梯度回波反相位上信号强度明显下降。

③肾上腺皮质癌：约半数肾上腺皮质癌伴有内分泌功能异常，其中又以 Cushing 综合症最多见。功能性和非功能性肾上腺皮质癌在 CT 上具有相似的表现，一般瘤体较大，直径可达 7～20 cm，呈卵圆、分叶或不规则形肿块，瘤内可有广泛出血、坏死或钙化致使肿块密度或信号不均。CT 和 MRI 增强检查可显示肿块呈不规则强化，还可显示肿瘤侵犯下腔静脉造成的瘤栓及淋巴结、肝、肾等处的转移灶。MRI 冠、矢状面检查有助于确定肿块来自肾上腺。

（2）Conn 综合征：

1）临床与病理表现：Conn 综合征即原发醛固酮增多症，是由于肾上腺皮质病变所致，其中 65%～95% 为肾上腺腺瘤（Conn 腺瘤），5%～35% 为肾上腺皮质增生。临床上以女性为多见，易发年龄为 20～40 岁，由于过量的醛固酮分泌造成水、钠潴留和血容量增加，表现为高血压、肌无力和夜尿增多。

2）影像学表现：

①CT 表现：CT 为主要检查方法，多表现为单侧肾上腺孤立性小肿块，瘤体一般较小，直径多在 2 cm 以下，呈圆形或椭圆形，边缘光滑，密度均匀，肿块与肾上腺侧支相连或位于两侧支之间，由于富含脂质，常近于水样密度，增强检查有轻度强化。

②MRI 表现：MRI 亦表现为肾上腺小肿块，信号强度类似或略高于肝实质，增强检查肿块发生强化。

（3）嗜铬细胞瘤：

1）临床与病理表现：肾上腺嗜铬细胞瘤是发生在肾上腺髓质、具有内分泌功能的一种少见的肿瘤，约占全身嗜铬细胞瘤的 90%。嗜铬细胞瘤也常称作"10% 肿瘤"，即 10% 为多发，10% 为恶性，10% 为双侧，10% 在肾上腺之外。肿瘤常较大，有完整包膜，易发生出血、坏死和囊变。临床上以 20～40 岁为多见，常有家族史。肿瘤能自主分泌儿茶酚胺，典型临床表现为阵发性高血压，伴有头痛、心悸、出汗等症状，发作数分钟后缓解，血和尿中儿茶酚胺升高。

2）影像学表现：

①CT 表现：为一侧肾上腺圆形或椭圆形肿块，瘤体较大，直径多在 3 cm 以上，边缘一般清楚，因肿瘤内常有陈旧性出血、坏死和囊变而致其密度不均，少数可有钙化。增强检查，肿瘤实体部分发生明显强化，而其内低密度区无强化（图 16-1）。

②MRI 表现：肿瘤在 T1WI 上信号强度类似软组织，而 T2WI 上呈明显高信号，有坏死或出血时，瘤内可有短 T1 或更长 T1、长 T2 信号灶。增强检查，肿瘤实体部分明显强化。

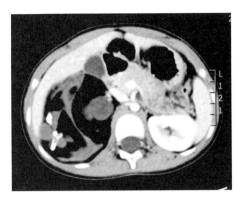

CT 显示右侧肾上腺区单发肿块,肿块直径大于 3 cm,边界清晰,含脂肪密度,伴钙化。

图 16-1　嗜铬细胞瘤 CT 表现

2. 肾上腺功能低下性病变

主要为慢性肾上腺皮质功能低下病变,即阿狄森(Addison)病,肾上腺结核为其主要原因之一。

(1)临床与病理表现:肾上腺结核是由于结核菌血行播散所致,常为双侧性,大多与体内其他部分的结核并存。病理上,肾上腺皮、髓质均遭破坏,形成干酪样坏死和肉芽肿病变,晚期可导致肾上腺萎缩并可发生钙化。临床上多有较长病史,主要症状有疲劳乏力,色素沉着和血压下降等。

(2)影像学表现:肾上腺结核的影像学表现与病期相关。在干酪化期,表现双侧肾上腺扩大,形成不规则肿块,CT 显示其密度不均,内有多发低密度区,代表干酪坏死灶,增强检查呈不均一强化;MRI 检查肿块呈混杂信号,T1WI 和 T2WI 像主要为低信号,其内可有长 T1 和长 T2 信号灶。晚期,双侧肾上腺萎缩,出现弥漫性钙化。X 线平片可显示双侧肾上腺区钙化影;在 CT 和 MRI 影像上,钙化灶分别呈高密度影和极低信号影,以 CT 检查最佳。

3. 肾上腺非功能性病变

肾上腺非功能性此类病变不影响肾上腺皮、髓质功能,类型较多,较常见的有肾上腺非功能性腺瘤和肾上腺转移瘤,其次为肾上腺囊肿、肾上腺髓脂瘤等。

(1)肾上腺非功能性腺瘤:

1)临床与病理表现:病理上,肾上腺非功能性腺瘤有完整包膜,细胞分化良好。临床上多无症状,亦无相关生化指标异常,多数为偶然发现。

2)影像学表现:CT 和 MRI 表现与功能性肾上腺腺瘤相似,无特异性。肿块多在 5 cm 以下,且同侧和对侧肾上腺无萎缩性改变,只能结合临床生化诊断。

(2)肾上腺转移瘤:

1)临床与病理表现:临床上较为常见,常见的原发部位是乳腺、肺、肾、胃和黑色素瘤。转移灶大多先停留在肾上腺髓质,形成早期的转移结节,而后再累及整个肾上腺。较大肿瘤内有坏死和出血。临床上主要为原发瘤的表现。

2)影像学表现:肾上腺转移瘤表现为双侧或单侧,多发或单发肾上腺肿块,呈圆形、椭圆形或分叶形,密度和信号可均一或不均一,大的肿瘤内可有坏死性低密度区。CT 和 MRI 增强检查,肿块呈均一或不均一强化。总之,肾上腺转移瘤的影像学表现无特异性,诊断在很大程度上依赖于临床资料。

4. 鉴别诊断

(1)Cushing 腺瘤:单侧肿块,直径 2~3 cm,密度类似肾实质,增强扫描快速强化和迅速廓清,同侧及对侧肾上腺变小。

(2)Conn 腺瘤:单侧孤立小肿块,直径<2 cm,富含脂质,似水样密度,快速强化和迅速廓清,同侧肾上腺无萎缩表现。

(3)肾上腺转移瘤:临床病史,双侧或单侧肿块,肿块均一强化。

Chapter 16

Adrenal gland

Section 1 Method of examination

1. CT examination

(1) Plain scan: No special preparation is needed, but it would be the best to make use of the rapid, high resolution CT instrument for CT scanning of adrenal glands. The patient is placed in supine position on the examinational table and the scanning is conventionally performed in body cross-section, with 4 to 5 mm thin slice and target scan technique. Range of scanning is from the diaphragmatic top to the level of renal hilum.

(2) Contrast scan: The conventional method is that the non-ionic iodine contrast agent 60-100 ml is rapidly injected intravenously, and the same scanning as plain scan is immediately performed. A majority of adrenal lesions, particularly mass lesions are required to administer CT contrast scan.

2. MRI examination

(1) Plain scan: The strong MR imaging system with middle, high magnetic fields is better for MRI examination of adrenal glands. MRI scanning is conventionally performed in cross-sectional (axial) plane with SE sequences, with 3 to 5 mm slice thickness. If necessary, coronal and (or) sagittal scanning may also be added. Using T1WI or T2WI with a fat inhibition technique will help to diagnose the lesions containing fat. Using gradient echo sequences "in-phase" and "out-of-phase" techniques may help to determine the lesions containing both water and lipoid in the cellular level. It is useful for differential diagnosis of adrenal adenoma.

(2) Contrast scan: After paramagnetic contrast medium Gd-DTPA is rapidly injected intravenously, T1WI scanning with a fat saturation technique is immediately performed. A majority of adrenal mass lesions are required to administer MRI contrast scan.

Section 2 Normal appearances

1. CT findings

The adrenal glands are located above the upper pole of each kidney and enclosed the same renal fascia capsule as the kidney. By plain scan, the normal adrenal glands may be clearly shown with the soft-tissue density shadows under contrast to the peripheral low-density fat tissue, with smooth margins, without node projecting laterally, with a CT number 30 to 50 Hu. Their shapes exist a great deal of variation according to different person and different CT level. The right adrenal gland appears commonly as the "oblique-line", inverted "V" or inverted "Y", the left is often the inverted "V", "arrowhead" or "triangular". The thickness and area of the collateral are usually used to estimate the size of adrenal gland. Normally, thickness of the collateral is less than 10 mm, the area is less than 150 mm^2. With contrast scan, the normal adrenal glands are uniformly enhanced. Generally, the cortex and the medulla can not be distinguished.

2. MRI findings

On plain scan in cross-sectional plane, the findings of normal adrenal glands are similar to that of CT. Their signal intensity in MRI depends on a variety of examinational sequences: On routine T1WI and T2WI images, the signal intensity is similar to normal hepatic parenchyma and obviously lower than the peripherical fat-tissue; On T1WI or T2WI with a fat inhibition technique, the signal intensity is obviously higher than the peripheral inhibited fat-tissue and presents with a relative high signal characteristic. By Gd-DTPA contrast scan, normal renal glands are enhanced.

Section 3　Basic pathologic changes

1. CT findings

Adrenal masses are common, and their size, shape and density are related to their histological types. The elliptic mass with water density may be seen in adrenal cyst containing fluid, also in adrenal adenoma with abundant lipoid; The uniform soft-tissue density mass followed by varying degrees of uniform enhancement is often found in adrenal adenoma, pheochromocytoma or metastatic tumor; Adrenal myololipoma is characterized as the mass with ununiform density and low-density fat focuses in it; Pheochromocytoma, adrenocortical carcinoma or neuroblastoma may present with the larger soft-tissue density mass, followed by the low density focuses caused by necrosis and cystic degeneration, appearing ununiform enhancement.

The diffuse enlargement of bilateral adrenal glands but maintaining normal density and shape are the findings of adrenal hyperplasia. The reduction of bilateral adrenal glands, representing adrenal atrophy, is often seen in pituitary hypofunction or idiopathic atrophy of adrenal glands, also found in Cushing adenoma.

2. MRI findings

Main abnormal finding is the adrenal mass. The size, shape, signal intensity and enhanced presentation of the mass are related to the histological type of the lesion. The elliptic mass with long T_1 and long T_2 signal and without enhancement is often the finding of adrenal cyst; The elliptic mass with the similar signal to hepatic parenchyma on both T_1WI and T_2WI images may be seen in adrenal adenoma and adrenal metastatic tumor. The former is characterized by an obvious decline of signal intensity on gradient echo sequences "out-of-phase" images; The peculiar finding of adrenal myelolipoma is the ununiform mass containing the high signal focus which can be inhibited by a fat inhibition technique; Pheochromocytoma, adrenocortical carcinoma or neuroblastoma may present with the larger ununiform signal mass, elliptic or lobulated, followed by the water or hemorrhagic signal focus in it, and appearing ununiform enhancement.

3. Comparative imaging

For imaging examination of adrenal diseases, conventional X-ray modalities such as abdominal plain film, urography and retroperitoneal gas contrast are basically of no value except that X-ray plain film may show abnormal calcifications of adrenal diseases (that a large number are occasionally found by X-ray plain film performing duo to other reasons), therefore these conventional modalities have been rarely used or disused at all. Currently, CT has been recognized to be the most efficient, firstly considered examination of adrenal diseases, whereas MRI is often a supplementary means after CT examination.

The advantages of CT for examination of adrenal diseases are that CT may show clear anatomical relation and has high density resolution, and easily detect small up to a few mm lesion, and may determine the side, number, size and range of lesions. The CT findings of adrenal diseases may also point out some histological features of the lesion, so this may help to determine the quality of the lesion. In observing and analysising the images of adrenal diseases offered by CT, one should know CT findings of normal adrenal glands and adjacent anatomical structure, understanding the classification of adrenal diseases and CT findings of elementary pathology, and on the basis of these, carefully observing the size, shape, density of adrenal lesion and the finding after enhancement and so on. A majority of adrenal diseases can be accurately diagnosed according to the CT findings of different types of lesions and further by combining with clinical symptoms, signs and experimental examination. Therefore, CT scanning should be performed for patient who is clinically suspected of adrenal diseases.

It should be indicated that there also is certain limitation for CT examination of adrenal diseases. For example, sometimes it is difficult to identify the origin of larger mass in adrenal regions; No all adrenaldiseases have abnormal findings in CT examination. For example, although about 50% of adrenocortical hyperplasia have functional abnormality, there are not obvious changes of adrenal shape and size in CT which is normal; In addition, CT difficultly distinguishes some nonfunctioning adrenal tumors from adrenal metastasis, thus the diagnosis depends on the clinical materials in great degree.

MRI is often a supplementary means after CT examination. The advantages of MRI for examination of adrenal diseases are that MRI may be imaged in multiple planes, multiple parameters and multiple sequences, and easily determine the origin of larger mass in adrenal regions, and has high soft-tissue resolution, and can more accurately demonstrate the mass and reflect histological feature of the lesion, thus helping the qualitative diagnosis of the lesion; Using gradient echo sequences "in-phase" and "out-of-phase" techniques can reliably differentiate adrenal adenoma containing abundant lipoid from adrenal metastasis without lipoid.

In observation and analysis of MRI images of adrenal diseases, one should carefully observe the number, size, side and shape of the mass, and signal intensity of different sequences and finding of enhancement to determine the origin of mass and infer the possible quality of mass. A majority of adrenal masses can be accurately diagnosed by combining with clinical manifestations and experimental examination.

The disadvantages of MRI are that MRI difficultly detects adrenal small mass (less than 1 cm) and can also not reliably show adrenal hyperplasia and adrenal atrophy.

Section 4 Diagnosis of common disease

The adrenal glands have complex histostructure and can produce a great number of hormones. The lesions of adrenal glands may be classified as three types according to their influence on adrenal function, that is hyperfunctioning adrenal diseases, adrenal insufficiency diseases and nonfunctioning adrenal diseases.

1. hyperfunctioning adrenal diseases

(1) Cushing's syndrome

1) Clinical and pathological manifestations: Cushing's syndrome may be divided into pituitarigenic, ectopicgenic and adrenogenic according to the causes of disease. The pituitarigenic and ectopicgenic account for 70 % to 85 % of all Cushing's syndrome and result in bilateral adrenal hyperplasia and diffuse enlargement of the glands because of an excess production of adrenocorticotropic hormone (ACTH) in pituitary tumor, hyperplasia and ectopic tumor; Adrenogenic Cushing's syndrome, accounting for only 15 % ~ 30 %, results from adrenal adenoma (Cushing adenoma) or adrenocortical carcinoma autonomously secreting cortisol, and may result in the atrophy of nontumor parts of adrenal glands duo to increase of cortisol level in blood causing feedback inhibition of ACTH

secretion of pituitary.

Clinically, Cushing's syndrome is most commonly taken place at mid-age women. The typical manifestations are central obesity, moon face, skin striae, acne, osteoporosis, hypertension and irregular menses etc.

2) Imaginal manifestations:

①adrenal hyperplasia

At present, adrenal hyperplasia is mainly diagnosed by CT and MRI in morphology, and presents with the diffuse enlargement of bilateral adrenal glands, thickening and extension of the collateral, whereas the shape and density of adrenal glands keep fixed. When obviously enlarged, the margins of adrenal glands may appear some small tubercles. It should be indicated that some of adrenal hyperplasias have not obvious change in shape and size, although they have the abnormality of function, so they can not be distinguished from normal adrenal glands.

② Cushing's adenoma

CT presents with the circular or elliptic mass of unilateral adrenal gland, with smooth margin and ununiform low density. By contrast scan, the mass appears as the light to middle enhancement. The adrenal areas of involved side beyond the lesion and contralateral adrenal gland appear the atrophy. In MRI examination, the signal intensity of the mass is similar to or slightly higher than hepatic parenchyma. On gradient echo sequences "out-of-phase" images, the signal intensity of the mass is obviously depressed because the adenoma cells contain abundant lipoid.

③ Adrenocortical carcinoma

About 50 % of adrenocortical carcinoma are accompanied by the abnormalities of endocrine function, and Cushing's syndrome is the most common one of them. Functional and non-functional adrenocortical carcinoma have the similar findings on CT scanning. Generally, the tumor is larger, up to 7 ~ 20 cm in diameter, and presents with elliptic, lobulated, or irregular mass probably followed by the ununiforem density or signal duo to vast hemorrhage, necrosis or calcification in it. CT and MRI contrast scan may show the mass appearing irregular enhancement, and may also demonstrate the tumor embolus resulting from the tumor invading inferior vena cava and metastatic lesions of the lymph nodes, liver and kidney etc. MRI examination in coronal and sagittal planes may help to determine the mass arising from the adrenal gland.

(2) Conn's syndrome

1) Clinical and pathological manifestations: Conn's syndrome, also called as primary Aldosteronism, results from the adrenocortical lesions. 65% ~ 95% of them are adrenal adenoma (Conn adenoma), whereas 5% ~ 35% are adrenocortical hyperplasia. Clinically, Conn's syndrome is most commonly taken place at women ages 20 to 40 years and presents with hypertension, muscle weakness and increase of nocturia because the hypersecretion of Aldosterone results in retention of water and sodium, and hypervolemia.

2) Imaginal manifestations:

①CT findings: CT scan is chief modality for the disease and is commonly manifested by the solitary small mass of unilateral adrenal gland. The tumor is usually smaller, less than 2 cm in diameter, circular or elliptic, with smooth margin and uniform density. The mass is connected with the collateral of adrenal gland or located between two the collateral, and often shown with approximately water density duo to containing abundant lipoid, and slightly enhanced on contrast scan.

②MRI findings: MRI examination presents also with the adrenal small mass, the signal intensity of the mass is similar to or slightly higher than that of hepatic parenchyma, and the mass is enhanced on contrast scan.

(3) Pheochromocytoma

1) Clinical and pathological manifestations: Adrenal pheochromocytoma is a rare tumor derived from the adrenal medulla and having endocrine function, accounting for about 90% of general pheochromocytomas. Pheochromocytoma is also often called as "10% tumor" which is described as that 10% are multiple, 10% are

435

malignant, 10% are bilateral, and 10% are extraadrenal. The tumor is usually larger, with perfect capsule, and readily occurs hemorrhage, necrosis and cystic degeneration. Clinically, the disease most commonly affects person ages 20 to 40 years and often has family history. The tumor can autonomously secrete catecholamines. Typical clinical manifestation is the paroxysmal hypertension followed by the symptoms such as headache, palpitation and sweating etc, tending to remit after attacking a few minutes. The levels of catecholamines in the plasma and urine are elevated

2)Imaginal manifestations:

① CT findings: CT may demonstrate the unilateral adrenal circular or elliptic mass which is generally larger and more than 3 cm in diameter, with smooth margin. The density of mass is often ununiform duo to remote hemorrhage, necrosis and cystic degeneration within it. There may be calcification in a small number of tumors. On CT contrast scan, the solid portion of tumor is obviously enhanced, whereas the low density areas within it does not occur enhancement (Figure 16-1).

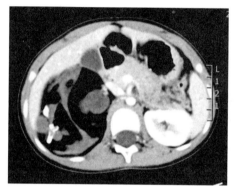

CT shows a single mass in the right adrenal region with larger than 3 cm in diameter, clear boundary, fat density and calcification.

Figure 16-1　CT findings of pheochromocytoma

②MRI findings: By MRI examination, the signal intensity of tumor is similar to that of soft-tissue on T1WI, whereas the tumor appears obvious high signal on T2WI. When occurring the necrosis or hemorrhage, there may be short T1 or longer T1, longer T2 signal focuses in the tumor. On MRI contrast scan, the solid portion of tumor is obviously enhanced.

2. Adrenal insufficiency diseases

Adrenal insufficiency diseases refer mainly to adrenocortical insufficiency diseases, that is Addison's disease. One of the primary causes is adrenal tuberculosis.

(1)Clinical and pathological manifestations: Adrenal tuberculosis results from the hematogenous spread of tubercle bacillus and is often bilateral, and commonly concurs tuberculosis of the other portions of body. Pathologically, both the adrenal cortex and medulla are destroyed, and produce caseous necrosis and granuloma lesion. In the later stage, the lesions may result in the atrophy of adrenal glands and produce the calcification. Clinically, the patient has usually the history of longer time. The chief symptoms include fatigue, hypodynamia, pigmentation and fall of blood pressure etc.

(2)Imaginal manifestations: Imaginal findings of adrenal tuberculosis are related to the phases of disease. In the caseous stage, CT may show the enlargement of bilateral glands and formation of irregular masses. The density of the mass is ununiform and followed by multiple low density areas within it, representing caseous necrosis focuses. On contrast scan, the lesions appear ununiform enhancement. By MRI examination, the mass presents with the mingled signal. On T1WI and T2WI images, the lesions are mainly low signal and followed by long T1 and long T2 signal focuses. In the later stage, bilateral adrenal glands may occur the atrophy and produce the diffuse calcification. X-ray plain film may show the shadows of calcification in bilateral adrenal regions. On CT and MRI images, the calcified focuses present separately with high density shadows and extreme low signal shadows, it is best for CT examination.

3. Nonfunctioning adrenal diseases

These diseases do not affect the functions of adrenal cortex and medulla, and have a great number of types including commonly the nonfunctioning adrenal adenoma and the adrenal metastasis, secondly the adrenal cyst and the adrenal myelolipoma.

(1) Nonfunctioning adrenal adenoma

1) Clinical and pathological manifestations: Pathologically, the nonfunctioning adrenal adenoma has the perfect capsule and good cell differentiation. Clinically, the patient has often not symptoms, and has also no related biochemical abnormalities. A vast majority of patients are found occasionally.

2) Imaginal manifestations: Findings of CT and MRI, without particularity, are similar to that of functioning adrenal adenoma. The most of masses are less than 5 cm in diameter, and collateral and contralateral adrenal glands do not occur the changes of atrophy. Diagnosis can be only based on the clinical and biochemical studies.

(2) Adrenal metastasis

1) Clinical and pathological manifestations: Adrenal metastasis is clinically common. Common sites of origin are female breast (most common), lung, kidney, stomach and melanoma. Metastatic focuses firstly stay at the adrenal medulla and form the metastatic tubercles of early stage, and then involve entire adrenal gland again. The larger tumors may occur the necrosis and hemorrhage within them. Clinically, adrenal metastasis is mainly manifested by the findings of the primary tumor.

2) Imaginal manifestations: Adrenal metastasis presents with the single or multiple, unilateral or bilateral, circular, elliptic or lobulated adrenal masses with uniform or ununiform density and signal. The larger tumor may appear the necrotic low density areas within it. On CT and MRI contrast scan, the mass appears as uniform or ununiform enhancement. In general, imaginal findings of Adrenal metastasis have no the particularity. In great degree, diagnosis depends on the clinical materials.

4. Differential diagnosis

(1) Cushing adenoma: unilateral mass, 2 ~ 3 cm in diameter, similar in density to renal parenchyma, enhanced scan for rapid enhancement and rapid clearance, ipsilateral and contralateral adrenal glands become smaller

(2) Conn adenoma: unilateral isolated small mass, diameter <2 cm, rich in lipids, water-like density, rapid enhancement and rapid clearance, no atrophy of ipsilateral adrenal glands

(3) Adrenal metastases: clinical history, bilateral or unilateral masses, uniformly enhanced masses.

(Chen Xiangyu, Chai Tian, Li Ya, Liu Meitao, Xiao Enhua, Liu Hui)

第十七章

女性生殖系统

影像学检查对女性生殖系统的疾病诊断有重要价值。女性生殖系统常见的疾病包括先天性畸形、炎症和肿瘤，影像学检查的目的是发现病变，确定其大小、范围乃至性质和分期。各种影像学检查有不同应用指征。MRI 检查对女性生殖系统先天性畸形及肿瘤分期有很高价值。由于性腺和胎儿对 X 线的辐射作用很敏感，故孕妇应慎用 X 线和 CT 检查。

第一节　检查方法

1. X 线检查

(1) X 线平片：通常摄取骨盆 X 线平片。检查前，需口服缓泻药，清洁肠道。

(2) 子宫输卵管造影：子宫输卵管造影是经子宫颈口注入对比剂以显示子宫和输卵管内腔的检查方法。对比剂为 40% 碘化油或有机碘制剂。在透视下注入对比剂，当子宫、输卵管充分充盈后，即摄片。对于输卵管显影者，还需 30 分钟后复查，以观察输卵管通畅情况。子宫输卵管造影应于月经后 5~7 天进行。以下情况禁用，即生殖器急性炎症、月经期、子宫出血和妊娠期。

(3) 盆腔动脉造影：方法是经皮穿刺行股动脉插管，将导管顶端置于腹主动脉分叉处、髂总或髂内动脉后，进行造影检查，可显示子宫动脉。如导管顶端置于肾动脉稍下方，则能显示卵巢动脉。

2. CT 检查

(1) 平扫检查：检查前一天需口服缓泻剂清洁肠管。检查前 2~3 小时，分多次口服 1% 泛影葡胺或水 1000 mL，以充盈和识别盆腔肠管。检查时，膀胱应在充盈状态下。扫描范围通常自髂峰水平至耻骨联合，层厚 5 mm 或 10 mm，连续扫描。

(2) 增强检查：常需进行，尤其是肿块性病变。方法是静脉内快速推注对比剂后，即对病变区进行扫描。对比剂为非离子型对比剂 50~100 mL。

3. MRI 检查

(1) 平扫检查：常规行 SE 序列的 T1WI 和 T2WI 检查。其中 T2WI 检查非常重要，能显示宫体宫颈、宫颈及阴道的各层解剖，并易于发现盆腔病变。通常使用相控阵线圈，检查层厚 10 mm 或 5 mm。

(2) 增强检查：平扫发现盆腔病变后，一般需行增强 MRI 检查。方法是静脉内注入顺磁性对比剂 Gd-DTPA，剂量为每千克体重 0.1 mmoL，注毕后，即对病变区行脂肪抑制前、后的 T^{1}WI 检查。

第二节　正常表现

女性内生殖器位于小骨盆内。子宫位于小骨盆中央，前邻膀胱，后方为直肠，两侧为输卵管、卵巢以及阔韧带。

1. X 线表现

（1）X 线平片：女性内生殖器呈软组织密度，与周围结构缺乏天然对比，不能显影。

（2）子宫输卵管造影：正常子宫腔呈倒置三角形，边缘光滑整齐；底边在上，为子宫底；下部与边缘呈羽毛状的长柱形宫颈管相连；子宫底两侧为子宫角，与输卵管相通。两侧输卵管自子宫角向外下走行，呈迂曲柔软的线状影。输卵管通入子宫壁内部分短而窄，为间质部，输卵管间质部外侧细而直，为峡部；远端粗大，为腹腔；输卵管末端开口于腹腔，呈漏斗状扩大，为伞端（图 17-1）。若输卵管通畅，则对比剂可进入腹腔内，呈多发弧线状或波浪状致密影，可分布于肠管之间、子宫直肠窝以及子宫膀胱窝内。

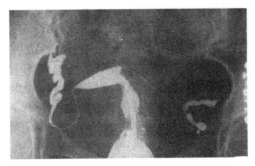

注入碘油后，宫腔显影为倒置三角形，边缘光整；宫颈管边缘呈羽毛
状；宫角两侧输卵管细长、迂曲；输卵管末端呈漏斗状扩大。

图 17-1　正常子宫输卵管造影表现

（3）盆腔动脉造影：正常子宫动脉发自髂内动脉，沿盆侧壁向前内下行，发出分支供应宫颈和阴道，其后在子宫侧缘迂曲上行，沿途发出螺旋状小分支进入子宫肌层及子宫内膜，这些小分支在肌层内形成丰富的血管网。卵巢动脉起自腹主动脉的肾动脉起始部稍下方，下行至骨盆上口处，跨越髂血管，向前下迂曲下行，分支经卵巢系膜供应卵巢。盆腔动脉造影能显示生殖系统恶性肿瘤的供血血管及肿瘤染色、出血血管、盆腔内动脉瘤以及动静脉畸形等，此外，造影后还可行介入性治疗。

2. CT 表现

（1）平扫检查：子宫体呈横置圆形或椭圆形的软组织密度影，边缘光滑，中心较小的类圆形或 T 形低密度区代表宫腔。子宫长径 7~8 cm，横径 4~5 cm，前后径 2~3 cm。宫颈显示在子宫体下方层面，呈梭形软组织密度影，外缘光滑，横径小于 3 cm。宫体与宫颈的比例，婴儿期为 1：2，成年人为 2：1。子宫旁组织位于宫体、宫颈及阴道上部的外侧，呈脂肪性低密度区，内呈细小条状或点状软组织密度影，代表宫旁血管、神经和纤维组织。子宫圆韧带呈条带状自宫底向前外侧走行。子宫前方为膀胱，呈水样低密度；后方为直肠，内常有气体。正常卵巢显示为双侧子宫旁低密度影，与相邻肠管不易区分，故 CT 检查时卵巢与输卵管均难以识别。

（2）增强检查：子宫肌层呈明显均匀强化，表明子宫壁血供丰富，中心低密度宫腔显示更为清晰，呈不强化。宫颈强化程度低于子宫壁。

3. MRI 表现

（1）平扫检查：T1WI 上，宫体、宫颈和阴道在周围高信号脂肪组织的衬托下，可清楚呈现为均匀低信号。高信号脂肪组织中可见成对的低信号影，代表子宫圆韧带与子宫骶骨韧带。T2WI 上，尤其是在矢状位，可清晰显示宫体、宫颈和阴道的解剖结构呈分层表现：①宫体自内向外有三层信号：中心高信号影代表子宫内膜及腔内分泌物，中间薄的低信号带为子宫肌内层，又称结合带，周围中等信号即为子宫肌外层（图 17-2）；②宫颈自内向外分四层信号：即高信号的宫颈管内黏液，中等信号的宫颈黏膜皱襞，低信号的宫颈纤维化基质，中等信号的宫颈肌层；③阴道分两层信号：即高信号的阴道内容物和低信号的阴道壁。T2WI 上的这种信号分层表现与生理状态有关，绝经后分层信号不再明显。绝经前常可识别正常卵巢，T1WI 上，为卵圆形均匀低信号；T2WI 上，其内卵泡呈高信号，中心部为低至中等信号(图 17-2)。

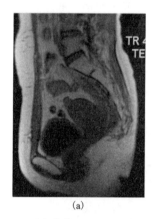 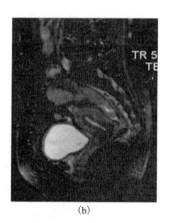

(a) (b)

(a)正中矢状位 T1WI 上，子宫呈均匀一致的较低信号，膀胱内呈明显低信号；(b)正中矢状位 T2WI 上，子宫内膜和宫腔内分泌物呈高信号，结合带呈低信号，子宫肌外层为中等信号。

图 17-2 正常子宫 MRI 表现

(2)增强检查：子宫强化表现与检查方法有关。常规增强检查，子宫内膜和子宫肌层强化，而结合带强化程度较低；动态增强检查，子宫各层强化程度随检查时间而异。

第三节 基本病变

1. X 线表现

(1)子宫输卵管造影异常表现：①宫腔异常：宫腔大小、形态有改变，但充盈良好，边缘光整，见于各种类型子宫畸形；宫腔变形，不规则并边缘不整，见于炎性病变，也可见于恶性肿瘤；宫腔内圆形光滑的充盈缺损，见于黏膜下肌瘤或息肉；②输卵管异常：可表现输卵管粗细不均、串珠样改变、僵硬、狭窄、边缘不整、梗阻和扩大积水，为非特异性炎症或结核所致。

(2)盆腔动脉造影：子宫动脉或卵巢动脉增粗，并出现异常的病理血管，见于女性生殖系统恶性肿瘤；对比剂外溢，提示新鲜出血；盆腔内动脉瘤和动静脉畸形可通过造影后行介入治疗。

2. CT 表现

女性盆腔 CT 检查异常表现包括子宫大小、密度改变及盆腔肿块。子宫增大并密度异常，常见于子宫肌瘤和子宫癌，前者子宫多呈分叶状增大，边缘清楚，可有钙化灶；后者表现为对称性或分叶状增大，内有坏死性低密度灶，并可累及宫旁组织。女性盆腔肿块常来自卵巢，也可为盆腔炎性肿块或其他来源的肿瘤。其中某些肿块具有特征性表现，不但能确定其起源，还可推断其性质，例如含多种组织成分的卵巢畸胎瘤，水样低密度的卵巢囊肿和卵巢囊腺瘤，含有气体的盆腔脓肿等；另一些盆腔肿块则少有特征，诊断困难。

3. MRI 表现

女性盆腔异常 MRI 表现包括子宫大小、形态和信号异常及盆腔肿块。子宫腔有形态改变，但子宫信号正常，见于各种类型先天性子宫畸形；子宫增大并信号异常，主要为各种类型良、恶性肿瘤所致，并可根据信号特征和增强表现，判断其范围与性质。MRI 检查易于发现盆腔肿块，其信号特征反映了肿块的组织构成。例如与尿液信号强度相似的长 T_1 和长 T_2 肿块信号灶，常为各种类型卵巢囊性病变；含有脂肪信号灶的不均质肿块，是卵巢畸胎瘤的表现特征。因此，当盆腔肿块的信号具有特征时，可判断其性质。

第四节　常见疾病诊断

目前影像学检查广泛用于妇科疾病诊断，包括先天性畸形、炎性病变及良性、恶性肿瘤。合理地运用影像学检查方法能对不同病变作出正确诊断。

1.子宫输卵管炎

（1）临床与病理表现：子宫输卵管炎为非特异性炎症或结核所致。急性子宫输卵管炎表现高热、下腹痛、白带多或子宫出血，慢性期为腰背痛、坠胀感和月经失调。结核性者多无明显症状和体征，或表现为一般感染症状，常有不育。病理上，急性子宫输卵管炎显示充血、水肿，继而形成积脓；慢性期发生宫腔粘连、输卵管粘连和闭塞；子宫输卵管结核，首先累及输卵管，由伞端至壶腹部，并逐渐蔓延至宫体和宫颈，形成干酪性坏死和溃疡，进而产生输卵管僵直、变硬、狭窄和粘连及宫腔狭窄、粘连和变形，还可有钙质沉着。

（2）影像学表现：子宫输卵管造影是检查子宫输卵管炎的主要方法，还有分离粘连的作用。

1）子宫输卵管结核：造影显示宫腔边缘不规则，严重时宫腔狭小、变形。双侧输卵管狭窄、变细、僵直、边缘不规则，可呈狭窄与憩室状突出相间。由于多数溃疡形成小的瘘道，形如植物根须状，是结核的重要征象。若输卵管完全闭塞，闭塞端圆钝，其近端局限性膨大，但很少形成囊状积水。

2）慢性输卵管炎：多为双侧性，炎症造成管腔粘连与闭塞。闭塞近侧输卵管扩大，形成输卵管积水，可粗如拇指，如碘油进入其中，显示多数油珠的集合，这种改变是非结核性炎症的重要征象。

2.卵巢肿瘤

（1）临床与病理表现：卵巢肿瘤是较为常见的病变，也是女性盆腔肿块的重要原因。卵巢肿瘤有良性或恶性、囊性或实质之分。其中常见良性肿瘤有囊腺瘤和畸胎瘤，此外，还有非肿瘤性的卵巢囊肿；恶性肿瘤以浆液性和黏液性囊腺癌多见。

（2）影像学表现：

1）卵巢囊肿：卵巢囊肿有多种类型，包括滤泡囊肿、黄体囊肿、黄素囊肿和多囊卵巢等。CT检查表现为边缘光滑、薄壁的圆形病变，呈水样密度。MRI检查，视囊内成分，T1WI上可表现为低、中或高信号，而T2WI上信号强度明显增高。表现典型的卵巢囊肿诊断不难，但多不能鉴别其类型。部分囊肿壁较厚或为多房性，不能与卵巢囊腺瘤鉴别。

2）浆液性囊腺瘤和黏液性囊腺瘤：CT和MRI检查，浆液性囊腺瘤和黏液性囊腺瘤一般较大，直径常超过10 cm。浆液性者壁薄而均一，可为单房或多房性；粘液性者壁较厚，通常为多房性。肿瘤的密度和信号强度均类似于卵巢囊肿（图17-3）。

3）囊性畸胎瘤：由三个胚层组织构成。CT和MRI检查均能显示肿瘤特征，分别表现为混杂密度或混杂信号肿块，内有脂肪性密度或信号灶，CT还可发现钙化、牙或骨组织。因而，卵巢囊性畸胎瘤易于诊断。

4）浆液性囊腺癌和黏液性囊腺癌：是最常见的卵巢恶性肿瘤。肿块边缘不规则，多同时具有囊性和实性部分；CT和MRI增强检查，实性部分发生强化；此外，肿瘤可产生腹水和大网膜转移，后者表现为扁平状实性肿块。有时可见腹膜和肠系膜多发结节状肿块，从而显示肿瘤的范围和转移情况。

3.子宫肌瘤

（1）临床与病理表现：子宫肌瘤是子宫最常见的良性肿瘤，在绝经期前妇女发生率为20%~60%。临床表现为月经过多和盆腔肿块。病理上，肿瘤由蜗状排列的平滑肌细胞组成，并含有不等量的胶原、间质和纤维组织。子宫肌瘤易发生玻璃样变性、黏液瘤样变性、囊性变和出血等。根据位置，子宫肌瘤分为浆膜下、肌壁间、黏膜下型和阔韧带肌瘤。

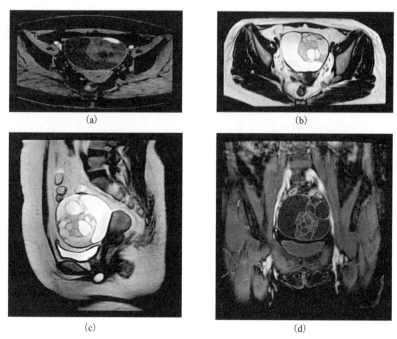

(a)横断位 T1 加权像；(b)同层面 T2 加权像；(c)矢状位 T2 加权像；(d)冠状位 T1 增强序列，子宫前方见多房囊样肿块影，壁薄而均匀，T1WI 呈低信号、T2WI 呈高信号，部分囊腔呈更高信号，增强扫描囊壁呈轻度强化，囊内容物未见强化。

图 17-3　右侧黏液性囊腺瘤 MRI 表现

(2)影像学表现：子宫肌瘤的主要影像学检查方法是超声和 MRI 检查，偶会用到 CT 检查。

1)超声表现：超声检查是诊断子宫肌瘤的常用方法，具有较高的敏感性和特异性；肌瘤多呈类圆形或椭圆形低回声的实性结节，单发或多发，大多界限清。较大肌瘤的内部回声不均，可见片状低回声。

2)CT 表现：显示子宫增大，可呈分叶状。肌瘤的密度等于或低于正常子宫肌，增强检查有不同程度强化。如发现瘤内有钙化，则能确诊为子宫肌瘤。

3)MRI 表现：能发现小至 3 mm 的子宫肌瘤。肌瘤在 T1WI 上信号强度类似子宫肌，然而在 T2WI 上呈明显均一低信号，边界清楚，具有特征。较大的肌瘤在 T2WI 像上，低信号瘤体内有代表退变的高信号灶（图 17-4）。注射 Gd-DTPA 后增强检查，肌瘤常为不均一强化。

4. 子宫癌

(1)临床与病理表现：子宫癌是女性生殖器官最常见的恶性肿瘤，分为子宫内膜癌和宫颈癌，以后者多见。临床上，子宫癌表现为不规则阴道出血，白带增多并血性和脓性分泌物，晚期发生疼痛。病理上，宫颈癌多为鳞状上皮癌，而子宫内膜癌常为腺癌，肿瘤晚期均可侵犯邻近组织、器官并发生盆腔淋巴结转移。

(2)影像学表现：子宫内膜癌和宫颈癌的诊断尤其早期诊断主要依赖组织病理学检查，影像学检查主要用于显示肿瘤侵犯范围和转移情况，以利于分期与治疗评估。

1)子宫内膜癌：子宫内膜癌又称宫体癌。其早期病变限于内膜时，无论超声、CT 或 MRI 检查均难以发现病变。当肿瘤侵犯肌层后，表现子宫对称性或局限性增大。超声检查呈不均质回声肿块，难以区分内膜及肌层。CT 增强，病变强化程度低于周围正常子宫肌。MRI 的 T2WI 像上，肿块呈不均匀高信号，并致邻近正常低信号联合带中断，DWI 上呈明显高信号，注射 Gd-DTPA 后检查肿块呈不均一强化。其中，MRI 检查对肿瘤侵犯肌层深度要优于 CT 检查。当肿瘤侵犯宫旁组织和邻近器官时，CT 和 MRI 检查均可显示宫旁组织和器官的密度和信号发生改变，代之以肿块影，此外，还可发现盆腔淋巴结转移。

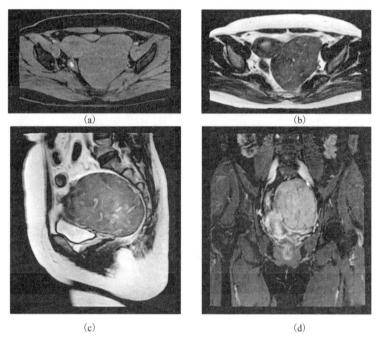

(a)横断位 T1 加权像；(b)同层面 T2 加权像；(c)矢状位 T2 加权像；(d)冠状位 T1 增
强序列，肿瘤位于子宫左侧，子宫受压向右侧推移，病变 T1WI 呈等信号，T2WI 呈等、
高混杂信号，增强扫描呈中度不均匀强化。

图 17-4 左侧阔韧带平滑肌瘤 MRI 表现

2）宫颈癌：宫颈癌时，CT、MRI 检查均可发现宫颈增大，甚至形成不规则肿块，分别呈不均匀稍低密度或 T2WI 稍高信号病变，增强早期明显强化，晚期呈低密度或低信号改变。当肿瘤侵犯阴道、宫旁组织、膀胱或直肠时，这些结构的密度和信号强度随之发生改变(图 17-5)。

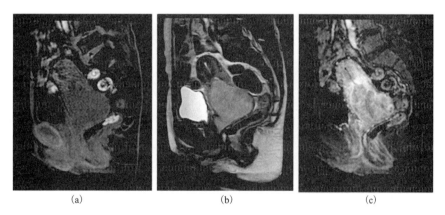

图 17-5 宫颈癌 MR 表现

(a)矢状位 T1 加权像；(b)同层面 T2 加权像；(c)同层面 T1 增强序列，宫颈肿大，T1WI 呈等信号、T2WI 呈稍高信号，增强扫描呈轻度不均匀强化

5. 盆腔炎性肿块

女性内生殖器及周围结缔组织、盆腔腹膜发生细菌性感染时，可形成盆腔炎性肿块。CT 和 MRI 检查，早期可无异常表现，发生盆腔脓肿时，可见圆形低密度区或长 T1、长 T2 信号灶，磁共振扩散加权成像表现为弥散受限的高信号，常位于子宫直肠陷窝内，增强检查呈周边环状强化。如内有气体，是诊断脓肿的有力佐证。

6. 先天性异常

女性生殖系统的先天性异常有多种类型，其中包括：①双子宫、双宫颈、双角子宫、纵隔子宫、半隔子宫、鞍状子宫、单角子宫、子宫发育不良（图 17-6）；②单侧或双侧卵巢发育不良或缺如；③输卵管重复畸形、先天性憩室和管腔闭塞等。

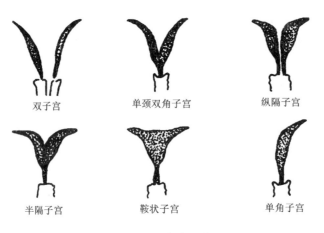

双子宫 单颈双角子宫 纵隔子宫

半隔子宫 鞍状子宫 单角子宫

图 17-6 子宫先天畸形

子宫输卵管造影可显示子宫输卵管畸形并能确定其类型，但不能发现卵巢异常；CT 和 MRI 检查能清楚显示各种类型子宫畸形并能发现卵巢异常。

（肖运平，欧幼宽，王小业，张敏萍，肖恩华，刘辉）

Chapter 17

Female reproduction system

The image examination has the important value to the disease diagnosis of the female genital system. The familiar diseases in the female genital system include the congenital abnormality, inflammation and tumor. The purpose with imaging examination is to detect the lesion and to make sure of its size, range, nature and stage. Various imaging examinations have different application range. MRI has high value to the diseases of the female genital system. Because sex gland and foetus are sensitive to the X-Ray, we should use X-ray and CT carefully.

Section 1 Method of examination

1. X-ray examination

(1) X-ray photography: Plain film of pelvis is usually taken. It requires patient take purgative in order to clean intestines before examination.

(2) Hysterosalpingography: Hysterosalpingography is a kind of imageology examination showing the lumen of womb and fallopian tube after injection of contrast medium from cervix. The contrast medium is 40% iodinated oil or organic iodine agent. Under clairvoyance photo, at once womb and fallopian tube are filled well after injection of contrast medium. It will take another 30 minutes for the patients with fallopian tube developing to re-examine so that the easy and smooth state of fallopian tube may be observed. Hysterosalpingography should proceed 5-7 days after menstruation. It is forbidden to do under the following states: acute genital organ inflammation, menstruation, metrorrhagia and gestation period.

(3) Pelvic arteriography: Pelvic arteriography is a kind of contrast imageology examination. The womb artery can be showed after injection of contrast medium by placing the catheter tip to abdominal aorta crotch, common iliac artery or internal iliac artery through femoral artery. Ovarian artery arising from aorta under kidney artery slightly inferior also can be showed if the catheter tip is catherized in it.

2. CT examination

(1) Plain scan: Laxative purgative should orally be taken in order to clean intestines on the day before the examination. 1%~2% iodine contrast medium or water 1000 ml should orally be taken in the 2-3 hours before check in order to fill and identify pelvic intestines. While checking, bladder should be filled well. CT examination should be undertaken using contiguous 5 mm or 10 mm slices from iliac crest level to pubic symphysis.

(2) Contrast-enhanced CT: Contrast-enhanced CT is usually necessary, specially to the tumor. An unenhanced (pre-contrast) series is performed followed by a post-contrast series by injecting intravenously contrast medium. The contrast medium is non-ionic contrast medium 50~100 mL.

3. MRI examination

（1）Plain scan: T1-weighted image and T2-weighted image with spin-echo sequence are routinely acquired. T2-weighted image is very important to show various dissections of cervix, corpus uteri, vagina and pelvic lesion easily. Phased-array coil are normally used. Section thickness is 5 mm or 10 mm.

（2）Contrast-enhanced MRI: Contrast-enhanced MRI is necessary after pre-contrast series, especially when the disease has been revealed with plain scan. The lesion area are scanned respectively to obtain T1-weighted image and T1-weighted fat-suppressed image after injecting intravenously Gd-DTPA, The dosage is 0.1 mmol per kilogram of body weight.

Section 2　Normal appearances

The uterus is located in the center of the small pelvis, adjacent to the bladder in the front, and rectum at the back, with fallopian tubes, ovaries and broad ligaments on both sides.

1. X-Ray findings

（1）X-Ray plain film: Female internal genitalia can not be shown and can not compare naturally with peripheral tissue because it's soft tissues density.

（2）Hysterosalpingography: Normal uterine cavity shows the inversive triangle with smooth and neat edge: Base is on the top, it is called fundus of uterus; inferior extremity is connected to the long cylindrical cervical canal with feathery edges; Superior two sides are uterine corner, mutually connect with fallopian tube. Bilateral fallopian tubes walk outwardly and downwardly, show winding and velvet line. The part of the fallopian tube that passes into the wall of the uterus is short and narrow, called interstitial portion. The outer side of the interstitial portion is thin and straight, called the isthmus. The distal of the fallopian tube opens in the abdominal cavity and expands in a funnel shape, it is called fimbriae (Figure 12-1). The contrast agent can enter abdominal cavity, distribute among intestines, uterine rectal fossa, and uterine bladder fossa, showing multiple arc-like or wavy dense lines if the fallopian tubes are unobstructed.

（3）Pelvic arteriography: Normal uterine artery originates from the internal iliac artery, descends anteriorly and inwardly along the lateral wall of the pelvis, sends out branches to supply cervix and vagina, then walks upwardly at uterine lateralarea, and unceasingly sends out small helical branches into the myometrium and endometrium, these small branches form abundant vascular network in myometrium. Ovarian artery comes from

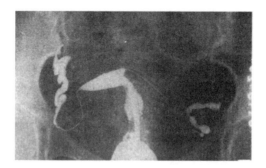

After injecting lipiodol, the uterine cavity shows the inversive triangle with smooth edge. The edge of the cervical canal is feathery. The fallopian tubes on both sides of uterine corner are slender and tortuous. The distal of the fallopian tube expands in a funnel shape.

Figure 17-1　Normal hysterosalpingography

slightly below the beginning of the renal artery of the abdominal aorta, descends to the upper mouth of the pelvis, crosses the iliac blood vessels, runs tortuously forward and downward, and branches through the mesangium to supply the ovaries.

Pelvic arteriography can show the blood supply vessels, tumor staining, bleeding vessels, intrapelvic aneurysms and arteriovenous malformations of malignant tumors of the reproductive system. In addition, interventional treatments can be performed after the angiography.

2. CT findings

(1) Plain scan: The uterine body shows transverse round or ellipsoidal soft tissues density with smooth margin, and a small round or T-shaped low-density area in the center represents uterine cavity. The long diameter of the uterus is about 7~8 cm, the transverse diameter is about 4~5 cm, and the thickness is about 2~3 cm. Cervix under uterine body, showing a fusiform soft tissue density with a smooth margin, transverse diameter less than 3 cm. The ratio of uterine body to cervix is 1:2 in infancy and 2:1 in adults. The parauterine tissue locates on the lateral of the uterine body, cervix, and vagina. It is a fatty low-density area, with small strips or punctate soft tissue density, representing parauterine blood vessels, nerves and fibrous tissue. The round ligament of the uterus runs from the fundus anterior to the outside in a strip shape. Bladder in front of the uterus shows watery low density; rectum behind the uterus often contains gas. Normal ovaries show bilateral low-density near the uterus, which are not easily to distinguish from the adjacent intestinal tubes. Therefore, it is difficult to identify the ovaries and fallopian tubes during scanning.

(2) Enhancement scan: Myometrium is obviously and uniformly strengthened, indicating that the blood supply of the uterine wall is abundant, and the central low-density uterine cavity shows more distinctly, without enhancement. The degree of cervical enhancement is lower than the uterine wall.

3. MRI findings

(1) Plain scan: On T1WI, normal uterine body, cervix and vagina may appear under contrast with peripheral high signal intensity adipose tissues, show uniform lower signal intensity. Pairs of low signals, representing the uterine round ligament and the hysterosacral ligament, can be seen in high-signal adipose tissue. On T2WI, especially in the sagittal position, the anatomy of the uterus, cervix and vagina can be shown clearly: 1) Uterine body shows three-tier signal from inside to outside, that is central area with high signal represents endometrium and intraluminal secretion; the thin low signal in the middle is the inner myometrium, also known as combining girdle, and the surrounding moderate signal is the outer myometrium. (Figure 17-2); 2) Cervix shows four kinds of signals from inside to outside, they are high signal endocervical mucus, moderate signal cervical mucosal folds, low signal cervical fibrosis matrix, and moderate signal myometrium; 3) Vagina only possess two kinds of signals, they are endovaginal contents with high signal and vaginal wall with low signal. On T2WI, This signal delamination is related to physiological status and is no longer obvious after menopause. Normal ovaries can often be identified before menopause. On T1WI, oval and uniform low signal; On T2WI, follicle shows high signal, with low to moderate signal in the center (Figure 17-2).

(2) Enhancement scan: With contrast-enhanced MRI, uterine enhancement images is related to the check methods. In conventional enhanced scanning, the endometrium and myometrium show enhancement, while combining girdle shows a lower enhancement; In dynamic enhanced scanning, the degree of enhancement of each layer of the uterus varies with the scanning time.

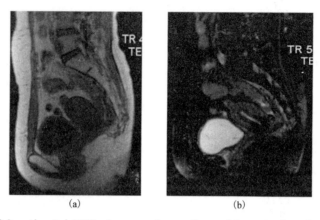

(a) On mid-sagittal T1WI, the uterus shows uniform and lower signal, and, the urine inside urine bladder shows obvious low signal; (b) On mid-sagittal T2WI, the endometrium and intrauterine secretions show high signal, the combining girdle shows low signal, and the outer layer of uterine myometrium has moderate signal.

Fig. 17-2   MRI image of normal uterus

Section 3   Basic pathologic changes

1. X-Ray findings

(1) The abnormal appearances for hysterosalpingography include: 1) The abnormality of uterine cavity: The size and the form of uterine cavity change, but the uterine cavity fills well, the margin of uterine cavity is smooth and regular, various uterine deformities may find these changes. Uterine cavity is deformed, irregular and the margin of uterine cavity is not smooth, these changes indicate adhesions of uterine cavity. Submucous myoma or polyp of uterine cavity may show round and smooth filling defect; 2) The abnormality of fallopian tube: Fallopian tube may appear disproportion for size, stiffness, constriction, irregular margin, obstruction, enlarged dropsy, these alterations indicate nonspecific inflammation or tuberculosis.

(2) Pelvic arteriography: Uterine artery or ovarian artery thickening, and abnormal pathological vessels, seen in female reproductive system malignant tumor. Contrast agent overflow, indicating fresh bleeding. Pelvic aneurysm and arteriovenous malformation can be treated by interventional therapy after angiography.

2. CT findings

The abnormal appearances of female pelvic include the changes of uterine size and density, and the pelvic masses. Hysteromyoma and cancer of the womb often show uterine enlargement and density abnormality. The uterus with hysteromyoma usually shows lobulated enlargement with distinct margin, may show calcification. The uterus with cancer of womb shows symmetrical or lobulated enlargement, containing necrotic lesion with low density, may also invade parametrium. The female pelvic lumps often originate from ovary, and it also is pelvic inflammatory tumor or other original tumor. Among them some lumps have characteristic images, not only can make sure their origins, but also can predict their pathologic statuses. For example, ovarian teratoma with various tissues, ovarian cyst and ovarian cystadenoma with watery low density, pelvic abscess with gas and so on. Other some pelvic lumps rarely show characteristic images, diagnosis is difficulty.

3. MRI findings

The abnormal MRI appearances of female pelvic include the changes of uterine size, form and signal, also the pelvic masses. Uterine cavity has morphologic alteration, but uterine signal is normal, various congenital teratisms of uterus may show these appearances. Uterine enlargement and abnormal signal are mainly caused by various benign tumors and malignant tumors, according to the characteristic signals and enhanced appearances, may judge their scope and kind. MRI is easy to detect pelvic lumps, their characteristic signals may represent the constitution of pelvic lumps. For example, the tumors with long T1 signal and long T2 signal as well as urine signal intensity, usually imply various cystic diseases of ovary. The lumps with various signal intensity which contain fat signal imply ovarian teratoma. Therefore, we can judge pelvic lump's kind when it shows characteristic signal.

Section 4　Diagnoses of common disease

Now medical imageology examination is used widely for gynecology disease diagnosis, including the congenital abnormality, inflammatory lesion and benign, malignant tumors. Making use of reasonably the medical imageology examination can make exactitude diagnoses to the different diseases.

1. Metrosalpingitis

(1) Clinical and pathological manifestations: Metrosalpingitis is resulted from nonspecific inflammation or tuberculosis. Clinical manifestations of acute metrosalpingitis include hyperpyrexia, lower abdominal pain, leukorrihagia or metrorrhagia. Its chronic period is characterized by lumbago, distending pain and menstrual disorder. Tubercle metrosalpingitis has no obvious symptom and physical sign, or has general infecting symptom, often has infertility. In pathology, acute metrosalpingitis shows hyperemia, dropsy, empyema subsequently. The intrauterine adhesions, adhesion and obstruction of fallopian tube take place in its chronic period. Uterotubal tuberculosis, first infects fallopian tube from umbrella to ampulla, then spreads to invade uterine body and cervix, results in caseous necrosis and ulcer, in the last fallopian tube becomes stiff, rigid, narrow and adhesion, uterine cavity becomes narrow, adhesion and deformation, calcinosis can also be showed sometime.

(2) Imaging manifestation

Hysterosalpingography is the main method to examine metrosalpingitis, which still has an effect on separating adhesion.

1) Uterotubal tuberculosis: Hysterosalpingography can reveal that the edge of uterine cavity is irregular. The uterine cavity is narrow and deformation when uterotubal tuberculosis is serious. Double fallopian tubes are narrow, thin, stiff and rigid, the edge of fallopian tube is irregular, fallopian tube can show narrow and protrusion with the shape of diverticulum in turn. The shape of plant root which is caused by small fistula is resulted from many ulcers and an important characteristic image for tuberculosis. If fallopian tube is obturated completely, the obturated terminal is round and blunt, its proximal portion is localized bulge, but seldom comes into being cystiform hydrocele.

2) Chronic metrosalpingitis: It is almost bilateral, the inflammation results in adhesion and obstruction for lumen. The out-of-the-way near side fallopian tube extends, becoming fallopian tube hydrocele, can augment such as thumb, if iodized oil enter them, shows that most oils bead gathers, it is an important symptom for non-tuberculous inflammation.

2. Ovarian tumor

(1) Clinical and pathological manifestations: Ovarian tumor is a familiar pathologic change, is also an important reason of female pelvic mass. Ovarian tumor may be benign or malignant, cystic or solid. Among them familiar benign tumors have cystadenoma and teratoma, in addition, have still ovarian cyst for non-tumor; familiar malignant tumors have serous and mucous cystadenocarcinoma.

（2）Imaging manifestations

1）Ovarian cyst: Ovarian cyst have various types, including follicular cyst, lutein cyst, flavin cyst and polycystic ovary etc. CT scan shows circular pathological change of the smooth and thin mural edge, it shows water kind density. On T1WI it shows low, medium or high signal, but on T2WI the signal increases obviously. Ovarian cyst with typical images is not difficult to diagnose, but can't discriminate its type more. Some ovarian cysts with thicker wall or multilocula body can't discriminate with cystadenoma.

2）Serous cystadenoma and mutinous cystadenoma: Serous cystadenoma or mutinous cystadenoma is generally big, its diameter is often over 10 cm. The wall of serous cystadenoma is thin and uniform. It is probable unilocular or multilocular. The wall of mutinous cystadenoma is thicker, usually multilocular. The internal density and the signal of the tumor are all similar to ovarian cyst (Figure 17-3).

3）Cystic teratoma: Cystic teratoma is constituted with three blastodermic tissue. CT and MRI all can show the characteristic images. CT and MRI show respectively lump with mixed density or signal, which contains fat density or signal, CT can also reveal calcification, tooth or bone organizing. As a result, ovarian cystic teratoma is easy to diagnose.

4）Serous cystadenocarcinoma and mucinous cystadenocarcinoma: Serous cystadenocarcinoma and mucinous cystadenocarcinoma are the most familiar ovarian malignant tumors. Medical imageology examination shows that the edge of lump is irregular, and the lump contains cystic and solid component at the same time. Enhanced CT scan and MRI, the solid part shows enhanced images, it can be used as the basis for diagnoses. In addition, the tumor can produce ascites and transfer to greater omentum, the latter shows a flat solid lump. Sometimes multiple nodular mass is seen in peritoneum and mesentery, so CT and MRI can reveal the scope of tumor and the transferred state.

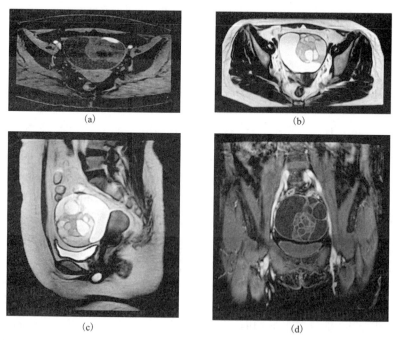

(a)　　　　(b)

(c)　　　　(d)

Axial T1WI(a), Axial T2WI(b), Sagittal T2WI(c), Coronal T2WI(c). There is a huge cystic mass with long T1 signal long T2 signal in pelvic right side. There is obvious compartmentation in it.

Figure 17-3　MRI findings of right mucinous cystadenoma.

3. Uterine leiomyoma

（1）Clinical and pathological manifestations: Uterine leiomyoma is the most familiar benign tumor of womb, morbidity is 20% ~ 60% in women before menopause. Clinical manifestation is excessive menstruation and pelvic mass. In the pathology, the tumor is constituted by smooth muscle cell with cochlear arrangement, and contains different quantity of collagen, mesenchymal and fiber tissue. Uterine leiomyoma easily causes vitreous degeneration, myxomatous degeneration, cystic degeneration and bleeding etc. According to the position, uterine leiomyoma is divided into subserous, intermuscular, submucous, and intraligamentary myoma.

(2) Imaging manifestations: The main medical imageology examination of uterine leiomyoma is ultrasound and MRI, and sometimes CT.

1) Ultrasonographic findings: Ultrasound is a common method for the diagnosis of uterine leiomyoma with high sensitivity and specificity. Uterine leiomyomas are mostly round or elliptic hypoechoic solid nodules, single or multiple, mostly with clear boundaries. The internal echogenicity of the larger uterine leiomyoma is not uniform, patchy hypoechogenicity can be seen.

2) CT findings: CT scan can show womb enlargement with lobulated shape. The density of uterine leiomyoma is equal to or lower than the normal womb muscle, enhanced CT scan can show different degree of enhancement. If the calcification is discovered in tumor, uterine leiomyoma can be distinctly diagnosed.

3) MRI findings: MRI can discover the uterine leiomyoma with the small diameter to 3 mm. The signal of uterine leiomyoma on T1WI is similar to the womb muscle, and uterine leiomyoma shows obvious uniform low signal on T2WI, its boundary is clear, it is characteristic images. Bigger uterine leiomyoma on T2WI shows low signal lump with high signal area which represents degeneration (Figure 17-4.). when we use enhanced MRI examination with Gd-DTPA, uterine leiomyoma is often unequal enhancement.

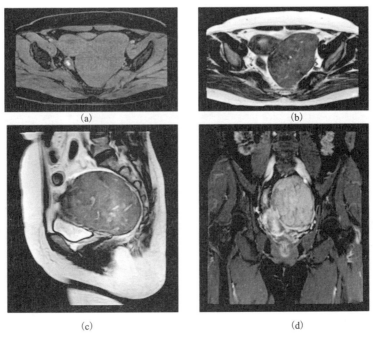

(a)　　　　　　　　　　(b)

(c)　　　　　　　　　　(d)

Axial T1WI(a), axial T2WI(b), sagittal T2WI(c), coronal T1 enhanced sequence (d). The tumor is located on the left side of the uterus, and the uterus is pressed to the right side. The lesions showed equal signal on T1WI, high mixed signal on T2WI, and moderate heterogeneous enhancement on enhanced scan.

Figure 17-4　MRI findings of uterine leiomyoma

4. Carcinoma of uterus

(1) Clinical and pathological manifestations: Carcinoma of uterus is the most familiar malignant tumor in

female reproduction system. It is divided into carcinoma of uterine body and carcinoma cervix. The latter is often met clinically. Clinical manifestation of carcinoma of uterus is the irregular vagina bleeding, leukorrhagia with blood and purulent secretion, late tumor causes ache. In the pathology, carcinoma cervix is almost squamous epithelial carcinoma. But carcinoma of uterine body is often adenocarcinoma. In the late stage, the tumor may invade the adjacent tissues and organs and have pelvic lymph node metastasis.

（2）Imaging manifestations：

Diagnosis of carcinoma of corpus uteri and carcinoma of cervix, particularly in the earlier diagnosis, mainly depends on histopathological examination. The medical imageology examination is used mainly to show the invasive scope of the tumor and the transferred state for the convenience of stages and treatment evaluation.

1）Carcinoma of uterine body：Carcinoma of uterine body is namely endometrial carcinoma. Its earlier pathological area is limited in mucous membrane. Both CT and MRI examinations are all hard to detect lesion. After the tumor infringes muscular layer, it shows womb symmetrical or local enlargement. Enhanced CT scan, the enhanced degree for the pathologic changes is lower than normal womb muscle. On MRI T2WI, the mass shows unequal high signal, and the nearby normal combining girdle with low signal has been interrupted. When we use enhanced MRI examination with Gd-DTPA, the mass shows unequal enhancement. Among them, MRI examination is better than CT to estimate the depth which the tumor infringes upon uterine muscle layer. When the tumor infringes upon parametrial tissues and nearby organs, CT and MRI all can reveal the alterations of density and signal for parametrial tissues and nearby organs which shows lumps, in addition, can also discover transferred pelvic lymph node.

2）Carcinoma of cervix：Both CT and MRI examinations showed enlargement of the cervix and even irregular masses, which were uneven with slightly lower density or slightly higher signal intensity on T2WI, with obvious enhancement in the early stage of enhancement and low density or low signal intensity change in the late stage. The density and signal intensity of these structures change when the tumor invades the vagina, paravertebral tissue, bladder or rectum (Figure 17-5).

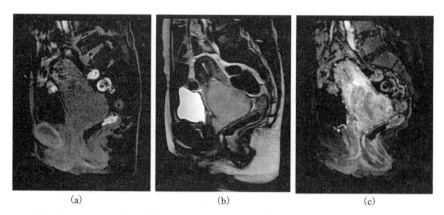

(a)   (b)   (c)

Sagittal T1WI(a), sagittal T2WI(b), T1 enhanced sequence(c). It shows cervical enlargement which shows equal signal on T1WI, slightly high signal on T2WI, mild uneven enhancement on enhanced scan.

Figure 17-5 MRI findings of carcinoma of uterus

5. Pelvic inflammatory lump

When female internal genital organs, surrounding connective tissue and pelvic peritoneum are infected by bacteria, they may cause pelvic inflammatory lumps. With CT and MRI examination, there is not abnormal appearance in the early period, When there is pelvic abscess, the lesion may show round low density or long T1 and long T2 signal, diffusivity weighted magnetic resonance imaging (DWI) showed high signals with limited dispersion, often locates in Diuglas' cul-de-sac, enhanced examination can show peripheral annular enhancement. If the lesion contains air, it is a potent evidence of diagnosing abscess.

6. congenital abnormality

Congenital abnormality of female reproduction system has various types, including: (1) Double womb, double neck of uterus, uterus bicornis, uterus septus, half-isolated uterus, bicorbate uterus, uterus unicornis, hypoplasia of uterus (Figure 17-6); (2) Unilateral or bilateral ovarian agenesis or anovaria; (3) Fallopian tube duplication deformity, congenital diverticulum and lumen emphraxis etc.

Hysterosalpingography can show uterotubal deformity and make sure its type, but can't detect abnormality of ovary; CT and MRI examination can distinctly show various deformities of womb, also can show abnormality of ovary.

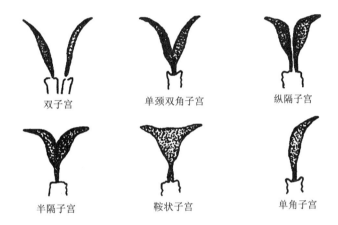

双子宫　　　　　单颈双角子宫　　　　　纵隔子宫

半隔子宫　　　　　鞍状子宫　　　　　单角子宫

Figure 17-6　Congenital abnormality of womb

(Xiao Yunping, Ou Youkuan, Wang Xiaoye, Zhang Minping, Xiao Enhua, Liu Hui)

第十八章

男性生殖系统

影像学检查对于男性生殖系统疾病有较好的诊断价值。前列腺增生，前列腺癌，睾丸肿瘤是男性生殖系统常见疾病，影像学检查的目的是发现病变，进行定性诊断，明确疾病的范围及确定有无转移，已便于肿瘤的分期和治疗。

第一节 检查方法

1.X 线检查

(1)普通 X 线：患者仰卧，X 线球管向足侧倾斜 20°，中心射线从耻骨上缘投入，以避开耻骨重叠影。

(2)输精管、精囊造影：外阴局部麻醉，在患侧或双侧阴囊外上方切开皮肤，找出输精管，游离出 1~2 cm 提起并行远端穿刺，注入 1.5~2 mL 非离子型碘对比剂，摄片时，X 线球管向足侧倾斜 15°拍正位片，须将两侧输精管包括于片内。若患者有碘过敏，急性炎症或一般情况不佳时不宜行此检查。

(3)膀胱造影：将导管经尿道插入膀胱，注入非离子型碘对比剂 100~200 mL，摄正位或左斜位、右斜位片。

2.CT 检查

男性生殖系统的 CT 检查同盆腔 CT 扫描。

(1)一般准备：为获得高质量 CT 图像，扫描前应常规做如下准备。

1)检查前四天开始进少渣饮食或流质饮食。

2)检查前两晚各口服一次缓泻剂(番泻叶泡茶饮)。

3)扫描前 12 小时及 3 小时各口服 1%泛影葡胺 250 mL 或水，以充盈小肠与结肠。

4)检查前 2 小时不排小便，使膀胱处于充盈状态，或请患者饮水 600 mL。

(2)平扫：患者取仰卧位，平静呼吸，自耻骨联合下缘开始向上至髂前上嵴做连续轴位扫描，层厚 10 mm，对较小的病变可加作 5 mm 薄层扫描。必要时采用俯卧位及直接冠状位扫描。

(3)增强：盆腔内有些病变在 CT 平扫后仍需静脉注射含碘对比剂再次扫描检查才能明确诊断，即增强扫描。其方法包括：静脉推注法、静脉注射点滴法、静注与静脉滴注合用及动态扫描。

(4)适应证及禁忌证：

1)发现病变：盆腔内的肿瘤、脓肿、血肿、囊肿、肿大淋巴结。

2)确定病变部位：通过轴位、直接冠状位及重建图像可以清楚显示病变的准确部位，以利穿刺活检及制定放疗计划。

3)确定病变的性质：CT 平扫及增强扫描可做出病变的良恶性诊断，并可鉴别病变是囊性、实性、脂肪性、血性等。

4)了解邻近器官侵犯情况以及有无淋巴结转移及转移的范围,有利于肿瘤的分期。

5)观察疗效:某些不易手术治疗的肿瘤,采用全身化疗或介入治疗后,可通过 CT 比较治疗前后肿瘤的变化,从而评价疗效。

6)对不能合作的患者以及早孕(3 个月内)者不宜做 CT 检查。

7)对碘过敏者不能做 CT 增强扫描。

3. MRI 检查

(1)一般准备:扫描前必须除去所有的金属物品,以免发生金属伪影,影响诊断。检查前 2 小时憋尿,使膀胱充盈 1/2 以上,以便更清楚的显示盆腔诸脏器的解剖关系。有人提议必要时可放置阴道栓,或经直肠充气,或给予小肠解痉剂,这些措施从理论上讲有助于提高图像质量,但同时也增加了患者的不适,因此没有常规使用。检查时患者取仰卧位,平静呼吸,并做好解释工作以消除患者对幽闭及射频噪声的恐惧感。

(2)参数选择:常规采用自旋回波(SE)序列即可获得满意的图像。完整的盆腔检查应包括矢状位、冠状位和轴位,并分别作 T1 及 T2 加权像(T1WI,T2WI)以获得足够的诊断信息,但因扫描时间过长,患者难以接受,故有作者认为除非特别需要,一般只需做三个方位的 T1 加权像及一个方位的 T2 加权像即可。盆腔扫描一般采用体部线圈,FOV:36 cm~40 cm,Tl WI:TR500msec、TEl5msec,4 次采集,T2WI:TR2000ms、TE90msec,2 次采集,层厚 10 mm,矩阵 128×256。

(3)适应证及禁忌证:

1)MRI 具有很高的软组织对比度,具有多方位、多参数成像等优点,因此,对显示盆腔病变比 CT 更为敏感,但在骨骼方面逊于 CT。MRI 主要用于发现病变,显示病变的准确位置,尤其是对于肿瘤的定性、了解有无转移及观察疗效有重要意义。

2)凡是体内置有金属物品者如人工关节、金属避孕环等不宜做 MRI 检查。这些金属物可改变磁场均匀性,并产生明显金属伪影掩盖整个盆腔,从而影响诊断。带有心脏起搏器的患者是 MRI 检查的绝对禁忌证。

第二节　正常表现

1. 普通 X 线表现

普通 X 线照片精囊及输精管不能显示,精囊及输精管区域无钙化或阳性结石。

2. X 线造影表现

(1)输精管、精囊造影表现:正常精囊蜿蜒弯曲,位于耻骨联合上方两侧。精囊的上方为扭曲膨大的输精管壶腹部,向外上伸延,然后向两侧沿精索行走至阴囊部。两侧射精管在两侧精囊内下方,相当于耻骨联合处,对比剂可进入膀胱,使膀胱同时显影(图 18-1)。

(2)膀胱造影表现:正常前列腺在膀胱造影片中,不造成对膀胱的压迹,膀胱下部边缘亦光滑整齐。

3. CT 表现

(1)前列腺:在耻骨联合下缘以上 CT 层面,可见前列腺表现为圆形或卵圆形均匀软组织密度影,边缘光整,CT 值为 30~75 Hu,无论平扫或是增强,均无法分辨其组织学区域。前列腺大小随年龄增加而增大,30 岁以下男性前列腺平均上下径、左右径和前后径分别为 30 mm、31 mm 和 23 mm,而 60~70 岁男性则分别为 50 mm、43 mm 和 48 mm。并且随年龄增加,前列腺钙化或结石的发生率也相应增高,50~70 岁年龄组可达 60%,CT 上呈散在点状或圆形的致密影。前列腺前方为耻骨后间隙,其内充填脂肪,呈低密度影,其后方为直肠膀胱间隙,其内亦为脂肪和纤维结缔组织,前列腺两侧为肛提肌。

(2)精囊:精囊位于前列腺上缘,膀胱的后方。在 CT 上表现为两侧对称性椭圆形软组织密度影,CT 值 30~75HU,双侧共长 6~8 cm。正常成人精囊体积最大,呈囊状,而老年人精囊萎缩变小。CT 检查的目

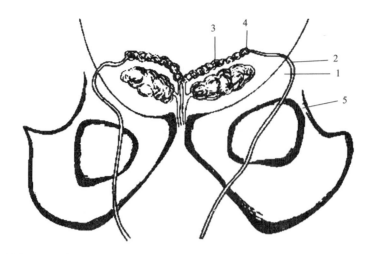

1—精囊；2—输精管；3—输精管壶腹部；4—输精管壶腹部结合部；5—射精管。

图 18-1　正常精路

的主要是观察精囊大小、形态、密度、两侧是否对称、精囊是否存在。仰卧时精囊外侧部分与膀胱后壁间形成 20°~40° 的夹角，称膀胱精囊角。俯卧位时由于精囊前移而贴近膀胱，使膀胱精囊角消失。因此在判断前列腺或膀胱肿瘤侵犯精囊时，可仰卧位扫描观察膀胱精囊角。

4. MRI 表现

（1）前列腺：MRI 可以多方位扫描并且能清楚分辨前列腺各区，故对显示前列腺的价值比 CT 更为优越。MRI 矢状位及冠状位对观察前列腺的毗邻关系效果较好，横轴位则适合观察前列腺的内部结构。T1WI 上，前列腺呈均匀一致的低信号，不能区分解剖带。T2WI 上，前列腺的中心区和外围区的信号强度存在较大差别，表现为中心区短 T2 低信号，外围区长 T2 高信号，这是由于前列腺中心区含有较短 T2 的肌纤维成分，而外围含有较长 T2 的腺体分泌液，所以两者容易区分。移行区的信号强度与中心区相似，两者不易区分。在前列腺的前侧方可见点状或线条状长 T1 长 T2 信号，为血流较慢的静脉丛。

（2）精囊：MRI 横轴位显示精囊效果较好，其大小、形态及部位与 CT 轴位所见相同。由于精囊内含精液，故在 T1WI 上表现为长 T1 低信号，T2WI 上表现为长 T2 高信号，其壁为短 T2 低信号。膀胱精囊角内为脂肪充填，故 T1WI 上呈明显高信号之锐角，两侧对称。在精囊周围可见点状或条状长 T2 高信号，为静脉丛。

（3）睾丸及附睾：目前公认 MRI 对人体生殖器官无损害，故可用于睾丸及附睾疾病的诊断，但其费用昂贵一般都首选采用物理检查或 B 超检查，MR 检查仅作为一种重要的补充手段。正常睾丸在 MR T1WI 上表现为低信号，在 T2WI 上表现为高信号。正常睾丸呈卵圆形结构，轮廓光滑整齐，信号均匀一致，睾丸周围的白膜由纤维组织构成，故呈长 T1 短 T2 低信号。附睾呈"逗点"状，位于睾丸背侧，呈长 T1 长 T2 信号，强度低于睾丸。阴茎各部在 T1WI 及 T2WI 均能显示。

5. 比较影像学

观察前列腺和精囊以 CT 及 MRI 检查为主，而 X 线检查，仅输精管造影还偶有应用。CT 能确切显示前列腺大小和形态，但无法分辨其各解剖区。而 MRI 可以进行多方位扫描并且能清楚分辨前列腺各区，所以对显示前列腺的价值比 CT 更为优越。MRI 矢状位及冠状位对观察前列腺的毗邻关系效果较好，横轴位则适合观察前列腺的内部结构。MRI 横轴位显示精囊效果较好，其大小、形态及部位与 CT 轴位所见相同。观察睾丸及附睾时首选 B 超检查，考虑到 X 线辐射，一般不主张用 CT 检查内生殖器。现已公认 MRI 对人体生殖器官无损害，故也可用于睾丸及附睾疾病的诊断，但其费用昂贵，所以仅作为一种重要的补充手段。生殖管道可在普通 X 线下作造影检查，显示其内腔情况，主要用于寻找不孕症的原因。

第三节　基本病变

1. CT 表现

（1）前列腺：前列腺增大常见。

1）大小：前列腺增大最常见，分为对称性增大及非对称性增大。对称性增大主要见于良性前列腺增生，也可见于炎症及前列腺癌，表现为前列腺横径>5 cm 或在耻骨联合上方 2 cm 层面仍可见前列腺。非对称性增大主要见于前列腺癌，表现为前列腺局部增大。

2）形态：前列腺呈分叶状或局部结节状膨隆，多为前列腺癌。

3）密度：前列腺内低密度灶多为脓肿、囊肿、肿瘤囊变坏死；前列腺内高密度影为腺体内结石或钙化；增强扫描前列腺内异常强化灶，见于脓肿或肿瘤。

（2）精囊：以精囊肿块多见。

1）大小：双侧精囊增大多为液体潴留所致，单侧精囊增大见于囊肿、脓肿、肿瘤等。

2）形态：精囊角消失，通常见于前列腺癌或膀胱癌累及精囊；精囊肿块，常见于精囊囊肿、脓肿、原发或继发肿瘤。

3）密度：精囊内水样密度灶，多见于囊肿及脓肿；精囊内软组织密度影并强化，多见于精囊原发或继发肿瘤。

（3）阴囊：阴囊增大并睾丸前方或左右方水样密度影，见于睾丸鞘膜积液。

（4）睾丸：睾丸肿块常见，多为睾丸肿瘤。

2. MRI 表现

（1）前列腺：

1）大小：前列腺对称性增大，常见于前列腺增生，表现为移行带增大为主，周围带受压变薄；前列腺非对称增大，多见于前列腺癌。

2）形态改变表现及意义同 CT 改变。

3）信号：①周围带于 T2WI 上见低信号灶，多见于前列腺癌，不除外慢性前列腺炎、肉芽肿性病变、活检后出血等。②移行带增大并 T2WI 内多发不均匀中、高信号结节，提示为良性前列腺增生，以移行带腺体增生为主。

4）DWI：前列腺内病灶 DWI 高信号，ADC 低信号，提示前列腺癌。

5）MRS：良性前列腺增生的移行带 Cit 峰明显升高，Cho、Cre 峰变化不明显，Cit/Cho 比值升高；前列腺癌外周带病灶区 Cit 峰明显下降和（或）（Cho+Cre）/Cit 比值显著升高。

6）PWI：分为三型。Ⅰ型：早期快速强化，随后快速廓清，多见于恶性病变。Ⅱ型：早期快速强化后仍持续缓慢强化，可见于良性及恶性病变。Ⅲ型：早期快速强化后出现平台期，多见于良性病变。

（2）精囊：

1）大小形态改变同 CT 改变。

2）信号：精囊肿块在 T1WI 上呈低信号，T2WI 上呈高信号，多为精囊囊肿；精囊肿块与前列腺肿块相连，并于 T2WI 上呈低信号，DWI 呈高信号，提示前列腺癌累及精囊。

（3）阴囊：阴囊增大并睾丸前方或左右方水样信号影，见于睾丸鞘膜积液。

（4）睾丸：睾丸肿块常见，多为睾丸肿瘤。睾丸肿瘤比正常睾丸信号的 T2WI 信号低。其中精原细胞瘤信号均匀，非精原细胞瘤信号不均。

第四节　常见疾病诊断

1. 前列腺炎

前列腺炎可分为细菌性与非细菌性。前列腺炎一般临床即可诊断，在影像学诊断中以超声为首选，但CT可显示脓肿的液化部分。

2. 前列腺结石和钙化

前列腺结石常见于40~70岁，罕见于儿童。原发性结石发生在前列腺的腺泡和导管，大小1~5 mm，可多发，常无症状，结石可通过前列腺排入尿道。继发性结石多较原发性结石大而不规则，常与感染、阻塞等有关，可伴有前列腺癌或结核。前列腺钙化或结石常为CT检查偶然发现，表现为前列腺实质内散在分布的点状和圆形高密度影，CT值100 Hu以上，少数患者可见到较大的钙化或结石。

3. 前列腺增生

(1)临床与病理表现：与男性激素失调有关，在组织学上主要为腺体增殖而间质增殖较少，腺体增殖可为弥漫性，亦可为局限性，其中以尿道周围腺体弥漫性增殖为主，这与我们在日常工作中见到的前列腺增生以中叶多见相一致。由于前列腺位于特殊的解剖部位，故增生的腺体可压迫膀胱颈部，在临床上主要表现为下尿路梗阻症状，由于尿路不畅可继发膀胱扩张甚至肾积水及肾功能损害等。直肠指检可触及增大的前列腺，表面光滑、富有弹性、中央沟变浅或消失。

(2)影像学表现：

1)CT表现：正常前列腺上界在CT图像上一般不超过耻骨联合上缘10 mm，如果在耻骨联合以上20~30 mm层面仍可见到前列腺组织即可诊断为前列腺增生，可为弥漫性或结节性增生，其密度与软组织相似，增大的前列腺可向上突入膀胱，CT轴位可误诊为膀胱肿瘤，此时采用冠状位或矢状位重建可见突入膀胱内的肿块呈宽基底或球形，且与增大的前列腺相连，膀胱壁向上受压推移，界限清楚。

2)MRI表现：MRI显示前列腺增生比CT更为直观全面，绝大多数前列腺增生结节发生在前列腺的正中叶，使前列腺体积逐渐增大，并可突入膀胱，使前列腺失去正常形态(图18-2)。增生的前列腺结节在T1加权像上表现为均匀的稍低信号，在T2加权像上呈均匀的或不均匀的高低相间的混杂信号，这是由于增生的结节内所含组织学成分不同之故，如以肌纤维成分为主则为短T2低信号，如以腺体成分为主则为长T2高信号，增生的结节周围常见一环形低信号假包膜。值得注意的是单凭前列腺形态的改变和信号异常难以鉴别前列腺肥大与前列腺癌，关键在于显示结节是位于前列腺的中央带是外周带，因为绝大多数前列腺癌起源于外周带，而前列腺增生绝大多数发生在中央带，这是二者的主要鉴别点。

4. 前列腺癌

(1)临床与病理表现：前列腺癌是我国男性老年人常见的恶性肿瘤之一，其发病率约占所有恶性肿瘤的1%，在欧洲，前列腺癌的发病率占15%。病因目前尚不清楚，早期前列腺癌的临床症状多为隐匿性，晚期可出现与前列腺肥大类似的下尿道梗阻症状、局部浸润或远处转移症状。绝大多数前列腺癌(约70%)发生在前列腺后叶周边带，其次为两侧叶，中叶较少发生。所以直肠指检仍然是目前能够比较容易发现病变的最简单的方法，但对判断肿瘤的侵犯程度及其分期无能为力，对此CT及MRI检查颇有价值，以下是前列腺癌的TNM分期(表18-1)。

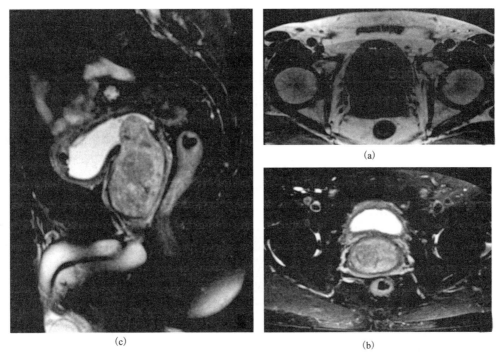

横断位 T1WI(a)呈大致均匀的中等信号，T2WI-FS(b)呈高信号伴中央叶多发小结节状低信号及外周带高信号区
受压萎缩，但信号正常，低信号包膜环清楚完整，矢状位 T2WI-FS(c)见前列腺明显突入膀胱，膀胱压迹光滑。

图 18-2　MRI 示前列腺均称性增生，前后径 49 mm，横径 59 mm，上下径 73 mm

表 18-1　前列腺癌的 TNM 分期

T1：临床和影像检查没发现肿瘤而病理检查有癌

T1a：组织学检查偶然发现肿瘤占≤5%

T1b：组织学检查偶然发现肿瘤占>5%

T1c：血清 PSA 升高，针刺活检发现癌

T2：肿瘤局限在前列腺内

T2a：肿瘤侵犯前列腺一叶的 1/2 或更少

T2b：肿瘤侵犯前列腺一叶的 1/2 以上，但小于两叶

T2c：肿瘤侵犯前列腺的两叶

T3：肿瘤穿透前列腺包膜

T3a：一侧包膜外扩展

T3b：两侧包膜外扩展

T3c：肿瘤侵及精囊腺

T4：肿瘤侵犯精囊以外的邻近组织并与之固定侵犯其中之一：膀胱颈、外括约肌、直肠肿瘤侵犯肛提肌和(或固定)盆壁

N 指有无淋巴结转移

N0 无局部淋巴结转移

N1 单个淋巴结转移，最大直径≤2 cm

N2 单个淋巴结转移，最大直径 2~5 cm；或有多发淋巴结转移，最大直径小于 5 cm

N3 单个淋巴结转移，最大直径>5 cm

M 指有无远处转移

M0 无远处转移

M1 远处转移

M1a 远处转移但无区域淋巴结转移

M1b 骨转移

M1c 其他器官转移

（2）影像学表现：

1）CT 表现：CT 检查的目的除明确诊断外，更重要的是对前列腺癌进行分期，特别是对Ⅲ期、Ⅳ期病灶的显示效果较好，遗憾的是对Ⅰ期、Ⅱ期病灶的显示并不十分令人满意，对Ⅲ期、Ⅳ期有时也易出现低估现象，即分期偏低，这是因为 CT 不易显示轻微的包膜外浸润或癌肿已侵犯至精囊或淋巴结，而其形态及大小仍保持正常之故。当癌肿位于包膜内时，CT 可见前列腺外周带有边界模糊的稍低密度的癌结节或前列腺外形出现不对称性隆起，此时癌结节的 CT 密度与正常前列腺组织差别不明显，故应调整适当的窄窗宽观察方可显示。当癌灶向外侵犯超出前列腺时，则容易为 CT 所发现，一个很重要的外侵征象是膀胱精囊角消失及精囊增大，提示癌灶细胞累及精囊与膀胱，此时绝大多数患者已有盆腔淋巴结转移。此外，前列腺癌易导致成骨型骨转移，在 CT 上表现为高密度。

2）MRI 表现：众所周知，由于 MRI 具有诸多优点，在前列腺癌的诊断及分期方面均优于 CT。有人对此作过对比研究，结果 MRI 的分期准确性为 83%，CT 为 65%。尽管如此，早期前列腺癌的 MRI 诊断仍存在困难。MRI 很难区别处于Ⅰ～Ⅱ期的前列腺癌与前列腺增生。T1 加权像上其信号无明显差异，有时可见外形隆起，T2 加权像上为中高混合信号。70%的前列腺癌发生在外周带，有人认为若高信号的前列腺外周带发生破坏、中断现象，应高度怀疑前列腺癌。前列腺癌的典型表现为在 T2WI 上见外周带孤立、多发或弥漫低信号结节，DWI 表现为高信号，ADC 值降低，DCE 呈流出型和平台型，T1W1 上与正常及增生的前列腺组织信号近似。文献报道 MRI 诊断前列腺癌敏感度为 77%～81%，特异度为 46%～61%，磁共振目前被公认为是前列腺癌诊断分期的最佳影像学方法。膀胱受累在 T2WI 可见膀胱壁的低信号环中断，膀胱精囊角消失。盆腔肌肉中出现高信号或中等信号，提示癌肿侵及邻近肌肉。骨转移常见于骨盆、椎体、股骨等，MRI 较敏感，T1WI 表现为低信号，T2WI 呈高信号。MRI 也可以发现盆壁及其他部位的淋巴结转移。

5. 输精管炎症

输精管炎是阴囊内炎症中少见的疾病，常与附睾炎同时存在，临床表现为患侧阴囊坠痛，可放射至下腹部及同侧大腿根部，以致行动不便。输精管炎症可选 X 线造影检查。

（1）非特异性炎症：输精管边缘模糊，粗大，严重者可扩大，扭曲，精囊扩大。

（2）结核：可见输精管狭窄、增厚和变硬，边缘呈虫蚀状，串珠状，晚期可有钙化。

6. 精囊病变

（1）临床与病理表现：精囊病变不多见，精囊炎相对较多见，临床表现有疼痛、血精、下腹疼痛及尿路刺激症状。精液检查可见大量红细胞和白细胞，精液培养可发现典型致病病原体。

（2）影像学表现：一般不需做 MRI 检查。在 T1 加权像上，精囊可增大，与周围脂肪界面模糊。在 T2 加权像上呈高信号，但不均匀，可有纤维组织增生或肉芽肿形成的低信号。精囊原发肿瘤很少见，包括乳头状瘤、乳头状癌及囊肿。肿瘤在 T1 加权像上呈中低信号，T2 加权像上信号较正常精囊组织明显减低，且信号不均匀。若向外侵犯或有远处转移，则提示精囊癌。囊肿在 T1 加权像上常显示不清，质子密度加权像和 T2 加权像第一回波上常表现为低于正常精囊腺的稍高均匀信号区。

7. 睾丸及附睾炎症

（1）临床与病理表现：分特异性或非特异性两类，特异性多为结核。一般先有附睾炎，再蔓延至睾丸。临床上可有红、肿、热、痛，结合实验室检查和临床表现诊断不难。

（2）影像学表现：

1）超声表现：睾丸炎的典型超声图像是睾丸体积增大，回声低且杂乱。彩色多普勒能量图能区分睾丸炎和肿瘤，因为炎症时睾丸内血流增加，急性附睾炎 B 超检查可发现附睾肿大，回声变低及内部回声不均匀，彩色超声可见丰富的血流信号。

2）MRI 表现：为睾丸体积增大，附睾及睾丸界限模糊，在 T1 加权像上信号降低或与正常侧信号相似，T2 加权像上信号呈不均匀升高或较正常侧信号降低。局限性睾丸炎，在 T2 加权像上表现为增大的睾丸中局限性不均匀低信号区，要与肿瘤鉴别。

8. 睾丸鞘膜积液

（1）临床与病理表现：睾丸鞘膜积液较常见，分原发性及继发性两类。体检睾丸呈球形或梨形，触诊有囊性波动感，透光试验阳性。

（2）影像学表现：液体的MRI信号因其成分不同而不同，一般的积液T1加权像上为低信号，T2加权像上为高信号。若积液中蛋白含量高（如脓液），则T1加权像上信号高于一般积液。若伴有出血，则T1和T2加权像均为高信号。MRI矢状面和冠状面还可更直观地判断积液是否为交通性，积液的量，有无合并畸形及睾丸萎缩等情况。

9. 睾丸损伤

（1）临床与病理表现：睾丸损伤是泌尿外科急诊，多发生于青少年，损伤可分为闭合性损伤和开放性损伤两大类，按损伤程度可分为睾丸挫伤、睾丸血肿、睾丸破裂（包括粉碎伤）、外伤性睾丸脱位、外伤性睾丸扭转等。

（2）影像学表现：

1）超声表现：彩色超声检查可准确判断是否为单纯阴囊血肿、睾丸破裂、睾丸白膜是否完整，有无睾丸组织突出白膜外，并且能够准确鉴别睾丸破裂与睾丸挫伤以及睾丸内血肿的存在。

2）MRI表现：睾丸挫伤在MRI上表现为T1加权像上可呈较低信号，T2加权像上显示不清。若有出血，则在T1和T2加权像上均呈高信号。睾丸裂伤，白膜撕裂，在T2加权像上可见白膜的低信号线中断。睾丸脱位极少见，睾丸可脱至腹股沟管甚至腹腔，也可脱至耻骨前、会阴部或股内侧皮下。

10. 睾丸肿瘤

（1）临床与病理表现：睾丸肿瘤较少见，仅占男性肿瘤的1%～1.5%，占泌尿系统肿瘤的5%。然而在15～34岁的年轻男性中其发病率列所有肿瘤之首。在睾丸肿瘤中绝大多数为恶性生殖细胞瘤，包括精原细胞瘤、胚胎性瘤、畸胎瘤、绒毛膜上皮癌。其中以精原细胞瘤最为多见，好发于30～40岁。睾丸肿瘤早期症状不明显，表现为患侧阴囊内单发无痛性肿块，20%～27%患者出现阴囊钝痛或者下腹坠胀不适。体检可见睾丸肿大，质地坚硬、表面不平、透光试验阴性。精原细胞瘤的治疗及预后取决于确诊时的临床分期，一般将其分为三期。

Ⅰ期：肿瘤局限在一侧睾丸内，临床及影像学检查未发现转移征象者为ⅠA期，如有腹膜后淋巴结转移者属ⅠB期。

Ⅱ期：临床及影像学检查发现有膈下转移，或主动脉旁淋巴结转移，但无膈上转移及内脏转移。

Ⅲ期：临床或影像学检查发现有膈上转移或远处转移。

（2）影像学表现：

1）超声表现：超声检查是睾丸肿瘤首选检查，不仅可以确定肿块位于睾丸内还是睾丸外，明确睾丸肿块的特点，还可以了解对侧睾丸的情况，敏感性几乎为100%。

2）CT与MRI表现：虽然CT及MRI扫描对睾丸肿瘤的检出及分期诊断很有帮助，但由于睾丸恶性肿瘤容易引起淋巴结转移，使许多患者在就诊时已属中晚期，因此，CT及MRI扫描往往先发现淋巴结转移，然后才明确睾丸肿瘤的诊断。由于CT对生殖器有一定损害，加上MRI对本病的诊断已能取代CT，故重点叙述MRI表现，睾丸体积较小，扫描层厚以3-5 mm为宜，最好采用特制的表面线圈，以保证较高的信噪比。典型睾丸肿瘤的MRI表现为一侧睾丸肿块，边缘清楚，可起自隐睾。睾丸肿块在MRI之T1加权像上表现为与正常睾丸相比近似等信号。在质子加权像上亦呈等高信号，在T2加权像上正常睾丸信号增高，而肿瘤信号相对较低，多较均匀。如果肿瘤内有出血，液化或坏死，其信号强度不均匀。如果睾丸白膜信号消失或中断，常提示肿瘤向睾丸外侵犯。睾丸精原细胞癌多沿精索静脉上行转移至髂内动脉、髂总动脉、主动脉旁、肾门附近淋巴结，甚至转移至纵隔及锁骨上淋巴结，MRI显示肿大的淋巴结效果较好，一般表现为直径大于15 mm的软组织信号影。

11.精索静脉曲张

精索静脉曲张是指精索静脉蔓状丛的伸展，扩张迂曲，分为原发性精索静脉曲张，亚临床型精索静脉曲张和继发性精索静脉曲张三类。有时输精管静脉与提睾肌静脉也有此改变，常见于青壮年，发病率占男性疾病的10%-15%，是导致男性不育的主要原因之一。以往用手术结扎；现用漂浮导管的可脱落硅胶囊栓塞治疗精索静脉曲张，效果良好。如无脱落胶囊导管也可用明胶海绵加不锈钢圈栓塞。

精索静脉曲张90%发生于左侧，因左侧精索内静脉垂直进入左肾静脉，血流受阻较大，且左侧精索静脉位于乙状结肠后面易受肠道压迫影响其通畅，行程稍长，临床症状表现为阴囊扩大，疼痛，有下坠感。

精索静脉曲张如有明显症状，久婚不育并且精液异常者应做栓塞治疗。有20%的精索静脉曲张是因左侧髂总静脉梗阻所致，故此需行手术治疗。该方法是通过导管选择性或超选择性向精索内静脉注入栓塞物如明胶海绵、弹簧钢丝或硬化剂等以达到闭塞曲张静脉的目的。该法既是一种诊断手段，又是一种良好的治疗方法。

用一般内脏导管插入靶血管内5~10 cm，也可用可控芯导丝引导插入，用医用明胶海绵切成2 mm大的小块，泡在10 mL 30%泛影葡胺内，搅拌后徐徐注入，使细小静脉栓塞，再推入5 mm直径不锈钢圈2枚于主干内，加强栓塞效果。10分钟后将导管退至肾静脉内再造影，观察是否完全栓塞。栓塞前见精索静脉曲张如蚯蚓状，网状。栓塞后再注入对比剂时，精索静脉即不通畅，曲张的静脉即不显影。

（肖运平，廖秋玲，张邢，戴生珍，吕敏，肖恩华，刘辉）

Chapter 18

Male reproduction system

For the disease of male reproduction system, medical imageology examination is of great value. Hyperplasia of prostate, prostate cancer and testis tumors are commonly encountered diseases of male reproduction system, the purpose of medical imageology examination is to discover pathologic changes, offer qualitative diagnosis, and define the range of the disease and make sure whether metastases have occurred in order to stage and treat it.

Section 1 Method of examination

1. X-rayexamination

(1) Ordinary X-ray photograph: Patient in dorsal position, X-ray ball pipe is askew 20°to foot, central ray is put in from pubis upper edge in order to avoid pubis shadow.

(2) Vas deferens and seminal vesicle contrast examination: In vulva local anesthesia, besides in affected side or double side of scrotum top cut open skin, find out vas deferens, dissociate 1 ~ 2 cm after, lift its far end to puncture, inject into 1.5 ml—2 ml nonionic iodine contrast agent, when taking X-ray, X-ray ball pipe is askew 15°to foot, take orthophoria position film, must include the vas deferens of two sides in film. The patient of iodine hypersensitivity, acute inflammation and poor general condition is unsuitable for the examination.

(3) Bladder contrast examination: After pipe is inserted from urethra into bladder, and nonionic iodine contrast agent 100~200 mL is injected, orthophoria or left, right oblique position film are taken.

2. CT examination

CT examination of male reproduction system is the CT scan of pelvic cavity.

(1) General preparation

Before scan, it should be conventional to make following preparation to get the CT image of high quality.

1) Four days before examination begin to eat few dregs food or liquid diet.

2) Two nights before examination take mild purgative once(make tea to drink with senna).

3) Twelve hours and Three hours before scan each take 1% meglucamine diatrizoate 250 ml or water, in order to fill small intestine and colon.

4) Two hours before examination do not urinate, make bladder full, or ask patient to drink 600 ml water.

(2) Plain CT scan

Plain CT scan, patient in dorsal position, in calm breath, scan range from pubis joint lower edge upward to anterior superior iliac spine make axial scan, thickness is 10 mm, it can add some slinces with 5 mm for less pathological changes. Necessity adopting in lie position and directly in coronal section scan.

（3）Enhancement CT scan

After some pathological changes in pelvic cavity plain CT scan still need venous inject to contain iodine contrast-medium again field calibration talent definite diagnosis, enhancement scan. Its method includes: it is used that intravenous injection, intravenous drip, intravenous injection with intravenous drip and development scan.

（4）Indication and contraindication

1）Discovery of pathological changes: Tumor, abscess and hematoma, cyst and swelling lymph node in pelvic cavity.

2）The location of pathological changes: Through axle position, direct coronal section and reconstruction image can show the accurate position of pathological changes for aspiration biopsy and establishing radiotherapy plan.

3）Determining the quality of disease: It can make the good and malignant diagnosis of pathological changes with plain CT scan and enhancement scan, and distinguish pathological changes that it is cystic, entity, fattiness and blood etc.

4）Understanding neighboring organ invasion condition, the scope of the metastases and infiltration of lymph nodes, that is of value for the staging of tumor.

5）Observation of treatment effects: some tumors that are not suitable for operation, with the whole body chemotherapy or interventional treatment, CT scan can compare the change of tumor, to judge treatment effect.

6）The patient that cannot cooperate and early pregnant (within three months) are unfit for CT scan.

7）Iodine allergic patient is not fit for CT enhancement scan.

3. MRI examination

（1）General preparation

Before scan, the metal goods should be removed, in order to avoid metal artifacts, 2 hours before examination, not to urinate, make bladder full, at least filling 1/2 more than, the purpose is judging accurately the dissect relation of organ in pelvic cavity. Having person suggestion necessity, can place vagina bolt or by rectum inflation, or give in small intestine to antispasmodic, these measures are helpful to improve image quality theoretically, but at the same time also increased the discomfort of patient, so it is not routinely used. When in examination, patient in dorsal position, in calm breath, make explanation so as to eliminate patients' sense of confinement indoors and the fear of the noise of radio frequenecy.

（2）Parameter option

We can get satisfactory image with spin echo (SE) routinely. The complete examination of pelvic cavity should include sagittal plane, coronal section and axle position, and is cubes T1WI and T2WI respectively to get enough diagnostic information, but scan time is longer, patient is hard to accept, so, author thinks foundation on T1WI in 3 positions, unless needing especially, normally it need only T2WI in a position. The scan of pelvic cavity adopts body department coil normally, FOV: 36~40 cm, T1WI: TR500msec, TE15msec, 4 times of collection, T2WI: TR2000ms, TE90msec, 2 times of collection, layer thick 10 mm, matrix: 128×256.

（3）Indication and contraindication

1）In MRI there is the very high contrast ratio of soft tissue, there is in many ways position and multi-parameter imaging such as the advantages, therefore it is more sensitive than CT to show the pathological changes of pelvic cavity, but the reverse is true in terms of skeleton imaging. MRI is mainly used in discovering pathological changes, showing the accurate location of pathological changes, especially tumor, judging the kind of pathological changes, and making sure whether metastasis has occurred and observing curative effect.

2）All body built-in metal goods as artificial joint and metal intrauterine device etc. are unfit for MRI examination, since these metal things can change the uniformity of magnetic field, produce obvious metal artifact to cover entire pelvic cavity, so affecting diagnosis, especially the patient with pacemaker, are the absolute contraindication for MRI examination.

Section 2　Normal appearances

1. General X-ray findings

Seminal vesicle and vas deferens cannot be shown in the ordinary X-ray photograph, having no calcification or positive calculus in seminal vesicle and vas deferens area.

2. X-ray radiography findings:

（1）Angiographic findings of vas deferens and seminal vesicle: Normal seminal vesicle is bent wriggledly on both sides above the symphysis pubis. The top of seminal vesicle is the twisty and inflated ampullar region of vas deferens, it expands outward on stretch to prolong, then walks along the spermatic cord on both sides to the scortum. The ejaculatory duct of double sides is under the seminal vesicle of double sides, is equivalent to the symphysis pubis. Contrast agent can enter the bladder, making bladder developed simultaneously (Figure 18-1).

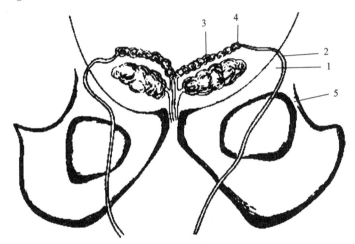

1—seminal vesicle; 2—vas deferens; 3—ampulla region of vas deferens; 4—combining site of ampulla region of vas deferens; 5—ejaculatory duct.

Figure 18-1　Angiographic findings of vas deferens and seminal vesicle

（2）Cystography findings: The bladder can't be compressed by normal prostate in the cystography, and the lower edge of bladder is smooth and neat.

3. CT findings:

（1）Prostate: Prostate tissue can be seen above the lower margin of the symphysis pubis in CT images, showing round or oval soft tissue shadow with homogeneous density and smooth edges. CT value is 30-75 HU. Plain CT scan or enhancement scan can not distinguish different histological area. Size of Prostate is increased with the age, the average vertical, transverse and anteroposterior diameter of the prostate in men under 30 years old is 30 mm, 31 mm, 23 mm respectively, while for the men between 60-70 years old is 50 mm, 43 mm and 48 mm respectively. With the increase of the age, the incidence rate of prostate calification or stones increases correspondingly. For the men aged 50 to 70 years old, it can reach 60 %. CT scan manifests scattered dots or round dense shadow. In front of prostate is the retropubic space, which is filled with fat and presents a low-density shadow. Behind it is the rectovesical space, which is also filled with fat and fibrous connective tissue, the levator ani muscleon is on the both sides of the prostate.

465

（2）Seminal vesicle：The seminal vesicle is located at the upper margin of the prostate and behind the bladder. It presents symmetrical and elliptical soft tissue density shadow in CT examination. The CT value is 30~75 HU and total length of bilateral sides is 6~8 cm. The volume of seminal vesicle in normal adult is the largest, showing cystic, and the seminal vesicle in elder tend to atrophy and become smaller. The purpose of CT examination is to observe the size, shape and density of seminal vesicle, bilateral symmetry and existence of seminal vesicle. An angle of 20°~40° is formed between the outer part of the seminal vesicle and the posterior wall of the bladder when keep in a supine position, which is called the vesicoseminal angle. In prone position, the seminal vesicle is close to the bladder as the seminal vesicle moves forward, which make the vesicoseminal angle disappeared. Therefore, we can observe whether prostate or bladder tumor invades the seminal vesicle through the vesicoseminal angle by scanning in supine and prone position.

4. MRI findings

（1）Prostate

MRI is superior to CT because it can scan the prostate in multiple directions and distinguish different regions of the prostate clearly. The sagittal and coronal MRI images is used to observe the adjacent structures of the prostate, while the axial MRI images is suitable for the observation of the internal structure of the prostate. In the Tl-weighted image, the prostate shows uniform hypointense and could not distinguish anatomical zones. In the T2-weighted image, there is a significant difference in signal intensity between the central zone and the peripheral zone of the prostate, the central zone presents hypointense whereas the peripheral zone is hyperintense, this is because there are many myofibers presenting hypointense in the central zone and glandular secretions presenting hyperintense in the periphery zone, so we could easy to distinguish them. The signal intensity in the transition zone is similar to that in the central area, so it is difficult to distinguish them. In the front of the prostate, there are long T1 and Long T2 signals in the shape of dots or lines, which are venous plexus with slow blood flow.

（2）The seminal vesicle：The axial position suits to observe the seminal vesicle. The size, shape and location of the seminal vesicle in MRI is the same as the CT. Due to the semen in the seminal vesicle, the seminal vesicle shows hypointense in the Tl-weighted image and hyperintense in the T2-weighted image, but it's tube wall presents hypointense in the T2-weighted image. The vesicoseminal angle is filled with fat, so the Tl weighted image showed an acute angle with significantly higher signal and bilateral symmetry. There are spots or strips hyperintense around the seminal vesicle in the T2-weighted image, which are the venous plexus.

（3）Testis and epididymis：Currently, it is generally accepted that MRI has no damage to human reproductive organs, so it can be used for the diagnosis of testicular and epididymal diseases. However, due to its high cost, physical examination or B-ultrasound examination are generally preferred, and MRI is only applied as an important supplementary means. Normal testis shows hypointense in the Tl-weighted image and hyperintense in the T2-weighted image. The normal testicle presents an oval structure with smooth and regular margin and homogeneous signal. The white membrane around the testicle is composed of fibrous tissue, so it presents long Tl and short T2 low signal. Epididymis manifests the "comma" form, located in the dorsal testicle, and presents long Tl and long T2 signals, whose intensity was lower than that of the testis. All parts of the penis can be seen in TlWI and T2WI.

5. Comparative imaging

CT and MRI are used mainly to observe the prostate and seminal vesicle, while X-ray is only used occasionally for vas deferens angiography. CT images can show the size and shape of the prostate accurately while can't distinguish the different anatomical areas. MRI can scan in multiple directions and can identify the zonal anatomy clearly, so it is more valuable than CT in showing the prostate. The sagittal and coronal MRI images is used to observe the adjacent structures of the prostate, while the axial MRI images is suitable for the observation of the internal structure of the prostate. The axial position also suits to observe the seminal vesicle. The size, shape and location of the seminal vesicle in MRI is the same as the CT. B-ultrasonic examination is usually chosen as the first methods to examine the testis and epididymis. Considering the X-ray radiation, CT examination of internal genitalia is generally not recommended. It has been recognized that MRI has no damage to human reproductive organs, so it can also be used for the diagnosis of testicular and epididymal diseases. However, due to its high cost, MRI is only applied as an important supplementary means. An ordinary X-ray radiography of the reproductive pipeline shows the cavity condition of the lumen, which is mainly used to investigate the cause of infertility.

Section 3　Basic pathological changes

1. CT findings

(1)Prostate: prostatic enlargementis more common.

1)Size: Prostatic enlargement was the most common. It was divided into symmetrical enlargement and asymmetrical enlargement. The symmetrical enlargement is mainly seen in benign prostatic hyperplasia, but also in inflammation and prostate cancer, which is manifested as a prostate with a lateral diameter of >5 cm or 2 cm above the pubic symphysis. The asymmetrical enlargement is mainly seen in prostate cancer, which manifests as a local enlargement of the prostate.

2)Morphology: The prostate is lobulated or partially nodular, most ofwhich are prostate cancer.

3)Density: Most of the low-density foci in the prostate are abscesses, cysts, and tumor necrosis. The high-density shadow in the prostate was intraglandular calculus or calcification. Abnormal enhancement in the prostate of enhanced scanning is seen in abscesses or tumors.

(2)Seminal vesicles: Seminal vesicle mass is more common

1)Size: The enlargement of bilateral seminal vesicles is mostly caused by fluid retention. Unilateral enlargement of seminal vesicles is seen in cysts, abscesses and tumors.

2)Morphology: The disappearance of seminal vesicle angleis usually seen in prostate cancer or bladder cancer involving the seminal vesicles; the seminal vesicle mass is common in the seminal vesicle cyst, abscess, primary or secondary tumor.

3)Density: water-like density foci in the seminal vesicles are more common in cysts and abscesses. The seminal vesicles manifest soft tissue density and is enhanced in enhanced scanning which is more common in the primary or secondary tumors of the seminal vesicles.

(3)Scrotum: The scrotum is enlarged and the water density in front of or to the left and right of the testis, which is seen in the testicular hydrocele.

(4)Testis: Testicular lumps are common, which mostly is testicular tumors.

2. MRI findings

(1)Prostate:

1)Size: The symmetrical enlargementof prostate is common in benign prostatic hyperplasia, manifesting as an increase in size in the transition zone, and the size of surrounding zone is compressed and thinned; the asymmetric enlargement of the prostate is more common in prostate cancer.

2)The appearance and significance of morphological changes are the same as CT changes.

3)Signal: ①Low signal focus is seen on T2WI, and it is more common in prostate cancer, not except chronic prostatitis, granulomatous lesions, bleeding after biopsy, etc. ②The transition zone is enlarged and there are multiple non-uniform medium or high-signal nodules in T2WI, suggesting benign prostate hyperplasia, which mainly is the transition zone gland hyperplasia.

4) DWI: DWI high signal and low ADC signal in prostate lesions suggest prostate cancer.

5) MRS: The transition zone of benign prostatic hyperplasia: the Cit peak is significantly increased, the changes of Cho and Cre peaks are not obvious, and the Cit/Cho ratio is increased; the peripheral zone of prostate cancer: The Cit peak is significantly decreased and (or) (Cho+Cre)/Cit ratio increased significantly.

6) PWI: It is divided into three types. Type I: Early rapid strengthening is followed by rapid clearance, more common in malignant lesions. Type II: It continues to slowly strengthen after early rapid strengthening, which can be seen in benign and malignant lesions. Type III: Plateau period occurs after early rapid enhancement, which is more common in benign lesions.

(2) Seminal vesicles

1) The change of size and shape is the same as that of CT.

2) Signal: seminal vesicle mass showed low signal on T1WI, high signal on T2WI, mostly suggesting seminal vesicle cyst; seminal vesicle mass connected with prostate mass, and low signal on T2WI, high signal on DWI, suggest that prostate cancer involves seminal vesicles.

(3) Scrotum: The scrotum is enlarged and the watery signal in front of or to the left and right of the testis, which is seen in the testicular hydrocele.

(4) Testis: Testicular lumps are common, which mostly is testicular tumors. The T2WI signal of testicular tumor is lower than that of normal testis. Among them, the signal of seminoma is uniform and the signal of non-seminoma is uneven.

Section 4　Diagnosis of common diseases

1. Prostatitis

Prostatitis can divide into germ and non-germ. Prostatitis can be diagnosed by ordinarily clinical manifestation, ultrasound examination is first selection in medical imageology examination, but CT scan can show the liquefied part of abscess.

2. Calculus and calcification of prostate

Prostate calculus is common at 40-70 years old, rare to children. Primary calculus occurs acinus and conduit in prostate, sizeof which is about 1~5 mm, can be multiple and frequently no symptom, and calculus can emit into urethra through prostate. Secondary calculus is bigger and anomalous than primary calculus, it generally be relate to infection, obstruction etc, it appear probably with prostate cancer or tuberculosis. Prostate calcification or calculus is accidental discovered by CT scan, which manifest the circular and the scattered punctate shadow of high density in prostate, CT value is more than 100 Hu, a few patients have bigger calcification or calculus.

3. Prostatic hyperplasia

(1) Clinical and pathological manifestations: Prostatic hyperplasia is also called hyperplasia of prostate, the majority think that the disease is relate to imbalance of male hormone, Prostatic hyperplasia mainly manifest as body of gland hyperplasia and mesenchyme hyperplasia lose comparatively in histology, body of gland hyperplasia can be diffuse and limitative, which is mainly body of gland urethra around diffuse hyperplasia, it is consistent in this and most prostate hyperplasia occur in center leaf that we see in daily work. Because prostate locates in special dissect position, so the body of gland of hyperplasia can oppress neck of urinary bladder, clinical manifestation primary is lower urinary tract obstruction, since urinary tract is not smooth, it can expand bladder even urinary infection and calculus etc. Digital examination of rectum can touch the increased prostate, its surface is smooth and

flexible, central ditch becomes shallow or disappear.

（2）Imaging manifestations:

1）CT findings: Normal prostate on CT image is generally not more than the upper bound on the pubic symphysis edge 10 mm, if it is still visible above the pubic symphysis 20 mm to 30 mm level, we can diagnose it as prostate hyperplasia, which is diffuse or nodular hyperplasia, its density is similar to soft tissue, the enlarged prostate gland can be upward into the bladder, CT axis can be misdiagnosed as bladder cancer, then using coronal or sagittal bits into bladder reconstruction, we can see a broader which is wide base or spherical, and connected to the enlarged prostate, bladder wall goes up due to pressure, but boundaries is clear.

2）MRI findings: MRI is more visual and overall than CT in manifesting prostate hyperplasia, most prostate hyperplasia tubercle occur center leaf in prostate, make a crescent prostate in volume and stick out in bladder, and can make prostate lose normal form (Figure 18-2). The prostate tubercle of hyperplasia in T1WI shows even low signal, in T2WI shows even or heterogeneous difference in degree appearance between mix signal, the reason is that the histology composition that contained in the tubercle of hyperplasia is difference. If muscle fiber composition is more in the tubercle, for short T2 low signal; if body of gland hyperplasia composition is more, for long T2 high signal and can see a annular low signal false capsule around the tubercle increased. What deserve to be noticed is that it is hard to distinguish prostatic hyperplasia and prostate cancer only rely on the changes of prostate form and signal, the key is to manifest tubercle locates in peripheral leaf or the central leaf of prostate, because the most prostate cancer orginates in peripheral leaf, and prostate hyperplasia most occur in central leaf, this is the main distinction.

4. Prostate cancer

（1）Clinical and pathological manifestations: Prostate cancer is one of the most common malignant tumors of man elderly people in China. The incidence rate is about 1% of all malignant tumors. The prevalence of prostate carcinoma is calculated with 15% in Europe. The cause of prostate carcinoma is still unclear. The clinical symptoms of early prostate cancer are mostly insidious, and symptoms of lower urethral obstruction similar to prostate hypertrophy, local infiltration, or distant metastasis may appear in the late stage. The majority of prostate cancer (about 70%) arises in the peripheral zone of posterior lobe of prostate, followed by the bilateral lobe, and less in the middle lobe. Therefore, digital rectal examination is still the easiest way to find lesions, but it is incapable of judging the degree of tumor invasion and its staging. CT and MRI examinations are valuable. Local staging of prostate cancer is as follows table regarding the current TNM classification(Table 18-1).

（2）Imaging manifestations:

1）CT findings: The purpose of CT scan isnot only to beside pinpointing diagnosis, but also the more important thing is to stage prostate cancer, especially stage Ⅲ, Ⅳ which is better in display of focus effect, what regret is that, stage Ⅰ, Ⅱ display of focus effect is not very much satisfactory, and stage Ⅲ, Ⅳ display of focus, sometimes are also easy to be underestimated, which is low by stage, because CT scan is not easy to show slight infiltration outside capsule, soak or the mass which has intruded to seminal vesicle or lymph nodes, and its form and size still keep normal. If the mass locates in capsule of tumor, CT scan manifests evidently cancerous nodes with the low density of vague boundary or the appearance of prostate appearance asymmetricalness bulge in the periphery prostate, at this time, the difference in the CT density of cancerous nodes and normal prostate organization are not obvious, so, it need adjust proper narrow window width to observe it. If cancer intrude outward to overstep prostate, it is easy to be discovered by CT scan, one very important intrude outward symptom is bladder seminal vesicle angle disappear and seminal vesicle increase, suggesting the cancer cell range to implicate seminal vesicle and bladder, most patient have had metastasis of pelvic cavity of lymph nodes at this moment. In addition, prostate cancer is easy to cause osteoblastic metastasis, in CT scan image, its manifestation is high density shadow.

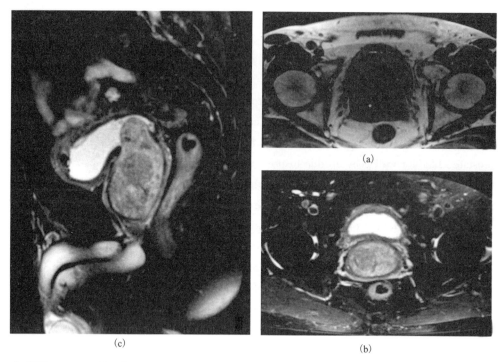

(a)

(c)   (b)

In MRI prostate manifests homogeneity aggrandizement, anteroposterior diameter is 49 mm, transverse diameter is 59 mm, superio-inferior diameter is 73 mm. Cross section in T1WI (a) mostly manifests even middling signal, in T2WI −FS (b) manifests high signal with majority tuberculous low signal in central leaf and high signal areas in outer leaf for atrophy, low signal of circularity capsule is clarity and integrity, Sagittal plane in T2WI−FS (c) manifests prostate inburst into bladder obviously, impression of bladder is smooth.

Figure 18-2   MRI findings of hyperplasia of prostate

Table 18-1）   TNM classification of prostate cancer

T1：Clinical and with imaging procedures not detectable tumour but pathological examination have tumour lesions
T1a：Accidentally histopathological finding in less than 5% of resected tissue
T1b：Accidentally histopathological finding in more than 5% of resected tissue
T1c：Elevated serum PSA, Tumour diagnosis by fine needle biopsy T1c
T2：Tumour is confined to the prostate
T2a：Tumour in half of one lobe or less
T2b：Tumour in more than a half of one lobe, but less than two lobe
T2c：Tumour in both lobes
T3：Tumour crosses the prostate capsule
T3a：Unilateral or bilateral extracapsular extension
T3b：Infiltration of seminal vesicles
T3c：Tumour invade the seminal vesicle gland
T4：Tumour is fixed or infiltrates different adjacent structures than seminal vesicles
T4a：Violation of one of them: bladder neck, external sphincter, rectum
T4b：Tumour invade the levator ani muscle and (or fixed) pelvic wall
N：With or without lymph node metastasis
N0：No regional lymph node metastasis
N1：Single lymph node metastasis, maximum diameter ≦2 cm
N2：Single lymph node metastasis, with a maximum diameter of 2~5 cm; or multiple lymph node metastases, maximum diameter < 5 cm
N3：Single lymph node metastasis, maximum diameter>5 cm
M：With or without distant metastasis
M0：No distant metastasis
M1：Distant metastasis
M1a：Distant metastasis but no regional lymph node metastasis
M1b：Bone metastasis
M1c：Other organ metastasis

2）MRI findings: As everyone knows, because MRI has many advantage, in the diagnosis andmake stage of prostate cancer aspect, it is superior to CT scan. Somebody has made contrast research for this, as a result accuracy of MRI by stage is 83%, CT is 65%. Though it is such, in early stage, the MRI diagnosis of prostate cancer still is difficult. Is it very difficult for MRI to distinguish prostate hyperplasia from prostate cancer in stage I – II. In T1WI its signal have no obvious discrepancy, sometimes its appearance is bulge. In T2WI it is mixed high signal. 70% of prostate cancers occur in the peripheral zone, Somebody thinks that if the prostate peripheral areas of high signal is destroyed and discontinuous, we should suspect prostate cancer highly. The typical manifestations of prostate cancer are isolated, multiple or diffuse low-intensity nodules in the peripheral zone on T2WI, high-intensity on DWI, low ADC value, outflow and plateau in DCE, and the signals on T1W1 normal and hyperplastic prostate tissue is approximate. It is reported in the literature that the sensitivity of MRI in diagnosing prostate cancer is 77%~81%, and the specificity is 46%~61%. Magnetic resonance is currently recognized as the best imaging method for the diagnosis and staging of prostate cancer. Have intruded to outside capsule of tumor, bladder is infringed, the low signal ring of bladder wall shows evidently discontinuous in T2WI, bladder seminal vesicle angle disappears. In the muscle of pelvic cavity, arise high signal or medium signal areas, refer to cancer invade near muscle. Bone metastasis usually betides pelvis, vertebra and thigh etc. , MRI is more sensitive, its manifestation is low signal in T1WI. MRI can also discover the metastasis of lymph nodes of basin wall and other positions.

5. Vas deferens inflammation

Vas deferens inflammation is a rare disease in the inflammation of the scrotum and often coexists with epididymitis. The clinical manifestation is pain in affected scrotum, which can radiate to the lower abdomen and the root of the thigh on the same side, causing inconvenience in mobility. Vas deferens inflammation take ordinary X-ray vas deferens contrast examination.

（1）Nonspecific inflammation: Edge of vas deferens is vague and it is thick, Serious is twisted, enlarges, seminal vesicle enlarges.

（2）Tuberculosis: Displaying vas deferens is narrow, thickened and hardened, its edge is vermiform, beaded, it can calcify in later period.

6. Seminal vesicle pathologic changes

（1）Clinical and pathological manifestations: Seminal vesicle pathologic changes are rare, seminal vesiculitis is relatively more common, its clinical manifestation is pain, hemospermia, lower abdominal pain and urinary irritation. The examination of sperm can see red blood cell and white blood cell and semen cultivation can find typical pathogenic pathogen.

（2）Imaging manifestations: Seldom need MRI examination. In T1WI, seminal vesicle can increase and be vague interface with around fat. In T2WI manifests high signal, but is heterogeneous, and low signal which is caused by fiber organization hyperplasia or granuloma. Primary tumour of seminal vesicle is rare, include papilloma, papillary carcinoma and cyst. Tumour in T1WI manifests low or medium signal, in T2WI its signal is lower obviously than the signal of the normal seminal vesicle, and signal is heterogeneous. If there is intrude outward or distant metastasis, refer to carcinoma of seminal vesicle. In T1WI tumor shows blurry frequently, in proton density image and in T2WI first wave shows the higher even signal areas below normal seminal vesicle frequently.

7. Testis and epididymis inflammation

（1）Clinical and pathological manifestations: Divide into specific or nonspecific inflammation two kinds, the majority of specific inflammation is tuberculosis. Normally epididymis inflammation appear first, stretch again to testis. Its clinical manifestation is red, swelling, hot, pain, and it is not difficult to diagnose with laboratory examination and clinical manifestations.

(2) Imaging manifestations:

1) Ultrasonographic findings: The typical ultrasound image of orchitis is an enlarged testicle with low echo and disorder. Color Doppler energy image can distinguish orchitis and testicular tumor. Because blood flow in the testis increases during inflammation, B-ultrasound examination of acute epididymitis can reveal epididymis swelling, low echo and heterogeneous internal echo. Color ultrasound shows abundant blood flow signal.

2) MRI findings: The volume of testis increases, limit of epididymis and testis is vague, and in T1WI the signal is lower or with signal of normal side similar, the signal is higher but heterogeneous or lower than signal of normal side in T2WI. Circumscribed orchitis manifests the increasing of circumscribed heterogeneous low signal areas in the testis in T2WI, it need be differentiated from tumor.

8. hydrocele testis

(1) Clinical and pathological manifestations: Hydrocele testis is more common, divides into primary and secondary two kinds. Somatoscopy find testis is spherical or pyriform, palpation find cystic undulatory sense, its transillumination is positive.

(2) Imaging manifestations: The MRI signal of liquid is distinguishing with its difference of the composition, general hydrops in T1WI is low signal, in T2WI is high signal. Hyperproteosis hydrops (such as pus liquid) in T1WI is higher signal than normally hydrops. If hydrops with bleeding, in T1WI and T2WI is both high signal. MRI arrow form surface and coronal-plane can still more judge product hydrops visually whether is traffic, amass the quantity of hydrops, whether merging deformity and atrophy of testis etc.

9. Testis hurts

(1) Clinical and pathological manifestations: Testis hurt is an emergency thing of urology, mostly occurs in adolescents. The injury can be divided into two categories: closed injury and open injury. According to the degree of injury, it can be divided into testis contusion, hematoma, rupture (including comminuted injury), and traumatic testis dislocation, testicular torsion, etc.

(2) Imaging manifestations:

1) Ultrasonographic findings: Color ultrasonography can accurately determine whether it is simple scrotal hematoma, testis rupture, testis albuginea intact, whether there is testis tissue protruding outside the albuginea, and can accurately distinguish the presence of testis rupture, testis contusion, and intratestis hematoma.

2) MRI findings: In MRI, contusion of testis in T1WI manifests lower signal, in T2WI manifests blurry. If having bleeding, in T1WI and T2WI manifests high signal. Lacerated testis, its tunica albuginea is lacerated, in T2WI the low signal line of tunica albuginea manifest discontinuity. Dislocation of testis is very less, testis can be dislocated to inguinal canal even to abdominal cavity, can also be dislocated before pubis, perineum or medial femiral subcutaneous part.

10. Testis tumors

(1) Clinical and pathological manifestations: Testis tumors are rare, accounting for only 1%~1.5% of male tumors and 5% of urinary system tumors. However, its incidence rate ranks first among all tumors in young men aged15-34. In testis tumor, the most is malignant germinoma, including seminoma, embryonal tumor, teratoma and chorioepithelioma. Among them, seminoma is the most familiar, occur easily at 30-40 years old. In testis tumor early stage, symptom is not obvious, manifestation is a single painless mass in the affected scrotum, and 20%~27% of patients have scrotum dull pain or discomfort in the lower abdomen. Physical examination find testis is tumescent evidently, very hard, and its surface is asperous, transillumination is negative. Prognosis and treatment of seminoma depend on clinical stage when definite diagnosis, normally divide it into three stages.

Stage I: Tumor is limited in a side of the testis, clinical and medical imageology examination do not discover metastasis that is stage I_A; if having metastasis of retroperitoneal lymph nodes, it belong to stage I_B.

Stage II: It is clinical and medical imageology examination discovery inferior phrenic metastasis, or metastasis of paraaortic lymph nodes, but no superior phrenic metastasis and metastasis of internal organs.

Stage III: It is clinical and medical imageology examination discovery superior phrenic metastasis and forane metastasis.

(2)Imaging manifestations:

1) Ultrasonographic findings: Ultrasound examination is the first choice for testis tumor. It can not only determine whether the mass is inside or outside testis, clarify the characteristics of the testis mass, but also understand the condition of the contralateral testis, the sensitivity is almost 100%.

2) CT and MRI findings: CT and MRI is very helpful for detection and diagnose by stage of testis tumor, but since testis malignant tumor bring the metastasis of lymph nodes easily, a lot of patients have been in later period when examining, therefore CT and MRI often discover metastasis of lymph nodes first, then just make clear the diagnosis of testis tumor. Since CT scan has the surely damaged for genitals and MRI can already replace CT for the diagnosis of this disease for genitals, so, this section narrate mostly MRI manifestation, volume of testis is less, scanning layer is thick with 3~5 mm that is advisable, had better adopt specially made surface coil in order to guarantee higher signal-to-noise ratio. The MRI manifestation of typical testis tumor is the mass of one side of testis, its edge is clear, can be from undescended testis. Mass of testis in T1WI is approximate equivalent signal compare with normal testis, in proton add right image also equivalent or high signal, in T2WI signal of the normal testis heighten, and tumor signal is relatively lower, even. If having bleeding, liquefied or thanatosis in tumor, its signal strength is heterogeneous. If signal of tunica albuginea of testis disappeares or discontinues, frequently refer to tumor intrude besides testis. Testis seminoma mostly transfer along spermatic fascia to internal iliac lymph nodes, common lymph nodes, paraaortic lymph nodes, renal hilus nearby lymph nodes, even transfer to mediastinum and supraclavicular lymph nodes. MRI manifests the effect of tumescent lymph nodes better, normally its manifestation is the signal of soft tissue larger than 15 mm for diameter.

11. Varicocele

Varicocele is that pampiniform plexus extend, ecstatic and tortuous, divided into three categories: primary varicocele, subclinical varicocele and secondary varicocele. Sometimes vas deferens vein and cremasteric vein have these changes too. It is much seen in youth adults, about 10% to 15% of male diseases, and is one of the main causes of male no procreate ability. Before, make operation binding; At present, use deciduous silicic capsule of float conduit to embolism to treat varicocele, its effect is good. If no having deciduous capsulet, can also use gelfoam with steel coil to embolism. Varicocele of 90% is in left side, because left spermatic vein vertically enter kidney vein, its resistance of blood flow is more, and the left spermatic vein is located behind the sigmoid colon, which easily affected by intestinal compression, and its route is slightly longer. Its clinical manifestation has enlarging for scrotum, pain and straining sense.

Varicocele has obvious symptom, those people that marry for a long time but can not procreate and sperm is exceptional, which should embolism treatment. Varicocele of 20% is owing to left common iliac vein obstruction, so, it still need operate. The method is to selectively or superselectively inject embolism such as gelfoam, spring steel wire or hardener into spermatic vein through a catheter to achieve the purpose of occluding the varicose vein. It is not only a diagnostic method, but also a good treatment method.

Insert with general organs conduit into target blood vessel 5~10 cm, can also use controllable core guide line to guide and insert, cut medical gelfoam with the pieces of 2 mm, dunk them in 30% meglucamine diatrizoate of 10 ml, inject slowly after stiring, make small vein embolism, push again two steel coils of the diameter of 5 mm into trunk, strengthen embolism effect. After 10 minutes return conduit in kidney vein again radiography, observe whether completing embolism. Before embolism see varicocele such as earthworm and reticular. When inject into contrast-medium again after embolism, spermatic fascia is not unobstructed, the crooked vein do not display.

(Xiao Yunping, Liao Qiuling, Zhang Xing, Dai Shengzhen, Lv Min, Xiao Enhua, Liu Hui)

中枢神经系统

中枢神经系统包括脑和脊髓，深埋于颅腔和椎管内。现代影像技术如DSA、CT 、MRI 等的迅速发展为其提供了高质量的图像，极大地提高了中枢神经系统疾病的诊断能力。

Part 5

Central nervous system

Central nervous system (CNS), including brain and spinal cord, embeds in the skull and the spinal canal. With the recent advances in imaging diagnosis of the newer modalities, such as digital subtraction angiography (DSA), computer tomography (CT), and magnetic resonance imaging (MRI), the high quality images can be performed. The ability of diagnosis to the diseases of CNS has been improved significantly.

第十九章

脑

第一节 检查方法

1. 颅骨 X 线平片

颅骨 X 线平片方法简单、经济、无创。常用后前位和侧位。

2. 脑血管造影

脑血管造影是将有机碘对比剂引入脑血管使脑血管显影的一种有创的检查方法，包括颈动脉造影和椎动脉造影。通常经股动脉穿刺和直接颈动脉穿刺，采用 DSA 技术，分别摄取脑动脉期、静脉期和静脉窦期图像。总并发症发生率为 8.5%，包括穿刺局部并发症，系统性并发症（包括造影剂过敏）和神经系统并发症，可以是暂时也可以是永久性的。

3. 脑 CT

脑 CT 包括平扫、增强扫描、CT 血管成像和 CT 灌注成像等。

（1）CT 平扫：头部常规扫描以横断位为主，有时加扫冠状位。头部固定，常规以听眦线（眼外眦与外耳孔中心的连线）为基线，依次扫描 10~12 层，层厚 10 mm。检查垂体则可取直接冠状切面行高分辨扫描。如遇小的病变可行薄层扫描。检查后颅窝时则取与听眦线成 20° 层面。

（2）CT 增强扫描：静脉注射碘对比剂后观察血管结构，在血脑屏障异常区域，静脉内的对比剂直接进入脑实质内，因此增强后病灶可显示更为清晰，并且增强扫描还可以显示平扫未能显示的病灶。用法：非离子型碘对比剂，剂量 1.5~2.0 mL/kg，静脉内快速注入。碘过敏是 CT 增强扫描的禁忌证。

（3）CT 血管成像（CTA）：静脉团注碘对比剂，当对比剂流经脑血管时进行螺旋 CT 扫描，三维重建得到脑血管图像。CT 血管成像可观察病变与血管的关系。

（4）CT 灌注成像（DWI）：快速静脉团注碘对比剂后，对受检部位同一层面进行连续快速扫描，计算机三维重建得到半定量的脑实质血流灌注图像。它反映了脑实质的微循环和血流灌注情况。常用的评价指标有平均通过时间（MTT），脑血流速度（CBF），脑血容量（CBV），其关系是 CBF=CBV/MTT。

4. 脑 MRI

脑 MRI 包括 MRI 平扫、增强 MRI 扫描、MR 血管成像和功能性磁共振等。

（1）平扫 MRI：常规扫描采用横断位扫描，也可根据病变部位选择冠状位和（或）矢状位扫描。常用自旋回波（SE）序列 T1WI 和 T2WI，层厚 8~10 mm，薄层则可用 2~5 mm。快速自旋回波序列（FSE）、梯度回波序列、脂肪抑制和水抑制成像也常在颅脑中应用。

（2）增强 MRI：对比剂常用 Gd-DTPA，剂量 0.1~0.2 mmol/kg（0.2~0.4 mL/kg）。增强后病灶显示更清晰，还有助于显示平扫未能显示的细小或多发病灶，明确病变的部位和范围，鉴别肿瘤与水肿，肿瘤术后复发与术后改变等。还用于脑血管病的诊断。

（3）MR 血管成像（MRA）：是唯一无创性脑血管成像技术，通过比较血管内流动的血液与相对静止组织之间的信号差异，计算机后处理抑制背景静态组织信号，可仅显示脑血管和血流信号图像，无需造影剂就可较好的显示颅脑和颈部的大血管。临床最常用的 MRA 方法是时间飞越法（TOF）和相位对比法（PC）。

（4）功能性磁共振：是基于 MR 技术基础之上的脑功能性成像，反映脑的生理、生化和物质代谢等功能变化，已应用于临床领域。包括：①MR 弥散成像（DWI）：反映局部环境中水分子的弥散情况。DWI 能在脑部不可逆损伤后几分钟内就反映出脑的缺血变化，所以常被用于早期脑缺血性疾病的诊断；②MR 灌注成像（DWI）：反映脑组织微循环的分布和血流灌注情况；③磁共振波谱（MRS）：无创性反映脑内生化环境，可用于对脑组织某一感兴趣区（体素）内代谢产物的定量分析，常用的有磷−31 和氢质子波谱。分为单体素和多体素 MRS；④脑功能成像（fMRI）：用于脑组织神经活动的功能定位，成像基础主要是血氧水平依赖对比法（BOLD）。

第二节　正常表现

1. 颅骨 X 线平片表现

正常颅骨 X 线平片表现因个体、年龄和性别而有明显的差别。颅骨分为内板、外板和板障，内板、外板是密质骨，呈高密度的线形影；板障居中，密度较低。颅板的厚度因年龄和部位不同。颅骨间有颅缝相连，包括冠状缝、矢状缝和人字缝，呈不规则锯齿状透亮影。婴儿颅缝很宽，额部和枕部分别有前囟和后囟。颅缝中可有缝间骨存在。侧位片可显示蝶鞍的大小、形态和结构，形状可为椭圆形、扁平形或圆形，正常前后径为 7~16 mm，平均 11.5 mm，深径 7~14 mm，平均 9.5 mm。生理性钙化最常见于松果体、大脑镰、床突间韧带和脉络丛等。生理性钙化的移位对颅内占位性病变仅起提示作用。

2. 脑 DSA 表现

颈动脉 DSA 的动脉期脑血管表现，如图 19-1 a，b。

颈内动脉上升至颅底经颈动脉管穿过海绵窦入颅，可分为四段：颈段、岩骨段、海绵窦段和颅内段。颅内段先后发出眼动脉、脉络膜前动脉和后交通动脉，终支为大脑前动脉和大脑中动脉。各分支又依次发出多个小分支，分支间相互重叠、交通，结合正侧位片可辨认。各分支位置较为恒定，并与脑叶有一定的对应关系。

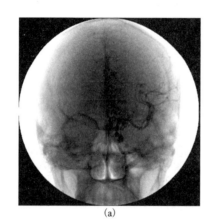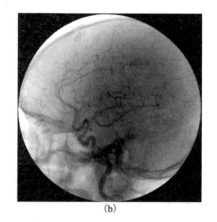

(a)　　　　　　　　　　　　　(b)

(a)后前位；(b)侧位。

图 19-1　正常颈动脉 DSA 的动脉期脑血管表现

3. 脑 CT 表现

正常脑 CT 表现见图 19-2 a, b, c, d, e, f。

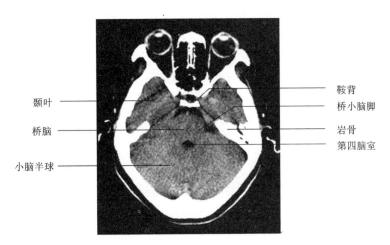

颞叶　　　　　　　　　　　　　　　　　　　　　鞍背
　　　　　　　　　　　　　　　　　　　　　　桥小脑脚
桥脑　　　　　　　　　　　　　　　　　　　　岩骨
　　　　　　　　　　　　　　　　　　　　　　第四脑室
小脑半球

图 19-2 （a）横断位桥脑层面

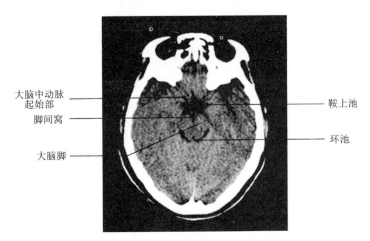

大脑中动脉
起始部　　　　　　　　　　　　　　　　　　　鞍上池
脚间窝
　　　　　　　　　　　　　　　　　　　　　　环池
大脑脚

图 19-2 （b）横断位鞍上池层面

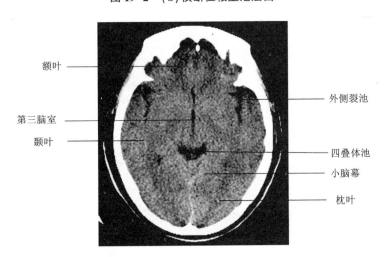

额叶
　　　　　　　　　　　　　　　　　　　　　　外侧裂池
第三脑室
颞叶　　　　　　　　　　　　　　　　　　　　四叠体池
　　　　　　　　　　　　　　　　　　　　　　小脑幕
　　　　　　　　　　　　　　　　　　　　　　枕叶

图 19-2 （c）横断位第三脑室层面

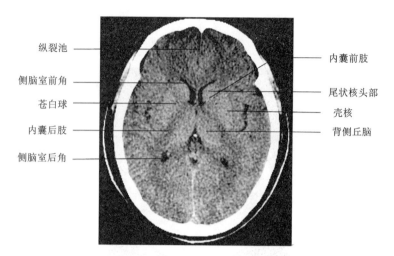

纵裂池 —————— 内囊前肢

侧脑室前角 ———— 尾状核头部

苍白球 ———————— 壳核

内囊后肢 ———————— 背侧丘脑

侧脑室后角 ——————

图 19-2　(d)横断位基底节层面

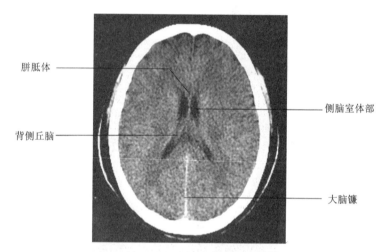

胼胝体 ———————— 侧脑室体部

背侧丘脑 ————————

大脑镰

图 19-2　(e)横断位侧脑室体部层面

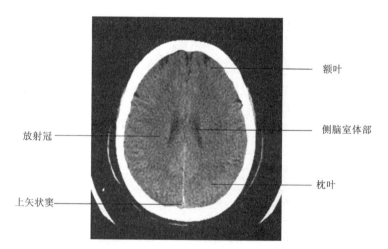

额叶

放射冠 ———————— 侧脑室体部

枕叶

上矢状窦 ————————

图 19-2　(f)横断位侧脑室顶部层面

（1）颅骨及空腔：颅骨表现为高密度，在颅底层面可以见到颈静脉孔、圆孔、卵圆孔和破裂孔等，呈低密度。乳突及鼻窦内气房气体呈低密度。

（2）脑实质：脑实质分为大脑额叶、颞叶、顶叶、枕叶以及小脑和脑干。皮质密度稍高于髓质，二者分界清楚。基底节是大脑深部的灰质核团，密度与皮质相近，包括三个部分：纹状体、屏状核和杏仁核。纹状体包括尾状核和豆状核，尾状核头部位于侧脑室前角后侧，体部沿丘脑的外侧面向后下行走。豆状核包括内侧的苍白球和外侧的壳核，位于尾状核和丘脑的外侧。屏状核呈带状，位于豆状核外侧和岛叶皮质之间。基底节可见钙化，表现为高密度。内囊是带状白质结构，位于尾状核、丘脑和豆状核之间，分为前肢、后肢和膝部。豆状核、屏状核和岛叶之间的条带状白质结构是外囊和最外囊。背侧丘脑紧邻第三脑室，外侧是内囊后肢和膝部。

（3）脑室系统：包括第四脑室、第三脑室、侧脑室和中脑导水管。其中侧脑室左右各一，两侧对称，分为前（额）角、后（枕）角、下（颞）角、体部和三角区五部分。脑室系统内充满脑脊液，呈均匀水样低密度。体部、后角和下角的交界区称为三角区。

（4）蛛网膜下腔：包括脑沟、脑裂和脑池等，内含脑脊液，故呈均匀水样低密度。脑池主要有小脑延髓池、鞍上池、环池、桥小脑角池、大脑外侧裂池、大脑纵裂池、脚间池和四叠体池等。小脑延髓池是其中最大的一个。鞍上池位于蝶鞍上方，多呈五角或六角型。

（5）增强扫描：正常脑组织呈轻度强化，血管结构直接强化。正常硬脑膜、垂体和松果体无血脑屏障，明显强化。

4.脑 MRI 表现

正常脑 MRI 表现见［图 19-3(a)～(d)］。

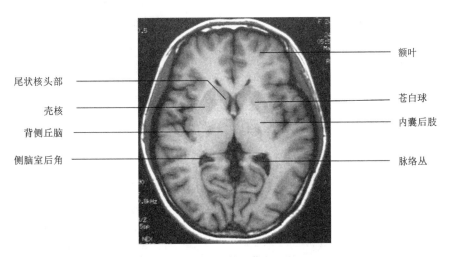

图 19-3　（a）横断位基底节区层面 T1WI

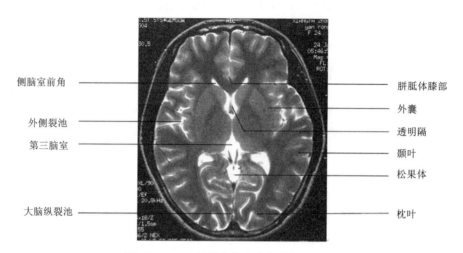

侧脑室前角
外侧裂池
第三脑室

大脑纵裂池

胼胝体膝部
外囊
透明隔
颞叶
松果体

枕叶

图 19-3　（b）横断位基底节区层面 T2WI

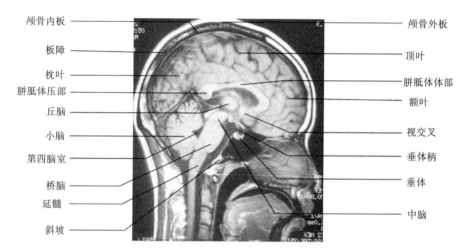

颅骨内板
板障
枕叶
胼胝体压部
丘脑
小脑
第四脑室
桥脑
延髓
斜坡

颅骨外板
顶叶
胼胝体体部
额叶
视交叉
垂体柄
垂体
中脑

图 19-3　（c）正中矢状位 T1WI

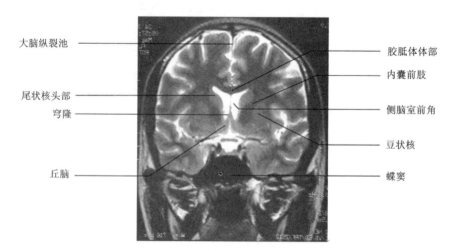

大脑纵裂池

尾状核头部
穹隆

丘脑

胼胝体体部
内囊前肢
侧脑室前角
豆状核
蝶窦

图 19-3　（d）冠状位 T2WI

（1）颅骨和软组织：颅骨内外板、颅内生理性钙化和脑膜由于所含质子数很少，T1WI 和 T2WI 为低信号。板障和头皮软组织则 T1WI 和 T2WI 均呈高信号。

（2）蛛网膜下隙和脑室系统：内含脑脊液，信号均匀，主要成分是水。脑脊液是长 T1 长 T2 物质，故蛛网膜下隙和脑室系统在 T1WI 上呈低信号，T2WI 呈高信号。水抑制序列则为低信号。

（3）脑实质：MRI 图像上皮质、髓质对比清晰。脑髓质 T1 和 T2 值均较短，故 T1WI 脑髓质的信号稍高于皮质，T2WI 则稍低于皮质。大脑深部灰质核团的密度与皮质相近。

（4）脑血管：由于流空效应，MRI 能直接显示血管结构，T1WI 和 T2WI 上均呈低信号。当血液流速较慢时则为高信号。

（5）颅神经：高场强 MRI 可以清楚显示颅神经的走行，T1WI 上呈等信号。

（6）增强扫描：虽然 MRI 使用的对比剂与 CT 不同，但其组织强化的情况与 CT 相似。

第三节　基本病变

1.颅骨 X 线平片表现

（1）颅内压增高：较常见，可见于多种颅内疾病，只表明颅内有病变，但无助于病变的定位和定性诊断。儿童常表现为头颅增大、颅缝增宽、颅板变薄和脑回压迹增多。成人则主要表现为蝶鞍的改变，如蝶鞍增大、鞍底和鞍背骨质模糊或消失等。

（2）颅内肿瘤定位征：①局限性颅骨改变，可表现为颅骨的局限性增生、硬化或骨质破坏，多见于邻近颅骨或脑表面的肿瘤，如脑膜瘤；②蝶鞍改变，邻近蝶鞍的肿瘤可引起蝶鞍的改变。鞍内的肿瘤，使蝶鞍呈气球样扩大，见于垂体瘤；鞍上肿瘤造成鞍背缩短，蝶鞍扁平；鞍旁肿瘤，鞍底受压下陷，甚至形成双鞍底，患侧前床突上翘或破坏；③钙化，包括肿瘤钙化和生理性钙化的移位。根据肿瘤钙化的位置和形态可大致推断肿瘤的位置和性质，松果体钙化移位可大致估计肿瘤的位置。

2.DSA 表现

脑 DSA 是诊断脑血管疾病的金标准。可见脑血管的移位、血管形态和血循环的改变。颅内占位性病变、水肿等推压脑组织使脑血管移位、聚集或分离、牵直或扭曲变形。某些肿瘤动脉造影可显示异常血管生成和肿瘤染色。

3.脑 CT 表现

（1）平扫密度改变：①高密度病灶，密度高于正常脑组织者为高密度，可见于新鲜血肿、钙化和富血管性肿瘤；②低密度病灶，常见于某些肿瘤、炎症、水肿、梗死、囊肿、脂肪瘤和脓肿等；③等密度病灶，密度与正常脑组织相同，可见于某些肿瘤、血肿吸收期和血管性病变等；④混杂密度病灶，见于多种成分，如钙化、出血、低密度脂肪、囊变和坏死等并存的病变，多见于肿瘤、血管性病变、脓肿等。

（2）增强扫描表现：颅内病变的强化特征是由于血脑屏障形成不良、异常血管增生引起的。①均匀性强化：见于脑膜瘤、转移瘤、生殖细胞瘤、神经鞘瘤、动脉瘤和肉芽肿等；②非均匀性强化：见于血管畸形、胶质瘤、脱髓鞘病变和炎症等；③环形强化：见于脑脓肿、转移瘤、胶质瘤和结核瘤等；④无强化：见于脑炎、囊肿和水肿等。

（3）脑结构改变：①占位效应，为颅内占位性病变如肿瘤和出血等以及水肿所致，表现为中线结构的移位，局部脑沟、脑池、脑室受压变窄或闭塞，中线结构移向对侧等；②脑积水，分为交通性脑积水和阻塞性脑积水。前者是由于脑室外脑脊液循环通路受阻或吸收障碍所致，表现为脑室系统普遍性增大，脑池增宽；后者为第四脑室出口以上部位发生阻塞造成，仅见梗阻近侧脑室增大，脑池无增宽；③脑萎缩，可分为局限性或弥漫性。皮质萎缩显示脑沟和脑裂增宽，脑池扩大；髓质萎缩则显示脑室扩大。

（4）颅骨改变：①颅骨本身病变，如外伤性骨折、炎症和肿瘤等；②颅内病变累及颅骨，如蝶鞍、内耳道和颈静脉孔扩大以及局部骨质增生和（或）破坏，常见于相应部位的肿瘤性病变。这些征象可协助颅内病变的定位和定性诊断。

4. 脑 MRI 表现

(1)出血:因血肿时期而异。①超急性期(24 小时内):血肿内主要为含氧合血红蛋白的红细胞,血肿在 T1WI 和 T2WI 上呈等信号;②急性期(1~2 天):血肿内红细胞主要为脱氧血红蛋白。T1WI 和 T2WI 呈等或稍低信号,不易发现;③亚急性期(3 天~3 周):红细胞溶解变性,血肿周围脑白质水肿达到高峰,脱氧血红蛋白进一步变性为正铁血红蛋白以及含铁血黄素,后者在血肿周围沉积。早期(3~5 天),血肿 T1WI 信号由周围向中心逐渐增高,T2WI 呈低信号;中期(6~10 天),T1WI 高信号区域由外周向中心扩大,T2WI 也为高信号;晚期(11 天~3 周),T1WI 和 T2WI 均呈高信号,血肿周围可出现含铁血黄素沉积形成的 T2WI 低信号环;④慢性期(3 周以后):随着血肿进一步演变,在血红蛋白分解同时产生大量含铁血黄素和铁蛋白,形成一类似脑脊液的囊腔,T1WI 呈低信号,T2WI 呈高信号,周围含铁血黄素沉积形成的 T2WI 低信号环更加明显。

(2)脑梗死:急性脑梗死早期(超急性期梗死)在 T1WI 和 T2WI 上信号多正常。病变沿各动脉血供区分布,可见占位效应。慢性期占位效应减轻,以脑萎缩性改变为主。急性期和慢性期由于脑水肿、坏死和囊变,T1WI 上呈低信号,T2WI 上呈高信号。

(3)肿块:一般肿块由于含水量高,T1WI 上呈低信号、T2WI 呈高信号;含顺磁性物质的黑色素瘤 T1WI 呈高信号,T2WI 呈低信号;钙化和骨化性肿块则 T1WI 上呈低信号、T2WI 上呈低信号;脂肪类肿块 T1WI 上呈高信号、T2WI 呈高信号。

(4)囊肿:含液囊肿 T1WI 上呈低信号,T2WI 上呈高信号,而含黏蛋白和类脂性囊肿时 T1WI 上呈高信号,T2WI 上呈高信号。

(5)水肿:脑组织发生水肿时,T1 和 T2 值均延长,T1WI 上为低信号,T2WI 上为高信号。可见占位效应。

5. 比较影像学

综上所述,从脑部影像学正常和基本病变表现可以看出,各种检查技术,包括 X 线平片,DSA,CT 和 MRI 等,各具优缺点。在设计某种疾病的影像学检查程序时,应做出合理选择,制定个性化的解决方案,首要原则是针对要解决的问题选择创伤最小的检查技术,其次就是选择能提供最多信息的检查方法。

随着 CT 和 MRI 技术的不断发展,颅骨 X 线平片已很少使用。脑 CT 和 MRI 已成为脑部影像学检查中最常用的手段,MRI 的出现使 CT 的在脑部的应用减少,但并不能完全取 CT,二者各有所长。对于颅骨本身的病变或颅内病变对颅骨的侵犯,X 线平片仅能大致反映颅骨骨质的改变,CT 和 MRI 能更敏感而详细的显示颅骨骨质的异常,并且有利于观察到与其相关的颅内病变。颅骨 X 线平片对颅内占位性病变的诊断价值也极为有限。

对于脑血管病的诊断,DSA 虽然是金标准,但因其属于有创检查,价值有限,单独应用已大为减少。近年来无创性 MRA 和微创性 CTA 技术发展迅速,已作为常规脑血管成像技术,与常规 MRI 和 CT 的联合应用逐步取代了传统的动脉造影技术。

CT 诊断对于骨质的改变和钙化特别是某些中枢神经系统肿瘤中的钙化具有特异性。而 MRI 在这两方面均劣于 CT。颅内炎症和脱髓鞘病变只能行 CT 和 MRI 检查,并且 MRI 优于 CT。结合增强扫描 CT 可对大部分颅内病变作出定位和定性诊断,而 MRI 则对中线结构、后颅窝和近颅底等病变的诊断敏感性高于 CT。对于脑出血性疾病,CT 对急性期出血的诊断价值优于 MRI,故通常行 CT 检查,但对于 CT 上呈等密度的慢性期血肿,MRI 则更有意义。CT 对蛛网膜下腔出血的显示优于 MRI,但当出血量较少时,MRI 比 CT 更敏感。

功能性磁共振成像反映了脑部的生理、生化和物质代谢,为颅内占位性病变的诊断、鉴别诊断和治疗提高了重要依据。DWI 已常用于早期脑梗死的诊断。

第四节　常见疾病诊断

1.头部外伤

头部外伤发病率高，为小儿及成人致残及致死的首位原因。它分为轻度、中度、重度及严重脑外伤。头部外伤的影像表现包括脑挫裂伤、颅内血肿、硬膜外血肿、硬膜下血肿及蛛网膜下腔出血。在严重头部外伤患者发病及治疗时，头颅平片作用有限，往往仅用于确定是否存在颅骨线形骨折。CT 扫描是头部外伤最有效的检查方法，能迅速检测急性出血（平扫表现为高密度），常常非常准确。CT 对评估面部及颅骨骨折很有帮助。CT 检查头部外伤时应常规包括脑组织窗及骨窗。CT 检查不易显示脑外颞下部出血、额下部出血及后颅窝出血。在检测弥漫性轴索损伤及血管损伤方面，CT 不如 MRI 敏感。

（1）脑挫裂伤：

1）临床及病理表现：脑挫伤时，颅内有散在出血灶、颅内血肿及脑组织肿胀。如果伴随脑、脑膜及脑血管的撕裂，定义为脑裂伤。脑挫伤合并脑裂伤，称为脑挫裂伤。

2）影像学表现：低密度水肿区，散在高密度出血灶（图 19-4）。但出血灶较小，诊断较容易。

（2）硬膜外血肿：

1）临床及病理表现：颅骨内板与硬脑膜之间的潜在腔隙称为硬膜外腔。硬膜外血肿最常见的原因是头部外伤合并颞骨骨折，骨折跨过脑膜中动脉或静脉区域。脑膜中动脉或静脉的撕裂导致血液外溢和急性硬膜外血肿。血肿常常位于颞顶叶部位。

2）影像学表现：

①CT 上表现为颅内脑外的高密度肿块，呈梭形（图 19-5）。采用骨窗发现有无颅骨骨折。慢性硬膜外血肿（3 周以上）常表现为低密度，硬膜下包膜有强化，可呈凹面形。

②MRI 上，根据血肿发生时间不同，有不同的影像表现，急性期血肿（3 天以内），T1 等信号，T2 低信号。几天后，亚急性血肿表现为 T1 与 T2 均为高信号。慢性期血肿，T1 低信号，T2 高信号。在所有脉冲序列上，硬脑膜组成血肿边缘表现为低信号。

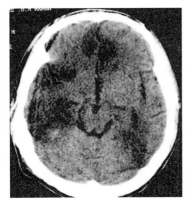

CT 平扫示多发低密度灶及散布的斑片状高密度出血灶。

图 19-4　脑挫裂伤 CT 表现

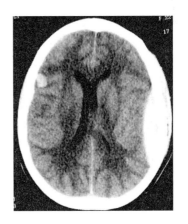

CT 示左颞部高密度血肿，梭形改变。

图 19-5　急性硬膜外血肿 CT 表现

（3）硬膜下血肿：

1）临床及病理表现：硬膜下隙为蛛网膜与硬脑膜之间的潜在腔隙。严重的头部外伤和桥静脉撕裂造成硬膜下血肿。硬膜下血肿见于近 30%严重头部闭合外伤的患者。3 天内为急性硬膜下血肿；3 天至 3 周为亚急性硬膜下血肿，3 周以上为慢性硬膜下血肿。

2)影像学表现:

①急性硬膜下血肿,CT表现为高密度新月形脑外肿块[图19-6(a)],血肿的厚度可大可小,向内凹陷。与硬膜外血肿相比较,硬膜下血肿不受颅缝限制,并且占位效应明显。亚急性硬膜下血肿表现为等密度或低密度。亚急性或慢性硬膜下血肿边缘可以强化,这是由硬膜下血管形成所致。如果灰白质交界面可见,并从正常的位置内移,应考虑颅内脑外的肿块性病变。增强扫描,皮质静脉内移有助于诊断等密度硬模下血肿。

②MRI上,硬膜下血肿的信号与血液的信号一致。急性硬膜下血肿T1等信号,T2低信号;亚急性硬膜下血肿T1、T2高信号。但是,随着时间的延长,T1高信号逐渐减低,与脑实质一样呈等信号,容易与硬膜下积脓相混淆。此时,临床特征相当重要。慢性硬膜下血肿T1上表现为低信号、T2为高信号[图19-6(b)、(c)]。

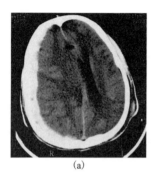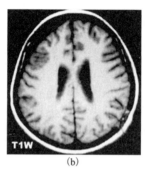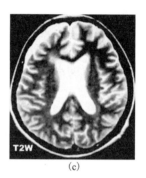

(a)CT平扫显示高密度病灶呈新月状,占位效应明显;(b)T1WI显示右额部病灶呈低信号;(c)T2WI显示右额部病灶呈高信号。

图19-6 急性硬膜下血肿CT和MRI表现

2.颅内感染及非感染性疾病

(1)软脑膜炎:

1)临床及病理表现:软脑膜炎常由远处感染性病灶直接血性扩散而来。病原菌也可通过没有血脑屏障的区域进入,如脉络丛、脑室周围的器官。直接由鼻窦炎、眼内蜂窝织炎、乳突炎、中耳炎蔓延相对少见。随着脑脊液流动的停滞,细菌便有机会侵犯脑膜并繁殖。感染早期阶段,软脑膜与蛛网膜充血。蛛网膜分泌物覆盖在脑组织上,特别是脑沟及基底池内。软脑膜增厚。临床特征包括发烧、头痛、呕吐、癫痫发作以及克尼格氏征等。

2)影像学表现:病变早期或及时治疗在影像上可表现正常。除此之外,急性脑膜炎的表现如下:蛛网膜下隙扩大,特别是基底池和沿大脑纵裂的部位,压水像(FLAIR)序列上为高信号,急性脑肿胀和交通性脑积水,伴颞角扩大,基底池消失。

(2)脑脓肿:

1)临床及病理表现:脑脓肿常由原发感染病灶通过血性传播形成。病因包括耳部炎症、鼻窦炎、穿透性外伤、手术后感染、心源性感染、药物滥用、脓毒血症等。最常见的发病部位是沿大脑中动脉分布的额叶及顶叶脑实质内。脓肿可单房或多房,可单发或多发,脓肿的形成分为4个阶段:①脑炎早期(1~3天);②脑炎晚期(4~9天);③脓肿形成早期(10~13天);④脓肿形成晚期(14天以后)。

2)影像学表现:

①CT上,脑炎阶段病变表现为低密度,有占位效应,斑片状或脑回样强化。2~3周后,成熟的脑脓肿形成,CT上表现为病灶中心低密度,周围低密度水肿围绕。化脓性脑脓肿可见均匀的环形强化[图19-7(c)]。

②MRI上,脑炎阶段病变T1表现为低信号,T2/FLAIR表现为高信号,病灶中心位于皮质与髓质交界处,呈斑片状强化。脑炎晚期,环行强化可见。2~3周后,成熟的脑脓肿形成,T1表现为圆形边界清晰的

低信号肿块［图19-7（a）］，占位效应明显，周围有低信号水肿带围绕。T2/FLAIR 上病灶腔内及周围可见高信号灶［图19-7（b）］，可见厚度不等的同心圆征。化脓性脑脓肿可见均匀的环形强化［图19-7（d）］。

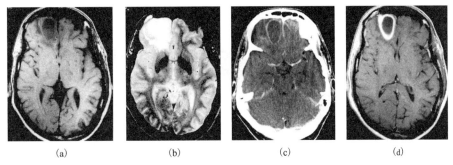

(a)　　　　(b)　　　　(c)　　　　(d)

（a）T1WI 示右额叶卵圆形低信号灶；（b）T2WI 示高信号病灶；（c）CT 增强扫描示环行强化；（d）MRI 增强示环行强化。

图 19-7　脑脓肿 CT 和 MRI 表现

（3）结核：

1）临床及病理表现：近年来结核的发病率显著升高，特别是随着耐药菌株及艾滋病的出现。有 5%～10% 的结核病累及中枢神经系统。颅内结核有两种病理学过程：结核性脑膜炎和颅内结核瘤。临床特征包括昏迷、发热、头疼、嗜睡、假性脑膜炎。腰穿脑脊液检查糖分减少，蛋白质增加，淋巴细胞增多，涂片阴性。

2）影像学表现：影像特征依赖于感染的阶段。脑膜炎期，平扫时由于渗出物密度增加，基底池与外侧裂池显示不清。增强时，可见明显强化。由于基底池蛋白质分泌物增加，FLAIR 信号增高。脑池明显强化，延伸至大脑半球的沟裂及皮质的表面。基底部脑膜较少有钙化。病变晚期可见交通性脑积水。脑内结核瘤呈结节状，可以单发但常为多发，有占位效应及瘤周水肿，钙化不常见（少于 20%）。典型结核瘤表现为病灶中心 T2 上为高信号，CT 上为低密度，结核瘤壁在 T1 上为高信号但在 T2/FLAIR 为低信号。结节周围 T2/FLAIR 为高信号，CT 上为低密度，这代表水肿合并占位效应。增强扫描为环形或结节状强化（图19-8）。

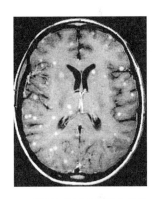

T1WI 增强扫描示多发强化结节，部分病灶周围有水肿。

图 19-8　结核瘤 MR 表现

3. 脑肿瘤

（1）脑膜瘤：

1）临床和病理表现：脑膜瘤为颅内脑外最常见的肿瘤。由于脑膜瘤起源于蛛网膜粒帽细胞，它能出现在蛛网膜存在的任何地方。脑膜瘤最常见发病位置是矢状窦旁、脑凸面、蝶骨嵴、桥小脑角池、嗅沟、蝶窦平面。90% 发生在幕上。据 2016 年世界卫生组织（WHO）中枢神经系统肿瘤分级标准，脑膜瘤分为三级，脑膜瘤（WHO I 级）、非典型性脑膜瘤（WHO II 级）和间变型脑膜瘤（WHO III 级）。

2）影像学表现：

①CT 平扫，约 75% 的脑膜瘤表现为稍高密度［图19-9（a）］。20% 的病例可见钙化、囊变、骨化、软骨化及脂肪退变相对少见。CT 增强脑膜瘤明显强化［图19-9（b）］。通过 CT 检查，可见"脑膜尾征"，增强的新月形硬膜由病灶向远处延伸形成。骨质改变有增生肥厚或骨质溶解，邻近病灶的骨质可以增厚。

②MRI 在显示脑膜瘤的范围、窦性侵犯或血栓、病变的血供、颅内水肿、骨质侵犯方面优于 CT。脑膜瘤的典型 MRI 特征为 T1 上相对灰质呈等或稍低信号［图19-9（c）］，T2 为等或稍高信号。可见"裂隙征"。通过 MRI 检查，可见"脑膜尾征"，增强的新月形硬膜由病灶向远处延伸形成［图19-9（d）］，这种征象为脑

膜瘤的典型表现，可见于大多数病例。脑膜瘤的实质水肿程度各不相同，尽管大的脑膜瘤有较大范围的水肿，小的脑膜瘤也能引起较大范围的白质水肿。水肿的程度与病变的位置相关，靠近脑皮质的脑膜瘤比基底池或此平面的脑膜瘤更容易引起水肿。脑膜瘤的水肿可能与压迫性缺血，静脉血液淤滞、病变的侵袭性生长或软脑膜血管的寄生物感染有关。静脉窦阻塞或静脉血栓形成也可引起脑实质的水肿。

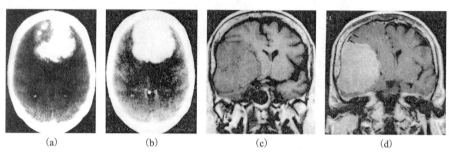

（a）CT平扫示大脑镰旁高密度肿块，钙化明显；（b）CT增强示病灶明显强化；（c）MRI冠状位T1WI示右颞部等、稍低信号肿块；（d）MRI冠状位T1WI增强扫描示右颞部肿块明显强化，可见脑膜尾征。

图19-9　脑膜瘤CT和MR表现

（2）胶质瘤：

1）临床及病理表现：胶质瘤占颅内肿瘤的35%~55%。脑胶质瘤包括星型细胞瘤、胶质母细胞瘤、少突胶质细胞瘤、室管膜瘤、室管膜下瘤、髓母细胞瘤、神经母细胞瘤、神经节细胞瘤、神经节神经胶质瘤。WHO中枢神经系统肿瘤分类将脑胶质瘤分为Ⅰ-Ⅳ级，Ⅰ级、Ⅱ级为低级别脑胶质瘤，Ⅲ级、Ⅳ级为高级别脑胶质瘤。弥漫性胶质瘤包括WHOⅡ级和Ⅲ级星形细胞瘤、Ⅱ级和Ⅲ级少突胶质细胞瘤、Ⅳ级胶质母细胞瘤以及儿童相关的弥漫性胶质瘤。WHOⅡ级弥漫星形细胞瘤、WHOⅢ级间变星形细胞瘤以及胶质母细胞瘤都分为异柠檬酸脱氢酶（IDH）突变型、IDH野生型和无特殊指定（NOS）三类。

2）影像学表现：CT扫描胶质瘤表现为低密度［图19-10（a）］。T1为低信号［图19-10（b）］，T2/FLAIR表现为高信号［图19-10（c）］，肿瘤囊变的部分在T1和T2上有类似脑脊液的信号改变［图19-10（d）］，但由于含有大量的蛋白，PDWI或FLAIR序列上信号高于脑脊液。病灶边界清晰。病灶的实性部分强化明显。Ⅰ-Ⅱ级胶质瘤没有或者轻微强化，Ⅲ-Ⅳ级胶质瘤明显强化［图19-10（e）］。胶质瘤囊变很常见，但少见钙化。Ⅰ-Ⅱ级胶质瘤占位效应较轻，Ⅲ-Ⅳ级胶质瘤占位效应明显。

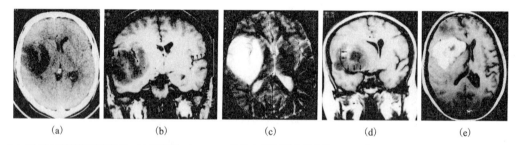

（a）CT示右颞部低密度肿块，边界清晰；（b）T1WI显示右颞部低信号肿块，边界清晰；（c）T2WI呈高信号，信号均匀，病理分级为Ⅱ级胶质细胞瘤；（d）T1WI显示右颞部低信号肿块，信号不均匀；（e）T1WI增强扫描示病灶环行强化，病理分级为Ⅳ级胶质细胞瘤。

图19-10　脑胶质瘤CT和MRI表现

（3）转移瘤：

1）临床及病理表现：转移瘤是成人幕上最常见的肿瘤，占颅内肿瘤的20%。70%~80%为多发，其中

20%的病例有 2 个病灶。转移到幕上的原发肿瘤有肺癌(50%)，乳腺癌(15%)，黑色素瘤(11%)，肾及胃肠道的原发肿瘤。病变的特征是位于灰白质交界部位，因为小血管直接延伸至皮质或白质区域。这些病变随着血液的动态流动，多见于颈内动脉系统分布区域，椎基底动脉系统少见(80%比 20%)，特别是大脑中动脉分布区域。80%的转移瘤位于灰白质交界区，3%位于基底神经节区，15%位于小脑部位。

2)影像学表现：转移瘤常表现为边界清晰，强化明显，中度水肿。如果不合并出血，CT 平扫表现为低密度，T1 表现为低信号，T2 信号的高低取决于有无出血、瘤内坏死、囊变、高核质比及顺磁性物质含量。几乎所有转移瘤都有一定程度的强化，强化形式可以是实性强化、环行强化、规则强化、均匀或不均匀强化(图 19-11)。相对胶质瘤，转移瘤定位明确，边界清晰。除了皮质区的转移瘤极少水肿或无水肿，其他部位的血管源性水肿往往与转移瘤的大小不成比例。无水肿时，T2 可能会遗漏病变。在这种情况下，增强扫描对病变的鉴别诊断相当重要。

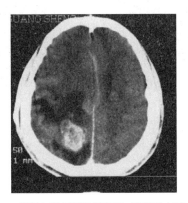

CT 增强扫描显示脑转移瘤，脑实质内可见多个结节灶，强化明显，伴周围水肿。

图 19-11 脑转移瘤 CT 表现

4.脑血管性病变

(1)脑梗死：

1)临床及病理表现：大动脉的粥样硬化、心血管栓塞和腔隙性梗死为缺血性脑卒中最常见的原因。复发性卒中在心源性卒中患者中最为常见，1 个月病死率也最高。缺血性脑卒中最主要的原因是栓塞，但栓塞的来源多种多样，可能是颈动脉的狭窄或阻塞、粥样硬化斑块、溃疡、心源性病变(来自心源性的栓子占缺血性卒中的 15%~20%)。分水岭梗死发生在主要动脉远端分布供应的区域。主要的分水岭梗死发生在大脑前动脉、中动脉和大脑中动脉、后动脉之间。腔隙性梗死是微小的发生囊变的脑梗死，由小的终末动脉阻塞形成。病变好发于基底节、内囊、桥脑和放射冠部位，病灶直径一般为 5 mm 左右，不超过 15 mm。出血性梗死为梗死的过程中合并有出血。

2)影像学表现：

①CT 技术的进步，在显示急性脑卒中的细微病变方面变得越来越敏感。部分梗死在 6 小时内可见灰白质界限模糊。大脑中动脉近端的高密度为脑梗死的早期征象，代表大脑中动脉内的急性血栓或钙化的栓子。12~24 小时内，在相应的血管分布区域可见分界不清的低密度病灶[图 19-12(a)、(b)]。起初占位效应不明显，24 小时后病灶边缘清晰，占位效应明显。可见脑沟的不对称及一侧脑室的轻微压迫。病变发生后的 2~5 天，占位效应达到顶峰。梗死前 3 天强化不明显，强化出现后使梗死的低密度区模糊。占位效应在 5 天后开始减退，常常 2~4 周后消失。占位效应持久出现超过 6 周强烈提示有其他病变的存在，肿瘤应最常考虑。大约 50%的病例，在第 2~3 周，梗死灶由低密度变为等密度。CT 上称之为"雾化"效应，常因坏死脑组织充血、重新灌注、淤血性出血以及巨噬细胞的作用所致。这些病变在 4 周后，恢复为边界清晰的低密度病灶。此时，在受影响的血管分布区域脑实质缺乏，常常不强化，占位效应不明显。

②DWI 和 PWI 为 MRI 的新技术，比 T2 敏感。DWI 在梗死发生后的 2~3 分钟即可检测到脑缺血（在大鼠），人类发生梗死 30 分钟内即可检测。如果恰好在脑梗死后的几个小时内，可以将其与常规 MRI 进行比较，这具有积极的意义。PWI 不同于 DWI 的在于它的目的是检测毛细血管水平的微小灌注情况。PWI 联合 DWI 已被提倡用来治疗急性脑卒中。在这种情况下，灌注与弥散异常征象的差别越大，越需要进行急性血管内介入溶栓治疗。如果没有灌注的异常，或者灌注与弥散病变的面积相等，进行溶栓治疗的效果就不大。

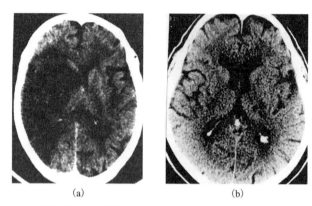

(a) CT 右额颞枕部大片低密度病灶，为大脑中动脉梗死所致；(b) CT
显示左侧丘脑可见直径约 10 mm 低密度灶，为腔隙性梗死。

图 19-12　脑梗死 CT 表现

（2）脑出血：

1）临床及病理表现：颅内脑实质出血仅占脑卒中的 10% 左右，平均发病年龄为 65 岁。70%~90% 的病例中，高血压是非创伤性脑实质出血的原因。脑实质出血也可由血管病变引起，包括淀粉样血管病、微动脉瘤、纤维动脉炎，这些加重了高血压的影响。不仅仅是高血压，实际上血压的快速变化也容易引起出血。这也是可卡因和其他药物与颅内出血发生率增加有关的原因之一。大概有 1/2 至 2/3 的脑出血发生在基底神经节-丘脑部位（特别是壳核），但脑出血的位置并不确定。近似 10%~50% 的脑出血发生在脑叶内，10%~15% 的脑出血发生在脑干，5%~10% 的脑出血发生在小脑。

2）影像学表现：脑出血的不同阶段有不同的 CT 和 MR 表现。超急性期出血（24 小时内），CT 表现为高密度病灶 [图 19-13（a）]，MRI 上，T1 表现为低信号，T2 上中心高信号外周低信号，因为病变为氧合血红蛋白而外周为脱氧血红蛋白。急性期出血（1~7 天），CT 表现为高密度病灶，T1 表现为等信号到低信号，T2 上由于脱氧血红蛋白的影响表现为明显的低信号。红细胞内脱氧血红蛋白氧化为正铁血红蛋白，这与高蛋白浓缩引起 T1 的缩短相一致，使正铁血红蛋白在 T1 上表现为高信号。因为顺磁性的正铁血红蛋白位于红细胞内，T2 上也表现为明显的高信号。亚急性期出血（1 周至 1 个月），正铁血红蛋白不如脱氧血红蛋白稳定，亚铁血红蛋白自发从蛋白质分子上丢失，游离的亚铁血红蛋白和（或）其他的外源性化合物（包括过氧化物和超氧化物）使红细胞溶解。伴随着蛋白质的分解及剩余的细胞外正铁血红蛋白的稀释，尽管蛋白质浓度下降，由于正铁血红蛋白的亚铁血红蛋白的 T1 缩短效应，即使蛋白浓度相对较低，T1 上仍表现为高信号 [图 19-13（b）]。由于红细胞分解局部磁场的不均匀性的损失及蛋白质浓度的下降，在 T2 上血肿信号增强 [图 19-13（c）]。慢性期出血（1 个月后），几个月后血块内液体和蛋白质几乎完全分解和吸收，代谢的血红蛋白分子中的铁原子沉积在含铁血黄素和铁蛋白分子中，由于血脑屏障的恢复而不能离开脑实质。T1 和 T2 上均表现为低信号，CT 图像上为低密度。

（3）动脉瘤：

1）临床及病理表现：动脉瘤为动脉的局限性扩张。动脉瘤形成的主要原因有动脉夹层、动脉粥样硬化、真菌或霉菌感染、肿瘤、外伤等。动脉瘤的形状有粟粒状、梭形和囊状。中枢神经系统最常见的动脉

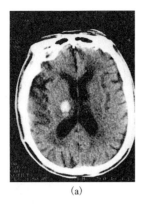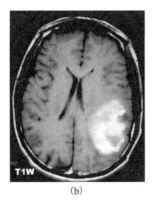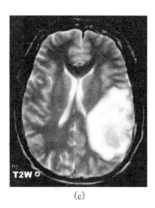

(a)   (b)   (c)

(a)CT平扫显示右侧丘脑区圆形的高密度灶，为丘脑血肿；(b)T1WI显示左颞枕叶不均匀高信号占位，亚急性血肿；(c)同一病例T2WI呈高信号改变。

图19-13 脑出血CT和MRI表现

瘤为粟粒状动脉瘤。梭性动脉瘤是粥样硬化动脉的扩张，多发生在椎基底动脉。夹层动脉瘤常发生在外伤后或自发出现。血管破裂出血引起的机化性血肿称为假性动脉瘤。假性动脉瘤没有真正的瘤壁，血肿由血管外膜限制。霉菌性动脉瘤常常由心内膜炎引起，可以是梭形或囊状，多位于大脑中动脉分布的外围区。多发性外周动脉瘤提示该病。成人尸检动脉瘤的发病率为1%~6%。尽管大部分动脉瘤为散发病例，但也有家族发病倾向，其子孙发病率偏高。动脉瘤会随着时间推移增大，较大的动脉瘤更容易出血。动脉瘤破裂出血的平均发病年龄近50岁。50%~70%的蛛网膜下隙出血由动脉瘤破裂引起。蛛网膜下腔出血的其他原因有原发性脑实质出血引起的继发出血、外伤、脑内动静脉畸形等。

2)影像学表现：CT能够诊断蛛网膜下隙出血，通过显示出血量最大的位置，大致判断出血性动脉瘤的位置。大脑纵裂及侧脑室的出血常由大脑前交通动脉的动脉瘤所致，外侧裂池的出血多由大脑中动脉的动脉瘤所致[图19-14(a)]，如果出血位于第四脑室常提示小脑后下动脉瘤。MR相当有价值，当蛛网膜下隙出血在CT消退时，T1上出血呈高信号改变。T1及T2上瘤腔呈圆形低信号改变，瘤内血栓呈低信号或高信号[图19-14(b)]。CTA和MRA为新技术。通过CTA、MRA和/或DSA[图14-14(c)]，能够清晰显示动脉瘤、瘤内血栓、瘤颈、瘤体及载瘤动脉。这对于治疗非常有用。

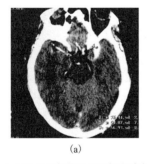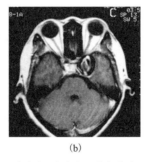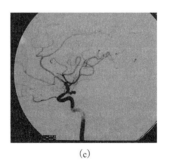

(a)   (b)   (c)

(a)CT增强扫描显示左侧海绵窦区动脉瘤，瘤内未强化部分为血栓；(b)MRI显示动脉瘤，T1上血栓呈高信号；(c)DSA显示后交通动脉瘤，可见瘤体、瘤颈及载瘤动脉。

图19-14 脑动脉瘤CT、MRI和DSA表现

(4)动静脉畸形：

1)临床及病理表现：动静脉畸形为先天血管畸形，起源于胎儿时期，但常在30或40年后产生症状。常由一根或多根增粗的供血动脉和增粗的早期引流静脉组成。有出血倾向，常导致蛛网膜下隙出血或脑实质出血。窃血现象是动静脉畸形的并发症。这种情况下，血液优先供应动静脉畸形，正常脑实质相对供血

不足。窃血会引起局部神经症状，癫痫，最终导致受影响区域脑功能的丧失。供血动脉、瘤巢和引流静脉为诊断动静脉畸形的主要因素。

2）影像学表现：CT 平扫显示脑实质中杂乱的高密度血管影，外表呈弯曲状、点状或不规则状。可见曲状或斑点状钙化，强化明显[图 14-15（a）]。MR 上，大多数脉冲序列上可见继快速流动后曲状的流空效应，可见扩张的供血动脉。MRA 在描述动静脉畸形的外形时作用较大[图 14-15（b）]。三维时间飞跃法和三维相位对比技术有一定作用，增强扫描使动静脉畸形显示更清楚，特别是静脉。脑血管造影是诊断动静脉畸形的金标准。通过显示扩大的供血动脉、瘤巢及引流静脉诊断动静脉畸形[图 14-15（c）]。

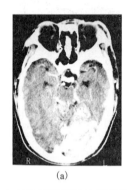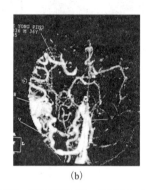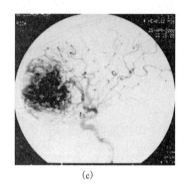

| (a) | (b) | (c) |

（a）CT 增强扫描显示动静脉畸形，瘤巢清晰可见；（b）MRA 显示 AVM 扩大的供血动脉、瘤巢及扩大的引流静脉；（c）DSA 显示 AVM 扩大的供血动脉、瘤巢及引流静脉。

图 19-15 脑动静脉畸形 CT、MRI 和 DSA 表现

（谭艳，胡瑟，孙祥茹，江浩茹，田大伟，肖恩华，刘军）

Chapter 19

Brain

Section 1　Method of examination

1. Plain Films

This technique is simple、 economical and noninvasive. Skull radiography is usually performed in posteroanterior (PA) and lateral projections.

2. Cerebral Angiography

Iodinated contrast is injected into the cerebral vessel to show the cerebral vessel, including carotid arteriography and vertebral arteriography. Cerebral angiography is usually performed by the transfemoral artery technique or direct percutaneous carotid puncture. Digital subtraction angiography(DSA) is usually performed to get the images of the arterial phase, the venous phase and the sinus venosus phase. The incidence of all complications was 8.5%. The complications are classfied into local, systemic (including contrast sensitivity), and/or neurologic complications and may be transient or permanent.

3. Head CT

Head CT scan includes unenhanced CT, contrast-enhanced CT, CT angiography and CT perfusion.

(1) Unenhanced CT: The standard slice orientation in most brain imaging is transaxial, and another standard plane of view is coronal. CT sections paralleling orbitomeatal baseline(the line connects the lateral canthus with the center of external acoustic) are the most common orientation for routine visualization of the brain. The number of the slices is 10 to 12 and the thickness of one standard slice is 10 mm. Direct coronal scan and high-resolution scan are preferred to show the pituitary gland. Thin-section CT scan can be used to reveal small lesions. A CT scanning plane angled approximately 20° to orbitomeatal baseline is often used to display the posterior fossa.

(2) Contrast-Enhanced CT: Intravenous iodinated contrast is often used in cranial CT to opacify blood vessel and detect lesions of abnormal blood-brain brain barrier, where iodinated contrast of intravenous enter into the parenchyma directly. Thus the lesions may be shown clearlier or the lesions which cannot be shown on unenhanced CT can be seen. The non-ionic iodine contrast agent is injected intravenously quickly. The dose is 1.5~2.0 mL/ kg. Hypersensitivity to iodine is the contraindication of contrast-enhanced CT.

(3) CT Angiography (CTA): After intravenous iodinated contrast, the contrast flows into the cerebral vessels and spiral CT scans are performed. If computer three-dimensional reconstruction is performed, CT angiograms can be produced. With CT angiography, the relationships of lesions and cerebral vessels can be detected.

(4) CT Perfusion: Iodine-based CT perfusion has been introduced recently. A large rapid iodinated contrast is

infused during continuous rapid scanning of the same slice and the wash-in and wash-out of the cerebral flow can be analyzed by a computer reconstruction to generate semi-quantitative images of brain perfusion. It is used to assess the microcirculation and perfusion of brain parenchyma. Commonly measured parameters are mean transit time (MTT), cerebral blood volume (CBV), and /or cerebra blood flow (CBF). The relationship is that CBF = CBV/MTT.

4. Head MRI

Head MRI includes unenhanced MRI, contrast-enhanced MRI, MR angiography and functional magnetic resonance imaging.

(1)Unenhanced MRI: The standard slice orientation in most brain imaging is transaxial, and other standard planes of view are coronal and sagittal according to the locations of the lesions. Spin-echo imaging remains the mainstay of the routine examination, T1-weighted and axial T2-weighted whole-brain images are routinely obtained. The thickness of one slice is 8 to 10 mm, or 2 to 5 mm in thin-section scan. Fast spin echo (FSE), gradient echo scanning, fat saturation and fluid attenuated inversion recovery (FLAIR) play an important roles in cranial MR imaging.

(2) Contrast-Enhanced MRI: Contrast-enhanced MR neuroimaging is performed with the gadopentetate dimeglumine (Gd-DTPA) and the recommended dose of the agent for routine uses is 0. 1~0. 2 mmol/kg (0. 2 mL~ 0. 4/kg). The lesions may be shown more clearly after contrast。 The small and/or multiple lesions which is unable shown in unenhanced MRI can be seen and the locations and dimension can be defined. This technique is used to discriminate the neoplasm and edema and distinguish postoperative relapse and postoperative changes. It is also used to the intracranial vascular diseases.

(3)MR angiography (MRA): MRA is the only method to produce noninvasive angiographic projectional images. MRA capitalizes on creating intensity differences between flowing (or intravascular) tissue and stationary tissue without contrast medium. By suppressing background stationary tissue and focusing only on the flowing blood, a data set that depicts only vascular structures can be obtained. MRA can produce images that is satisfactory to visualize the intracranial circulation and cervical vessels. The most commonly used clinical MRA techniques are time-of-flight (TOF)MRA and phase-contrast (PC)MRA.

(4)Functional Magnetic Resonance Imaging: The neuroimaging methods based on MRI technology focused on the brain function—physiology, biochemistry, and metabolism—have entered the clinical realm and are routinely applied in a variety of situations. The functional MRI methods that we employ are diffusion-weighted imaging, perfusion MRI, MR spectroscopy and brain activation studies using BOLD (blood oxygen level detection) fMRI. ① Diffusion-weighted imaging (DWI), which assesses the local environment of the cell to reflect the water molecules diffusion. DWI can show cerebral ischemia within minutes of irreversible damage. So DWI is commonly used to detecting the acute ischemic diseases of brain. ②Perfusion MRI (PWI): PWI is often combined with DWI, which allows the evaluation of the microcirculation and the cerebral blood perfusion. ③MR spectroscopy(MRS): MRS attempts to interrogate the biochemistry environment of the brain, and identifies the metabolites and their amount within a volume of interest region or voxel noninvasively. Two flavors of MRS dominate ^{31}P and ^{1}H spectroscopy. Single voxel MRS and multivoxel MRS can be obtained. ④fMRI of brain: Noninvasive techniques that can localize the neuronal activation of brain. In the most widely used fMRI method, the fMRI signal is modulated by blood oxygenation, known as the BOLD contrast technique.

Section 2　Normal appearances

1. Plainfilm findings

Normal skull appearances are variable of body, age and sex. The skull bones possess an outer and an inner layer made up of compact bone separated by a variable thickness of cancellous bone usually referred as the diploe. The outer and inner tables displays hyperdense lines and the diploe is low density. The thickness of the layer is variable of age and position. The skull bones are joined together by sutures. The sutures, including coronal suture, sagittal suture and lambdoid suture, are irregular and bright. Infant has a fairly wide separation between the bones and large fontanelles (one frontal, the largest, and one occipital). Sutural bones may exist between the bones. The lateral plain films generally gives an demonstration of the configuration of the sella turcica which may be elliptical、 flat or round. The width of the sella turcica is 7－16 mm (mean 11.5 mm), and height is 7 ~ 14 mm (mean 9.5 mm). The most frequent sites of physiological intracranial calcifications are pineal body, falx cerebri, petroclinoid ligaments and choroid plexus. The shift of the physiological intracranial calcifications may suggest the possibility of the intracranial space occupying lesions.

2. Cerebral DSA findings

The arterial phase of carotid DSA[see Figure 19-1(a), (b)]

Afterascending to the base of the skull, passing through the carotid canal of the temporal bone and running forward within the cavernous sinus, the internal carotid artery terminates intracranially at its bifurcation into the anterior and middle cerebral arteries. The internal carotid artery may be divided into four portions: Cervical, petrous, cavernous, and cerebral portions. The branches of the cerebral portion are the ophthalmic artery, the anterior choroidal artery and the posterior communicating artery. A number of small branches arise from the branches. Numerous anastomoses and overlaps of the branches may be observed. These artery and their branches are best seen in the AP and lateral projections. In spite of the various origins and branching patterns of the arteries, the territory of supply by each artery is fairly constant together with the constant relationship to the lobes.

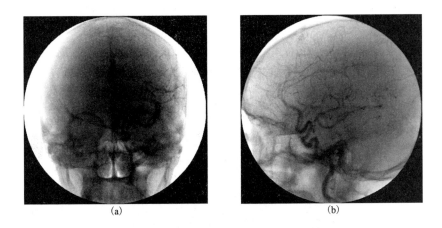

(a)　　　　　　　　　　　　　　(b)

(a) AP projection; (b) lateral projection.

Figure 19-1　The arterial phase of carotid DSA

3. Head CT findings

The normal appearances of head CT[see Figure 19-2(a) ~ (f)]

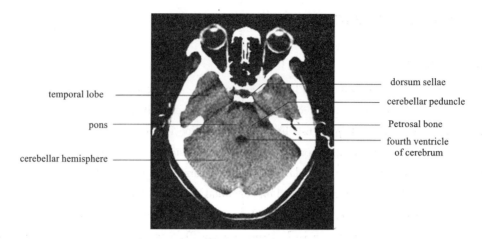

temporal lobe

pons

cerebellar hemisphere

dorsum sellae

cerebellar peduncle

Petrosal bone

fourth ventricle
of cerebrum

Figure 19-2 （a）**Transverse CT image at the level of the pons**

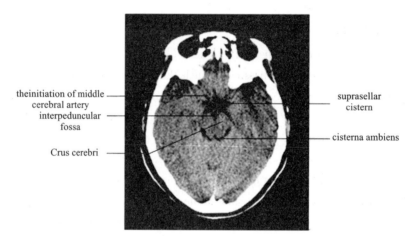

theinitiation of middle
cerebral artery
interpeduncular
fossa

Crus cerebri

suprasellar
cistern

cisterna ambiens

Figure 19-2 （b）**Transverse CT image at the level of the suprasellar cistern**

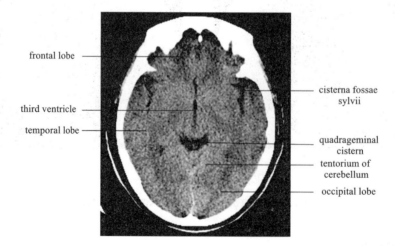

frontal lobe

third ventricle

temporal lobe

cisterna fossae
sylvii

quadrageminal
cistern

tentorium of
cerebellum

occipital lobe

Figure 19-2 （c）**Transverse CT image at the level of the third ventricle**

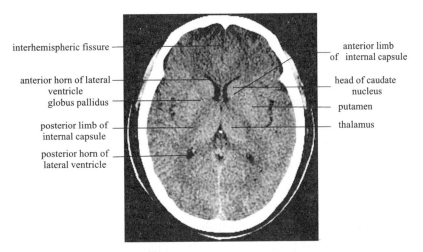

Figure 19-2 （d）Transverse CT image at the level of the basal ganglia

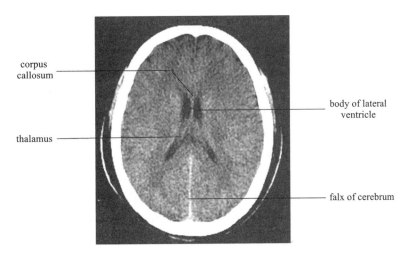

Figure 19-2 （e）Transverse CT image at the level of the body of lateral ventricle

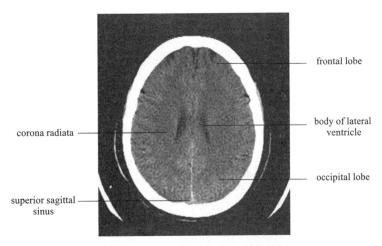

Figure 19-2 （f）Transverse CT image at the level of the top of the lateral ventricle

（1）Skull and the foramina: Skull is high density. Jugular foramen, foramen rotundum, foramen ovale and foramen lacerum are usually seen at the level of skull base and they are all low density. Mastoid and paranasal sinuses are also low density because of their air cells.

（2）Brain parenchyma: The brain parenchyma may be divided into cerebrum (frontal lobe, temporal lobe, parietal lobe, occipital lobe), cerebellum and brain stem. The density of cortex is higher than medulla can be identified clearly. Basal ganglia are the deep gray nuclei. Its density is similar to cortex. Basal ganglia have three parts: corpus striatum (caudate nucleus and lenticular nucleus), claustrum and amygdaloid body. The head of the caudate nucleus is at the posterolateral aspect of the frontal horn. The body of caudate nucleus makes a descent along the superolateral surface of the thalamus. The lenticular nucleus (globus pallidus and putamen, former inside and latter outside) is at the lateral aspect of the caudate nucleus and the thalamus. The grey nucleus between the lenticular nucleus and the insula is the claustrum. Hyperdense calcification may be seen in the basal ganglia. The white matter band area where the caudate nucleus, the thalamus and the lenticular nucleus join together is known as internal capsule(anterior limb, posterior limb and genu). The white matter between the lenticular nucleus, the claustrum and the insula are the external capsule and extreme capsule. The thalamus is bounded medially by the third ventricle and laterally by the posterior limb and genu of the internal capsule。

（3）The ventricular system: The ventricular system consists of cavities in the brain containing cerebrospinal fluid. They are all low density as water. There are four ventricles including fourth ventricle, third ventricle, lateral ventricles and aqueduct. The lateral ventricle may be divided into five parts: Frontal (anterior) horn, posterior (occipital) horn, and inferior (temporal) horn, central(middle) part and collateral trigone. The area where the central part, occipital horn, and temporal horn join together is known as the collateral trigone.

（4）Subarachnoid space: The subarachnoid space consists of sulcus, cisterna and fissure of the brain containing cerebrospinal fluid. They are also low density as water. The important cisterns are cisterna magma, suprasellar cistern, cisterna ambiens, cerebellopontine angle cistern, cisterna fossae sylvii, interhemispheric fissure, interpeduncular cistern and quadrageminal cistern. Cisterna magma is the biggest one. Suprasellar cistern is above the sella turcica and may be pentagonal or hexagonal.

（5）Contrast-enhanced CT: The normal brain parenchyma reveals slight enhancement. The vessels show obviously enhanced directly. The obvious enhancement may be seen in the dura, the pituitary body and the pineal body owing to the absence of the blood-brain barrier.

4. Head MRI finding

The normal appearances of head MRI [see Figure 19-3(a) ~ (d)]

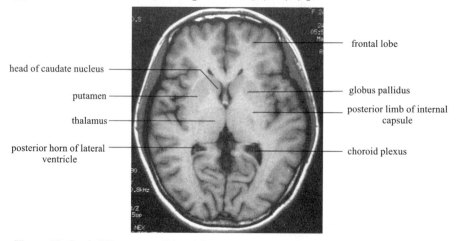

Figure 19-3　(a) Transverse T1-weighted MR image at the level of the basal ganglia

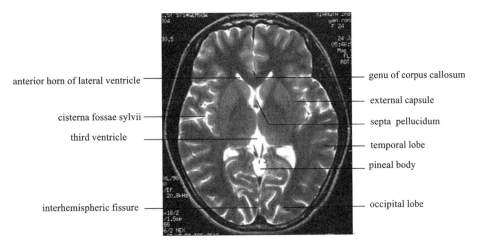

anterior horn of lateral ventricle

cisterna fossae sylvii

third ventricle

interhemispheric fissure

genu of corpus callosum

external capsule

septa pellucidum

temporal lobe

pineal body

occipital lobe

Figure 19-3 （b）**Transverse T2-weighted MR image at the level of the basal ganglia**

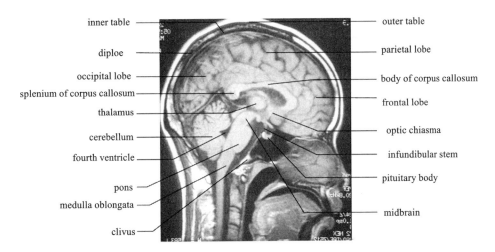

inner table

diploe

occipital lobe

splenium of corpus callosum

thalamus

cerebellum

fourth ventricle

pons

medulla oblongata

clivus

outer table

parietal lobe

body of corpus callosum

frontal lobe

optic chiasma

infundibular stem

pituitary body

midbrain

Figure 19-3 （c）**Midline sagittal T1-weighted MR image.**

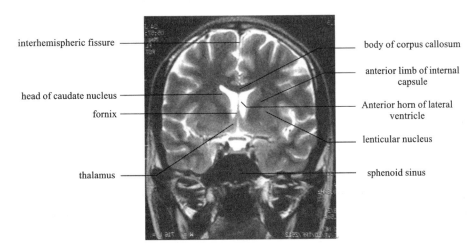

interhemispheric fissure

head of caudate nucleus

fornix

thalamus

body of corpus callosum

anterior limb of internal capsule

Anterior horn of lateral ventricle

lenticular nucleus

sphenoid sinus

Figure 19-3 （d）**Coronal T2-weighted MR image**

499

（1）Skull and soft tissues：The inner and outer tables are compact bone which contain few water and proton. There is few proton in the normal calcifications and the meninges. So they are all hypointense on T1WI and T2WI. The diploe and the soft tissues of the scalp are hyperintense on T1WI as well as on T2WI.

（2）Subarachnoid space and the ventricular system：These cavities are full of cerebrospinal fluid, which is homogeneous. The T1WI shows low signal while the T2WI shows high signal in the cavities owing to the very long T1 and T2 of the cerebrospinal fluid. On FLAIR sequence MRI they may be low signal.

（3）Brain parenchyma：The contrast of the medulla and cortex in MRI is clearer. The T1WI shows slight higher signal in medulla than cortex and the T2WI shows slight lower signal in medulla owing to the shorter T1 and T2 of medulla. The signal of the deep gray nuclei is similar to cortex.

（4）Brain Vessels：Owing to the flowing void effect, the vessels may be seen directly and they are hypointense either on T1WI or on T2WI. However, the signal is high when the flow is slow.

（5）Cranial nerve：Using a high-field MRI system, cranial nerves can be shown clearly, which are isointensity on T1WI.

（6）Contrast-enhanced MRI：Intravenous iodinated contrast medium administration on CT examination and Gadolinium-associated enhancement on MR scanning is similar.

Section 3　Basic pathological changes

1. Plain film findings

（1）Increased intracranial pressure：It appears in many intracranial lesions. It only demonstrates the possible existence of the abnormalities, while it cannot determine the localization and qualitative of the lesions. In children, it can be seen that the enlargement of head, the widening of the sutures, the thinness of the layers and the increase of impressions gyrorum. In adults, the abnormal of the sella turcica is more common, such as the enlargement of the sella turcica and the thinness of the floor of the sella and dorsum.

（2）Localization of the Neoplasms：1）Local abnormal of the skull, includes the localized proliferation, sclerosis or bone destruction of the skull. It is often seen in the tumors adjacent to the skull or the surface of brain, such as meningioma. 2）Abnormal of the sella turcica, indicates the presence of neoplasms near by the sella turcica. Sellar neoplasms can enlarge the sella turcica, such as pituitary tumor；Suprasellar neoplasms may short the dorsum sellae and make the sella turcica flat；Parasellar neoplasms oppress the floor of the sella and even result in the "double floor". The anterior clinoid may be raised or destructed. 3）Abnormal calcification, includes calcification of the tumor and the displacement of the normal intracranial calcification. The position and configuration of the calcification in tumor can possibly indicate its location and quality. The displacement of the pineal body calcifications may suggest the possible location of the intracranial neoplasms.

2. DSA findings

Brain DSA isthe gold-standard vascular imaging technique for qualitatively diagnosing of the intracranial vascular disease. Displacement of the brain vessel and abnormal of vessel formation and circulation may be observed. Intracranial space-occupying lesions and edema may oppress the brain tissue to cause vascular displacement, aggregation or separation, straighten and distort. Angiography of some neoplasms may show abnormal vascularity and tumor stain.

3. Head CT findings

（1）The density of unenhanced CT changes：1）Hyperdensity lesions：Density of the lesions is higher than normal brain parenchyma. Fresh hematoma, calcification, multi-vascular tumor, et al, are manifested by high-density area. 2) Hypodensity lesions: It is shown in some tumors, inflammation, edema, infarction, cyst, lipoma, abscess, and so on. 3) Isodensity lesions: Density of the lesions is similar to normal brain parenchyma. It may be seen in some neoplasms, hematoma in absorption period, vascular disease, and so on. 4) Mix-density lesions: When the lesion consists of variety of patterns, such as calcification, hemorrhage, fat, cystic change and necrosis, it may be mix-density. Mix-density is commonly shown in many kinds of tumors, vascular lesions, abscesses, and so on.

(2) Appearances of contrast-enhanced CT: The enhancement in lesions is due to disruption of the blood-brain barrier and abnormal vascularity. 1) Homogeneous enhancement: It can be seen in meningioma, metastatic neoplasm, germinoma, neurinoma, aneurysm, granuloma, and so on. 2) Hetrogeneous enhancement: It can be seen in vascular malformation, glioma, demyelination, inflammation, and so on. 3) Ring enhancement: It can be seen in brain abscess, metastatic neoplasm, glioma, tuberculoma, and so on. 4) Nonenhancement: It can be seen in encephalitis, cyst, edema, and so on.

(3) Abnormal of brain constitution: 1) Mass effect: Intracranial space-occupying lesions (such as tumor and hemorrhage) and edema may result in mass effect. We can find the midline structure constitution is displaced, and the local sulci, cistern and ventricle are compressed to narrow or occluded, and the midline structure moves to the opposite side, and so on. 2) Hydrocephalus: It includes communicating hydrocephalus and obstructive hydrocephalus. The former is caused by obstruction or absorption of external ventricular CSF circulation, and it widens the ventricular system and cisterna generally. The latter is caused by obstruction above the outlet of the fourth ventricle and results in enlargement of the obstruction proximal ventricular, but the cisterna is normal. 3) Brain atrophy: It can be divided into local and diffuse atrophy. Atrophy of the cortex shows the widening of sulci and fissure, and enlargement of cistern. While in patients of medulla atrophy, only cerebral ventricles are enlarged.

(4) skull abnormal: 1) Skull disorders: Such as traumatic fracture, inflammation and tumor. 2) Intracranial lesions involving the skull: Such as sella turcica, jugular foramen or internal acoustic meatus widens, and local hyperosteogeny and/or destruction, are common in neoplastic lesions at the corresponding sites. The skull abnormal may be helpful to the localization and qualitative diagnosis of the intracranial lesions.

4. Head MRI findings

(1) Hemorrhage: It varies with the period of the hematoma. 1) In the hyperacute stage (within 24 hours): The red blood cells (RBCs) in the hematoma are oxyhemoglobin. The hematoma shows isointense on T1WI and T2WI. 2) In the acute stage (1-2 days): RBCs in the hematoma are deoxyhemoglobin. The acute hematoma is isointense to slightly hypointense on T1WI and T2WI. It is hard to find it with MRI. 3) In the subacute stage (3 days to 3 weeks): Erythrocytic degeneration and white matter edema arround the hematoma peaks. Deoxyhemglobin deoxidized to orthemoglobin and hemosiderin. The latter is deposited around the hematoma. In the early stage (3-5 days), the signal of T1WI increases gradually from the surrounding to the center, and the signal of T2WI is low. In the middle stage (6-10 days), the T1WI high signal area expands from periphery to center, T2WI also shows high signal. In the late stage (11 days-3 weeks), both T1WI and T2WI shows hyperintensity, and the T2WI hypointensity ring formed by hemosiderin deposition could be seen around the hematoma. 4) In the chronic stage (after 3 weeks): As the hematoma evolves, the hemoglobin is broken down and large amounts of hemosiderin and ferritin are produced, forming a CSF-like sac, the hematoma shows hypointensity on T1WI and hyperintensity on T2WI. The hemosiderin ring of the brain immediately adjacent to the hematoma is markedly hypointense on T2WI.

(2) Cerebral Infarction: In early acute infarction (hyperacute infarction), signals are mostly normal on T1WI and T2WI. The lesions are distributed along the blood supply area, and mass effect can be seen. The mass effect is reduced in chronic period, mainly with cerebral atrophy. Due to brain edema, necrosis, and cystic degeneration,

501

the infarction shows hypointensity on T1WI and hyperintensity on T2WI in acute and chronic stages.

(3) Mass: The mass always shows hypointense on T1WI and hyperintense on T2WI owing to its high water content. Some tumors show hyperintense on T1WI and hypointense on T2WI because of the paramagnetic component, such as melanoma. Mass with calcification or ossification shows hypointense on both T1WI and T2WI. Fatty tumors such as lipoma may show hyperintense on both T1WI and T2WI.

(4) Cyst: Generally the cyst full of fluid shows hypointense on T1WI and hyperintense on T2WI. But the cyst with mucoprotein or lipoid may shows hyperintense on both T1WI and T2WI.

(5) Edema: The change of edema is long T1 and long T2 relaxation times on MRI, so the edema shows hypointense on T1WI and hyperintense on T2WI. Mass effect is present.

5. Comparative imaging

Based on the normal and abnormal appearances of the plain film, DSA, CT and MRI, we can find that there is superiority as well as deficiency. When designing imaging procedures for certain diseases, reasonable choices should be made and personalized solutions should be developed. The least invasive examination should be chose first, and if we have more than one equally noninvasive methods, then we should carry out the examination that will likely yield the most information.

Skull radiographshave played a decreasing role in neuroimaging since the advancing of CT and MRI. CT and MRI have become the most commonly used method in neuroimaging. MRI may have reduced the application of CT in the brain, but it will not replace it completely. In skull primary lesions or the invasions from the intracranial disorders, skull plain film may be useful only in demonstrating skull bone abnormal, but CT and MR are much more sensitive than the plain film and they have also greatly improved the discovery of the intracranial diseases. The role of plain film is also limited for the intracranial space-occupying lesions.

Although brain DSA is the gold standard for diagnosing of the intracranial vascular diseases, it is invasive and its value is limited. So it is not usually applied alone. Recently, noninvasive MRA and microinvasive CTA have developed rapidly and have become the most routinely method for cerebral vascular imaging. The combination with conventional MRI and CT has gradually replaced the traditional arteriography. Today, MRA and CTA are most commonly performed as an adjunct to conventional MRI and CT imaging.

CT is the bestmethod for bony lesions and calcification, especially in some central nervous system tumors. MRI is less sensitive to the bone and calcification. Intracranial inflammation and demyelination can only be detected with CT and MRI, and MRI is better than CT. Combined with contrast-enhanced CT, We can get locational and qualitative diagnosis for most of intracranial lesions. However, MRI is more sensitive to the lesions located in the midline structure, the posterior fossa and near skull base. CT is much more sensitive than MR for detecting hemorrhage in the acute stage. But MRI is more sensitive than CT for detecting the chronic hematoma which is isodense on CT. CT is the more sensitive imaging method for the detection of subarachnoid hemorrhage than MRI, but if the volume of hemorrhage is small, MRI is better.

Functional MRI may increase our understanding of the physiology, biochemistry and metabolism correlates of intracranial lesions, which is helpful to the diagnosis, differential diagnosis and treatment of the space-occupying lesions. DWI has been commonly used to detect acute infarction.

Section 4　Diagnosis of common diseases

1. Head trauma

Traumatic brain injury (TBI) is the leading causes of disability and death in child and young adults. It is classified into mild, moderate, severe, or very severe brain injury. Imagingmanifestations of TBI include cerebral contusion, laceration, intracerebral hematoma, epidural hematoma, subdural hematoma and subarachnoid hemorrhage. Skull films have little role in the diagnosis and treatment of patient with significant head trauma. They are useful only to ascertain whether linear skull fracture is present. The most efficient method of examination of TBI is CT. It is fast and usually very accurate to detect acute hemorrhage (high density on unenhanced scan). CT is also excellent for assessing facial and skull fractures. When trauma is evaluated with CT, imaging should include brain and bone windows routinely. CT does not easily detect extracerebral hemorrhages of the infratemporal region, subfrontal region, or posterior fossa. It is also less sensitive than MRI in detecting diffuse axonal injury and vascular injury.

(1) Cerebral contusion and laceration of brain

1) Clinical and pathological manifestations: In cerebral contusion, there are scattered hemorrhage lesions, intracerebral hematoma and swelling of brain. If it is companied with lacerating of brain, meninges and brain vessel, it is defined laceration of brain. Cerebral contusion, combined with the laceration of brain, are called cerebral contusion and laceration of brain.

2) Imaging manifestations: Low density hydrocephalus and scattered high density hemorrhages can be seen (Figure 19-4). But the size of hemorrhage lesions is small. It can be diagnosed easily.

(2) Epidural hematoma

1) Clinical and pathological manifestations: The potential space between the inner table of the skull and the dura is the epidural space. The most common cause of epidural hematoma is head trauma with skull fracture of the temporal bone crossing the vascular territory of the middle meningeal artery or vein. Tears of the middle meningeal artery or vein structures result in the extravasation of blood and acute epidural hematoma. Most frequently, hematomas are observed in the temporal parietal region.

2) Imaging manifestations:

①CT (Figure 19-5) reveals a high density acute intracranial and extracerebral mass. The shape is fusiform. In these cases, bone window is used to look for fractures. Chronic epidural hematomas (after 3 weeks) reveal low density. The subdural capsule is enhanced. They may be concave.

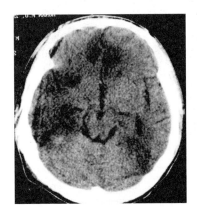

low density lesions and scattered high density hemorrhages can be seen on CT plain scan.

Figure 19-4 CT findings of cerebral contusion and laceration of brain

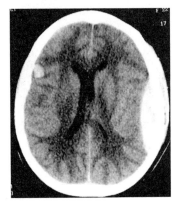

CT demonstrates high density extraaxial mass in the left temporal region. The lesion is fusiform.

Figure 19-5 CT findings of acute epidural hematomas

②On MR, the epidural hematoma has different appearances depending on the interval between the traumatic event and imaging. Acute hematoma (in 3 days) demonstrates low intensity on T2WI and isointensity on T1WI. After a few days (subacute hematoma), it demonstrates high intensity on T1WI and T2WI. Chronic epidural hematoma reveals low intensity on T1WI and high intensity on T2WI. One may visulize the medial dural margin as a hypointense rim on all pulse sequences.

(3) Subdural hematoma

1) Clinical and pathological manifestations: The potential space between the pia-arachnoid and the dura is the subdural space. Acute subdural hematomas result from significant head injury and are caused by the shearing of bridging veins. Subdural hematomas are seen in approximately 30% of patients with severe closed head trauma. In 3 days, they are considered acute, 3 days to 3 weeks are subacute, and after 3 weeks are considered chronic subdural hematomas.

2) Imaging manifestations:

①Acute subdural hematomas on CT are high-density crescent extracerebral masses [Figure 19-6(a)]. The thickness of the hematoma can range from pencil-thin to large and can be convex inward at times. As opposed to epidural hematomas, subdural hematomas are not confined by the cranial sutures and mass effect is significant. Subacute subdural hematomas may be isodense to low density. The edge of subacute and chronic subdural hematomas can be enhanced resulted from the vascularization of the subdural membranes. If the gray matter-white matter interface is visualized and buckled inward from its normal position, then an intracranial and extracerebral mass should be considered. Contrast is helpful in diagnosis isodense subdural hematoma by visualized the inwardly displaced cortical veins.

②On MR, subdural hematomas follow the intensity of blood. Acute subdural hematomas are isointense on T1WI and hypointense on T2WI. Subacute subdural hematomas generally have high intense on T1WI and T2WI. However, the high intensity on T1WI gradually diminishes over time and the extracerebral collection becomes isointense to brain. Such a collection can be confused with an extracerebral abscess such as a subdural empyema. At this time, the clinical correlation would be important. Chronic subdural hematomas reveals low intensity on T1WI and high intensity on T2WI[Figure 19-6(b), (c)].

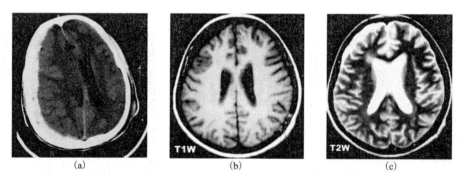

(a)   (b)   (c)

(a) Acute subdural hematoma: non-enhanced CT shows high density and crescent. Mass effect is significant;

(b) Chronic Subacute subdural hematoma: T1WI shows low intensity lesion of the right frontal region;

(c) Chronic subacute subdural hematoma: T2WI shows high intensity lesion of the right frontal region.

Figure 19-6   CT and MRI findings of subdual hematoma

2. Infectious and noninfectious diseases of the brain

(1) Leptomeningitis

1) Clinical and pathological manifestations: Leptomeningeal inflammation most often occurs following direct hematogenous dissemination from a distant infectious focus. Pathogens can also passing through regions that may not

have a normal blood-brain barrier, such as choroid plexus or circumventricular organs. Direct extension from sinusitis, orbital cellulitis, mastoiditis, or otitis media is much less common. With stagnation of CSF flow, bacteria are offered the opportunity to invade the menings and indulge. Early in the course of infection, there are congestion and hyperemia of the pia and arachnoid mater. Then exudates cover the brain, especially in the dependent sulci and basal cisterns. The leptomeninges become thickened. The clinical features include fever, headache, vomiting, seizures, Kernig's sign, and so on.

2) Imaging manifestations: Imaging findings in early stage of infection are normal if treated successfully. The manifestation in acute meningitis are as follows: Visualization of distended subarachniod space, particularly noted in the based cisterns and along the interhemispheric fissure; high intensity of subarachniod fluid on FLAIR; acute cerebral swelling and communicating hydrocephalus, with enlargement of the temporal horns and disappearance of the basal cisterns.

(2) Pyogenic brain abscess

1) Clinical and pathological manifestations: Cerebral abscess is most often the result of hematogenous dissemination from a primary infectious site. The various causes include otitis, paranasal sinusitis, penetrating injury, postsurgical infection, cardiac infection, drug abuse, sepsis and so on. The most frequent locations are the frontal and parietal lobes along the distribution of the middle cerebral artery. Abscess may be unilocular or multilocular, solitary or multiple. Abscess formation has been divided into four stages: ①Early cerebritis(1 to 3 days); ②Late cerebritis(4 to 9 days); ③Early capsule formation(10 to 13 days); ④Late capsule formation(14 days and later).

2) Imaging manifestations:

①In the cerebritis phase, CT reveals low-density abnormalities with mass effect. Patchy or gyriform enhancement is present. After 2 to 3 weeks, a mature brain abscess is formed, CT shows low density in the center of the lesion, surrounded by low density edema. The suppurative brain abscess shows homogeneous annular enhancement [Figure 19-7(c)].

②On MRI, low signal on T1WI and high signal on T2WI/FLAIR may be observed, with a typical epicenter at the corticomedullary junction and patchy enhancement. In the late cerebritis, ring enhancement may be present. After 2 to 3 weeks, a mature abscess appears on T1WI[Figure 19-7(a)] as a round, well-demarcated low-signal region with mass effect and peripheral low-signal (edema)beyond the margin of the lesion. On T2WI/FLAIR[Figure 19-7(b)], high signal can be seen in the cavity and in the parenchyma surrounding the lesion. Concentric bands of various thickness on T2WI/FLAIR have been observed in abscesses. Uniform ring enhancement is always present in pyogenic brain abscess. The suppurative brain abscess shows homogeneous annular enhancement[Figure 19-7(d)]

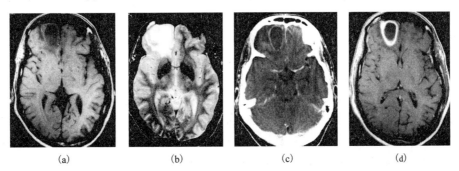

(a)　　　　　　(b)　　　　　　(c)　　　　　　(d)

(a)T1WI reveals low intensity lesion on the right frontal lobule. The margin is well-defined; (b)T2WI shows high intensity lesion; (c)Uniform ring enhancement can be seen on CT enhanced scan; (d)MRI reveals ring enhancement.

Figure 19-7　CT and MRI findings of cerebral abscess

（3）Tuberculosis

1）Clinical and pathological manifestations: The incidence of tuberculosis has markedly increased in recent years, particularly with the arise of drug-resistant strains of the bacillus and AIDS. Approximately 5% to 10% of cases of tuberculosis have CNS involvement. Intracranial tuberculosis has two related pathologic processes-the tuberculous meningitis and intracranial tuberculoma. Clinical features of tuberculosis include confusion, fever, headache, lethargy, and meningismus. Lumbar puncture reveals hypoglycorrhachia, increased protein, pleocytosis, and negative smears for organisms.

2）Imaging manifestations: Imaging features depend on the stage of the infection. In tuberculous meningitis, the basal and sylvian cisterns are poorly visualized without contrast because of the dense exudates. With contrast, it can be markedly enhanced. On FLAIR, the basal cisterns can have increased signal compared with normal, because of the thick proteinaceous exudates. The cisterns enhance markedly, and this enhancement can extend into the hemispheric fissures and over the cortical surfaces. Calcification are rarely seen in the basal meninges. Communicated hydrocephalus can be seen in the late stage. The intracranial tuberculoma shows as a nodule (Figure 19-8). It can be solitary but is commonly multiple and is associated with mass effect and edema. Calcification is uncommon (less than 20%). The typical tuberculoma would appear as a nodule with a small central area of high signal on T2WI or low density on CT. The wall of tuberculoma shows high signal on T1WI but low signal on T2WI/FLAIR. Surrounding the nodle is high signal on T2WI/FLAIR or low density on CT. This represents edema with mass effect. Enhancement is in rings or nodules.

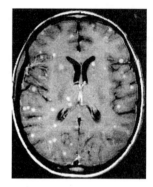

multi-nodules can be seen on T1WI enhanced scan. Enhancement is in nodules. Some lesions are surrounding with edema.

Figure 19-8　MR findings of tuberculoma

3. Neoplasms of the brain

（1）Meningiomas

1）Clinical and pathological manifestations: Meningiomas constitute the most common extraaxial neoplasm of the brain. Because meningiomas arise from arachnoid cap cells, they can occur anywhere that arachnoid exists. The most common locations for meningioma are the parasagittal dura, convexities, sphenoid wing, cerebellopontine angle cistern, olfactory groove, and planum sphenoidale. Ninety percent of meningioma originate supratentorially. According to the 2016 WHO classification standard for central nervous system tumors, meningiomas are divided into three grades, meningiomas (WHO grade I), atypical meningioma (WHO grade II) and anaplastic meningioma (WHO grade III).

2）Imaging manifestations:

①On unenhanced CT scans, approximately 75% of meningiomas are slightly hyperdense compared with normal brain tissue[Figure 19-9(a)]. One may see calcification with meningiomas in approximately 20% of cases. Cystic, osteoblastic, chondromatous, or fatty degeneration of meningiomas occurs rarely. On enhanced CT scans, they are markedly enhanced [Figure 19-9(b)]. Through CT examination, "meningeal tail sign" can be seen, which is the enhancement of the dura separate from the lesion in crescentic fashion, and the typical features of meningiomas and has been seen in most cases. Bony changes are associated with meningiomas of hyperostotic or osteolytic. The bone near the lesion is thickened.

②MR is superior to CT in detecting the extent of meningiomas, sinus invasion and/or thrombosis, vascularity, intracranial edema, and intra-osseous extension. The typical MR signal intensity characteristics of meningiomas are isointensity or slight hypointensity compared to gray matter on the T1WI[Figure 19-9(c)] and isointensity to hyperintensity compared to gray on the T2WI. The "cleft sign" can be seen. With MR, you may see the "Dural tail", enhancement of the dura separate from the lesion in crescentic fashion [Figure 19-9(d)], which is the typical features of meningiomas and has been seen in most cases. The degree of parenchymal edema is variable in meningiomas. Although it is true that larger meningiomas tend to have a greater degree of parenchymal edema, there are exceptions where small meningiomas result in a large amount of white matter edema. The degree of edema seems to correlate with location, because meningiomas adjacent to the cerebral cortex tend to cause greater edema than those along the basal cisterns or planum. Edema associated with meningiomas may be caused by compressive ischemia, venous stasis, aggressive growth, or parasitization of pial vessels. Venous sinus occlusion or venous thrombosis can also cause intraparenchymal edema from a meningioma.

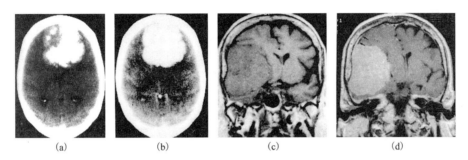

(a) (b) (c) (d)

(a) unenhanced CT shows hyperdense mass with calcification on the parasagittal dura; (b) the mass is markedly enhanced on enhanced CT scan; (c) T1WI reveals isointensity to slight hypointensity mass; (d) the mass is markedly enhanced and dural tail sign can be seen.

Figure 19-9   CT and MRI findings of meningioma

(2) Glioma

1) Clinical and pathological manifestations: Gliomas accout for 35% to 55% of all intracranial tumors. The category of gliomas of the brain includes astrocytomas, glioblastoma multiforme (GBMs), oligodendrogliomas, ependymomas, subependymomas,

medulloblastomas, neuroblastomas, gangliocytomas, and gangliogliomas. The WHO classification of central nervous system tumors classifies gliomas into grades I-IV, low-grade gliomas are grades I and II, high-grade gliomas are grades III and IV. Diffuse gliomas include astrocytoma (grade II and III), oligodendroglioma (grade II and III), glioblastoma (grade IV) and childhood-related diffuse glioma. WHO grade II diffuse astrocytoma, WHO grade III anaplastic astrocytoma and glioblastoma are all divided into isocitrate dehydrogenase (IDH) mutant type, IDH wild type and not otherwise specified (NOS) type.

2) Imaging manifestations: On CT scans, gliomas show hypodense [Figure 19-10(a)]. MR reveals hypointensity on T1WI and hyperintensity on T2WI/FLAIR [Figure 19-10(b)~(d)]. The cystic portion of the tumor has signal similar to CSF on T1WI and T2WI, but may be hyperintense to CSF on the PDWI or FLAIR because of large amount of protein. The lesion is very well defined. The solid portion of gliomas enhance strongly [Figure 19-10(e)]. Enhancement of glioma is very slight or nothing in graded I and grade II, but very strong on grade III and grade IV. In gliomas, cystic degeneration is very common, but calcification is very rare. Mass effect of gliomas graded I and grade II is slight, but markedly with gliomas grade III and grade IV.

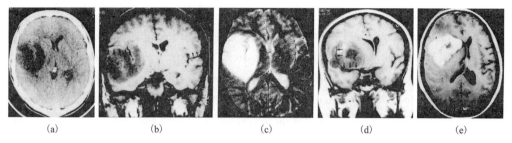

(a) the lesion shows hypodense on CT plain scan; (b) T1WI reveals hypointensity mass and the margin is clear; (c) the mass shows hyperintensity on T2WI and it is glioma graded Ⅱ; (d) T1WI reveals hypointensity mass and the signal is not even. Figure 19-10(e). Glioma: the lesion enhances strongly on enhanced scan and it is glioma graded Ⅳ.

Figure 19-10　CT and MRI findings of glioma

(3) Metastases

1) Clinical and pathological manifestations: Metastases are the most common masses in the supratentorial space in the adult, making up 20% of intracranial neoplasms. 70%~80% are multiple with just 20% having two lesions. The primary tumors that spread to the supratentorial part of the brain are lung (50%), breast (15%), melanoma (11%), kidney and gastrointestinal tumors. They are located at the gray matter-white matter boundary characteristically because of the small caliber of vessels in this region and may extend into the cortex or white matter. The lesions tend to follow vascular flow dynamically, being deposited in the carotid system more commonly than in the vertebrobasilar system (80% to 20%) and favor the middle cerebral artery distribution. Metastases lodge at the gray-white interface in 80% of cases, basal ganglia in 3%, and cerebellum in 15%.

2) Imaging manifestations: Metastases usually appear as relatively well-defined masses that accompanied with enhancement and moderate edema. They are typically hypodense on nonenhanced CT and hypointense on T1WI unless hemorrhage. On T2WI, the signal is various depending on the presence of hemorrhage, intratumoral necrosis, cyst formation, high nuclear/cytoplasm ratios, or paramagnetic content. Most of the metastases enhance at a variable degree, but the pattern may be solid, ringlike, regular, homogeneous, or heterogeneous (Figure 19-11). As opposed to gliomas, metastases are better defined and have sharper borders. The vasogenic edema is often out of proportion when compared to the size of the metastasis except in the cortical metastases, where edema may be minimal or absent. When edema is absent, T2WI may miss metastases. Contrast becomes essential for identification of lesions in this situation.

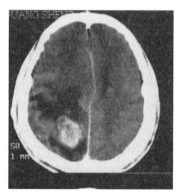

enhanced CT scan reveals markedly enhanced multi-nodule with hypodensity edema in the parenchyma.

Figure 19-11　CT findings of metastases

4. Vascular diseases of the brain

（1）Infarct of brain

1）Clinical and pathological manifestations: Large artery atherosclerosis, cardioembolism, and lacunar infarction account for the most common causes of ischemic stroke. Recurrent strokes are most common in patients with cardioembolic stroke, which also have the highest one month mortality. The principal causes of ischemic stroke are emboli, however, the sources of emboli are variable. They can arise from carotid arterial stenosis and occlusion, atherosclerotic debris and ulceration, or cardiac sources(an embolus from a cardiac source occurs in about 15% to 20% of ischemic strokes). Vascular watersheds are generally distributed as the most distal arterial territories, where communication between the principal arteries. Major watershed zones are found between the anterior and middle cerebral arteries and the middle and posterior cerebral arteries. A lacunar infarction is a small cerebral infarct that becomes cystic and is produced by occlusion of a small end artery. These lesions are always in the basal ganglia, internal capsule, pons, or corona radiata. The diameter of lesion is about 5 mm and less than 15 mm. Hemorrhagic infarct is infarct of brain with hemorrhage.

2）Imaging manifestations:

①As the development of CT, it become more sensitive in the subtle findings in acute stroke. Within 6 hours of some infarcts, loss of definition of gray-white border may be observed. High density in the proximal middle cerebral artery has been defined as an early sign of infarction representing either an acute thrombus or calcified embolus located in the middle cerebral artery. Within 12 to 24 hours, an indistinct area of low density is apparent in the appropriate vascular distribution [Figure 19-12(a), (b)]. Mass effect may be not obvious initially. The region starts to become circumscribed after 24 hours with more apparent mass effect. The asymmetry of the sulci and slight compression of one side of the ventricle can be observed. Mass effect peaks was usually between 2 and 5 days after ictus. Enhancement is not obvious in the first 3 days, the infarcted region reveals low density when then enhancement is present. Mass effect starts to decrease after about 5 days and usually disappears in 2 to 4 weeks. Persistence of mass effect beyond 6 weeks strongly implies that another lesion, most like tumor, should be considered. In about 50% of cases, between the second and third week, the infarct changes from low density to isodensity. This has been termed the CT "fogging" effect and appears to result from hyperemia from reperfusion, petechial hemorrhage, and extensive macrophage activity in the necrotic brain. These lesion reverts to a well-circumscribed region of low density after 4 weeks. At this time, there is usually absence of enhancement and no mass effect, and parenchymal loss is observed in the affected vascular territory.

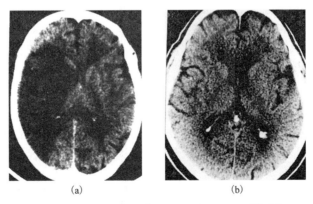

(a)　　　　　　　　　(b)

（a）Infarct of brain: low density of the infracted region can be seen on CT plain scan; （b）Lacunar infarction: a small cerebral infarct can be seen in the left thalamus and the diameter is about 10 mm.

Figure 19-12　CT findings of infarct of brain

②DWI and PWI are new techniques that are more sensitive than T2WI. DWI can detect cerebral ischemia within about $2\sim3$ minutes after its onset (on the rats) and about 30 minutes for humans. The DWI result can be compared to the conventional MR if the infarction is within a few hours after a cerebral infarction. PWI differs from DWI in which its aim is to characterise microscopic flow at the capillary level. PWI in combination with DWI has been advocated in the treatment algorithm for acute stroke. In such a scenario, the larger the difference between the perfusion and diffusional abnormalities, the greater the need for acute interventional with thrombolyticagents. If there is no perfusional abnormality, or it is equal to the diffusional lesion, then the effect of thrombolytic therapy is not great.

（2）Hemorrhage

1）Clinical and pathological manifestations: Intraparenchymal hemorrhage accounts for about 10% of strokes, which has a median age of about 65 years. Hypertension is the presumed cause of nontraumatic intraparenchymal hemorrhage in 70% to 90% of cases. Intraparenchymal hemorrhages may also result from vascular lesions including amyloid angiopathy, microaneurysms, and fibrinoid arteritis, which may be superimposed on hypertentive changes. It is not only hypertension but also the rapid change of blood pressure that can predispose to hemorrhage. It is one reason why cocaine and other drugs are associated with an increased incidence of intracranial bleeding. The location of intraparenchymal hemorrhage is variable, although approximately half to two thirds of intraparenchymal hemorrhage occurs in the basal ganglionic-thalamic (especially in the putamen) region. Approximately 10% to 50% of intraparenchymal hemorrhage may be lobar, 10% to 15% of hemorrhages occur in the brain stem, and 5% to 10% of hemorrhages occur in the cerebellum.

2）Imaging manifestations: In different stages of hemorrhage, there are different manifestations on MR and CT. Hyperacute hemorrhage ($\leqslant 24$ hours), CT reveals high-density [Figure 19-13(a)]. On MR, the lesion is low signal on T1WI, while the central of lesion is hyperintense with peripheral hypointense on T2WI. Because the central of lesion is oxyhemoglobin with peripheral deoxyhemoglobin. Acute hemorrhage (1 to 7 days), CT shows high-density. T1WI shows isointense to low signal and there is marked hypointensity on T2WI because of the susceptibility effects of deoxyhemoglobin. There is oxid ation of the deoxyhemoglobin to methemoglobin inside the RBC. This effect, in concert with the T1 shortening from the high protein concentration, gives methemoglobin its characteristic hyperintensity on T1WI. Because the paramagnetic methemoglobin remains encapsulated within the RBC, hyperintensity is also seen on the T2WI. Subacute hemorrhage (1 week to 1 month), methemoglobin is less stable than deoxyhemoglobin, and the heme group can spontaneously be lost from the protein molecule. The free heme and/or other exogenous compounds (including peroxide and superoxide) can produce RBC lysis. Concomitantly there is protein breakdown and dilution of the remaining extracellular methemoglobin. Hyperintensity [Figure 19-13(b)] persists on the T1WI despite the decrease in the protein concentration because of the T1-shortening effects of the hemo of methemoglobin even at relatively low concentrations. The hematoma signal intensity increases on T2WI [Figure 19-13(c)] because of a loss of local field inhomogeneity on RBC lysis and a decrease in the protein concentration. Chronic hemorrhage (>1 month), there is nearly complete breakdown and resorption of the fluid and protein within the clot after months. The iron atoms from the metabolized hemoglobin molecules are deposited in hemosiderin and ferritin molecules, which are unable to exit the brain parenchyma because of restoration of the blood-brain barrier. So the T1WI and T2WI demonstrates hypointensity and the CT image shows low density.

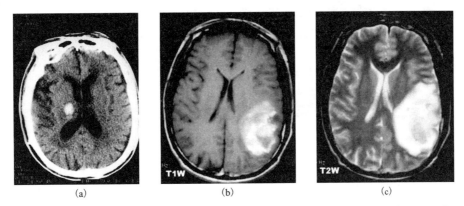

(a)unenhanced CT reveals a round high density lesion in the right thalamus; (b) Hemorrhage：T1WI shows a hyperintensity lesion. It is a subacute hemorrhage; (c) Hemorrhage：the lesion shows hyperintensity lesion on the T2WI.

Figure 19-13　CT adn MRI findings of hemorrhage

（3）Aneurysm

1）Clinical and pathological manifestations：An aneurysm is a focal dilatation of an artery. The principal causes of aneurysms are dissection of artery, atherosclerotic, mycotic infection, neoplasm, traumatic and so on. The shapes of aneurysm include miliary, fusiform, saccular. The most frequent aneurysm encountered in the CNS is miliary aneurysm. Fusiform aneurysms are atherosclerotic dilatations, mostly in the vertebral and/or basilar artery. Dissecting aneurysms may occur after trauma or may occur spontaneously. Organized hematoma resulted from vessel rupture is termed pseudoaneurysm. Pseudoaneurysm has no true vessel walls, and the hematoma is confined by the adventitia. Mycotic aneurysms are the result of endocardutis and may be saccular or fusiform and tend to be peripheral in middle cerebral artery distribution. Multiple peripheral aneurysms should suggest this diagnosis. The prevalence of intracranial aneurysms has been estimated to be between 1% to 6% in adult autopsy. Although most aneurysms occur sporadically, there is also a familial incidence, with siblings having higher incidence rate. Aneurysms may enlarge in time, the larger aneurysms tending to bleed more frequently. The average age of patients with an aneurysmal bleed is approximately 50 years. 50% to 70% of SAHs result from the rupture of intracranial aneurysms. Other causes of SAH include secondary leakage of blood from a primary intraparenchymal hemorrhage, trauma, intracranial AVM, and so on.

2）Imaging manifestations：CT confirms the diagnosis of SAH and can suggest the probable location of the bleeding aneurysm by showing where the greatest amount of hemorrhage lies. Blood in the interhemispheric fissure and lateral ventricle is most consistent with an anterior communicating artery aneurysm. Hemorrhage in the sylvian fissure is most compatible with a middle cerebral artery aneurysm [Figure 19-14(a)], whereas blood in the fourth ventricle suggests a posterior inferior cerebellar artery aneurysm. MR is particularly useful because it is able to show hemorrhage with hyperintensity on T1WI when the subarachnoid blood fades away on CT. On MR, the lumen of aneurysm is round hypointensity on T1WI and T2WI images. The thrombus of aneurysm show hypointensity and/or hyperintensity [Figure 19-14(b)]. CTA and MRA are new techniques. By CTA, MRA and/or DSA[Figure 19-14(c)], we can see aneurysm, thrombus of aneurysm, neck, body of aneurysm and aneurysm of artery clearly. They are very useful in the aneurysm treatment.

（4）Arteriovenous malformations

1）Clinical and pathological manifestations：Arteriovenous malformations (AVMs) are considered congenital anomalies of blood vessels that arise in fetal life but usually become symptomatic in the third or fourth decade of

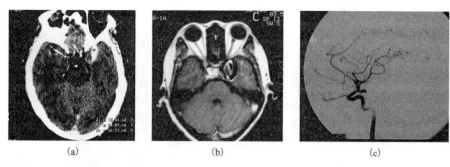

(a) enhanced CT demonstrates an aneurysm. The unenhanced part of the lesion is thrombus of aneurysm;
(b)T1WI shows the aneurysm. Thrombus of aneurysm is hyperintensity; (c)DSA demonstrates an aneurysm of
posterior communicating artery. Neck of aneurysm, body of aneurysm and aneurysm of artery can be seen clearly.

Figure 19-14 CT, MRI and DSA findings of aneurysm

life. They contain one or more enlarged feeding arteries and have enlarged early draining veins. They have a tendency to hemorrhage and result in SAH or hemorrhage of parenchyma. A recognized complication of AVMs is the steal phenomenon. In this situation, blood supply preferentially supply the AVMs and normal brain parenchyma is thus relatively undersupplied. Steal can produce focal neurologic symptoms, seizures, and ultimately result in a loss of brain function in the affected part of the brain. Feeding arteries, nidus, and draining veins are the most factors of diagnosis of AVM.

2)Imaging manifestations: On CT, the tangled vessels in the brain parenchyma are high density without contrast and have a serpentine, punctate, or an irregular mélange configuration [Figure 19-15(a)]. Curvilinear or speckled calcification may be present. These lesions enhance after enhancement. On MR, curvilinear flow voids resulted from the fast flow are observed on most pulse sequences, and dilated feeding arteries can also be observed. MRA is useful for mapping the AVM [Figure 19 - 15 (b)]. Both three-dimensional time-of-flight and three-dimensional phase-contrast techniques are useful. Enhancement increases the conspicuity of AVM, particularly the venous portion. The cerebral angiography is the gold-standard for the diagnosis of AVM. The diagnosis is made by demonstrating an enlarged feeding artery, the core or nidus, and the draining vein [Figure 19-15(c)]

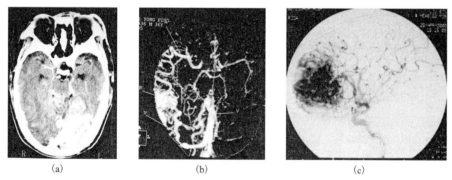

(a)enhanced CT demonstrates the tangled vessels in the brain parenchyma and the nidus can be seen clearly;
(b)Arteriovenous malformation: MRA shows the enlarged feeding artery, the nidus, and the enlarged draining
veins of AVM; (c)Arteriovenous malformation: DSA reveals the enlarged feeding artery, the nidus, and the
draining vein of AVM.

Figure 19-15 CT, MRA and DSA findings of arteriovenous malformation

(Tan Yan, Hu Se, Sun Xiangru, Jiang Haoru, Tian Dawei, Xiao Enhua, Liu Jun)

第二十章

脊髓

第一节　检查方法

1. 脊椎 X 线平片

常规摄取 X 线正位片、侧位片，如需观察椎间孔或椎弓，则加摄 X 线斜位片。

2. 脊髓造影

脊髓造影是将对比剂注入脊髓蛛网膜下隙，通过动态观察对比剂在椎管内的充盈和流动情况，以诊断椎管内占位性病变和蛛网膜粘连。

3. CT

CT 先扫描定位像，以确定扫描平面。观察椎骨和椎管病变，以层厚 8~10 mm 连续扫描病变区；观察椎间盘病变，对病变椎间盘及其上椎体、下椎体缘以每组 3~5 层，每层 2~5 mm 扫描；分别以骨窗和软组织窗显示。CT 增强扫描对诊断椎管内肿瘤和血管性病变有帮助。脊髓造影 CT（CTM）常与脊髓造影配合，在脊髓造影后 1~2 小时内进行扫描，具有 CT 和脊髓造影的双重优势。

4. MRI

MRI 矢状面成像非常重要，它可全面地观察脊髓的解剖和病变。横断面和冠状面成像可进一步确定病变与周围结构的关系。常规则采用自旋回波序列 T1WI 和 T2WI。注射 Gd-DTPA 增强的横断面及矢状面 T1WI 对病变的鉴别诊断有帮助。MRA 常用于诊断椎管内血管畸形。MR 脊髓成像（MRM）表现类似脊髓造影，可用于椎管内占位性病变的评价。

第二节　正常表现

1. 脊椎 X 线平片表现

脊椎 X 线正位片显示两侧椎弓根对称，上下椎弓根内缘连线平直，根间距即代表椎管的横径。侧位片显示上下椎体后缘和椎板前缘的连线各呈一条光滑的曲线，两线间距即代表椎管的前后径。斜位片显示椎间孔呈椭圆形，边缘光整。

2. 脊髓造影表现

脊髓造影是通过对脊髓、马尾和神经根在蛛网膜下腔中的表面解剖轮廓的显示，从而对其进行侧面描述。蛛网膜下隙表现为两侧对称的高密度，中间呈柱状充盈缺损的为脊髓。马尾位于脊髓圆锥以下，呈束带状低密度。神经根起源于脊髓，其根鞘清晰可见，呈带状充盈缺损位于外周蛛网膜下隙。

3. 脊椎 CT 表现

（1）骨性椎管：椎管的前界是椎体和椎间盘，侧面是椎弓根和椎间孔，侧后面是上下关节突，后界是椎板。正常椎管前后径和横径的下限分别为 11.5 mm 和 16 mm；侧隐窝宽度下限为 3 mm。椎间孔位于椎管的前外侧，脊神经和伴随的血管由此进出椎管。

（2）椎管内软组织：硬膜囊呈圆形或卵圆形，位于椎管中央，周围是低密度的脂肪。脊髓在硬膜囊内呈中等密度，两者之间是低密度的蛛网膜下隙，但是只有在上颈段才能区分脊髓和硬膜囊。黄韧带附于椎板内侧面，正常 2~4 mm 厚。CTM 在高密度的脑脊液衬托下可清晰显示脊髓、马尾和神经根。

4. 脊髓 MRI 表现

MRI 可直接显示脊髓及其他椎管内结构。在矢状面 T1WI 上，脊髓呈中等信号，周围为低信号的脑脊液，脊髓边缘光整、清晰可见；在旁矢状面上，由于椎间孔内高信号的脂肪衬托，神经根和神经节清晰可见。在 T2WI 上，脑脊液和脊髓的信号翻转，脑脊液明显高于脊髓。椎管的边缘由于骨皮质和韧带的信号特征，在 T1WI 和 T2WI 均呈低信号。在横断面上，脊髓和周围结构的关系显示更清晰。MRM 表现与脊髓造影相似。

第三节　基本病变

1. 脊椎平片表现

椎管内占位性病变表现为椎管扩大，如椎弓根内缘变平或凹陷、椎弓根间距增宽和椎体后缘凹陷。脊椎恶性肿瘤或结核可见椎骨破坏和椎旁软组织肿块，常侵及椎管。神经源性肿瘤常表现为椎间孔扩大伴边缘骨质硬化。

2. 脊髓造影表现

脊髓造影可明确椎管内占位性病变的部位，为疾病诊断提供有力证据。髓内病变表现为脊髓膨大、蛛网膜下隙对称性变窄或杯口状阻塞。髓外硬膜下病变表现为蛛网膜下隙内充盈缺损、邻近蛛网膜下隙增宽和脊髓受压向对侧移位。硬膜外病变表现为梳齿状阻塞、患侧蛛网膜下腔变窄和脊髓向对侧轻度移位。

3. 脊椎 CT 表现

脊椎 CT 采用软组织成像技术可在一定程度上显示椎管内病变，但由于与软组织对比差异小，病变显示不佳。CTM 可基本确定病变在椎管内的部位，并可清晰地显示软组织和骨性椎管的改变，优于脊髓造影。

4. 脊髓 MRI 表现

MRI 可直接显示椎管内病变的部位和范围，清晰显示肿块、出血、变性及坏死等病理改变，其 MRI 表现与头部病变相似。MRM 同脊髓造影和 CTM 一样可明确椎管内占位性病变的部位。

5. 比较影像学

脊椎 X 线平片对脊髓病变的观察非常有限。CT 检查侧重于骨性椎管，对椎管内软组织显示不及 MRI。脊髓造影和 CTM 是有创的检查方法，已逐渐被 MRM 所取代。MRI 可能是目前最好的脊髓检查方法，它不但能像 CT 一样轴位成像，而且还能以同样的分辨率冠状位和矢状位成像，从而无创地显示整个脊髓的长度和病变的纵向范围；另外，通过不同的脉冲序列成像可鉴别不同的组织学特征，提供其他成像方法所不能提供的信息。

第四节　常见疾病诊断

1. 椎管内肿瘤

（1）临床及病理表现：椎管内肿瘤包括髓内肿瘤、髓外硬膜下肿瘤和硬膜外肿瘤。前者以室管膜瘤和星形细胞瘤常见；髓外硬膜下肿瘤多为神经源性肿瘤和脊膜瘤；后者多为转移瘤。

（2）影像学表现：

1）X线表现：脊椎平片可提示椎管内占位性病变，但它提供的诊断信息非常有限。脊髓造影和CTM能确定肿瘤部位，给予一定的定性评价。

2）CT表现：CT能清晰地显示椎管内肿瘤导致的椎体骨质改变，但它对椎管内肿瘤的显示不及MRI。

3）MRI表现：MRI能对椎管内肿瘤作出定位、定量甚至于定性的诊断，已经成为首要的检查方法（图20-1）。椎管内肿瘤在T1WI上常表现为等或稍低信号，在T2WI上表现为等或高信号。由于肿瘤内的出血、坏死或囊性变可表现为混杂信号。注射Gd-DTPA后肿瘤实质出现不同程度和不同形式的强化。

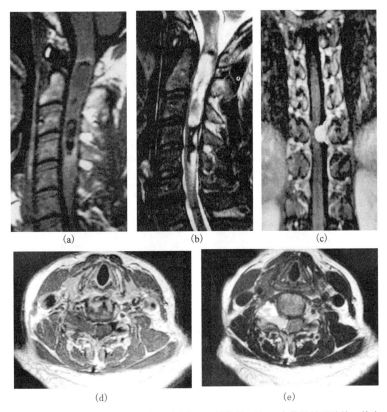

（a）、（b）脊髓室管膜瘤 颈1-4水平髓内长T1低信号、长T2高信号梭形肿块，其头、尾侧长T1、短T2低信号为含铁血黄素；（c）脊膜瘤 增强T1WI示胸11水平髓外硬膜下间隙均匀强化结节，伴脊膜尾征；（d）、（e）神经鞘瘤 稍长T1略低信号、长T2高信号亚铃状肿块，右侧椎管内、外联合受累。

图20-1　椎管内肿瘤MRI表现

2. 脊髓损伤

（1）临床及病理表现：脊髓损伤包括脊髓震荡、脊髓挫裂伤、脊髓横断和脊髓压迫。病理上，急性脊髓损伤可表现为局部的水肿，不同程度的脊髓出血，单纯的组织丢失或碎裂；当病变愈合后，可形成脊髓软化、囊性变、萎缩或粘连性蛛网膜炎。

(2)影像学表现:

1)X 线表现:脊椎 X 线平片能显示椎骨骨折和脱位。脊髓造影可显示硬膜囊撕裂和脊髓受压。

2)CT 表现:一般用于进一步地评价骨折的范围和检查碎骨片突入椎管的情况;也可显示脊髓内出血和硬膜外血肿。CT 三维重建和 CTM 可进一步提供如脊髓膨大、受压及断裂等有利信息。

3)MRI 表现:能直接显示损伤的类型、部位、范围和程度。脊髓挫裂伤在 T1WI 上见脊髓内低信号水肿区,也可无信号异常,但 T2WI 均可见不均匀高信号。脊髓水肿 T1WI 上表现为稍低信号,T2WI 上表现为高信号。脊髓血肿各时期的相关信号演变与脑出血相似。脊髓软化、囊性变及空洞形成 T1WI 上表现为低信号,T2WI 上表现为高信号。脊髓萎缩可以是弥漫性的或是局限性的,伴有或不伴有信号异常。

3.脊髓空洞症

(1)临床及病理表现:脊髓空洞症是一种慢性脊髓退行性疾病。可为先天性发育异常所致,也可继发于脊髓创伤、感染或肿瘤。病理上包括中央管扩张和脊髓内空洞形成。

(2)影像学表现:

1)CT 表现:平扫时,单纯的空洞表现为脊髓内边缘清晰的脑脊液样低密度囊腔。相应的脊髓外形可膨大、正常或萎缩。CTM 时囊腔显影提示囊腔与脑脊液相交通;而延迟 4~6 小时显影者,提示两者不相通。

2)MRI 表现:矢状位图像能清晰地显示脊髓空洞情况、流体动力学改变及进一步确定其病因。空洞在 T1WI 上表现为脊髓中央的低信号,T2WI 上表现为高信号(图 20-2)。当空洞与脑脊液相交通时,在 T2WI 上高信号的脑脊液中可出现由于脑脊液搏动所致的条状低信号影。注射 Gd-DTPA 后增强的 T1WI 可以进一步提高对单纯空洞与肿瘤并发空洞的鉴别。

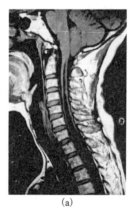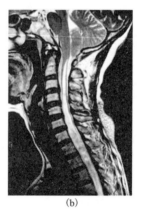

(a)   (b)

(a)T1WI 示脊髓增粗,呈脑脊液样低信号,边缘光滑;小脑扁桃体疝为合并的 Chiari 畸形;(b)T2WI 示脊髓中央呈不均匀高信号,提示空洞与蛛网膜下隙相通。

图 20-2 脊髓空洞症合并 Chiari 畸形 MRI 表现

4.椎管内血管畸形

(1)临床及病理表现:椎管内血管畸形的病理机制和分类与脑血管畸形相似。其中以动静脉畸形(AVM)最常见,分为硬膜内和硬膜外 AVM 两类。

(2)影像学表现:

1)CT 表现:平扫时,AVM 表现为椎管内软组织的局限性增粗,密度不均,有时可见点状钙化。增强扫描可不同程度地显示条状或团块状强化的畸形血管及供血动脉和引流静脉。CTA 检查能够较为清楚显示 AVM 全貌。

2) MRI 表现：MRI 可作为 AVM 的筛选检查方法，它能提供诸如病变的部位、范围、合并症和继发的出血、慢性缺血及梗塞等重要信息。椎管内的异常血管表现为条状或团块状流空信号。其他病理改变的 MRI 表现如前所述。注射 Gd-DTPA 后增强的 MRA 能检出小的 AVM。

3) 血管造影表现：仍然是诊断 AVM 的金标准。它能直接显示供血动脉、畸形血管和引流静脉。

（谭艳，刘泽，昌倩，肖恩华，刘军）

Chapter 20

Spinal cord

Section 1   Method of examination

1. Vertebral plain film

Anteroposterior and lateral projections are routine examination. Oblique views are necessary for intervertebral foramina and arch of vertebra.

2. Myelography

Myelography is used to diagnose intraspinal space occupying lesions and adhesive arachnoiditis after injection of a contrast medium into the spinal subarachnoid space and observing its filling and circulation in intraspinal space.

3. CT

A scout view is required so that each cut may be accurately localized. To observe the lesions of vertebra and spinal canal, continuous scanning, with a 8 ~ 10 mm section thickness, should be done. To observe the intervertebral disc lesions, scanning should include intervertebral disc and contiguous border of vertebral border, with 3–5 slices per series, 2~5 mm thick per sections; The images may then be displayed using bony and soft-tissue windows. Enhanced-CT-scanning is helpful to diagnosis intraspinal tumors and vascular lesions. CT myelography (CTM), which is usually combined with myelography and performed 1–2 hours after myelography, has the superiority of both CT and myelography.

4. MRI

Sagittal view is particularly important, which can observe completely the anatomy and pathology of spinal cord. Axial and coronal views can further determine the relationship between lesions and peripheral structures. Standard spin-echo T1WI and T2−WI are routine examination. When a lesion is identified, T1−WI with Gd-DTPA in the axial and sagittal plane are helpful. MR angiography (MRA) is usually performed to diagnose intraspinal vascular malformations. MR myelography (MRM) can be employed to assess intraspinal lesion, the manifestation of which is similar to myelography.

Section 2   Normal appearances

1. Findings of vertebral plain film

Anteroposterior view shows symmetrical structure of the amphi-pedicles, and the medial margin lines that connects the amphi-pedicles are smooth. Interpediculate distances represents the transverse diameter of the spinal canal. Lateral view displays the lines of posterior vertebral bodies and anterior laminaes, which should form smooth curves. Distances between the two lines suggest the anteroposterior diameter of the spinal canal. Oblique view demonstrate the foramina, which should have a ellipsoidal form with smooth margins.

2. Findings of myelography

Myelography delineates spinal cord, cauda equina and nerve root through the silhouetted images of their surface anatomy in the subarachnoid space. The subarachnoid space manifests as symmetric amphi-hypperdense and the columnar filling defect is spinal cord. Cauda equina is located below conus medullaris in the subarachnoid space, manifesting as band hypodensity. Nerve roots originate from the spinal cord and their sleeves are visualized clearly, manifesting as band filling defect in the peripheral subarachnoid space.

3. Findings of vertebra CT

(1) Osseous vertebral canal: The vertebral canal is bounded anteriorly by the vertebral bodies and their intervening discs, laterally by the pedicles and intervertebral foramina, posterolaterally by the articular processes, and posteriorly by the laminae. The lower limit of normal anteroposterior and transversal diameter of the vertebral canal is 11.5 mm and 16 mm, respectively, and the width of the lateral recess is 3 mm. The intervertebral foramina is located in anterolateral vertebral canal, from which the spinal nerves and their accompanying blood vessels enter and exit the vertebral canal.

(2) Intraspinal soft tissue: The dural sac has a round or ovale configuration and is located in the central of the vertebral canal surrounded by peripheral low density fat. The spinal cord manifests as mid-density in the dural sac, and between them is low densitysubarachnoid space. Only at the superior cervical region the spinal cord can be distinguished from dural sac. The ligamenta flava is located in the internal surface lamina, which is usually 2~4 mm thick. CTM can reveal spinal cord, cauda equinal and nerve root clearly under the hyperdensity cerebrospinal fluid(CSF).

4. Findings of spinal cord MRI

MRI can show directly spinal cord and other intraspinal constitution. On the sagittal images, T1WIs of the spinal cord shows an intermediate signal surrounded by low signal CSF. Its margins can be readily identified and the border are smooth. On the parasagittal images, the nerve roots and ganglia are well visualized due to the presence of hypersignal of intra-foramen fat. On T2WIs, there is an inversion of the intensity of CSF and spinal cord, the CSF becomes high intensity compared with spinal cord. The margins of the canal are low signal on both T1WI and T2WI due to the low signal characteristics of cortical bone and ligamentous structures. On the axial images, the relationship between spinal cord and peripheral structures can be displayed better. The manifestation of MRM is similar to that of myelography.

Section 3 Basic pathological changes

1. Findings of vertebral plain film

Intraspinal lesions manifest as expansion of the spinal canal, such as flattening or depressing of the medial margin of the pedicles, widening of the distance between the pedicles and depressing of posterior border of the body. Vertebral malignant tumor and tuberculosis may manifest as destruction of vertebra and para-vertebral mass of soft tissues, which usually lead to encroachment of vertebral canal. Neurogenic tumour usually present as enlargement of intervertebral foramen with marginal bony sclerosis.

2. Findings of myelography

Myelography can define the localization of intraspinal lesions and provide valuable information for diagnosis. Intramedullary lesions manifest as enlargement of the cord, symmetric narrow or coryloid occlusion of subarachnoid space. Extramedullary/intradural lesions present as filling defect in subarachnoid space, widening of the adjacent subarachnoid space, contralateral displacement of the spinal cord. Extradural lesions usually manifest as pectinate obstruction, narrowing of homonymous subarachnoid space, mild displacement to the contralateral of the spinal cord.

3. Findings of vertebral CT

Although vertebral CT images with soft-tissue technique may show intraspinal lesions in some degree, the contrast differences are very slight between lesions and soft tissue and the lesions visualization is usually not that good. CTM can define the localization of lesions in canal and reveal the change of soft tissues and vertebral canal clearly caused by lesions, which is superior to myelography.

4. Findings of spinal cord MRI

MRI can show the localization and dimension of intraspinal lesions exactly and describe basic pathological changes clearly, such as mass, hemorrhage, degeneration and necrosis, whose manifestation on MRI is similar to brain. MRM can also define the localization of intraspinal lesions in canal like myelography and CTM.

5. Comparative imaging

Vertebral plain film is very limited in observing spinal disorders. CT examinationlays emphasis on osseous vertebral canal and it is not ideal in the intraspinal soft tissue displaying. Myelography and CTM are invasive examination method, which have been gradually replaced by MRM. MRI are considered arbitrary examination method of the spinal cord because that it can generate images in the axial plane as CT, or coronally and sagittally with the same degree of resolution, where the entire length of the spinal cord and the longitudinal extent of pathology can be imaged non-invasion directly, and the alterations in the pulse sequence can enhance various tissue characteristics and provide information that is not available with other imaging methods.

Section 4　Diagnosis of common diseases

1. Intraspinal tumors

(1) Clinical and pathological manifestations: Intraspinal tumors include intramedullary tumors, extramedullary/intradural tumors and extradural tumors. Ependymoma and astrocytoma are the predominant type of intramedullary tumors; Neurogenic tumor and meningioma are mainly extramedullary/intradural tumors; Metastatic tumors are extradural tumors.

(2)Imaging manifestations:

1)X-ray findings: Vertebral plain film may indicate intraspinal lesions, but diagnostic information provided by plain film is quite limited. Myelography can define the localization of tumor and give some qualitative evaluation.

2)CT findings: CT can display the change of vertebral bone matrix clearly caused by intraspinal tumors, while MRI can provide much more information in the manifestation of tumors.

3)MRI findings: MRI can define the positioning of the tumors, and make a quantitative and even qualitative diagnostic for intraspinal tumors and has become the prominent examination method for it (Figure 20 - 1). Intraspinal tumors usually manifest as equal-or slightly low-signal on T1WI and equal-or high-signal on T2 - WI compared to spinal cord. Sometimes, mixed-signal occurs because of hemorrhage, necrosis and or cystic degeneration in tumors. With the administration of Gd-DTPA, the nidus of tumor enhances by means of various degree and patterns.

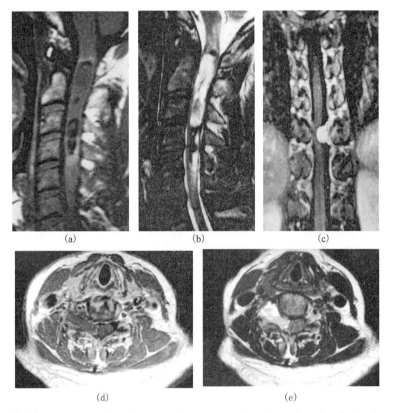

(a)(b)Ependymoma of spinal cord. Fusiform mass with long T1 signal and long T2 signal at 1-4 level of the neck. The long T1 and short T2 in the head and tail of the tumor is hemosiderin. (c)Meningioma. On contrast-enhanced T1WI, the tumor shows homogeneous enhancement nodules in the epidural space at the level of thoracic 11, accompanied by the tail sign of meninges. (d)(e)Neurilemmoma. The tumor shows sub-bell shaped mass with slightly long T1 and slightly long T2, the right side of the spinal canal was involved.

Figure 20-1　MRI findings of intraspinal tumors

2. Spinal cord injury

(1)Clinical and pathological manifestations: Spinal cord injury involves cord concussion, contusion and laceration, transection and compression. Pathologically, acute injury to the spinal cord may manifest as a focal area of edema, variable amounts of hematomyelia, frank tissue loss or crushing. As the lesion heals, malacia, cystic degeneration or atrophy of spinal cord or adhesive arachnoiditis develops.

(2)Imaging manifestations:

1)X-ray findings: Vertebral plain film can show vertebral fracture and dislocation. Myelography can display dural laceration and spinal cord compression.

2)CT findings: CT is commonly obtained to further evaluate the extent of the fracture and detect fragments projecting into the spinal canal. It can also show intramedullary hemorrhage and epidural hematomas. CT three-dimensional imaging and CTM can provide additional useful information such as spinal cord swelling, compression or disruption.

3)MRI findings: MRI can reveal the injury types, injury location, injury dimension and injury degree directly. Low signal or no abnormal signal edema area in spinal cord is found on T1WI in spinal cord contusion and laceration injury, but heterogeneous high signal could be seen on T2WI. The spinal cord edema is present as slightly diminished signal on T1WI and increased signal on T2WI. The time-related signal changes of intramedullary hematomas proceed as described in the brain. The malacia, cystic degeneration and cavity formation manifest as very low signal on T1WI and very high signal on T2WI. Spinal cord atrophy may be diffuse or localized, displaying with or without signal abnormality.

3. Syringomyelia

(1) Clinical and pathological manifestations: Syringomyelia is a kind of chronic degenerative spinal cord disease. The presence of syringomyelia may be due to congenital dysplasia and/or following cord trauma, infection or tumor. On pathology, syringomyelia involve expansion of the central canal and formation of intramedullary cavity.

(2) Imaging manifestations:

1) CT findings: On plain scans, simple syrinx cavities generally have smooth internal margins, contain fluid signal as the CSF. The configuration of corresponding spinal cord may be expansion, normal or decreased. On CTM, visualization of cavity suggests communication between the cavity and CSF, whereas delaying visualization after 4-6 hours indicates no communication.

2) MRI findings: Sagittal view can demonstrate clearly the condition of cavities and the change of fluid dynamics, and further determine its etiological factor. The cavity manifests as diminished signal in the central spinal cord on T1WI and increased signal on T2WI (Figure 20-2). When there is some communication channel between the cavity and CSF, low-signal zonale generated by CSF pulsation may occur in high-signal of cavity on T2WI. The addition of T1WI with Gd-DTPA may further improve the distinction between "simple syrinx" and those associated with tumor.

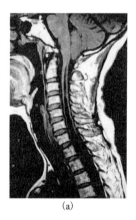 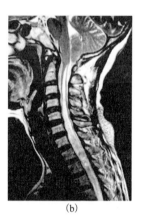

(a)   (b)

(a) On T1WI, the spinal cord is thickened with low signal like cerebrospinal fluid and smooth edge; cerebellar tonsillar hernia is associated with Chiari malformation. (b) T2WI shows inhomogeneous high signal in the center of spinal cord, suggesting that the cavity communicates with subarachnoid space.

Figure 20-2 MRI findings of syringomyelia with Chiari malformation

4. Intraspinal vascular malformations

(1) Clinical and pathological manifestation: The pathologic mechanisms and the classification of intraspinal vascular malformations are similar to that of cerebral. Arteriovenous malformation (AVM) is the most common intraspinal vascular malformations, classified as intramedullary or extramedullary, and is discussed below.

（2）Imaging manifestations：

1）CT findings：On nonenhanced scans, AVM may manifest as localized expansion of intravertebral soft tissue, and accompanied with calcification. On enhanced scans, the deformed vessel as well as feeding arteries and draining veins can be shown in different degree as the zonale or agglomerative under contrast enhancement. CTA can clearly show the whole picture of AVM.

2）MRI findings：MRI is the screening method and gives important information about its location and extent, as well as evidence for hemorrhage, chronic ischemia and infarction. Intraspinal abnormal vessel presents as zonale or agglomerative flow void signal. Manifestation of other pathological changes on MRI is similar to previous brain disease. Gd-DTPA enhanced MRA can detect micro-AVM.

3）Findings of angiography：Angiography remains the gold standard for AVM. It can demonstrate directly deformed vessel, feeding arteries and draining veins.

（Tan Yan, Liu Zeliang, Chang Qian Xiao Enhua, Liu Jun）

第六篇

头颈部

头颈部疾病包括眼、耳、鼻和鼻窦、喉、鼻咽、口腔颌面部、颈部疾病。疾病种类繁多，影像学检查在临床疾病诊断中起着关键作用，不仅能显示头颈部精细解剖及其变异，而且显示头颈部病变的部位、大小和范围，还可对大部分病变作出定性诊断。X线平片主要检查口腔颌面部和鼻窦病变。X线造影用于检查涎腺和泪道病变。CT是头颈部大多数疾病的主要影像检查技术，用于头颈部先天性、肿瘤性、炎性和外伤性等疾病检查。MRI目前已成为头颈部疾病的常规检查技术，MRI对软组织分辨力高，加上动态增强、脂肪抑制技术、扩散加权成像(DWI)、磁共振波谱(MRS)、灌注加权成像(PWI)等功能成像，有利于病变的检出和定性诊断，MR水成像技术可清楚显示膜迷路的三维结构。

Part 6

Head and neck

Head and neck diseases include eye, ear, nose and sinuses, larynx, nasopharynx, oral and maxillofacial diseases, neck diseases. There are many kinds of diseases. The imaging examination plays a key role in the clinical diagnosis of many kinds of diseases. It can not only show the fine anatomy and its variation of the head and neck, but also show the location, size and range of the lesions in the head and neck, qualitative diagnosis can also be made for most lesions. X-ray plain film mainly examines the oral and maxillofacial region and the paranasal sinuses pathological changes. X-ray radiography is used to examine salivary gland and lacrimal duct lesions. CT is the main imaging technoque for most diseases of head and neck. It is used for congenital, neoplastic, inflammatory and traumatic diseases of head and neck. MRI has become a routine examination technique for head and neck diseases, high soft tissue resolution, fat suppression technique, diffusion-weighted imaging (DWI), magnetic resonance spectrscopy (MRS), perfusion-weighted imaging (PWI), and other functional imaging are helpful for the detection and qualitative diagnosis of the lesions, the three-dimensional structure of membrane labyrinth can be clearly displayed by water imaging.

第二十一章

眼

第一节　检查方法

1. X 线平片检查

眼部 X 线平片能提供有价值的诊断信息有限，但仍是常用检查方法，主要应用于外伤骨折、异物插入等。常用摄影位置包括枕额位投照、侧位投照以及视神经孔位投照。此外眼眶血管造影，通常采用选择性的插管造影，然后侧位及前后位投照或者颌下垂直投照。泪腺造影检查通常在泪囊联合处注入适量局部麻醉药，将一根柔韧的导管插入泪小管，持续注入少量水溶性碘离子对比剂，再断层成像，用于观察泪囊泪道功能和形态。

2. CT 检查

CT 是眼部疾病的主要影像检查技术，适用于检查眼部先天性、肿瘤性、炎性、血管性及外伤性等病变。通常采用常规容积扫描，薄层多方位重建技术，再行软组织窗和骨窗观察。高空间分辨率 CT 能很好地显示眼眶及其内部结构，尤其是视神经和眼外肌。显示视神经病变时，常用血管内对比剂做增强扫描。此外与 MRI 相比，CT 能更好地检查和监视躁动不合作的患者，并且能检测到钙化灶，这在视网膜母细胞瘤的诊断中特别重要。同时，CT 也是眼眶外伤和骨折成像的首选方法。

3. MRI 检查

MRI 在眼眶疾病诊断方面的应用是一重要进展，其优势在于直接多平面成像和获得超清晰的眼眶结构影像，可显示视神经和眶尖的解剖学细节，可以进行血管成像，并可以检测不同的血液降解产物以及含黑色素的病变，同时它还没有射线辐射以及由邻近骨骼和牙质所造成的假影。但与 CT 相比，其缺点在于发现钙化和骨质破坏的能力较差。其次如果眼眶外伤伴有怀疑具有磁性的异物时，需禁用 MRI 检查。

4. 超声检查

超声检查是眼球疾病的首选检查技术，常规选用 5MHz 以上高频专用探头。超声影像可多角度投照，能有效的显示肌锥内外病变，同时可检测视网膜脱离，此外多普勒超声检查还可用于评估眼眶血管，特别是在存在瘘管或血管肿瘤的情况下。但是对比高分辨 CT，超声图像的征象更具有主观性。

第二节　正常表现

1. 眼眶的壁

眼眶是一个类似金字塔的窦腔，它的底部在前方，以坚固的骨性边缘包围；它的顶部易碎，因为脑回压迹而显得不规则。额窦的眶上切迹通过它的前部，上斜肌的滑车处于眶顶的内前方。内壁或者叫纸板，它很薄，在前方把眼眶和鼻窦分开，在后方把眼眶与筛窦及蝶窦的前部分开，前下方有泪窝，泪房，泪囊。眶底部也很薄，从后至前通过眶下神经开始走行于槽内，然后进入开口于上颌窦前上边缘的管内，后者被眶底将其与眼眶分开。

眼眶的外壁是最坚固的，由颧骨和蝶骨翼组成，它把眼眶和颞骨分割开来。视神经管处于蝶骨小翼的2个根部之间，其内走行着视神经和眼动脉，视神经管通常是两侧对称的。位于蝶骨大小翼之间的眶上裂与海绵窦的前部相连。其内有动眼神经，第五颅神经第一分支的泪腺支、鼻支和额支，眼静脉和一支连接脑膜和眼睛的动脉。眶上裂轻微不对称是常见的。眶下裂位于侧壁和下壁之间，它把中颅窝与上颌窦分开。

2. 眼的构成

眼包括眼球、视神经、眼外肌、泪腺、血管和神经。所有这些结构被眶内脂肪包绕着。眼球近似一个球体，其前后径通常约 22 mm，由富血管的脉络膜和视网膜覆盖，眼球包括晶状体、睫状体、虹膜。前房以虹膜的前部角膜为界，中心为晶状体，后房在晶状体和虹膜之间，这些房包含房水。眼晶状体后房充满了玻璃体。视神经较粗传输纤维直径约 4 mm，是脑组织的外延，因此它被充满脑脊液的脑膜包围着。四个眼直肌从腱环由腱膜相连，分为内外间隙，这些肌起自 Zinn 总腱环。上下斜肌与斜视密切相关，眼睑上提肌位于上直肌的上方。

泪腺位于眼球前外上侧表面，在内眦处，后上方微小泪管汇集成小管，开口在泪囊，再通过鼻泪管排空至鼻腔(窦)。

第三节　基本病变

1. 大小与形态异常

CT，MRI 检查均可观察眼眶，眼球，眼外肌，视神经形态及大小改变。

(1)眼眶增大主要见于占位性病变；眼眶缩小见于无眼球，小眼球或婴幼儿期行眼球摘除术后；眶周病变向眶内膨隆或侵入也可使眼眶变小。眼眶形态改变见于先天发育畸形或骨纤维异常增殖，额窦或筛窦黏液囊肿等。

(2)眼球增大见于眼球占位，青光眼晚期，高度近视眼，巩膜葡萄肿等；眼球缩小见于先天发育畸形，眼球肿瘤放疗后等。

(3)眼外肌增粗见于炎性病变，外伤，甲状腺眼病等；眼外肌变细见于各种原因引起的眼球运动神经受损。

(4)视神经增粗见于肿瘤，炎症等；视神经变细见于视神经萎缩。

2. 密度(信号)异常

(1)CT 表现：眼眶密度增加是眶内占位性病变的常见表现。眶内钙化灶见于视网膜母细胞瘤，眶内静脉畸形。密度减低见于外伤后眶内积气，表皮样囊肿等。病变内钙化表现为高密度，坏死表现为低密度，病变密度不均匀提示病变构成成分复杂。

(2)MRI 表现：眶内大部分病变成 T1WI 低信号，T2WI 高信号；脉络膜黑色素瘤呈 T1WI 高信号，T2WI 低信号；表皮样囊肿或皮样囊肿因含脂类成分，T1WI 及 T2WI 均呈高信号，脂肪抑制扫描后信号强度减低；硬化性炎性假瘤或陈旧性出血呈低信号。病变信号不均匀提示病变有坏死，钙化或多种成分存在。

3. 位置异常

眼球突出见于球后占位性病变，外伤后出血，甲状腺眼病及颈动脉海绵窦瘘等，体位性眼球突出见于脉管性病变。眼球内陷多见于暴裂性骨折或眶内静脉曲张。眼外肌或视神经位置异常时，可根据移位方向

判断病变的位置或来源

4.眼眶骨质异常

骨质破坏见于眶内,眶周恶性病变或转移瘤;泪腺肿瘤可致骨质吸收,神经纤维瘤病可致蝶骨大小翼骨质缺损。骨纤维异常增殖症,脑膜瘤及眶周骨髓炎可致眼眶骨质增生。

5.眼眶通道异常

视神经管扩大见于视神经胶质瘤,视神经鞘瘤,脑膜瘤或神经纤维瘤病;视神经管缩小见于骨纤维异常增殖症,蝶骨嵴脑膜瘤等。眶上裂增大见于视神经鞘瘤和颈动脉海绵窦瘘;眶上裂缩小见于骨纤维异常增殖症。

6.肿块

密度中等,均匀,边界清楚光整的软组织肿块多为良性肿瘤;密度不均,边界不清,提示炎性病变,如伴有骨质破坏多为恶性肿瘤。病变强化明显提示血供丰富,见于炎性病变、恶性肿瘤、血管瘤等;强化不明显提示乏血供,见于黏液囊肿,表皮样囊肿等。

7.邻近解剖结构改变

发现眼部病变需注意观察邻近结构,如鞍区,颅底,鼻窦是否受累,以利于眼部病变的鉴别诊断。

第四节 常见疾病诊断

1.特发性眶部炎症

(1)临床及病理表现:特发性眶部炎症常被称为炎性假瘤。从组织学上讲,是指眼眶内一个或者多个结构受淋巴细胞或者浆细胞浸润。发生部位频率依次为泪腺、眼外肌、巩膜、视神经和脂肪。一般只发生于一侧,患者临床体征为眼痛、眼球突出,伴或者不伴视力障碍。视力下降不常见。

(2)影像学表现:X线片通常不能显示病变。CT显示泪腺肿胀和眼外肌模糊肿胀,眼外肌肌腱也受累。巩膜及视神经可以看见类似的改变。由于眶内脂肪的密度增加,眼后结构和眶内脂肪的对比度降低。所有受累组织在增强扫描时显示明显异常强化。炎性浸润期T1WI呈等低信号,T2WI呈高信号;纤维化期T2WI呈低信号,增强后中度至明显强化。

2.视网膜母细胞瘤

(1)临床及病理表现:视网膜母细胞瘤是小儿眼部最常见的恶性肿瘤,通常在发生于3岁以下的儿童。临床表现为"白瞳症",即瞳孔区黄光反射。病变多为散发,少数可呈常染色体显性遗传。可累及单眼或双眼。

(2)影像学表现:典型CT表现为眼球内不规则肿块,95%发生钙化,钙化呈团块状、斑片状或点状,大小不一。肿瘤生长可突破眼环,球后见软组织密度肿块,累及视神经时表现为视神经增粗、扭曲及视神经管扩大。肿瘤继续生长可侵及视交叉并于颅内形成肿块。与正常玻璃体信号相比,肿块呈T1WI稍高信号,T2WI低信号,信号可不均匀,肿块实性成分明显强化。本病需要与渗出性视网膜炎、硬化性眼内炎及永存性原始玻璃体增生症鉴别。上述病变一般无钙化斑,眼球大小正常或变小。

3.眼眶外伤

(1)临床及病理表现:经典的眼眶爆裂性骨折累及眶下壁,通常可见眶内组织经骨折处疝出。眼眶下壁骨折常累及眼眶内壁,眼眶内壁骨折也可孤立地发生。骨折常常引起邻近鼻窦骨折。眶内气肿通常与眼眶内壁骨折有关。眼眶骨折可能引起颅内积气、脑脊液瘘和颅内并发症。

(2)影像学表现:CT能较好地显示眼眶骨壁及眶内软组织形态异常。磁共振成像可以评估颅内并发症。视神经管、眶上裂和眶尖骨折可能导致视神经损伤。CT扫描是定位骨折的最佳方法,MRI成像是评估视神经损伤的必要手段。视神经管的骨碎片移位、撞击导致视神经压迫。视神经压迫也可能继发于视神经蛛网膜下隙出血、骨膜下出血或球后出血。对这些可治疗的病因进行快速诊断和早期外科治疗，可以极大地挽救视力。

（谭艳，李秋云，骆永恒，刘欢，韦勇，肖恩华，刘军）

Chapter 21

The eye

Section 1   Method of examination

1. Plain film

Plain film can provide limited valuable diagnostic information, but it is still a common examination method, mainly used for traumatic fractures, foreign body insertion, etc. Commonly used photography positions include occipital-frontal projection, lateral projection, and optic nerve projection. In addition, orbital angiography usually uses selective intubation, followed by lateral and posterior anterior projection or submandibular vertical projection. Lacrimal angiography usually injects an appropriate amount of anesthetic at the joint of the lacrimal sac, inserts a flexible catheter into the lacrimal canaliculus, and continuously injects a small amount of water-capacity iodine ion contrast agent, and then tomographic imaging is used to observe the function and shape of the lacrimal duct.

2. CT examination

The main imaging techniques of checking ocular disease, it was used to check congenital, neoplastic, inflammatory, vascular ocular diseases and other traumatic lesions. Commonly used is conventional volume scanning and thin multi-faceted recombinant techniques, and soft tissue and bone window are used to observe. High spatial resolution CT can show good orbital and internal structure, particular the outer extraocular muscles and optic nerve. When displays optic neuropathy, vascular contrast agents are used in the enhanced MRI. In addition, compared with MRI, CT can better check and monitor the uncooperative and restless patient . What's more, calcification can be detected, which is especially important in the diagnosis of retinoblastoma. Meanwhile CT is the preferred imaging method of orbital trauma and fractures.

3. MRI examination

The application of MRI in the diagnosis of orbital diseases is an important progress. Its advantage lies in direct multi-plane imaging and super-clear orbital structure images, which can display the anatomical details of the optic nerve and orbital apex, perform vascular imaging, and detect different blood degradation products and melanin-containing lesions, and it has no radiation and artifacts caused by adjacent bones and dentine. However, compared with CT, its disadvantages are its poor ability are to detect calcification and bone destruction. In addition, if the orbital trauma is accompanied by a foreign body suspected of being magnetic, MRI should be disabled.

4. Ultrasound

Ultrasound examination is the preferred examination technique for eye diseases, and special probes for high frequency above 5MHz are routinely used. Ultrasound images can be obtained from multiple angles, which can effectively show the internal and external lesions of the muscle cones, and detect retinal detachment. In addition, Doppler ultrasound can also be used to evaluate orbital blood vessels, especially in the presence of fistulas or vascular tumors. Compared with high-resolution CT, the signs of ultrasound images are more subjective.

Section 2　Normal appearances

1. The walls of the orbit

The orbit is a pyramidal cavity, with its base lying anteriorly, surrounded by a strong bony rim in continuity with the walls. The roof is fragile, and irregular, due to the convolutional impressions of the meninges. The supraorbital recess of the frontal sinus invaginates its anterior part, and the trohclea, or pulley, of the superior oblique muscle lies anteromedially on the orbital roof. The medial wall, or lamina papyracea, which is very thin, separates the orbital contents from the nasal fossa anteriorly, and the ethmoid air cells and the anterior portion of the sphenoid sinus posteriorly. An anterior depression, the lacrimal fossa, houses the lacrimal sac. The floor of the orbit is also thin; it travels from posterior to anterior by the infraorbital never, which runs in a groove at first and then in a canal which opens at the anterosuperior border of the maxillary antrum. This is separated from the orbit by the orbit floor latter.

The lateral, strongest wall of the orbit, formed by the malar and the greater wing of the sphenoid, separates the orbital contents from the temporal fossa. The optic canal, lies between the two roots of the lesser wing of the sphenoid, The optic nerve and ophthalmic artery pass through the optic canal, which are usually bilaterally symmetrical. The superior orbital fissure, between the greater and lesser wings of the sphenoid bone, communicates with the anterior part of the cavernous sinus, which contains the ocular motor nerves, the lacrimal, frontal and nasal branches of the first division of V, the ophthalmic veins and an arterial connection between the middle meningeal and ophthalmic arteries. Slight asymmetry of the superior orbital fissures is frequent. The inferior orbital fissure lies between the lateral and inferior walls, separating the middle cranial fossa from the maxillary antrum.

2. The orbital contents

These include the eye (or globe), the optic nerve, extraocular muscles (including the levator palpebrae superioris), lacrimal gland, vessels and nerves, all of which are surrounded by orbital fat.

The globe is approximately spherical, with a normal anteroposterior diameter of 22 mm. It is covered with the richly vascular choroid and the retina. Its contents include the lens, iris and ciliary body. The anterior chamber is bounded by the cornea, the anterior surface of the iris and the central portion of the lens, while the posterior chamber lies between iris and lens; These chambers contain the aqueous. The retrolental portion of the globe is filled with the vitreous. The thick optic never, with a transverse diameter of about 4 mm, is a direct anterior extension of the brain and is thus covered by meninges, with a subarachnoid space containing cerebrospinal fluid. Four rectus muscles, connected by an aponeurosis, form the muscle cone, divide into extra-and intraconal spaces. These muscles originate on the annulus of Zinn. Superior and inferior oblique muscle are associated with oblique gaze; The levator palpebrae superioris muscle lies directly above the superior rectus.

The lacrimal gland lies anteriorly on the superolateral surface of the globe. At the inner canthus, posterioroinferior lacrimal canaliculi run into a common canaliculus, which opens into the lacrimal sac and drains via the nasolacrimal duct into the nasa cavity.

Section 3　Basic pathological changes

1. Abnormal size and shape

CT and MRI examination can observe the change of orbital, eyeball, extraocular muscle, optic nerve shape and size.

（1）Orbital enlargement is mainly found in space-occupying lesions. Orbital reduction is observed after enucleation of small eyeball or infant eyeball. Orbital enlargement or invasion of periorbital lesions can also make the orbital smaller. Orbital morphologic changes are found in congenital developmental malformations or abnormal proliferation of bone fibers, frontal sinus or ethmoid sinus mucocele, etc.

（2）Ocular enlargement is found in ocular space occupying, advanced glaucoma, high myopia, scleral staphyloma, etc. Eyeball shrinkage is seen in congenital malformation, eyeball tumor after radiotherapy and so on.

（3）Extraocular muscle thickening can be seen in inflammatory lesions, trauma, thyroid ophthalmopathy, etc. Thinning of the extraocular muscles is seen in a variety of causes resulting in damage to the oculomotor nerve.

（4）Thickening of optic nerve can be seen in tumor and inflammation. Thinning of the optic nerve is seen in optic atrophy.

2. Density（signal）anomaly

（1）CT findings：Increased orbital density is a common manifestation of space-occupying lesions in the orbit. Orbital calcification are seen in retinoblastoma, orbital venous malformations. Reduced density is seen in orbital gas accumulation and epidermoid cysts after trauma. The calcification in the lesion shows high density, the necrosis shows low density, and the uneven density suggests complex composition of the lesion.

（2）MRI findings：Most orbital diseases is low signal in T1WI and high signal in T2WI. Choroidal melanoma shows high signal on T1WI and low signal on T2WI. Epidermoid cysts or dermoid cysts contain fatty components, both T1WI and T2WI show high signal, and the signal decreases after fat suppression scanning. Sclerosing inflammatory pseudotumor or old bleeding shows low signal. The inhomogeneous lesion signals indicate necrosis, calcification or the presence of multiple components.

3. Abnormal position

Exophthalmopathy is found in space-occupying lesions after bulb, hemorrhage after trauma, thyroid ophthalmopathy and carotid cavernous fistula, etc. Postural exophthalmopathy is found in vascular lesions. Enophthalmos are more common in blowout fractures or orbital varicose veins. When the position of the extraocular muscle or optic nerve is abnormal, the location or source of the lesion can be determined according to the direction of displacement.

4. Abnormal orbital bone

Bone damage is found in the orbital, periorbital malignant lesions or metastatic tumors. Lacrimal neoplasms may lead to bone resorption, and neurofibromatosis may lead to bone defects of the sphenoid bone and the winged bone. Abnormal hyperplasia of bone fiber, meningioma and periorbital osteomyelitis may cause orbital bone hyperplasia

5. Abnormal orbital passage

Enlargement of optic canal is seen in optic glioma, optic sheath meningioma or neurofibromatosis. Optic canal shrinkage is seen in abnormal hyperplasia of bone fiber, sphenoid ridge meningioma and so on. Enlargement of supraorbital fissure is found in optic schwannoma and carotid cavernous sinus fistula. Reduction of supraorbital fissure is seen in bone fibrous dysplasia.

6. Lumps

Soft tissue masses with moderate density, uniform and clear boundary are mostly benign tumors. The uneven density and unclear boundary suggest the inflammatory lesions, those accompanied with bone destruction are mostly malignant tumors. The enhancement of lesions obviously indicates rich blood supply, which can be seen in inflammatory lesions, malignant tumors, hemangiomas, etc. Enhancement is not obvious in the absence of blood supply, in mucoid cysts, dermoid cysts, etc.

7. Changes in adjacent anatomical structures

To detect ocular lesions, it is necessary to observe the adjacent structures, such as saddle area, skull base and sinus involvement, so as to facilitate the differential diagnosis of ocular lesions.

Section 4　Diagnosis of common diseases

1. Idiopathic orbitalinflammation

(1) Clinical and pathological manifestations: Idiopathic orbital inflammation is usually referred as inflammatory pseudotumor. Histologically, there is infiltration by lymphocytes and plasma cells in one or more of the orbital structures. The origination are as follows: The lacrimal gland, extraocular muscles, sclera, optic nerve and fat. An only one side is usually affected. The patient presents with a painful proptosis and/or opthalmoplegia, decreased visual acuity is not uncommon.

(2) Imaging manifestations: Plain films are usually normal. Typically, CT shows swelling of the lacrimal gland, and swelling and loss of definition of the extraocular muscles, including their anterior portion. The sclera and optic nerve may show similar changes, and the contrast between the retrobulbar structures and the orbital fat is reduced, due to an increase in the density of the latter. All the involved structures may show intense abnormal contrast enhancement. In inflammatory infiltration stage, it was isohypointense on T1WI and hyperintense on T2WI. In fibrosis stage, it is hypointense on T2WI, moderate to obvious enhancement.

2. Retinoblastoma

(1) Clinical and pathological manifestations: Retinoblastomas are the most common malignant tumor of the eye in infants. They usually occur in children under 3 years old. The clinical manifestation is leukocoria, that is, yellow light reflection in the pupil area. Most of the lesions are sporadic, and a few can be inherited in an autosomal dominant manner. It can affect one or both eyes.

(2) Imaging manifestations: The typical CT findings are irregular lumps in the eyeball, 95% of which are calcified. The calcifications are in the form of lumps, patches or spots, with different sizes. The tumor can break through the eye ring, and a dense mass of soft tissue is observed behind the bulb. When the optic nerve is involved, the optic nerve is enlarged and twisted and the optic canal is enlarged. The tumor can invade the optic chiasm and form masses in the skull. Compared with normal vitreous, the tumor shows slightly higher signal on T1WI and lower signal on T2WI. The signal is uneven, and the solid component of the mass is obviously enhanced. This disease needs to be differentiated from Coat's disease, sclerosing endophthalmitis and permanent primordial vitreous hyperplasia. No calcification is found in the above lesions, and the size of the eyeball is normal or smaller.

3. Orbital trauma

(1) Clinical and pathological manifestations: The classic blow-out fracture involves the floor of the orbit.

Frequently, orbital tissues are incarcerated in the fracture site. Orbital floor fractures are always involved the medial wall of the orbit. Isolated fracture of the medial orbital wall may also occur. Orbital emphysema is commonly associated with medial orbital wall fractures. These fractures may be associated with pneumocephalus, CSF leak, and intracranial complications. The frontal sinus fractures may be present.

（2）Imaging manifestations: CT has an advantage in the delineating the soft tissue along with the bony deformity of the orbit. MR imaging is indicated to evaluate possible intracranial complications. Fractures of the optic canal, superior orbital fissure, and orbital apex may be associated with optic nerve damage. CT scan is best to localize the fracture, and MR imaging is necessary to evaluate damage to the optic nerve. Compression of the optic nerve can develop when bony fragments impinge on the nerve within the optic canal. Optic nerve compression may also occur due to hemorrhage within the optic nerve sheath or subperiosteal hemorrhage or retrobulbar hemorrhage. Rapid diagnosis and surgical treatment of treatable causes may result in significant visual recovery.

（Tan Yan, Li Qiuyun, Luo Yongheng, Liu Huan, Wei Yong, Xiao Enhua, Liu Jun）

第二十二章

耳

第一节 检查方法

1.X 线平片检查

目前 X 线平片很少用于耳的检查，其主要用于人工耳蜗植入术后观察电极的形态及位置以及颞骨的特殊解剖结构等。在临床上可行不同方向投影的常规照射，以研究颅底及其周围结构。此外除了标准的 X 线照片外，还有一些以 Schüller, Stenvers 和 Mayer 命名的特殊投影。

2.CT 检查

耳部病变的主要影像学检查技术。常规行容积扫描，多方位高分辨率重组，也可行其他多种后处理，包括三维表面遮盖显示、迷路成像和听骨链成像等。特别是近年来随着软件的快速发展，耳的解剖结构包括听小骨和骨迷路的解剖断层影像可以很详细的显示，此外 CT 仿真内镜技术也日益成熟，可观察鼓室、乳突窦、迷路及内耳道结构。

3.MRI 检查

MRI 在软组织成像方面具有无可比拟的优势，是桥小脑角听神经瘤、转移瘤、神经瘤、面神经以及软组织病变的常规检查方法。MRI 水成像技术可清楚显示膜迷路的三维结构；高分辨率三维采集的源图像可观察桥小脑角区的脑神经与血管的关系；MRI 增强检查则常用于肿瘤性病变及炎性病变的诊断与鉴别诊断等。

第二节 正常表现

耳由内耳、中耳和外耳三个部分构成。包含复杂的听觉与平衡器官。

1.内耳

内耳由前庭、耳蜗管和半规管组成。前庭在 Stenver's 投照上显示好。表现为一个小卵圆腔，紧邻内听道外侧的末端，半规管之下和耳蜗之上。

外侧半规管在经眶位投照上显示好，从前庭水平延伸，在锤砧关节，突入中耳腔的上部。上半规管在 Stenver's 投照上显示好，从前庭向上呈一突出在岩骨的前后表面。后半规管从前庭水平向后，它的外侧边缘经入口与小房紧连。

耳蜗呈顶在前的蜗牛状形状的结构，它可见于 Stenver's，上眼眶和经眼眶投照，轴位亦可显示。

2. 中耳

中耳由鼓室、咽鼓管、乳突组成，是含气的空间，其内容纳听小骨并通过咽鼓管与鼻咽部相通，通过鼓室入口与乳突气房相连。鼓膜将外耳与中耳鼓室分隔。中耳在其与鼓膜的鼓室环关系的基础上可以分为5个部分。鼓室上隐窝位于环的上方，中鼓室与环和鼓膜紧邻，下鼓室位于环的下方，正鼓室位于环的前方，后鼓室位于环的后方。另外，中耳与内耳外耳紧密相联系。鼓室上隐窝位于内听道的水平，中鼓室位于耳蜗的水平，下鼓室位于耳蜗和外听道的下方。

3. 外耳

外耳在鼓膜的外侧，由外听道和耳廓组成。外侧半由软骨构成，内侧半由颞骨的骨质构成。

4. 内听道

内听道是一个狭窄的管形、壶腹形和喇叭形结构，两侧对称，前后径及垂直径多在4~6 mm，冠状面可见底部之镰状嵴。

5. 面神经管

一个复杂弯弯曲曲的面神经走行和管道，可能与其演变发展过程相关。因为神经容易染病，而面神经又与颞骨的大多数重要结构紧邻。除了面神经麻痹外，还有许多其他不同的临床病理症状。面神经症状可来自临近的病变，它的行程可以方便地按相应耳的三个部分分为三个部分：迷路段、鼓室段、乳突段。

6. 乳突气房

起自鼓室上隐窝后份，为一小通道成为至小房的入口，进入乳突小房内，构成乳突气房系统第一部分不同大小的腔。正常小房最大横径约6 mm，最大高度约11 mm。

第三节　基本病变

1. CT 表现

（1）颞骨结构与形态异常：外耳与中耳的先天性畸形，可表现为颞骨正常结构和形态的改变，如外耳道狭窄、闭锁，听小骨畸形、融合，鼓室腔狭窄等。内耳的先天性畸形，可表现为前庭半规管及耳蜗的结构异常、内耳道狭窄等。内耳道单侧或双侧扩大提示内耳道占位性病变，常见于听神经瘤。

（2）颞骨骨质异常：CT 可以清晰地显示有无骨质破坏，及其骨质破坏的部位、范围及分界，以及骨破坏区内有无软组织密度的肿物。

（3）乳突窦与乳突气房异常：乳突窦与乳突气房的发育与密度，是急性和慢性中耳与乳突炎症和胆脂瘤所造成的改变之一。

（4）骨质连续性异常：颞骨骨折时可表现为平行（纵行）或垂直于（横行）岩骨的骨折线，有时合并听骨链脱位及面神经管骨折。

2. MRI 表现

（1）信号异常：鼓室骨壁、听小骨及其中气体等，MRI 均无信号。如鼓室内积液、积血、炎症、肉芽肿、新生物及胆脂瘤，可出现异常 MRI 信号。

（2）结构异常：内耳畸形在内耳水成像中显示结构异常。听神经瘤显示内耳道内等信号占位病变及向脑桥小脑角蔓延。

（3）中耳乳突炎的并发症：如硬膜外脓肿、乙状窦栓塞性静脉炎等均可在 MRI 上显示。

第四节　常见疾病诊断

1.感染和炎性疾病

浆液性中耳炎是咽鼓管系统病变的常见并发症，表现液体积聚在中耳和乳突。它常发生在幼儿，可能是腺样体增大所致。如果成年人出现浆液性耳炎的征象，提示放射科医生须警惕更严重的疾病，如鼻咽癌。

(1)急性浆液性中耳炎和乳突炎：急性浆液性中耳炎是中耳黏膜的炎症，通常并发积液和咽鼓管功能障碍。在CT和MRI上可以看到在中耳和乳突的含气间隙变得浑浊，并可以看见气液平面。在MRI可以看到颞骨气房信号增高。随着病变进入亚急性期，乳突小房系统的分隔可以出现骨质疏松征象。

(2)慢性化脓性中耳炎和乳突炎：慢性化脓性中耳炎可以导致合并症，如颞骨岩部骨髓炎、脑炎和脑脓肿形成、骨质破坏、横窦或者乙状窦血栓，甚至死亡。长期慢性炎症的并发症包括岩尖炎、鼓室硬化和胆脂瘤形成。可能有中耳黏膜增厚和气液平面，这在CT上可以清楚地显示。肉芽肿、肉芽组织和/或胆脂瘤可表现为局限性的肿块样病变。这些软组织肿块都可以导致内耳和听小骨的破坏。CT能发现骨质破坏，有助于鉴别肉芽组织和胆脂瘤，而MRI难以显示骨质破坏。

2.颞骨骨折

颞骨骨折通常发生在颅脑外伤，也经常伴发在脑、颅畸形。颞骨骨折可根据在颞骨岩部的长轴的征象分为两类：纵向和横向骨折。有些骨折呈粉碎状，不能简单分类。这两类骨折多并发其他颅底骨折。颞骨骨折合并症包括：面瘫、听小骨脱位继发听力损伤、脑脊液耳漏、颈动脉夹层或颈动脉瘤、迷路积血或积气、鼓膜破裂、耳聋、脑挫伤和脑膜炎。这些并发症的发生率因骨折类型而异。纵向骨折可能累及颈动脉管，可以在CT上看到它的细微改变。骨折也可以横过蝶骨到达对侧颞骨。在这种情况下可考虑通过MR血管造影或者常规血管造影来探查有否动脉夹层、损伤或假性动脉瘤。横向骨折常横贯内听道、耳囊状结构，是神经损伤的高发原因。骨折能累及枕骨、颈静脉窝，甚至枕骨髁。颈静脉窝受损时可能出现第Ⅸ，第Ⅹ，第Ⅺ和第Ⅻ颅神经症状。

听骨链中断有时能在常规脑部CT扫描中发现，但最好行颞骨高分辨率CT检查。

3.原发和继发恶性肿瘤

鳞状细胞癌最常见，但是基底细胞癌和淋巴瘤也通常发生。大多数发生在靠近鼓室环处，并迅速侵犯骨质。这些征象在CT和MRI中很容易看到，有利于给肿瘤分期。

4.耳的先天畸形

耳的先天畸形被是头颈部第二常见的先天性畸形，仅次于唇裂和腭裂。耳畸形分为外耳畸形、中耳畸形和内耳畸形。

(1)外耳闭锁：骨性外耳道的发育不全或者畸形通常合并耳郭的畸形；骨性外耳道可能完全缺失或者部分由不同厚度的软组织填充。当骨性耳道完全缺失的时候在原处鼓膜的位置可以看到一个较厚的外侧闭锁的骨板。听小骨可以融合到外侧的骨板或者互相融合。鼓室壁也可以表现为不同程度的发育不全，而且常常畸形。

(2)中耳畸形：中耳畸形很少单独发生，通常合并外耳发育畸形。听小骨互相融合常见，锤骨和砧骨与鼓室壁融合也是常见的。镫骨常常畸形。镫骨的底板可以和卵圆窗(前庭窗)融合。这些情况下面神经常常前移，或与蹬骨异常关联。中耳畸形的患者行中耳重建术前必须明确面神经的位置和走行。如果不清楚面神经走行而进行外科探查很容易损伤面神经。

(3)内耳畸形：内耳畸形可发生在耳蜗，前庭，半规管，导水管或者内听道。这些畸形可能孤立或者联合发生。小的外侧半规管畸形最常见。

1) Michel 畸形是最严重的内耳畸形,内耳和颞骨岩部完全未发育。Mondini 畸形指耳蜗的部分发育不全,仅出现基部圈(没有顶圈和中圈),耳蜗呈球形,通常伴发前庭和半规管异常。Michel 畸形通常双侧出现;Mondini 畸形可为单侧或双侧,但是两侧畸形程度可不同。

2) 前庭和半规管发育不全可能孤立发生。内听道变窄或者膨大可能孤立或者合并其他内耳畸形发生。大前庭导水管综合征是先天性耳聋的最常见原因。表现为前庭导水管合扩大,并先天性耳聋或者轻微伤后的突聋。必须综合 CT 和 MRI 的影像才能了解前庭导水管的大小和形状。

(谭艳,李秋云,骆永恒,刘欢,韦勇,肖恩华,刘军)

Chapter 22

The Ear

Section 1 Methods of examination

1. Plain film

X-ray plain films are rarely used for ear examinations now, and are mainly used to observe the shape and position of electrodes after cochlear implantation and the special anatomical structure of temporal bone. The conventional irradiation is used clinically to study the skull base and its surrounding structures in different directions. In addition to standard radiograph methods, there are also special projection methods named after Schüller, Stenvers and Mayer.

2. CT examination

CT is the main imaging technique for ear lesions. Conventional volume scanning and multi-directional high-resolution reorganization are used. Other post-processes are also feasible, including three-dimensional surface masking display, labyrinth imaging and ossicular chain imaging. Especially in recent years, with the rapid development of software, the anatomical tomographic images of the anatomical structure of the ear, including the ossicles and bony labyrinth, can be displayed in detail. In addition, the CT virtual endoscopy technology has become increasingly mature, which can observe the tympanic cavity, mastoid sinus, labyrinth and inner ear canal structure

3. MRI examination

MRI has unparalleled advantages in soft tissue imaging. It is a routine examination method for cerebellopontine angle acoustic neuroma, metastasis, neuroma, facial nerve and soft tissue lesions. MRI water imaging technology can clearly show the three-dimensional structure of the membrane labyrinth. High-resolution three-dimensional source images can be used to observe the relationship between the cranial nerves and blood vessels in the cerebellopontine angle. Enhanced MRI is often used for the diagnosis and differential diagnosis of tumors and inflammatory lesions.

Section 2 Normal appearances

The ear consists of three major parts: the inner, the middle, and the external. It contains the complex transducers for hearing and balance.

1. The inner ear

It consists of three components, the vestibule, cochlea and semicircular canals.

The vestibule is well seen on Stenver's projections as a small oval cavity lying close to the lateral end of the internal auditory meatus below the semicircular canal and above the cochlea.

The lateral semicircular canal, seen on perorbital projections extends horizontally from the vestibule and project into the upper part of the middle ear cavity at the junctions of the cavity properand the epitympanic recess. The superior semicircular canal, seen on Stenver's projection, extends upwards from the vestibule to produce a prominence on the anterosuperior surface of the petrous. The posterior semicircular canal, seen on the supraorbital projection extends horizontally backwards from the vestibule, its lateral limb is close to the aditus ad antrum.

The cochlea is a snail-shaped structure with its apex placed anteriorly. It is seen in Stenver's, supraorbital, and perorbital projections and may also recognized on the axila view.

2. The middle ear

The middle ear consist of the tympanic cavity, the eustachian tube and the mastoid. It is an air-filled space that contains the ossicles and communicates with the nasopharynx through the eustachian tube and the mastoid antrum through the aditus ad antrum.

The tympanic membrane separates the external ear from the middle ear or tympanic cavity.

The tympanic cavity communicates anteroinferiorly with the nasopharynx by the pharyngotympanic tube and posterosuperiorly with the mastoid air cell system by the aditus ad antrum. The middle ear can be divided into five parts on the basis of its relationship to the tympanic annulus of the tympanic membrane. The epitympanum lies above the annulus, the mesotympanum lies adjacent to the annulus and tympanic membrane, the hypotympanum lies below the annulus, the protympanum is anterior to the annulus, and the posterior tympanum lies posterior to the annulus. In addition, the middle ear has a close relationship to the inner and external ear. The epitympanum is at the level of the IAC, the mesotympanum at the level of the cochlea, and the hypotympanum below the cochlea and EAC.

3. The external ear

The external ear is lateral to the tympanic membrane. The external ear consists of the pinna and the external auditory meatus. The external meatus is cartilaginous in its lateral half, continuous with the cartilage of the pinna. The inner half is bony and lies within the petrous temporal bone.

The internal auditory canal (IAC) is a tubular narrow tube, ampullary and trumpet-shaped symmetrical structure. The anteroposterior and vertical diameters are mostly 4~6 mm, and the sickle crest located at the bottom of the coronal surface.

The facial nerve canal: The complex tortuous course of the facial nerve and canal may be related to its evolutionary development. Because of the susceptibility of the nerve to disease and its close proximity to almost every important structure in the temporal bone, it can be associated with many different clinical symptoms besides facial paralysis. Facial nerve symptoms may arise from adjacent pathologies. Its course can be conveniently divided into three parts, corresponding to the three parts of the ear that traverses: Labyrinthine, tympanic, and mastoid.

The mastoid air cells: Arising from the posterior aspect of the epitympanic recess is a short channel called the aditus ad antrum, leading to the mastoid antrum itself, which is a cavity of variable size forming the first part of the mastoid air cell system. The normal antrum is the shape of an inverted truncated cone with a "maximum" transverse diameter of 6 mm and a maximum height of 11 mm.

Section 3　Basic pathological changes

1. CT findings

（1）Abnormal structure and morphology of the temporal bone: They are congenital malformations of the external ear and the middle ear, which can be manifested as the changes of the normal structure and morphology of the temporal bone, such as the stenosis and atresia of the external auditory metaplasia, fusion, tympanic cavity stenosis, etc. Congenital malformation of the inner ear can be manifested as structural abnormalities of the vestibular semicircular canal and cochlea, and stenosis of the inner ear canal. Unilateral or bilateral enlargement of the inner ear canal indicates a space-occupying lesion of the inner ear, commonly seen in acoustic neuromas.

（2）Abnormal bone of the temporal bone: CT can clearly show the presence or absence of bone destruction, and the location, scope and boundary of bone destruction, as well as the presence or absence of soft tissue density masses in the bone destruction area.

（3）Abnormal mastoid sinus and mastoid air chamber: Development and density of mastoid sinus and mastoid gas chambers are one of the changes caused by acute and chronic middle ear and mastoid inflammation and cholesteatoma.

（4）Abnormal bone continuity: Abnormal bone continuity in temporal bone fracture can be presented as parallel（longitudinal）or perpendicular to（transverse）petrosal fracture line, sometimes combined with ossicular chain dislocation and facial nerve canal fracture.

2. MRI manifestations

（1）Abnormal signals: There is no signal on MRI in tympanic bone wall, auditory ossicle and gas etc. Abnormal MRI signals may occur, such as effusion, hematoma, inflammation, granuloma, neoplasm and cholesteatoma.

（2）Abnormal structure: Inner ear malformations show structural abnormalities in inner ear hydrography. Acoustic neuroma shows isotopic lesions in the inner ear canal and spread to the cerebellopontine Angle.

（3）Complications of otitis media and mastoiditis: Complications such as epidural abscess and sigmoid embolism phlebitis can be shown on MRI.

Section 4　Diagnosis of common diseases

1. Infective and inflammatory disease

Serous otitis is a common complication of malfunction of the eustachian canal system. Fluid accumulates in the middle ear and mastoid. It is very common in children, probably due to large adenoids. The presence of serous otitis in adults can alert the radiologist to the diagnosis of more serious pathology, such as nasopharyngeal cancer.

（1）Acute otitis media and mastoiditis

Acute otitis media is an inflammation of the mucosa lining the middle ear, usually associated with fluid production and Eustachian tube dysfunction. On CT and MRI, air space opacification associated with fluid levels are commonly seen in air spaces with any inflammatory change of the middle ear or mastoids. On MRI, there is a cast of the temporal bone air spaces that produces signal rather than the normal signal voids. As the disease progresses into the subacute stage, demineralization with loss of trabecular pattern of the mastoid air cells may occur.

（2）Chronic suppurative otitis media and mastioditis

Chronic suppurative otitis may lead to complications such as osteomyelitis of the temporal bone, cerebritis and brain abscess formation, bone destruction, transverse or sigmoid sinus thrombosis, and even death. Long-term complicationsare petrous apicitis, tympanosclerosis, and the formation of granuloma or cholesteatoma. There may be mucosal thickening and occasionally fluid levels, both can be readily appreciated on CT. Focal mass lesions can represent granuloma, granulation tissue, and/or cholesteatoma. All of these soft-tissue masses in the middle ear can also produce labyrinthine and ossicular destruction. CT, but not MRI, can detect bone destruction to help differentiate granulation tissue from cholesteatoma.

2. Fractures of the temporal bone

Fractures of the temporal bone are usually associated with major head trauma. There are commonly other associated brain and skull abnormalities as well. Temporal bone fractures can be classified into two main categories: Longitudinal (lateral to medial) and transverse (anterior to posterior) with respect to the long axis of the petrous temporal bone. Some temporal bone fractures are so comminuted that a simple classification is not possible. These two types of fractures that are frequently associated with other multiple skull base fractures. Complications of temporal bone fracture are facial nerve palsy, conductive hearing loss due to ossicular dislocation, CSF otorrhea, carotid dissection/aneurysm, blood or air within the labyrinth, membranous disruption, a dead ear, brain contusions, and meningitis. The incidence of these various complications varies with the type of fracture.

Longitudinal fractures may extend into the carotid canal and may be subtle on conventional CT. The fracture line may also extend across the sphenoid into the opposite temporal bone. MR angiography or conventional angiography may be considered to look for arterial dissection, injury, or pseudoaneurysm formation. Transverse fractures usually cross the IAC and otic capsule structures, accounting for a high incidence of neurologic injury. The fractures may also extend into the occipital bone, jugular fossa, and even the occipital condyles. With jugular fossa extension, there may be cranial neuropathies of nerves IX, X, XI, and XII.

Ossicular disruption can sometimes be seen on conventional CT of the brain, but is better evaluated with high resolution CT of temporal bone.

3. Primary and secondary malignant neoplasms

Squamous cell carcinoma isthe most common type, but basal cell carcinomas and lymphoma also occur. Most arise closely to the tympanic annulus and invade bone rapidly. These features can be readily appreciated on CT or MRI, which may help in the staging of the disease.

4. Congenital anomalies of the ear

Congenital malformations of the ear constitute the second most common congenital malformations of the head and neck after cleft lip and palate. They may be classified as (1)External ear atresia; (2)Middle ear aonmalies; and (3)Inner ear malformations.

(1)External ear atresia: Atresia or hypoplasia of the osseous external ear is usually associated with deformity of the pinna. The bony canal may be completely absent or partially formed with soft tissue with variable thickness to fill the canal. When there is complete absence of the bony ear canal, a thick lateral atretic bony plate is found in the location of the tympanic membrane. The ossicles can be fused with the plate laterally. The tympanic bone shows various degrees of hypoplasia and is frequently malformed.

(2)Middle ear aonmalies: Malformations of the middle ear rarely occur in isolation and are usually seen with external canal malformation. Fusion of the ossicles to each other is common, as the fusion of the malleus and incus with the atretic plate. The stapes is frequently malformed. The foot plate may be fused to the oval window. The location and course of the facial nerve must be identified in these patients prior to surgery if there will be an attempt to reconstruct the middle ear. The facial nerve always displaced anteriorly or associated with the stapes anomalously. The facial nerve can be easily damaged if its course is not identified prior to surgical exploration.

（3）Inner ear malformations: Malformations of the inner ear may affect the cochlea, vestibule, semicircular canals, aqueducts, or internal auditory canal. The malformations may occur together or in isolation. An anomalous small lateral semicircular canal is the most common inner ear anomaly.

1）The Michel anomaly is the most severe form, there is complete aplasia of the inner ear and the petrous pyramid in this case. Mondini described a deformity with partial aplasia of the cochlea and presence of only the basal turn (with absence of the apical and middle turns). The cochlea is frequently globular in shape. It may be associated with anomalies of the vestibule and semicircular canals. Whereas the Michel anomaly is usually bilateral, the Mondini deformity may be unilateral or bilateral, and the severity of deformity may vary from side to side.

2）Hypoplasia of the vestibule and semicircular canals may occur in isolation. Narrowing or ectasia of the internal auditory canal may occur alone or in combination with other inner ear anomalies. The giant vestibular aqueduct syndrome is the most common cause of congenital deafness. It consists of enlargement of the vestibular aqueduct and may be associated with congenital deafness or with sudden onset of deafness after only minor trauma. This anomaly may be present alone or in association with other inner ear abnormalities. Imaging may be accomplished with CT or MR to demonstrate the size and shape of the vestibular aqueduct.

（Tan Yan, Li Qiuyun, Luo Yongheng, Liu Huan, Wei Yong, Xiao Enhua, Liu Jun）

第二十三章

鼻和鼻窦

第一节 检查方法

1. X 线平片检查

X 线平片可用于检查鼻骨骨折和鼻窦病变，但敏感度较低，目前已较少应用。在少数情况下，可能会进行鼻窦检查，以排除具有气液平面或完全堵塞的急性鼻窦炎。临床上常见的如 Water's 位、Caldwell's 位等。

2. CT 检查

CT 是鼻和鼻窦病变的主要影像检查技术。常规行高分辨率 CT 检查，并进行多方位观察，从而能够以高空间分辨率和软组织高对比度对鼻旁窦进行非叠加显示，以检测鼻窦的炎性，创伤性和赘生性疾病；鼻窦的参考窗位 200 Hu、窗宽 2000 Hu，炎症和肿瘤性病变还需行软组织窗观察；部分病变尚要行增强扫描。此外仿真内镜可清楚显示鼻腔和鼻窦的开口以及鼻窦的黏膜面，并且 CT 导航技术已用于各种鼻窦病变的内镜手术治疗。

3. MRI 检查

鼻部病变的临床常规检查技术，标准检查方案应包括 T1WI、T2WI 和脂肪抑制序列，必要时辅以冠状位和矢状位检查。增强检查常在鼻腔、鼻窦肿瘤的诊断和鉴别诊断中具有重要价值；水成像技术可显示脑脊液鼻漏。在某些情况下，需进行 MR 血管造影评估血管结构的关系以及观察动脉、静脉侧支等。

4. DSA 检查

通常用于治疗不受控制的鼻出血以及术前评估和栓塞青少年鼻咽血管纤维瘤和其他颅底血管瘤。临床上常使用弹簧圈、球囊和快速聚合的液体物质闭塞目标血管。

第二节 正常表现

1. 上颌窦

成人上颌窦是一个位于上颌骨体部上的大腔，在前后位投照呈三角形，侧位投照呈四边形。

2. 额窦

成人额窦由位于额骨内外板间的不规则腔组成，可以向前或者向后不同程度地延伸。

3. 筛窦

筛窦位于筛骨两旁、在眼眶和鼻腔上半侧壁之间的多数筛泡，每侧可多达 20 余个，分为前后两组。

4. 蝶窦

蝶窦内隔膜常常不对称，正常成人的蝶窦上接垂体窝、前邻筛窦、下为蝶骨的底部和鼻咽部的顶部。考虑上述因素，正常鼻窦的放射影像表现为相对透亮的、边界清楚的区域，黏膜较薄不能显示。

5. 鼻腔

鼻腔由成对的鼻道组成，通过前面的外鼻和后面的鼻咽部之间。鼻中隔把鼻腔分为两半。从侧壁突向另一侧的三个管状物为鼻甲。最大者为下鼻甲，中鼻甲结构没有下鼻甲复杂。

第三节　基本病变

1. 黏膜增厚

正常状态下，黏膜呈细线状或不能显示。黏膜增厚在 CT 上为中等密度条状影，MRI 上为长 T1 长 T2 信号条带状影，常见于各种鼻窦炎性病变。

2. 肿块

软组织肿块，密度中等，均匀，边界清楚光整，轻至中度强化多为良性肿瘤；无强化或周边强化提示黏膜下囊肿或粘液囊肿；密度不均匀，边界不清楚，明显强化的病变多为恶性肿瘤；密度高且近似于骨密度，提示骨瘤或骨化性纤维瘤。

3. 窦腔积液

表现为窦腔内液体密度或信号影，可见气-液平面。常见于急性炎症，外伤出血等。窦腔内充满液体时，CT 不易与肿瘤或囊肿相区别，此时可行增强检查，液体不强化而肿瘤强化，或行 MRI 检查，两者信号强度有所不同。

4. 窦腔形态，大小异常

鼻窦窦腔个体发育差异很大，要注意鉴别。窦腔增大多提示病变原发于鼻窦或窦口阻塞，窦腔缩小提示病变来源于窦周结构。

5. 鼻腔大小形态异常

鼻腔狭小或闭塞见于先天发育畸形，鼻甲黏膜肥厚，鼻息肉及各种鼻腔肿瘤。

6. 骨质异常

骨质破坏见于各种恶性肿瘤，急性炎症，真菌感染及部分良性肿瘤。骨质增生见于长期慢性炎症，骨纤维异常增殖症，成骨性转移瘤。骨质中断，移位，粉碎见于外伤骨折，手术等。骨质吸收见于部分良性肿瘤。

8. 邻近解剖结构改变

鼻和鼻窦病变容易累及眼眶、颅底、颅内、口腔及鼻咽部，引起上述部位的形态、密度和骨质异常。

第四节　常见疾病诊断

1. 感染和过敏性炎症

（1）临床及病理表现：感染是迄今为止鼻和鼻窦最常见的疾病。非过敏性炎症常常继发于急性上呼吸道感染。炎症也可继发于过敏性鼻炎和鼻窦炎，由于黏膜水肿阻塞了鼻窦的引流。任何其他导致引流阻塞的病因，包括创伤、先天性鼻中隔偏曲等都易发感染。上颌窦感染有时由牙根的脓毒血症引起。牙根碎片丢失进入上颌窦后常导致感染。

（2）影像学表现：鼻窦 X 线片检查应包括眼眶正位、顶颏位和侧位扫描。CT 扫描在可疑病例中很有价值，怀疑感染向眼眶或颅内蔓延时应使用CT。基本征象是鼻窦透亮度的降低，其表现形式如下所述。需要注意的是，病变常常双侧同时出现，因此不能通过比较双侧鼻窦透亮度来判断鼻窦炎。

2. 急性鼻窦炎

急性鼻窦炎，无论是由感染还是过敏引起，都导致黏膜肿胀。上颌窦最常受累，其次是额窦。筛窦和蝶窦的孤立性炎症并不常见，通常并发于上颌窦炎和额窦炎。筛窦炎最常见于儿童和青少年，可能并发眼眶蜂窝织炎。

受累的上颌窦黏膜肿胀，感染性上颌窦炎的肿胀黏膜平行于窦壁。气液平面最常见于上颌窦炎，也可见于额窦炎。

3. 慢性鼻窦炎

一些病例表现为持续性的黏膜肿胀，偶尔伴随窦壁的增厚和骨质硬化。

4. 内翻性乳头状瘤

（1）临床及病理表现：这是一种少见的起自鼻腔黏膜的良性肿瘤，少见于男性。在手术切除后有复发的趋势，偶尔发生恶变。

（2）影像学表现：包括鼻内肿块和鼻窦密度增高模糊。鼻腔内肿块表现出与鼻息肉相似的特征，鼻腔扩张、骨壁变薄。通常没有骨质破坏。病变旁的鼻窦出口可被阻塞，导致受累的鼻窦密度增高。内翻性乳头状瘤可能发生在上颌窦，肿块完全占据上颌窦腔，易误诊为黏液囊肿甚至癌。

区分压迫性骨质萎缩和真正的上皮恶性病变的早期侵犯较为困难，因此活检很有必要。

5. 鼻窦恶性肿瘤

（1）临床及病理表现：鼻窦肿瘤多来源于上皮。大多数位于上颌窦，但筛窦癌也常见。很少见于额窦和蝶窦。鼻窦癌多发于中老年患者，男性发病率较高。鼻窦亦有来源于结缔组织和骨的恶性肿瘤，但少见，包括纤维肉瘤、黏液肉瘤和骨肉瘤。浆细胞瘤和黑色素瘤偶尔可见。鼻窦转移癌与原发性肿瘤在影像学上难以区分。上颌窦癌生长缓慢，表现为疼痛、鼻塞和鼻出血。

（2）影像学表现：影像学表现为软组织肿块，部分或者完全充满窦腔。破坏骨壁，累及临近结构。骨质破坏不规则，无骨质硬化。良性肿瘤和黏液囊肿常见的窦腔扩大很少见于上颌窦癌。骨质破坏在CT上显示较准确，尤其是前壁；但由于部分容积效应，可能无法检测到微小的骨质变化。肿瘤可能扩展到颞下窝、眼眶、翼腭窝、鼻咽、颅腔等重要部位，可通过CT检查判断是否有肿瘤侵犯。

放射学检查，包括CT，不能区分良性肿瘤和早期恶性病变，除非出现骨质侵蚀或者软组织向外蔓延。为此，活检仍是必不可少的。

（谭艳，李秋云，骆永恒，刘欢，韦勇，肖恩华，刘军）

Chapter 23

The nose and paranasal sinuses

Section 1　Method of examination

1. Plain film examination

X-rayplain films can be used to examine nasal bone fractures and sinus lesions, but the sensitivity is low, therefore it has been used rarely. In rare cases, sinus examinations may be performed to rule out acute sinusitis with gas-liquid levels or complete blockage. Clinical examination methods are commonly used, such as Water's position, Caldwell's position and so on.

2. CT examination

CT is the main imaging technique for nasal and sinus diseases. Routine high-resolution CT examination and multi-directional observation are used, so that the paranasal sinuses can be displayed non-superimposed with high spatial resolution and soft tissue high contrast to detect the inflammatory, traumatic and neoplastic diseases of the paranasal sinus. The reference window of the nasal sinuses is 200 HU and the window width is 2000 HU. Inflammation and tumor lesions need to be observed through the soft tissue window. Some lesions still need to be enhanced scanning. In addition, virtual endoscopy can clearly show the openings of the nasal cavity and sinuses and the mucosal surface of the sinuses, and CT navigation technology has been used for endoscopic surgical treatment of various sinus diseases.

3. MRI examination

MRI is the clinical routine examination techniques of nasal diseases. The standard examination plan should include T1WI, T2WI and fat-suppression sequence. It is supplemented by coronal and sagittal examinations when necessary. Enhanced examination often has important value in the diagnosis and differential diagnosis of nasal cavity and sinus tumors. MRI water imaging technology can show cerebrospinal fluid rhinorrhea. In some cases, MR angiography is required to evaluate the relationship between vascular structures and observe the collateral branches of arteries and veins, etc.

4. DSA examination

It is usually used to treat uncontrolled epistaxis andmake preoperative evaluation and embolization of juvenile nasopharyngeal angiofibroma and other skull base hemangioma. Coils, balloons, and rapid polymerizing liquid substances are often used clinically to occlude the target blood vessel.

Section 2 Normal appearances

1. Maxillary antra

The adult maxillary antrum is a large cavity lying in the body of the maxilla. It is triangular when in the posteroanterior projection and quadrilateral in the lateral projection.

2. Frontal sinuses

The frontal sinuses in the adult consist of irregular cavities lying between the inner and outer layer of the frontal bone with a variable extension anteriorly and posteriorly.

3. Ethmoid sinuses

The ethmoid sinuses lie in the lateral masses of the ethmoid bone between the orbits and the lateral wall of the upper half of the nasal cavity. There are up to 20 ethmoid cells in each side and classified into anterior and posterior groups radiologically.

4. Sphenoid sinuses

The intersinus septum is often asymmetrically placed. The normal adult sphenoid sinus is inferior to the pituitary fossa, posterior to the ethmoid sinus, and superior to the floor of the sphenoid bone and the roof of the nasopharynx.

When these factors have been taken into consideration, paranasal sinus shows an area of relative radiolucency with a clearly defined bony margin. The mucosal in the sinus is thin and is not usually visible.

5. The nasal cavity

The nasal cavity consists of paired routes located between the external nose anteriorly and the nasopharynx posteriorly. A central septum divides the nasal cavity into two halves.

The three tubinates on each side are projecting from the lateral wall. The largest is the inferior turbinate. The middle turbinate is less complex in structure than the inferior turbinate.

Section 3 Basic pathological changes

1. Mucosal thickening

Under normal conditions, the mucosa is fine line or cannot be shown. The thickened mucosa showed medium density bands on CT and long T1 and T2 signal bands on MRI, whichare commonly seen in various inflammatory sinus lesions.

2. A lump

Soft tissue mass, medium density, uniform, clear and smooth boundary, mild to moderate enhancementare mostly benign tumor. No enhancement or peripheral enhancement suggested submucosal cyst or mucocele. The lesions with uneven density, unclear boundary and obvious enhancement are mostly malignant tumors. High density and similar to bone density suggest osteoma or ossifying fibroma.

3. Sinus effusion

It is manifested as liquid density or signal shadow in the sinus cavity, with gas-liquid plane visible. It is commonly seen in acute inflammation, traumatic bleeding, etc. When the sinus cavity is filled with fluid, CT is not easy to be distinguished from tumor or cyst. At this time, enhanced examination is feasible, fluid is not enhanced but tumor is enhanced, or MRI examination is performed, and the signal strength of the two is different.

4. Abnormal shape and size of the sinus cavity

The ontogenesis of sinus cavity is very different, so we should pay attention to its differentiation. The enlargement of sinus cavity indicates that the lesion originates from the obstruction of nasal sinus or sinus orifice, while the narrowing of sinus cavity indicates that the lesion originates from the peri-sinusial structure.

5. Abnormal size and shape of nasal cavity

Narrow or occlusive nasal cavity is seen in congenital malformation, turbinate mucous membrane hypertrophy, nasal polyp and various nasal tumors.

6. Bone abnormalities

Bone destruction is seen in various malignant tumors, acute inflammation, fungal infections, and some benign tumors. Hyperosteogeny is found in chronic inflammation, abnormal proliferation of bone fibers, and metastases. Bone disruption, displacement, and comminution are seen in traumatic fractures, surgery, etc. Bone resorption is seen in some benign tumors.

7. Changes in adjacent anatomical structures

Lesions in the nasal and paranasal sinus can easily involve the orbital, skull base, intracranial, oral cavity and nasopharynx, causing the morphology, density and bone abnormalities in these areas.

Section 4　Diagnosis of common diseases

1. Infection, inflammation and allergy

(1) Clinical andpathological manifestations: The infection is by far the largest group of diseases of the nose and paranasal sinuses. Nonallergic infection is often following an actue upper espiratoryinfection. Infection may also occur in patients with allergic rhinitis and sinusitis, the oedematous muscosa cuasing obstruction to the drainage of the paranasal sinuses. Any other cause of obstruction, such as trauma or congenital deviation of the nasal septum may predispose to infection. Infection of the maxillary antrum sometimes occurs due to dental toot sepsis, and may follow dental extraction. Loss of a dental root fragment into the antrum is always followed by infection.

(2) Imaging manifestations: Radiological examination should consist of an occipitomental projection, with the addition of the occipiofrontal and lateral when necessary. Conventional tomography may be of value in doubtful cases, and CT is indicated where there is possibility of orbital or intracranial extension of the infective process. The principal finding is a loss of radiolucency of the affected sinus, the manifestation was described below. The loss of radiolucency cannot be resolved by comparison with the opposite side, since bilateral disease is often present.

2. Acute sinusitis

Acute inflammatory disease of the paranasal sinuses, whether precipitated by infection or by allergy, results in swelling of the mucosa. The maxillary antrum are most frequently affected, followed by the frontral sinuses. Isolated inflammatory disease in the ethmoid and sphenoid sinuses is uncommon, such infections usually accompanied with antral and frontal sinusitis. Ethmoid sinusitis is seen most in children and teenagers, and may be complicated by orbital cellulitis.

The affected maxillary antrum shows swelling of its mucosa, which tends to parallel the antral walls in simple infection. Fluid levels are most frequently seen in the maxillary antrum, but are also found in the frontal sinuses.

3. Chronic sinusitis

Some cases show persisting mucosal swelling, which are occasionally associated with some thickening or sclerosis of the bony walls of the sinus.

4. Inverted papilloma

（1）Clinical and pathological manifestations: This is an uncommon benign tumor arising from the mucous membrane of the nasal cavity and less commonly in males. There is a tendency to recurrence after removal and malignant change is occasionally found.

（2）Imaging manifestations: The radiological features usually consist of a nasal mass with opacification of the paranasal sinuses. The nasal mass tends to show features similar to those found in nasal polyposis with expansion of the nasal cavity and thinning of its wall. Bone destruction does not always occur. The ostia of the paranasal sinuses on the side of the lesion may be obstructed. In which cases the affected sinuses became opaque. An inverted papilloma may however arise in the maxillary antrum, producing a tumor which completely occupies the affected sinus with expansion and thinning of its walls. The features erroneously suggest a mucoele or even a carcinoma.

The difficulty of distinguishing pressure atrophy of bone fromtruly epithelial malignant invasion makes biopsy necessary in most cases to exclude malignancy.

5. Malignant tumors of the paranasal sinuses

（1）Clinical and pathological manifestations: The majority tumours of the paranasal sinuses are of epithelial origin. Most arise in the maxillary antrum, though ethmoid carcinoma is also quite common. Malignant tumours are rare in the frontal and sphenoid sinuses. Carcinoma of the paranasal sinuses tends to occur in middle-aged and elderly patients, affecting males more frequently. Tumors of the connective tissue and bony origin also arise in the paranasal sinuses, but occur much less frequently. They include fibrosarcoma, myxsarcoma, and osteosarcoma. Plasmacytoma and melanoma may be seen occasionally. Metastase may show features indistinguishable from primary tumors of the paranasal sinuses. Carcinoma of the maxillary antrum is a slow growing tumour presenting with pain, nasal obstruction and epistaxis.

（2）Imaging manifestations: The radiological features consist of a soft tissue mass which partly or completely fills the air space of the affected sinus. Bone destruction may occur followed by extension of the tumor into the adjacent structures. The bone destruction is irregular, and is not associated with sclerosis. Expansion of a sinus, as seen in benign tumors and mucoceles, is rarely present in carcinoma. The extent of bone destruction is better defined in CT, particularly of the anterior wall; but minimal bony changes may not be detected because of partial volume effect. Possible tumour extension into such important areas as the infratemporal fossa, the orbit, the pterygopalatine fossa, the nasopharynx and the cranial cavity, the nasopharynx and the cranial cavity may be assessed by CT.

Radiological methods, including CT, do not distinguish benigh tumours from early malignant lesions, before the development of bone erosion, or before soft tissue extension beyond the affected sinus has taken place. For this purpose biopsy remains essential.

（Tan Yan, Li Qiuyun, Luo Yongheng, Liu Huan, Wei Yong, Xiao Enhua, Liu Jun）

第二十四章

喉部

第一节 检查方法

1. X 线平片检查

观察喉部一般拍摄颈部侧位 X 线片，采用软组织条件拍摄，但是目前喉部病变较少应用 X 线平片检查。其可以显示部分喉室结构，但对于较小病变和周围软组织内部情况常难以显示。

2. CT 检查

喉部病变的主要影像检查技术。常采用薄层多方位重建技术，并行软组织窗观察，可清晰显示喉部及其周围结构的异常表现，明确病变部位、范围，对病变来源、性质及肿瘤的分期提供依据。此外增大宽窗有利于显示声带及喉室情况，若发现病变时需另行增强检查。

3. MRI 检查

可任意方向成像，具有高的软组织分辨率，因此是喉部病变的常规影像学检查。常规进行横断面、矢状位、冠状位 T1WI 和 T2WI 扫描，必要时增强扫描。可清楚显示喉腔、喉壁各层结构和喉周间隙改变，尤其在区分放疗后纤维化和肿瘤复发方面具有明显优势，对软组织受累程度和侵犯显示较为清楚。

第二节 正常表现

很多喉咽部的原发肿瘤位于黏膜表面，使用内窥镜容易证实临床诊断。但是，黏膜下肿瘤病变范围不能单独使用内窥镜证实。MRI 及 CT 扫描在检测临床的重要盲区的病变如黏膜下区域很有用。

咽部构成气道的上部，在上面的颅底和下面的环状软骨之间。喉咽部由三个独立的部分组成（指鼻咽部、口咽部和下咽部）。它们的分界线是舌会厌软骨、咽会厌软骨折叠、杓状软骨，其次是喉咽下部的环状软骨的下缘。鼻咽部位于鼻后孔后面及软腭的下缘之间。口咽部位于硬腭（鼻咽的底部）和舌骨（舌咽的上部）下面。其前部是舌底，它起自轮廓状的乳突后面；口咽部的结构包括舌底、由扁桃体腭弓包围的腭扁桃体和由五对肌肉（软腭肌、腭肌、悬雍垂肌、舌腭肌、腭咽肌、提腭肌）形成的。口咽部的其他结构包括口咽部黏膜，自软腭水平至会厌上部的咽部括约肌（大致在 $C_2 \sim C_3$ 椎体水平）和会厌谷。扁桃体的运动感觉神经窝，扁桃体柱的后部和舌底部走行着舌咽神经。

下咽部或者说咽的喉部，上起舌骨，下至环状软骨，这部分对应在 C_3 椎体的下部至 C_6 椎体的上部之间的区域。下咽部的结构包括下咽骨黏膜，小唾液腺和下咽括约肌。下咽部的三个主要部分是梨状窝，环状软骨区及咽后壁。

喉部分成三部分：声门上区，声门，声门下区。声门上区喉部自会厌顶部至喉室尾部。声门上区包括：前庭、会厌软骨、假声带、喉室、杓状软骨、会厌谷、前会厌软骨、喉旁区域。喉室是喉部声门上方的气道。声门区位于上部的真声带和下面的喉室侧壁下 1 cm 之间。声门区的侧壁是副声门区。声门区包括真声带及前、后联合。真声带由覆盖在甲状状肌的黏膜形成。这块肌肉起自甲状叶片中内部表面，附在杓状软骨的前外侧表面。声门韧带起自杓状软骨的声门全程至甲状软骨，它组成了真声带的边缘。在 CT 和 MRI 扫描时，声带突标志着真声带水平。平静呼吸状态下，真声带保持细小形态而且分开。在屏住气时，真声带却与此相反。在真声带水平的喉旁区域主要由肌肉和甲状叶片内部的狭窄带状松散蜂窝组织构成。声门下区上起喉室下 1 cm，下至环状软骨下表面。

第三节　基本病变

1. 形态学改变

声门区结构可出现肿胀，也可出现破坏、消失，或有真假声带分辨不清、软组织增厚或肿块，气道狭窄。局限性正常结构消失、紊乱而边界清楚者常为良性病变。广泛性结构消失、紊乱而边界不清者多为恶性病变。软组织增厚或肿块表面不光滑而伴有黏膜破坏者为恶性病变。

2. 密度和信号改变

囊性病变表现为低密度或长 T1、长 T2 信号，实性病变表现为软组织密度或等 T1、长或稍长 T2 信号。

3. 对称性与位置变化

喉部左右不对称，真声带、假声带、喉室及声门下间隙的任何不对称、歪曲、变形均为病理征象。喉内或喉外病变可引起整个喉部移位。

4. 喉软骨的破坏

软骨破坏是诊断肿瘤的一个重要征象，表示肿瘤已广泛浸润。CT 表现为骨质破坏或增生硬化；MRI 表现为 T1WI 上喉软骨中出现高信号或高信号骨髓中出现中、低信号。

5. 功能改变

可以扩张、活动的正常部位变僵硬，或不同呼吸相检查均不显示活动，表明肿瘤浸润、固定。是区别肿瘤性与非肿瘤性病变的重要征象。

6. 喉部周围脂肪间隙的改变

恶性肿瘤可侵犯喉旁间隙，CT 表现为低密度的脂肪消失，代之以等或略高密度的软组织影，MRI 表现为正常脂肪高信号中出现等信号软组织影。

第四节　常见疾病诊断

喉癌大约 95% 为鳞状上皮细胞癌，其发作年龄为 50~70 多岁。最重要的诱因是抽烟，饮酒过度也有促进作用。影像学检查的作用不是提供鉴别诊断，而是确定范围。喉癌分为声门上型、声门型和声门下型。声门型、声门上型、声门下型的发生率分别是 65%，30% 和 5%。声门上型和声门下型的肿瘤都能通过声门形成跨声门肿瘤，提示预后不良。

声门型是喉癌的最常见类型。它通常由于声嘶的原因能被早期发现，因此有较高的治愈率。早期声门型喉癌生长缓慢，容易鉴别。大多数累及声带前半部的肿瘤可能通过前联合延伸至对侧。通过前联合声门癌长至声门下区、声门上区、甲状软骨或环甲膜。肿瘤向后延伸至后联合、杓状软骨、环杓软骨关节。通过后联合，肿瘤可以扩散至声门下区或者环状软骨后区域。

声门上型喉癌分化低，预后差。声嘶是晚期症状，提示病变累及声带。颈部淋巴结转移发生率较高，根据原发病灶的大小，有30%~75%发生淋巴结转移。累及的淋巴结通常包括颈内静脉的颈静脉上淋巴结及颈静脉二腹肌淋巴结。25%~35%的患者发生双侧淋巴结转移。

（谭艳，李秋云，骆永恒，刘欢，韦勇，肖恩华，刘军）

Chapter 24

The larynx

1. Plain film examination

Observation of the larynx generally takes a lateral view of the neck, using soft tissue conditions, but currently larynx lesions are rarely examined by X-ray. It can show parts of the laryngeal structure, but it is often difficult to show the internal conditions of smaller lesions and surrounding soft tissues.

2. CT examination

CT examination is the main imaging technique for laryngeal lesions. The thin-layer multi-directional recombination technique is often used, and the soft tissue window is observed. It can clearly show the abnormal manifestation of the larynx and its surrounding structures, clarify the location and scope of the lesion, and provide a basis information for the source, nature and staging of the tumor. In addition, enlargement of the wide window is beneficial to display the vocal cords and laryngeal compartment. Additional enhancement scan is required if lesions are found.

3. MRI examination

MRI can be imaged in any direction and has high soft tissue resolution, so it is a routine clinical imaging examination for laryngeal diseases. Cross-sectional, sagittal, and coronal T1WI and T2WI scans are routinely performed, and the enhanced scan is needed if necessary. It can clearly show the changes in the structure of the laryngeal cavity, laryngeal wall, and the perilaryngeal space, especially in distinguishing fibrosis and tumor recurrence after radiotherapy, and it can show clearly the degree of soft tissue involvement and invasion.

Section 2 Normal appearances

Many of the primary neoplasms of the pharynx and larynx are located at the mucosal surface, and the clinical diagnosis is readily confirmed by endoscopic biopsy. However, submucosal tumor extension cannot be assessed reliably with endoscopy alone. Both MR imaging and CT scanning are helpful for detecting lesions in clinically important blind spots such as the submucosal spaces.

The pharynx forms the upper portion of the aerodigestive tract between the skull base superiorly and the cricoid cartilage inferiorly. The pharynx is composed of three separate sections (i. e. , the nasopharynx, the oropharynx, and the hypopharynx). The boundaries of the larynx are superiorly the glossoepiglottic and pharyngoepiglottic folds, inferiorly the lower border of the cricoid cartilage, laterally the aryeipglottic folds and the arytenoid cartilages, anteriorly the mucosa extending from the level of the hyoid bone to the thyroid cartilage, and posteriorly the posterior lamina of the cricoid cartilage in the lower portion of the larynx.

The nasopharynx lies between the posterior choanae and the lower border of the soft palate.

The oropharynx lies beneath the hard palate (lower margin of the nasopharynx) and the hyoid bone (upper margin of the hypopharynx), and posterior to the tongue base, which begins behind the circumvallate papillae; The contents of the oropharynx are the tongue base, the palatine tonsils, which are surrounded by the tonsillar pillars, and the soft palate, which is formed by five pairs of muscles (the tensor villae palatini, uvular, palatoglossal, palatopharyngeal, and levator villi palatini muscles). The other components of the oropharynx are the oropharyngeal mucosa, the pharyngeal constrictor muscles from the level of the soft palate to the top of the epiglottis (approximately at the level of C2−C3), and the valleculae. Innervation of the tonsillar fossa, the posterior tonsillar pillars, and the base of the tongue is the glossopharyngeal nerve.

The hypopharynx, or the laryngeal part of the pharynx, extends from the hyoid bone superiorly to the cricoid cartilage inferiorly. This portion of the pharynx corresponds to the region between the lower portion of C3 and the upper portion of C6. The contents of the hypopharynx are the hypopharyngeal mucosa, minor salivary glands, and inferior pharyngeal constrictor muscles. The three major subdivisions of the hypopharynx are the pyriform sinus, post cricoid area, and posterior pharyngeal wall.

The larynx is divided into three regions: the supraglotticc, glottic, and subglottic portions. The supraglottic larynx (supraglottis) extends from the tip of the epiglottis cephalad to the laryngeal ventricle caudad. The contents of the supraglottic larynx are the vestibule, epiglottis, false vocal cords, ventricle, arytenoid cartilages, aryepiglottic folds, and the pre-epiglottic and paraglottic (paralaryngeal) spaces. The vestibule is the air space within the supraglottic larynx.

The glottic region (glottis) lies between the true cords superiorly and a line 1 cm below the most lateral point of the ventricle inferiorly. The lateral boundaries of the glottic region are the paraglottic (paralaryngeal) spaces. The contents of the glottic region are the true vocal cords and the anterior and posterior commissures. The true vocal cords are formed by mucosa covering the thyroarytenoid muscle. This muscle originates from the median inner surface of the thyroid lamina and inserts on the anterolateral aspect of the arytenoid cartilage. The vocal ligament, which extends from the vocal process of the arytenoid to the thyroid cartilage, constitutes the free margin of the true vocal cord. On axial CT or MR scans, the vocal process marks the level of the true cord. With quiet respiration, the true cords remain slightly apart. During breath holding, the true cords are opposed. The paraglottic (paralaryngeal) spaces at the level of the true cords are formed mainly by muscle and a narrow band of lose areolar tissue medial to the thyroid laminae.

The subglottic larynx (subglottis) extends from a level 1 cm below the ventricle superiorly to the inferior surface of the cricoid cartilage inferiorly.

Section 3 Basic pathological changes

1. Morphological changes

Swelling, destruction and disappearance of glottis area may occur, or there may be indistinguishable true and false vocal cords, soft tissue thickening or mass, and airway stenosis. Local normal structure disappeared, disorder and clear boundaries are often benign lesions. Extensive structural loss, disorder and unclear boundaries are more likely malignant lesions. Soft tissue thickening or mass surface is not smooth accompanied with mucosal destruction is malignant lesions.

2. Density and signal changes

Cystic lesions show low density or long T1 and long T2 signals, solid lesions show soft tissue density or equal

T1, long or slightly long T2 signals.

3. Symmetry and position change

The left and right sides of the larynx are asymmetric, and any asymmetry, distortion and deformation of the true vocal cords, false vocal cords, laryngeal Chambers and subglottic Spaces are pathological signs. Lesions in or outside the larynx may cause displacement of the entire larynx.

4. Destruction of laryngeal cartilage

The destruction of cartilage is an important sign in the diagnosis of tumor, indicating that the tumor has been extensively infiltrated. CT shows bone destruction or proliferative sclerosis. MRI shows high signal in the upper laryngeal cartilage of T1WI or medium signal and low signal in the bone marrow.

5. Functional changes

Normal parts that can be expanded or moved become rigid, or different respiratory examination shows no activity, indicating tumor invasion and fixation. It is an important sign to distinguish neoplastic lesions from non-neoplastic lesions.

6. Changes in the fat space around the larynx

malignant tumors can invade the paratholaryngeal space. CT shows the loss of low-density fat, replaced by equal or slightly high-density soft tissue signal. MRI shows the appearance of equal signal soft tissue in the high signal of normal fat.

Section 4　Diagnosis of common diseases

Approximately 95% of epithelial malignancies of the larynx are squamous cell carcinomas. The age of onset is between the fifth and seventh decades. The most important risk factor is cigarette smoking. Excessive use of alcohol has a synergistic effect. The role of the radiologist in the workup of laryngeal cancer is not to offer a differential diagnosis, but to determine the extent of disease. The laryngeal cancer is divided in to supraglottic, glottic, or subglottic. The incidence of glottic, supraglottic, and infraglottic carcinomas are 65%, 30% and 5%, respectively. Both infraglottic and supraglottic tumors can extend through the glottis and become transglottic, accompanied with a worsened prognosis.

Carcinoma of the true vocal cord (glottic) is the most common form of laryngeal cancer. This tumor is usually discovered early, owing to the development of hoarseness, and is therefore highly curable. These early carcinomas of the true vocal cord are slow growing and well differentiated. Most tumors involve the anterior half of the vocal cord, with possible extension to the opposite side via the anterior commissure (horseshoe-shaped lesion). From the anterior commissure, glottic carcinomas may grow into the infraglottic or supraglottic regions or into the thyroid cartilage or cricothyroid membrane. Extension of tumor toward the posterior commissure, arytenoid cartilages, and cricoarytenoid joints may also occur. From the posterior commissure, tumor may spread to the infraglottic or postcricoid regions.

Carcinoma of the supraglottis carry a poor prognosis since they are usually poorly differentiated. Hoarseness is a late symptom that indicates extension of a lesion to the vocal cord. There is a high incidence of cervical lymph node metastasis — 30% ~ 75%, depending on the size of the primary lesion. The most commonly involved lymph nodes include the upper jugular and jugulodigastric lymph nodes of the internal jugular chain. Bilateral cervical lymph node metastasis occurs in approximately 25% ~ 35% of patients at the time of presentation.

(Tan Yan, Li Qiuyun, Luo Yongheng, Liu Huan, Wei Yong, Xiao Enhua, Liu Jun)

第二十五章

鼻咽部

第一节　检查方法

1. X 线平片检查

目前咽部病变较少应用 X 线平片检查，其一般只有在病变晚期出现骨质破坏和软组织改变时才显示出异常表现。咽部造影通常需要吞咽钡剂以观察咽腔形态和评估吞咽运动，这对于治疗计划很重要。

2. CT 检查

咽部的常规影像检查技术，通常先行 CT 平扫检查，层厚应在 2~4 mm，可以快速清晰显示咽腔、咽壁和咽周间隙改变。评估血管结构时必须使用对比剂，例如颈动脉及其分支的走向，静脉结构以及评估血管性病变的严重程度。此外 CT 图像引导活检可用于组织学诊断。

3. MRI 检查

MRI 软组织分辨率高，因此是临床咽部病变常规影像检查技术，常规行矢状位、冠状位、横断位 T1WI、T2WI 检查，在某些情况下，使用对比增强的脂肪抑制序列可优化对病变增强模式的评估。当疑为血管性病变、肿瘤侵入颅内或者需要确定肿瘤大小、形态、浸润范围时，需行增强检查。

第二节　正常表现

鼻咽部是呼吸系统的一部分，位于鼻腔后方，颅底和软腭水平之间。约有高 4 cm，宽 4 cm，前后径 2~3 cm。由 5 个壁围成并在悬雍垂下缘水平与口咽部为界。其前壁从内鼻孔的上表面和鼻中隔的后表面至软腭水平。鼻咽部和鼻腔通过内鼻孔相连。鼻咽上部由咽颅底筋膜牢固地附在颅底部。鼻咽的顶部和后部形成斜坡，它经由蝶窦底部，蝶骨体部，枕基底部及 C_1~C_2 颈椎。因为鼻咽顶部的黏膜下有淋巴组织因此形成许多折叠。鼻咽部的侧壁包括耳咽管的三角孔，它以后上方的咽鼓管圆枕为界。这个突出物后方是咽隐窝或者叫 Rosenmüller 窝。

在鼻咽水平上方的轴位扫描可以显示鼻咽部的双侧咽隐窝。更前部的切迹为耳咽鼓管开口，咽鼓管圆枕将前方的咽鼓管口和后方的咽隐窝分开，它由腭帆提肌的肌肉突出部及耳咽管的软骨构成。咽隐窝大小各不相同，通常不对称，其不对称通常由局部淋巴组织引起。在轴位层面，下颌骨的冠状突的前部及内侧部是颞肌的深部头。在下颌骨角及其伸支内侧是内侧翼肌、外侧翼肌。外侧翼肌起自外侧翼板通过颞下窝到下颌骨的骨节。内侧翼肌其自内外翼板之间的翼窝，延伸至下颌骨角的内侧。翼内肌下部变粗，上部内外侧翼肌被外侧翼板隔开。

第三节　基本病变

1. 咽腔狭窄或闭塞

咽腔狭窄或闭塞常见于肿瘤、外伤等，X线平片、CT、MRI均可观察咽腔形态改变。

2. 咽壁增厚或不对称

咽壁增厚或不对称见于炎症、肿瘤。咽后壁脓肿、肿瘤可见软组织增厚。脓肿形成时可见液平，肿瘤表面可凹凸不平。炎症常表现弥漫性软组织增厚，肿瘤表现为局限性软组织增厚。

3. 增强改变

增强扫描脓肿壁强化而中心液化区不强化，肿瘤可呈现不同程度强化。

4. 颅底骨质改变

鼻咽部恶性肿瘤可引起颅底骨质的溶骨性破坏，轻者孔道增大，重者整个骨块消失。少数可见颅底骨质增生。

5. 颈椎骨质改变

咽后壁脓肿可由颈椎结核引起，此时可见颈椎骨质、椎间隙及椎旁软组织的改变。

6. 咽旁间隙受累

咽旁间隙两侧对称，其位置和形态改变有助于肿瘤定位。来源于鼻咽部肿瘤，咽旁间隙向外移位；咀嚼肌间隙或腮腺深叶的占位病变，咽旁间隙向内或前内移位。颈动脉间隙内血管的移位方向，对鉴别肿瘤的部位和性质有帮助。淋巴结增大使血管向内前或内后深部移位；迷走神经源性肿瘤，常发生于颈动脉和颈内静脉之间，使其向两侧分离；交感神经源性肿瘤，常推挤这些血管共同向前外方移位；颈动脉体肿瘤位于颈动脉分叉处，可使颈内动脉与颈外动脉分离，并有受压变形。

第四节　常见疾病诊断

1. 青少年鼻咽纤维血管瘤

（1）临床及病理表现：青少年鼻咽血管纤维瘤是一种良性的、极富血管的肿瘤，见于青少年男性。起源于蝶腭孔的鼻侧，蝶腭孔是翼腭窝的内界。最常见的临床表现是鼻塞和鼻出血。尽管不会转移，青少年鼻咽血管纤维瘤具有局部侵袭性，并通过邻近的颅底孔道延伸。如果不完全切除，肿瘤经常复发。

（2）影像学表现：在影像学上，青少年鼻咽血管纤维瘤表现为CT/MRI的显著强化，中心位于鼻咽。随着肿块继续增大，常常向翼腭窝或眼眶延伸。青少年鼻咽血管纤维瘤有三大特征：①鼻咽肿块；②翼腭窝扩大；③上颌窦后壁向前弯曲或移位。

青少年鼻咽血管纤维瘤常在切除术前行栓塞治疗，以减少出血。

2. 鼻咽癌

（1）临床及病理表现：鼻咽癌与EB病毒感染相关，与吸烟或酗酒无关。最常见于40~60岁男性，但可出现20岁余和60岁余双峰。临床表现与鼻咽的各种结构受累有关，包括颅神经麻痹、咀嚼肌间隙功能障碍或咽鼓管功能障碍引起的中耳炎，也可能是隐匿性的。90%患者并发颈部淋巴结肿大，不少病例以颈部淋巴结肿大就诊。

（2）影像学表现：CT和MRI表现为以鼻咽为中心的侵袭性肿块。颅底部的骨质破坏是肿瘤的常见征象。鼻咽癌可通过岩斜裂向上延伸至颅骨，也可经神经周围扩散。

（谭艳，李秋云，骆永恒，刘欢，韦勇，肖恩华，刘军）

Chapter 25

Nasopharynx

Section 1　Method of examination

1. Plain film

X-rayplain films are rarely used for pharyngeal lesions now, because lesions generally show abnormal manifestations in the late stage of the disease when bone destruction and soft tissue changes occur. Pharyngography usually requires to swallow barium to observe the shape of the pharyngeal cavity and assess swallowing movement, which is important for the plan of treatment.

2. CT examination

CT is the conventional imaging examination technology for the pharynx, usually by unenhanced CT scan first, and the layer thickness should be about 2 ~ 4 mm, the changes in the pharyngeal cavity, pharyngeal wall and peripharyngeal space can be quickly and clearly showed. Contrast agents must be used to assess the vascular structure, such as the orientation of the carotid artery and its branches, the structure of the vein, and the severity of vascular disease. In addition, CT image-guided biopsy can be used for histological diagnosis.

3. MRI examination

The MRI is a routine imaging technique for clinical pharynx lesions since its high soft tissue resolution. Sagittal, coronal, and transverse T1WI and T2WI examinations are performed routinely. In some cases, contrast-enhanced fat-suppression sequences can optimize the evaluation of enhanced model of diseases. The enhanced scan examination is required when it is suspected of vascular disease, tumor invasion into the skull, or need to determine the size, shape, and infiltration range of the tumor.

Section 2　Normal appearances

The nasopharynx is the portion of the respiratory system located behind the nasal cavity and between the base of the skull and the level of the soft palate. It is approximately 4 cm in height, 4 cm in width, and 2 to 3 cm in the anteroposterior dimension. It is bounded by five walls and separated from the oropharynx at the level of the lower margin of the uvula. The anterior wall extends from the superior aspect of the choanae and the posterior surface of the nasal septum to the level of the soft palate. The nasopharynx and nasal cavities communicate through the choanae. The upper portion of the nasopharynx is firmly bound to the base of the skull by the pharyngobasilar fascia. The roof and posterior wall of the nasopharynx form a slope that extends over a portion of the floor of the sphenoidal sinus, the basisphenoid, the basiocciput, and the upper two cervical vertebrae. The contour of the mucosa of the nasopharyngeal roof forms numerous folds owing to the underlying lymphoid tissue. The lateral wall of the nasopharynx contains the triangular orifice of the eustachian tube, which is bounded superiorly and posteriorly by the torus tubarius. Behind this prominence is the pharyngeal recess, or the fossa of Rosenmüller.

The bilateral paired pharyngeal recesses of the nasopharynxcan be shown on the axial scan at the upper level of the nasopharynx. The more anterior indentation represents the orifice of the eustachian tube. This orifice is separated from the more posterior recess by the torus tubarius, which is composed of the muscular prominence of the levator veil palatini muscle and the cartilaginous portion of the eustachian tube. The pharyngeal recess is of variable size, which is always asymmetry in both sides; this asymmetry is often caused by regional lymphoid tissue. In the axial section, the deep head of the temporalis muscle is anterior and medial to the coronoid process of the mandible. The medial and lateral pterygoid muscles are between the condyle and ascending ramus of the mandible are. The lateral pterygoid muscle arises from the lateral pterygoid plates and extends horizontally across the infratemporal space to the mandibular condyle. The medial pterygoid muscle arises from the pterygoid fossa, which was located between the lateral and medial pterygoid plates, extends inferiorly and laterally and reaches the medial aspect of the angle of the mandible. The medial pterygoid muscle becomes larger at lower levels. Superiorly, the medial and lateral pterygoid muscles are separated by the lateral pterygoid plate.

Section 3　Basic pathological changes

1. Stenosis or occlusion of the pharyngeal cavity

It is commonly seen in tumor, trauma, etc. The pharyngeal cavity morphological changes can be observed by plain film, CT, MRI.

2. Thickening or asymmetry of the pharyngeal wall

It is seen in inflammation and tumors. The posterior pharyngeal wall abscess and tumor are seen with thickened soft tissue. The abscess can be formed with smooth fluid, and the tumor surface can be uneven. Diffuse soft tissue thickening is often seen in inflammation and localized soft tissue thickening is often seen in tumor.

3. Enhance change

The wall of abscessis strengthened by contrast-enhanced scan and the central liquefaction area is not enhanced.

4. Bone changes in the skull base

Nasopharyngeal malignant tumor can cause osteolytic destruction of skull base bone, in light cases, the pores are enlarged, and in heavy cases, the whole bone mass disappears. A small number of bony hyperplasia are seen in the skull base.

5. Bone changes in cervical vertebra

An abscess in the posterior pharyngeal wall may be caused by cervical tuberculosis, with changes in cervical bone, intervertebral space, and paraspinal soft tissue.

6. Parapharyngeal space involvement

The parapharyngeal space is bilaterally symmetrical, and changesof its position and morphology contribute to tumor localization. The tumor originates from nasopharyngeal, the parapharyngeal space displaces laterally. The lesions come from the masticatory muscle space or deep lobe of parotid gland, the parapharyngeal space moving inward or forward and inward. The direction of vascular migration in the carotid space is helpful to identify the location and nature of the tumor. Lymph node enlargement causes the vessel to shift inward or inward and deep; The vagus neurogenic tumor usually occurs between the carotid artery and the internal jugular vein, which separates them to both sides. Sympathetic neurogenic tumors often push these vessels forward and outward together; Carotid body tumor is located at the bifurcation of carotid artery, which can separate internal carotid artery from external carotid artery and cause compression and deformation.

Section 4　Diagnosis of common diseases

1. Juvenilenasopharyngeal angiofibroma

(1) Clinical and pathological manifestations: Juvenile nasopharyngeal angiofibroma (JNA) is a benign, highly vascular tumor seen in adolescent males. The most common clinical presentation is nasal obstruction and epistaxis. Despite the lack of metastatic behavior, JNA is very locally aggressive and insinuates through adjacent skull base foramina. Tumors frequently recur if resected incompletely. JNA arises from within the nasal aspect of the sphenopalatine foramen, which is the medial boundary of the pterygopalatine fossa.

(2) Imaging manifestations: On imaging, JNA enhances avidly and is centered in the nasopharynx. As the mass continues to grow, extension into the pterygopalatine fossa or the orbits is commonly seen. The three classic findings of JNA include: 1) Nasopharyngeal mass; 2) Expansion of the pterygopalatine fossa; 3) Anterior bowing or displacement of the posterior maxillary sinus wall. Pre-operative embolization is often performed to reduce the vascularity of the lesion prior to resection.

2. Nasopharyngeal carcinoma

(1) Clinical and pathological manifestations: Nasopharyngeal carcinoma is positive correlated with Epstein-Barr virus (EBV) infection, but unrelated to smoking or alcohol exposure. Most commonly seen in males 40-60 years old with bimodal peaks in the second and sixth decades. The manifestation of nasopharyngeal carcinoma is various, depending on the involvement of various structures in the nasopharynx, including cranial nerve palsies, masticator space dysfunction, or otitis media from eustachian tube dysfunction. 90% present with cervical adenopathy. Some cases present with enlargement of cervical lymphnodes.

(2) Imagingmanifestations: The features of CT and MRI are the aggressive mass lesion centered within the nasopharynx. Destruction of the skull base is a common feature and the tumor may extend superiorly into the cranium via the petroclival fissure. It may also spread along Perineural.

(Tan Yan, Li Qiuyun, Luo Yongheng, Liu Huan, Wei Yong, Xiao Enhua, Liu Jun)

第二十六章

口腔颌面部

第一节　检查方法

1. X 线平片检查

X 线平片检查是最常用、经济的检查方法，此外口腔曲面断层全景片检查是其特有检查方法，用于观察牙齿、牙槽骨、颌骨和颞颌关节等部位病变范围及程度，也可用于治疗前后的对比和疗效判断。X 线造影检查主要用于观察涎腺部位的病变，显示其导管及腺泡，为临床诊断提供有效信息。

2. CT 检查

目前临床检查口腔病变常用的是锥形束 CT，其优势在于低剂量、高分辨率等，但也存在穿透性差、信噪比低等缺点。此外多排螺旋 CT 检查也是临床常规检查技术，对于牙齿、牙槽骨、涎腺等病变的检出、诊断及鉴别具有重要价值。

3. MRI 检查

MRI 检查不受骨骼伪影影响，较 CT 图像有着较高的软组织对比度，常规行横断面、矢状位、冠状位 T1WI 和 T2WI 扫描，必要时行增强 T1WI 检查。可清晰显示颞颌关节囊内积液、粘连、关节盘穿孔、颌面部肿瘤等病变，故为临床常规影像检查，也是舌、颞颌关节病变的主要影像检查技术。

第二节　正常表现

每颗牙大部分由牙质组成，一种具有薄层骨的 X 线密度活性的物质，其 70% 的成分与无机钙盐相似。在牙冠部及牙表面覆盖着釉质，它是身体最坚固、最不透 X 线的组织，拥有 97% 的无机钙盐成分。牙根部覆有薄层粘合质，它有与牙质一样的 X 线密度，因为太薄而不能显示在影像中。它被牙周膜包围，后者可以看到围绕牙根部连续透亮线性结构。在这之外有一薄层不透 X 线包围齿根，并与临近牙齿在齿槽水平连续。牙髓为软组织，可透 X 线，每一牙齿的牙髓存在于牙冠，牙冠可与一个或者多个牙管相连。

下颚骨，像躯干的长骨一样，呈管状结构，以致密的皮质包围骨小梁。下颌骨双侧对称，当从上或者从下看时，形状类似马碲。从侧面看类似 L 型，由水平的体部和垂直的升部构成。

腮腺大小随患者不同而大小差别较大，但常常对称，它位于下颌骨的后面，胸锁乳突肌的前面，延伸至颅底，底部在下颌骨三角下方区域，前方部分突出一点覆盖在咬肌表面。

第三节 基本病变

1. 涎腺造影的改变

良性肿瘤可见涎腺导管的受压、移位与包绕。恶性肿瘤时可见导管的粗细不均、中断或断续充盈，腺泡不规则充盈缺损，对比剂外溢等征象。

2. CT 表现

（1）涎腺腺体形态、大小和密度的异常：借此可以判断病变的部位及蔓延范围，良性肿瘤与恶性肿瘤的鉴别，以及腮腺外肿瘤的侵犯。良性肿瘤的 CT 特征是肿块多呈类圆形，边缘光整，密度均匀，血管瘤有明显的强化。恶性肿瘤的形态多不规则，边界模糊，密度不均匀，肿块内常有出血、坏死或囊变，常侵犯周围软组织及脂肪间隙，颅底骨质破坏及淋巴结转移。

（2）颞颌关节的改变：颞颌关节形状的改变见于下颌及颅面骨发育障碍。骨质的改变见于类风湿性颞颌关节病变、肿瘤或化脓性炎症造成的髁状突骨质的破坏。外伤骨折可引起骨质连续性中断。

3. MRI 表现

（1）腮腺的改变：包括腺体大小、形态、信号的改变及其周围结构的位置与信号的改变。

（2）颞颌关节的改变：包括关节盘的移位与信号改变，髁状突及关节面下骨质的信号改变，关节腔内积液造成的信号改变。MRI 可显示颞颌关节紊乱的变化，MRI 增强扫描可显示异常增强信号。

第四节 常见疾病诊断

1. 牙源性囊肿

（1）临床及病理表现：牙源性囊肿是颌骨最常见的良性囊性病变，下颌骨较上颌骨常见。好发于 10~39 岁男性患者。可发生于颌骨任何部位。牙源性囊肿常见的类型有含牙囊肿和根尖囊肿。囊肿生长缓慢，早期无自觉症状，若继续生长则骨质逐渐向周围膨胀形成面部畸形。较大囊肿因骨板极薄，可有乒乓球感觉，压迫神经则可产生疼痛。

（2）影像学表现：含牙囊肿多为单房，边界清楚，囊腔内可含一个未萌出的牙冠。囊肿通常位于牙冠上方，囊壁附着于牙颈部。呈边界清楚的圆形或卵圆形低密度影，CT 值常在 20~45 Hu 之间。周围有骨硬化边包绕。MRI 上，含牙囊肿在 T1WI 上表现为低或中等信号；在 T2WI 上呈高信号。囊内容物无强化，囊壁可强化。

根尖囊肿 CT 上多为均匀的水液密度改变。根尖囊肿在 T1WI 上信号变化多样（囊内含铁血黄素和胆固醇晶体沉积）；在 T2WI 上呈均匀高信号。增强可见囊壁呈明显增厚的环形强化。

2. 成釉细胞瘤

（1）临床及病理表现：这种良性肿瘤起源于牙源性外胚层细胞，尽管这种细胞与有功能的成釉细胞生物学特征相似，却不能形成有效的牙釉质。成釉细胞瘤可发生于任何年龄，其平均发病年龄为 33 岁，其中 50% 的病例发生于 20~40 岁之间，没有性别差异。80% 的造釉细胞瘤源于下颌骨，主要是下颌骨体部后份及升支区域。大多数成釉细胞瘤是新生的，偶尔发生在牙源性囊肿的壁内（壁状成釉细胞瘤）。成釉细胞瘤隐匿而无疼痛，当它破坏下颌骨或牙齿时，以及偶然行 X 线片、CT 检查才发现。

（2）影像学表现：成釉细胞瘤的典型影像学表现是下颌骨内囊性透亮区，骨间隔将透亮区分成多个小房。但是它也可呈单个透亮区。病变边缘光滑，邻近的牙齿因牙根受压或者牙根部被吸收而病理性移位。造釉细胞瘤较大时可以看见下颌骨膨大，但是一般存有菲薄的皮质外壳。

3. 腮腺多形性腺瘤

（1）临床及病理表现：多形性腺瘤是目前最常见的腮腺肿瘤，又称混合瘤，占所有腮腺肿瘤的 80%。

肿瘤通常表现为中老年患者的小而坚固的肿块。女性较多。虽然多形性腺瘤是良性的，但完全手术切除是标准的治疗方法。如果不切除，肿瘤可以继续生长，并且恶变为多形性腺瘤癌的风险增加。此外，单凭影像学无法区分良性多形性腺瘤和恶性黏液表皮样癌。

（2）影像学表现：CT 表现为腮腺内圆形或椭圆形软组织密度肿块，边缘光滑，与正常低密度的腺体分界清楚，增强扫描呈均匀或环形强化。MRI 上，肿瘤较小时信号较均匀，T1WI 为等信号，T2WI 为高信号，周边常可见低信号薄壁包膜。发生坏死、囊变时 T1WI 及 T2WI 信号不均匀。

（谭艳，李秋云，骆永恒，刘欢，韦勇，肖恩华，刘军）

Chapter 26

Teeth, mandible and temporomandibular joints

1. Plain film

X-ray plain examination is the most commonly used and economical examination method. In addition, oral curved tomographic examination is the unique examination method, which is used to observe the scope and extent of lesions in teeth, alveolar bone, jaw and temporomandibular joint. It can be used for the efficacy judgment before and after treatment. X-ray contrast examination is mainly used to observe the lesions of the salivary glands, showing the ducts and acinars, and providing effective information for clinical diagnosis.

2. CT examination

Cone-beam CT is commonly used in clinical examination of oral lesions currently. Its advantages are low-dose and high-resolution, but it also has disadvantages, such as poor penetration and low signal-to-noise ratio. In addition, multi-slice spiral CT examination is also a routine clinical examination technique, which has important value for the detection, diagnosis and differential diagnosis of tooth, alveolar bone, salivary glands and other diseases.

3. MRI examination

MRI examination is not affected by skeletal artifacts, and has higher soft tissue contrast than CT images. The cross-sectional, sagittal, and coronal T1WI and T2WI scans are routinely performed, and enhanced T1WI examination is performed when necessary. It can clearly show the temporomandibular joint capsule effusion, adhesions, joint disc perforation, maxillofacial tumors and other diseases, so it is a routine clinical imaging examination for tongue and temporomandibular joint disease.

Section 2 Normal appearances

Each tooth is composed largely of dentine, a living material with the radiodensity of lamellar bone and a similar proportion of calcified inorganic material(70%). The intraoral part of the tooth or crown has a covering of enamel, the hardest and most radio-opaque tissue in the body. With a calcified inorganic content of 97%. The root is covered with a thin layer cementum, which has the same radiodensity as dentine, and is too thin to show on a radiography. It is surrounded by the periodontal membrane, which is clearly visible as a radiolucent line outlining the root, and beyond this lies the lamina dura which forms a continuous radio-opaque line around the root, which is continuous with the lamina dera of the adjacent teeth at the level of the alveolar crest. The pulp of the tooth appears radiolucent as consist of soft tissues. Each tooth contains a pulp chamber in the crown, and is continuous with one or more root canals.

The mandible, like the long bones of the body, is essentially a tubular structure with dense cortical walls filled with trabecular bone. The mandible is bilaterally symmetric and shaped like a horseshoe when viewed from above or below. In profile, it is L-shaped, with a horizontal body and a vertical ascending ramus on each side.

The parotid gland varies considerable in size from patient but is usually symmetrical. It lies posterior to the mandible and anterior to the strrnocleidomastoid muscle and extends from skull base to an area below the angle of the mandible and anterior to a point overlying the masseter muscle.

Section 3   Basic pathological changes

1. Changes in sialography

The benign tumor shows compression, displacement, and inclusion of the salivary duct. Malignant tumor can be seen in the uneven thickness of the duct, interrupted or interrupted filling, irregular filling defect of acinar, contrast extravasation and other signs.

2. CT findings

(1) Abnormalities in the morphology, size and density of salivary glands can be used to determine the location and spread of lesions, the differentiation between benign and malignant tumors, and the invasion of extra-parotid tumors. The CT features of benign tumors are mostly round, with smooth edges, uniform density and obvious enhancement of hemangioma. The morphology of malignant tumor is irregular, with fuzzy boundary and uneven density. There is often hemorrhage, necrosis or cystic degeneration in the tumor, which often invades the surrounding soft tissue and fat space, and the bone destruction in the skull base and lymph node metastasis.

(2) Changes in the shape of the TMJ are found in mandibular and facial cranial development disorders. Bone changes are seen in the destruction of condylar bone caused by rheumatoid temporomandibular joint lesions, tumors, or suppurative inflammation. Traumatic fractures can cause disruption of bone continuity.

3. MRI manifestations

(1) Changes of parotid gland include changes in gland size, shape, signal, position of surrounding structures and signal.

(2) The changes of TMJ include the displacement and signal change of articular disc, the signal change of condyle and bone under articular surface, signal changes caused by fluid accumulation in the lumen. MRI films can show the changes of TMJ disorder, and MRI enhanced scan can show abnormal enhancement signals.

Section 4   The diagnosis of common diseases

1. Odontogenic cyst

(1) Clinical and pathological manifestations: Odontogenic cysts are the most common benign cystic lesions of the jaw, and the mandible is more common than the maxilla. It occurs in male patients aged 10-39 years and occur in any part of the jaw. Common types of odontogenic cysts are dentinal cyst and apical cyst. Cysts grow slowly and have no symptoms in the early stage. If they continue to grow, the bone will gradually expand to the surroundings to form facial deformities. Larger cysts can feel like a table tennis ball because of the extremely thin bone plate, and they can cause pain when they compress nerves.

（2）Imaging manifestations：Most of the dentinal cysts are unicameral, with clear boundary, and an unerupted crown can be contained in the cavity. The cyst is usually located above the crown and attached to the neck of the tooth. The CT value was usually between 20~45 HU. There is a sclerotic edge around it. On MRI, dentinal cysts showed low or moderate signal intensity on T1WI and high signal intensity on T2WI. The contents of the capsule were not enhanced, but the wall of the capsule could be enhanced.

Most of the apical cysts showed homogeneous water density on CT. The signal intensity of apical cyst varied on T1WI (the capsule contained hemosiderin and cholesterol crystal deposition), and showed uniform high signal intensity on T2WI. The wall of the cyst was obviously thickened and annular enhanced.

2. Ameloblastoma

（1）Clinical and pathological manifestations：This benign tumor arises from odontogenic ectodermal cells that have not differentiated sufficiently to form enamel, despite a histologic similarity to functional ameloblasts. Ameloblastomas may arise at any age, but the mean age at time of discovery is 33 years, about 50% of all cases occurring at the ages of 20 and 40 years. There is no predilection for either sex. Eighty percent of ameloblastomas arise in the mandible, principally in the posterior body and ascending ramus area. Most ameloblastomas developed denovo but occasionally may occur within the wall of a cyst of dental origin (mural ameloblastoma). The ameloblastoma arises insidiously without pain. It is discovered only when it becomes disruptive of jaw architecture or the teeth, or when it is noted as an incidental finding on a radiograph.

（2）Imaging manifestations：The classic radiographic appearance of an ameloblastoma is that of a multilocular central radiolucent lesion in the jaw, with septa of bone dividing the lucent area into compartments. However, the lesion may present as a unilocular radiolucency as well. The periphery of the lesion has a smooth border, and adjacent teeth are displacement pathologically either may be resulted from the pressure on the roots or their roots may be resorbed. A large ameloblastoma may expand the mandible, but a thin cortical shell generally is preserved.

3. Pleomorphic adenoma of parotid gland

（1）Clinical and pathological manifestations：Pleomorphic adenoma is by far the most common parotid tumor, accounting for 80% of all parotid tumors. The tumor typically presents as a small firm mass in a middle-aged patient. There is a slight female predominance.

Although pleomorphic adenoma is benign, complete surgical resection is the standard treatment. The tumors will continue to grow without complete surgical resection, and there is an increasing risk for malignant transformation tocarcinoma pleomorphic adenoma. Additionally, it is not possible to distinguish between benign pleomorphic adenoma and malignant mucoepidermoid carcinoma by imaging alone.

（2）Imagingmanifestations：CT shows a round or oval soft tissue density mass in parotid gland with smooth edge and clear boundary with normal low-density gland. Enhanced scan showed homogeneous or circular enhancement. On MRI, when the tumor was small, the signal was homogeneous and isointense on T1WI, slightly hyperintense or hyperintense on T2WI, and low signal thin-walled capsule was often seen around the tumor. The signal intensity of T1WI and T2WI was uneven when necrosis and cystic degeneration occurred.

（Tan Yan, Li Qiuyun, Luo Yongheng, Liu Huan, Wei Yong, Xiao Enhua, Liu Jun）

第二十七章

颈部

第一节　检查方法

1. X 线平片检查

目前颈部病变较少应用 X 线检查，偶尔用于观察颈部气管和软组织。此外可应用 DSA 显示病变血管及血供情况。

2. CT 检查

颈部病变的主要影像学检查方法，同时还需常规进行增强扫描，并进行薄层多方位重建。先选用软组织窗观察软组织病变，必要时选用骨窗观察颈椎及其附件结构。但与超声检查相比，CT 对于甲状腺病变的显示和诊断稍有局限。

3. MRI 检查

软组织分辨率高，因此对于颈部软组织及脊髓病变、囊实性病变、肿瘤转移、术后改变及复发判断等具有很高的价值。若发现异常应行增强 T1WI 检查。

第二节　正常表现

甲状腺由于储藏碘化物，平扫时即容易识别。其上极位于甲状软骨下角之上，其后部以食管为界，它的峡部横过气管的前方。甲状旁腺通常在甲状腺后方，有可能异位。尽管正常甲状旁腺 CT 扫描看不见，但在肿大时却可能显示。

第三节　基本病变

1. CT 表现

（1）病变部位：对于确定病变性质非常重要。发生于颈前区的病变，多为甲状腺的病变，如甲状腺囊肿、甲状舌管囊肿、弥漫性甲状腺肿、甲状腺癌及甲状旁腺腺瘤等。来源于颈外侧区的病变，有鳃裂囊肿、淋巴管瘤、颈动脉瘤、颈动脉体瘤、颈静脉球瘤、神经鞘瘤或神经纤维瘤、淋巴结转移等。颈后区的病变较少见，可为颈椎骨质的病变如结核及其在颈后区形成的脓肿、动脉瘤样骨囊肿、骨巨细胞瘤及成骨细胞瘤等。神经源性肿瘤常呈哑铃状，部分位于椎管内，部分位于椎管外，伴有椎间孔扩大。

（2）病变的密度：对于区分囊性与实性肿物有重要价值。增强扫描对于区分病变为血管病变与非血管病变、富血管病变与乏血管病变也有重要作用。

2.MRI 表现

（1）颈部结构形态与大小的改变：许多病变可引起组织器官形态与大小的变化。如甲状腺腺瘤可出现局限性甲状腺增大，结节性甲状腺肿或甲状腺炎则表现为甲状腺弥漫性增大。

（2）异常肿块的出现：颈部原发性肿瘤与转移性淋巴结增大，均可表现为颈部异常肿块。

（3）颈部脂肪间隙的受压与推移：组织器官的增大与异常肿块，可造成相邻脂肪间隙的受压与推移。脂肪在 MRI 图像上显示为高信号，通过脂肪间隙的变化，易于对病变的大小、形态与侵犯范围作出准确评价。

（4）病变信号的表现：良性肿瘤多信号均匀，恶性肿瘤常信号不均匀且与周围结构分界不清。囊性病变 T1WI 为低信号，T2WI 为高信号。肿瘤出血则在 T1WI 上出现高信号。

第四节　常见疾病诊断

1.甲状舌管囊肿

（1）临床及病理表现：甲状舌管囊肿是由于甲状舌管持续存在引起的。甲状舌管沿着胚胎甲状腺从舌根的中线下降到颈部的正常位置。大多数甲状舌管囊肿在儿童时期表现为颈部肿块增大，并伴有舌突出。大部分甲状舌管囊肿（65%）位于舌骨下，其余位于舌骨水平或以上。大多数甲状舌管囊肿位于中线，但它们可能会稍微偏离中线，尤其是在舌骨下。

（2）影像学表现：CT 和 MRI 显示中线一个厚壁、周边强化的囊性结构，通常位于下颌舌骨肌下方。甲状腺乳头状癌是一种罕见的并发症，见于 1% 的甲状舌管囊肿。

2.甲状腺肿瘤

（1）临床及病理表现：甲状腺肿瘤多发于 20~40 岁的女性，表现为甲状腺区结节或肿块，可引起声音嘶哑、呼吸困难。恶性肿瘤半数左右发生颈部淋巴结转移而表现淋巴结增大。良性甲状腺肿瘤主要为腺瘤，占甲状腺肿瘤的 60%。恶性甲状腺肿瘤中绝大部分是癌，以甲状腺乳头状癌最多。

（2）影像学表现：腺瘤在 CT 上表现为圆形、类圆形境界清楚的低密度影。癌则表现为形态不规则、边界不清楚的不均匀低密度影，其内可有散在钙化及更低密度坏死区，病变多与周围组织分界不清，颈部淋巴结肿大。腺瘤不强化或轻度强化，癌则不均匀明显强化，转移淋巴结多呈环状强化。

对于已确诊为甲状腺癌的患者，CT 可以显示甲状腺癌是否侵犯喉、气管和食管，发现有无气管或食管旁淋巴结转移，判断喉返神经是否受累。也可显示颈部或上纵隔有无淋巴结转移。

腺瘤在 T1WI 上呈边界清楚的低、等或高信号结节，滤泡型腺瘤内胶样物多为高信号。腺癌呈边界不规则的低、中等信号。腺瘤和腺癌在 T2WI 上均呈高信号。

如果有所属淋巴结肿大、喉返神经麻痹、甲状软骨或其他喉软骨破坏等表现，则有利于诊断恶性。钙化不是鉴别良、恶性的依据。

3.颈动脉体瘤

（1）临床及病理表现：颈动脉体瘤（颈动脉体副神经节瘤）在颈动脉分叉处分开颈外动脉和颈内动脉。颈动脉体瘤通常是非分泌儿茶酚胺的肿瘤，由于局部效应而引起注意，表现为颈部肿块和/或伴有下颅神经麻痹。5% 的病例为双侧肿瘤，5% 至 10% 为恶性肿瘤。

（2）影像学表现：副神经节瘤是一种良性的、高度血管性的神经嵴细胞肿瘤，其特征是 CT/MRI 上的显著强化。由于肿瘤内的流动性空洞，MRI 上表现为明显的"盐和胡椒"征。副神经节瘤通常发生于颈动脉分叉部（颈动脉体瘤）、中耳（鼓室球瘤）和颈静脉窝（颈静脉球瘤）内。

颈动脉体瘤影像表现为一个极富血管的肿块，在磁共振成像上有血流空洞。较大的肿瘤可以看到典型的"盐和胡椒"征。"胡椒"代表 T1WI 小血流空洞，而"盐"则是 T1WI 高信号的小出血灶。

颈动脉体瘤的治疗通常是栓塞（使病变血管断流）和手术切除相结合。

（谭艳，李秋云，骆永恒，刘欢，韦勇，肖恩华，刘军）

Chapter 27

Neck

1. Plain film

X-ray plain examination is rarely used for cervical lesions now. It is used to observe the neck trachea and soft tissues occasionally. In addition, DSA can be used to show the blood vessels and blood supply of the lesions.

2. CT examination

CT examination is the main imaging examination method for neck lesions. At the same time, it is necessary to perform enhanced scan and thin-layer multi-directional reorganization routinely. The soft tissue window is selected firstly to observe the soft tissue lesions, and use the bone window to observe the cervical spine and its accessory structure if necessary. However, CT is slightly limited in the display and diagnosis of thyroid disease compared with ultrasound examination.

3. MRI examination

The high soft tissue resolution of MRI plays an important role in the diagnosis for cervical soft tissue and spinal cord disease, cystic and solid disease, tumor metastasis, postoperative changes and recurrence judgment. Enhanced T1WI should be performed if abnormalities are found.

Section 2 Normal appearances

The thyroid gland normally stores iodine and is easily seen on the non-enhanced scan. The superior poles of the thyroid gland is superior to the inferior cornu of the thyroid cartilage. Posteriorly, the thyroid gland is anterior to the esophagus, whereas the isthmus transverse in front of the trachea. The parathyroid glands are normally posterior to thyroid gland but may be ectopic. Although the parathyroid glands are not visible on the normal scan, it may be seen when enlarged.

Section 3 Basic pathological changes

1. CT manifestations

(1) Lesion location: It is very important to determine the nature of the lesion. The lesions located in the anterior cervical region are mostly thyroid lesions, such as thyroid cyst, thyroglossal duct cyst, diffuse goiter,

thyroid cancer and parathyroid adenoma. The lesions come from the lateral cervical region are mostly branchial cyst, lymphangioma, carotid aneurysm, carotid body tumor, bulbar jugular tumor, schwannoma or neurofibroma, lymph node metastasis, etc. Lesions in the posterior cervical region are relatively rare, which are always from the cervical bone lesions such as tuberculosis and abscess formed in the posterior cervical region, aneurysmal bone cyst, giant cell tumor and osteoblastoma, etc. Neurogenic tumors are always dumbbell-shaped, partly was in the spinal canal, and partly was out of the spinal canal, accompanied with intervertebral foramen enlargement.

(2) The density of lesions

The density of lesions is important in distinguishing cystic and solid masses. Contrast-enhanced scan also plays an important role in distinguishing vascular lesions from non-vascular lesions, vascularized lesions and hypovascular lesions.

2. MRI manifestations

(1) Changes in cervical structure, shape and size: Many lesions can cause changes in the shape and size of tissues and organs. A localized enlargement of the thyroid gland may be present in a thyroid adenoma, whereas nodular goiter or thyroiditis may present as a diffuse enlargement of the thyroid gland.

(2) The appearance of abnormal mass: Both primary neck tumor and metastatic lymph node enlargement can present as abnormal neck mass.

(3) Compression anddisplacement of fat spaces in the neck: The enlargement and abnormal mass of tissues and organs may cause compression and displacement of adjacent fat spaces. Fat shows high signal on MRI images, and it is easy to evaluate the size, shape and invasion pattern of the lesions accurately through the change of fat space.

(4) Manifestations of lesions signals: The signals in benign tumors are always uniform. However, signals in malignant tumors are often uneven and indistinguishable from surrounding structures. The signal of cystic lesion is low in T1WI and high in T2WI. The tumor bleeding showed high signal in T1WI.

Section 4　The diagnosis of common diseases

1. Thyroglossal duct cyst

(1) Clinical and pathological manifestations: A thyroglossal duct cyst is due to persistence of the thyroglossal duct. The thyroglossal duct descends to its normal position in the neck along the embryonic thyroid gland from the base of the tongue. Most thyroglossal duct cysts present in childhood as an enlarging neck mass accompanied with tongue protrusion. The majority of thyroglossal duct cysts (65%) are infrahyoid, the rest are found at the level of the hyoid or above. Most thyroglossal duct cyst are located in the midline, but may be slightly off from the midline, especially in the infrahyoid.

(2) Imaging manifestations: CT and MRI show a thick-wall and peripherally enhanced cystic structure in the midline, often inferior to the mylohyoid. Thyroid carcinoma (papillary type) is a rare complication, which is seen in 1% of thyroglossal duct cyst.

2. Thyroid tumor

(1) Clinical and pathological manifestation: Thyroid tumors usually occur in women aged 20-40 years old. They appear as thyroid nodules or masses, which can cause hoarseness and dyspnea. About half of malignant tumors have cervical lymph node metastasis and lymph node enlargement. Benign thyroid tumors are mainly adenomas, accounting for 60% of thyroid tumors. Most of the malignant thyroid tumors are cancer, and most of them are papillary thyroid carcinoma.

(2) Imaging manifestations: The adenoma shows round and round like low-density with clear boundary on CT.

Cancer is characterized by uneven low-density with irregular shape and unclear boundary. There may be scattered calcification and low-density necrosis in the tumor. The boundary between the lesions and surrounding tissues is unclear, and the cervical lymph nodes are enlarged. The adenoma shows no enhance or slightly enhance, but the carcinoma shows heterogeneous and obviously enhance, and the metastatic lymph nodes show ring enhancement.

For patients who have been diagnosed with thyroid cancer, CT can show whether the thyroid cancer invades the larynx, trachea and esophagus, find out whether there is tracheal or paraesophageal lymph node metastasis, and judge whether the recurrent laryngeal nerve is involved. It can also show whether there is lymph node metastasis in neck or upper mediastinum.

On T1WI, the adenoma shows low, isointense or hyperintense nodule with clear boundary. The colloidal substance in follicular adenoma is mostly hyperintense. Adenocarcinoma shows irregular low and medium signal. Adenoma and adenocarcinoma showed high signal intensity on T2WI.

Lymph node enlargement, recurrent laryngeal nerve paralysis, thyroid cartilage or other laryngeal cartilage damageare conducive to diagnosis of malignancy. Calcification is not the basis for differentiating benign from malignant.

3. Carotid body tumor

(1)Clinical and pathological manifestation: Paraganglioma of the carotid body (carotid body tumor) splays the external and internal carotid arteries at the carotid bifurcation. Carotid body tumors are usually non-catecholamine-secreting tumors and draw attention due to its local effects, presenting as a neck mass and/or with lower cranial nerve palsies. These tumors are bilateral in 5% of cases and malignant in 5 to 10%.

(2) Imaging manifestations: Paraganglioma is a benign, highly vascular neoplasm of neural crest cells, accompanied with intense enhancement and a characteristic salt-and-pepper appearance on MRI due to intra-tumoral flow voids. Paraganglioma was typically located within the middle ear (glomus tympanicum), jugular fossa (glomus jugulare), and carotid bifurcation (carotid body tumor). The imaging of paraganglioma shows as a vascular tumor with flow voids on MRI. Classic "salt-and-pepper" appearance can be seen with larger tumors. "Pepper" represents small T1 flow voids, whereas "salt" are areas of small hemorrhage which are hyperintense on precontrast T1 images.

The treatment of paraganglioma is usually a combination of embolization (to devascularize the lesion) with surgical resection.

(Tan Yan, Li Qiuyun, Luo Yongheng, Liu Huan, Wei Yong, Xiao Enhua, Liu Jun)

介入放射学

　　介入放射学作为微创性诊断亚专业，起源于诊断放射学。目前介入放射学已成为一门独立学科，它采用导丝、导管、栓塞剂、球囊、支架和其他介入器材，在影像引导下进行各种微创治疗、诊断操作、以及侵入性诊断成像。介入放射学诊疗操作所涉及的疾病或器官范围较广且仍在不断拓展，包括但不限于外周血管、心血管、胃肠道、肝胆、泌尿生殖、肺、肌肉骨骼和中枢神经系统等。介入放射科医师能够独立地或与其他学科医师合作下对介入诊疗相关患者进行评估和管理，介入放射学已成为现代医学的组成部分。

Part 7

Interventional radiology

Interventional radiology (IR) originated within diagnostic radiology as a minimally invasive diagnostic subspecialty. IR is now a therapeutic and diagnostic specialty that comprises a wide range of image-guided, minimally invasive therapeutic and diagnostic procedures as well as invasive diagnostic imaging by using puncture needle, guidewire, catheter, embolic agent, balloon, stent and other interventional equipment. The range of diseases and organs amenable to IR procedures are extensive and constantly evolving, and include, but are not limited to, diseases and elements of the peripheral vascular, cardiovascular, gastrointestinal, hepatobiliary, genitourinary, pulmonary, musculoskeletal and central nervous system. The interventional radiologists provide patient evaluation and management relevant to image-guided interventions independently or in collaboration with other physicians. IR has become an integral part of modern medicine.

第二十八章

血管介入技术

根据治疗领域,介入放射学可分为血管介入放射学和非血管介入放射学。基本的血管介入技术包括诊断性动脉造影、经导管动脉栓塞、化学栓塞、经皮腔内血管成形术和经导管血管内药物灌注术等。

第一节 Seldinger 技术

1953 年, Sven-Ivar Seldinger 医师首创了用套管针、导丝和导管经皮动脉插管的方法。该技术由穿刺动脉、引入导丝、通过导丝置入血管鞘和导管等步骤组成,被称为 Seldinger 技术。传统 Seldinger 技术穿刺血管前后壁,改良 Seldinger 技术仅穿刺血管前壁(图 28-1)。Seldinger 技术消除插管前手术暴露血管的需要,使血管造影从手术室转移到放射科。Seldinger 技术开辟了一个全新的医学领域,已成为所有血管和部分非血管介入操作的基础。

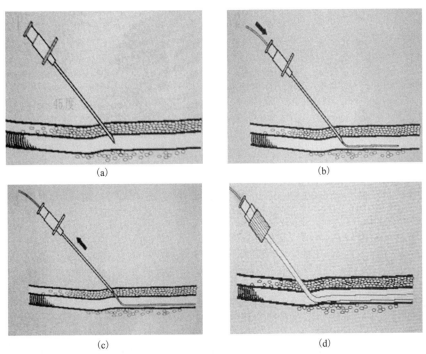

采用穿刺针穿刺动脉(a)通过穿刺针引入导丝;(b)撤出穿刺针,保留导丝;(c)通过导丝置入血管鞘,建立血管通道(d)。

图 28-1 改良 Seldinger 技术

第二节　经导管血管造影术

1. 概念

经导管动脉造影指在影像导向下采用穿刺针和(或)导管经皮插入动脉,然后注射对比剂对血管进行成像的介入诊断操作。随着科技的发展,部分经导管血管造影已被无创的 CT 血管造影或 MR 血管造影所取代。然而,经导管血管造影仍被广泛的运用于需行外科手术、血管成形术或血管内支架置入术的患者。经导管血管造影可以实时地提供清晰、准确和详细的血管图像。它对血管细节的显示是其他非创伤性血管造影技术无可比拟的。这对疾病的诊断与治疗很有帮助。因此,该技术仍然是诊断血管性疾病的金标准。

经导管血管造影技术可将导管插至人体特定部位的靶血管内。与 CT 血管造影和 MR 血管造影不同,经导管血管造影技术不仅可以进行造影诊断疾病,必要的时候还可以对疾病进行治疗。

2. 适应证

(1)诊断影响血管血流动力学的管腔狭窄或阻塞及其程度,如颈内动脉狭窄。

(2)动脉瘤或血管局部异常的扩张、膨大,如腹主动脉瘤。

(3)脑血管疾病如脑梗死、脑出血等。

(4)血管畸形如动静脉瘘等。

(5)用于判定出血的来源,如外科术后急性出血。

(6)用于判断肿瘤良恶性的辅助诊断。

(7)其他检查难以确诊的出血性疾病。

3. 禁忌证

(1)严重肝、肾或心功能不全。

(2)无法纠正的凝血功能障碍,或血小板降低($<50\times10^9/L$)。

(3)无法控制的全身感染或败血症。

(4)严重的碘对比剂过敏。

4. 器械

(1)穿刺针、导管鞘、导引导丝(如超滑导丝)。

(2)造影导管:有多种型号和管径(如 1.5F、1.8F、2F、3F、4F、5F、6F 等),根据术中目标血管的走行和直径选择合适导管。

(3)对比剂:非离子型对比剂最常用。

5. 患者准备

(1)术前 2 小时禁食,或术前 4~8 小时限制少许流质。

(2)术前检查:肝功能、肾功能、血常规、凝血功能、胸片、心电图等。

(3)建立静脉通道,留置针或中心静脉管。

(4)排空膀胱,必要时留置导尿管。

(5)根据所用对比剂说明是否做碘过敏试验。

(6)签订知情同意书。

6. 操作步骤

(1)患者进入介入手术室后,平卧检查床上。连接生命体征监测设备,必要时吸氧。

(2)根据需要选择手术穿刺部位(多为右侧股动脉)。

(3)对穿刺点进行局部麻醉(常用 1%~2%利多卡因);采用 Seldinger 技术穿刺所选血管,并置入导管鞘;通过导管鞘在导丝引导下将导管引入靶血管内。

（4）通过高压注射器经导管向血管内注入对比剂，同时进行一系列的 X 线图象采集、处理。可根据需要多角度造影或进行三维成像并重建，直到满足诊断要求。

（5）术后患者需行穿刺点局部加压包扎，且穿刺侧肢体制动 6~8 小时。

7. 并发症

（1）对比剂或局麻药过敏：其症状包括皮肤瘙痒不适、荨麻疹、严重者可能会出现血压下降、呼吸困难甚至昏迷。

（2）血栓形成：术中在导管的尖端附近形成血栓的可能性较小，一旦发生可阻塞血管，所以做好血管再通的准备也是必要的。导丝在导管内反复操作不能达到目的时，建议退出导丝，接注射器大力抽吸至血液返流至注射器内，再注入肝素盐水。然后重新插入导丝进行操作或换用其他形状导管。

（3）肾功能损伤：对比剂主要经肾脏排泄，如果肾脏有原发疾病存在则可能加重，部分患者可能导致对比剂肾病，因此术前需完善肾功能相关指标排查，对于术中大量使用对比剂者术后水化并利尿。

（4）出血：很少的情况下导管可损伤血管导致内出血，也有可能损伤血管内膜导致夹层或血管阻塞。

（5）穿刺部位假性动脉瘤形成。

（6）感染，对于操作部位存在潜在感染，且难以避免者，可预防性使用抗生素。

第三节　经导管血管栓塞术

1. 概念

经导管血管栓塞术（TAE）是指经导管血管内置入栓塞器械或注入栓塞剂，阻塞靶血管血流以达到治疗目的的介入治疗操作。该治疗技术已广泛应用于几乎所有血管分布区病变或器官，如控制出血、栓塞先天或获得性血管异常、控制肿瘤生长和使组织梗死。TAE 的栓塞水平小到毛细血管床大到大动脉，栓塞时间可以是暂时性或永久性，栓塞目的可以是治愈性或姑息性。根据适应证，TAE 可分为部分性或完全性栓塞，相应地导致局部病灶或整个靶器官的动脉血流不同程度减少或阻断。最后，栓塞术既可作为单独的治疗技术，也可作为组成部分与动脉内化疗灌注、放疗及其他介入治疗技术联合使用。

2. 适应证

（1）出血：TAE 可以被用来治疗急性或复发性出血，包括咯血、消化道出血、创伤性和医源性出血、产后出血以及肿瘤破裂出血。栓塞术通过输送栓塞材料到靶血管直接阻断出血动脉实现止血。它还包括置入覆膜支架，用以隔绝病变段血管的血流，或用以减少出血或瘘管部位供血分支的血流。

（2）肿瘤：TAE 通过肿瘤祛血管化，可用于肿瘤姑息治疗（如控制肿瘤生长、减轻疼痛或预防出血）或减少外科手失血。临床应用主要有原发性和转移性肝癌、肝血管瘤、肾血管平滑肌脂肪瘤、肾细胞癌、鼻咽血管纤维瘤、子宫肌瘤、盆腔和其他富血管恶性肿瘤等。

（3）血管疾病：TAE 可用于闭塞先天或后天性动脉瘤、假性动脉瘤、血管畸形或其他可能影响健康的血管异常。

（4）非肿瘤组织祛血管化：TAE 可通过阻断对机体造成不良影响的非肿瘤组织的血液供应，用于治疗某些疾病，包括脾功能亢进、顽固性肾血管性高血压、终末期肾蛋白尿、精索静脉曲张、盆腔充血综合征、阴茎异常勃起和异位妊娠。

（5）血流再分配：TAE 可用于重新分配血流以保护正常组织（如肝动脉栓塞术和放射栓塞术中预先栓塞胃十二指肠动脉和胃右动脉，使入肝动脉血流仅供应肝脏，避免误栓并发症）或便于后续的其他治疗（如肝脏手术切除前预先栓塞门静脉右支诱导左叶肥大）。

（6）Ⅱ型内漏：栓塞可用于治疗Ⅱ型内漏，包括直接囊内穿刺或侧支血管栓塞。

3. 禁忌证

（1）严重肝、肾或心功能不全。

（2）无法纠正的凝血功能障碍，或血小板降低（$<50×10^9/L$，部分性脾栓塞例外）。

（3）无法控制的全身感染或败血症。

（4）严重的碘对比剂过敏。

4. 器械

（1）穿刺针、导管鞘、导管、导丝、微导管系统等。

（2）TAE栓塞剂种类较多，其物理特性、输送方法和栓塞持久性各异。栓塞剂的选择主要取决于临床需求和介入操作的技术特点。常用的栓塞剂如下：

1）明胶海绵是最早和最常用的栓塞剂之一。该栓塞剂可被压缩，并在4~6周内吸收。栓塞用明胶海绵主要有无菌块状、颗粒（150~2000 μm）和粉末（约50 μm）。对暂时性栓塞，明胶海绵块和颗粒非常有用。明胶海绵通常与对比剂混合，使之悬浮并在透视下显影；悬浮后明胶海绵可被压缩经导管注入，到达靶血管后膨胀到比干燥时更大的尺寸，达到阻断血流作用。明胶海绵粉末体积小，常导致永久性闭塞。

2）聚乙烯醇（PVA）是一种廉价、惰性、永久性栓塞剂。PVA颗粒通过导管注入，然后被动脉血流输送至栓塞部位。PVA颗粒通常以不规则形的颗粒形式提供，以致栓塞时容易在血管内聚集，导致近端栓塞。PVA粒径大小的选择对于预防导管堵塞和达到理想的栓塞效果至关重要。栓塞过程中，PVA输送需在透视监视下通过轻柔的注射来完成，注意防止PVA返流进入非靶血管。

3）栓塞微球是一种血流导向的球形固体栓塞剂。经导管注入时，微球粒径可被压缩。与不规则PVA颗粒相比，微球的这些特性可导致更少的集聚和更有效的栓塞效果。载药微球除了阻断血流作用外，还具有装载和可控性释放药物的能力。

4）栓塞弹簧圈有多种尺寸、长度、形状，并由不同材质构成（通常是不锈钢或铂）。弹簧圈通过物理性栓塞管腔实现血管阻断。弹簧圈上可附着纤毛以促进血小板聚集和血栓形成。通过导管，弹簧圈可被精确地输送并释放于靶血管内，达到栓塞目的。推送式弹簧圈的输送可通过导丝推送或采用1~3 mL注射器注水推送完成。可分离式弹簧圈输送到位后通常需要通过电流熔断连接或采用机械技术释放弹簧圈。

5）液体栓塞材料包括乙醇、硬化剂、医用胶和聚合物。前两者可永久性破坏血管内皮，经导管注入动脉时后，可达到毛细血管水平实现远端栓塞。医用胶和聚合物是非常有用的血流导向性栓塞剂，可以通过微导管注入，然后凝固，实现较大空间的栓塞，这对动静脉畸形和静脉曲张的治疗有独特的价值。

5. 患者准备

（1）患者评估。

（2）实验室检查，主要包括肾功能、凝血功能和血液学参数等。

（3）胸片、心电图检查

（4）CT或MRI检查，尤其对于肿瘤栓塞。

（5）预防性使用抗生素，如脾动脉栓塞、耗时较长且需多次导管交换的TAE操作。

（6）排空膀胱，必要时留置导尿管。

（7）根据所用对比剂说明是否做碘过敏试验。

（8）签署知情同意书。

6. 操作步骤

（1）经皮穿刺右侧股动脉，置入5F动脉导管鞘。

（2）血管造影以明确病变的性质、部位、范围和程度［图28-2（a）］。

（3）采用优选的导管和（或）同轴微导管对靶动脉进行选择性插管。

（4）根据病变性质、栓塞目的和血管条件选择合适的栓塞剂。

（5）在透视引导下，通过导管或微导管准确地输送栓塞剂，控制栓塞的范围和程度，避免栓塞剂返流和误栓。

（6）血管造影复查以确保栓塞效果［图28-2（b）］。

（7）退出导管和导管鞘，手动按压穿刺部位完成止血。

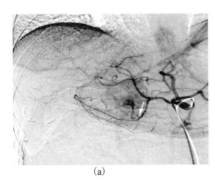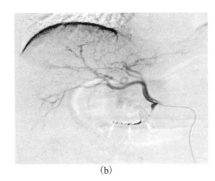

（a）腹腔干造影显示胃十二指肠动脉出血，局部对比剂外溢（箭）；（b）栓塞治疗后选择性胃十二指肠动脉造影显示胃十二指肠动脉出血段血管闭塞，注意出血点远、近端置入的微弹簧圈（箭头）。

图 28-2　坏死性胰腺炎组织清除术后出血的经导管动脉栓塞治疗

7. 栓塞后综合征与并发症

（1）栓塞后综合征由一系列症状组成，包括疼痛、发热、恶心、呕吐和因器官或病灶梗死局部缺血引起的白细胞增多。栓塞后综合征不应被视为并发症，而是栓塞的预期结果。这些症状通常在对症治疗后会缓解。

（2）TAE 相关并发症主要包括感染、靶组织缺血、非靶组织误栓、出血、脊髓梗死、操作相关性死亡等。并发症的发生率取决于患者临床状况、术者经验、栓塞血管范围、病变性质及围手术期处理等。

第四节　经导管动脉化疗栓塞术

1. 概念

经导管动脉化疗栓塞术（TACE）分为常规或载药微球 TACE。常规 TACE 是指经导管动脉内注入化疗药或化疗药与碘化油乳剂，再辅以明胶海绵、聚乙烯醇或空白微球等颗粒性栓塞剂进行栓塞的介入治疗技术。载药栓塞 TACE 是指经导管动脉内注入加载了化疗药物的载药微球的介入治疗技术。

TACE 是不可切除性原发性和转移性肝癌的主流疗法，并在过去 40 年中得以广泛应用。化疗栓塞的基本原理基于正常肝组织与肝脏恶性肿瘤的血流供应差异，正常肝组织大部分血液供应来自门静脉（75%），而肝脏恶性肿瘤大部分血供来自肝动脉（90%~100%）。因此，采用肝动脉作为治疗途径是合理的，在靶向治疗肿瘤的同时又可保护正常肝组织。动脉内注入细胞毒性药物，随后栓塞肿瘤供血动脉，可诱发显著的细胞毒效应和缺血效应，从而实现大量肿瘤坏死的目的。TACE 也可被用于治疗多种肝外恶性实体瘤。

2. 适应证

（1）肝细胞癌：TACE 是不可切除性肝细胞癌的主要治疗方法，也是巴塞罗那分期中期肝癌患者的一线治疗方法。

（2）肝内胆管细胞癌：肝内胆管细胞癌发病率仅次于肝细胞癌，是第二大常见的原发性肝脏恶性肿瘤。不可切除、转移或术后残留的局部肝内胆管癌患者可能会从 TACE 治疗中获益。

（3）肝转移：TACE 可用于治疗常规治疗失败的结肠癌、神经内分泌瘤、乳腺癌、卵巢癌、肉瘤、葡萄膜黑色素瘤和其他恶性肿瘤的肝转移瘤。

（4）其他恶性实体肿瘤：对于某些常规治疗无效的肝外恶性实体瘤，如肺癌、骨和软组织肉瘤、脊柱恶性肿瘤、肾恶性肿瘤、盆腔恶性肿瘤、腹膜后恶性肿瘤，TACE 也是一种有效的姑息性治疗方法。

3. 禁忌证

(1)严重肝功能障碍(Child-Pugh C)。

(2)门静脉主干完全闭塞。

(3)肿瘤负荷占全肝体积70%以上。

(4)体力状态差(体力状态评分>2)。

(5)无法纠正的凝血功能障碍或血小板减少($<50×10^9/L$)。

(6)无法控制的全身感染或败血症。

(7)严重的肾功能或心功能障碍。

4. 器械

(1)常规穿刺针、5F血管鞘、5F导管、0.035英寸导丝、2F~3F微导管系统。

(2)化疗药物(如阿霉素、顺铂、5-氟尿嘧啶、丝裂霉素和伊立替康)。

(3)碘化油(如Lipiodol)

(4)栓塞剂(如明胶海绵、聚乙烯醇、空白微球或载药微球)

5. 患者准备

(1)患者评估。

(2)实验室检查,主要为肝功能、肾功能、凝血功能和血常规及胸片、心电图。

(3)肝脏增强CT或MRI检查,以及用于评估可能的肝外转移的其他影像学检查[图28-3(a)、(d)]。

(4)术前禁食4~6小时。

(5)预防性止吐和预防性使用抗生素。

(6)排空膀胱,必要时留置导尿管。

(7)根据所用对比剂说明是否做碘过敏试验。

(8)签署知情同意书。

6. 操作步骤

(1)经皮穿刺右侧股动脉,置入5F动脉导管鞘。

(2)通过导丝引入5F导管,插管至腹腔干和肠系膜上动脉。进行选择性动脉造影,用于评估肝脏血管解剖、门静脉开放情况和检测潜在的富血管病变[图28-3(b)]。如有可能,应检查膈下动脉、胸内动脉和肋间动脉,以排除异位血供情况。

(3)通过5F导管同轴引入微导管,选择性插管至肿瘤的供血动脉。

(4)经导管动脉内注入化疗药或化疗药与碘化油乳剂,再注入颗粒性栓塞剂进行栓塞。如采用载药微球TACE,则经导管注入载药微球,可根据需要追加空白微球栓塞。栓塞终点为肿瘤供血动脉血流完全闭塞或近似停滞。

(5)动脉造影复查确认肿瘤供血动脉阻断[图28-3(c)]。

(6)撤出导管和导管鞘,手动按压股动脉穿刺点实现止血。

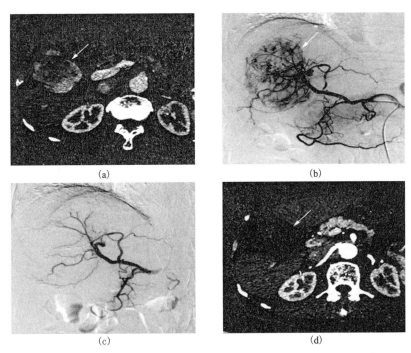

(a)增强 CT 动脉期图像显示肝内肿块,呈动脉期强化(箭)和门静脉期廓清(图像未展示),符合肝细胞癌改变;(b)TACE 术前肝总动脉造影证实肝内富血管肿瘤(箭);(c)TACE 术后血管造影显示肿瘤动脉血供阻断;(d)TACE 术后 1 个月增强 CT 动脉期图像显示靶病灶无强化(箭),提示肿瘤完全反应。

图 28-3 肝细胞癌患者的 TACE 治疗

7. 栓塞后综合征与并发症

(1)TACE 诱发的栓塞后综合征(发热、疼痛、恶心和白细胞增多)本身不是并发症,而是栓塞的预期结果。该综合征在治疗大体积肿瘤的病例中常见,通常具有自限性。

(2)TACE 相关并发症包括肝脓肿、胆汁瘤、缺血性胆囊炎、胃肠道溃疡/出血、骨髓抑制、肺或脑栓塞、肝衰竭、急性肾衰竭、肿瘤溶解综合征等。

第五节 血管成型术

1. 概念

血管成型术是介入治疗的基本技术之一,具体过程是:将球囊导管的球囊部分送至病变血管(冠状动脉、脑动脉、四肢动脉等)的梗阻处,充盈球囊扩张血管狭窄段后收缩球囊撤出球囊导管。这使得狭窄的血管可以恢复(或接近恢复)它本来的形状,血流重新畅通。血管狭窄或阻塞最主要的原因是动脉粥样硬化,当脂质沉积在动脉血管壁上并逐渐增大时就会使血管内腔不断受到挤占,导致血流逐渐减慢,最终该血管供血的器官会因缺血缺氧而功能受损。血管成型术通过恢复狭窄的血管管腔,使病变血管血流恢复正常或得到改善,阻断器官功能损害的进程。

在众多的血管成型术中,有 70%~90%需要用到支架,目的是为了使扩张后的血管保持通畅,否则狭窄血管弹性回缩或粥样硬化斑块再次增大突出于动脉管腔,都会导致血管再发狭窄。血管内支架通常是用金属丝编织成管状或以金属管激光雕刻而成。将支架在收缩状态下固定于球囊外称之为球扩式支架,球囊扩张后支架就会张开并紧贴在血管壁上,而后收缩球囊将支架留在病变血管区。靠自身弹性张开的支架称之为自膨式支架,以球囊扩张动脉狭窄部位后,将自膨式支架送至该处释放。

同外科手术(搭桥、切开取栓、内膜剥脱等)相比血管成型术创伤小得多,手术时只需在穿刺部位皮肤上留一小孔,术后无需做伤口缝合。且多数情况下,仅在局部麻醉下就可完成手术。患者恢复快,住院时间短,对生活影响小。即以极小的身体损伤代价得到较大的器官功能及生活质量的改善。

2.适应证

(1)冠脉狭窄:冠脉狭窄的患者的胸痛由心肌缺血所致。血管成型术常被用来替代冠状动脉血管移植术以预防心肌梗死或再发梗死。

(2)周围动脉疾病:动脉粥样硬化也是其常见病因,髂动脉是其好发部位。下肢血供不足常会导致其肌肉不能正常工作以及行走时疼痛。严重者只能静坐不能行走,血管成型术/支架放置术可使其恢复行走。这对老年患者尤为重要。

(3)肾动脉狭窄:用血管成型术可以控制由于一侧或双侧肾动脉狭窄导致的肾性高血压。

(4)颈动脉狭窄:对颈动脉狭窄的患者,用血管成型术,可以使颈动脉通畅,保证脑的血氧供应。对于不能行外科手术的患者可考虑行血管成型术。

(5)静脉系统:对于接受血液透析的肾衰竭患者,血管成型术可被用于保证行透析管的通畅。肾衰竭患者通常在手臂的动静脉之间建立一条通道以便利于血浆置换,一般情况下,这条通道保持畅通的时间约为1年。如果在其内放置支架可以使其通畅的时间延长至3~5年;可用于治疗布加综合征患者下腔静脉或肝静脉狭窄;也可用来治疗颅内静脉窦狭窄等。

3.禁忌证

(1)严重肝、肾或心功能不全。

(2)无法纠正的凝血功能障碍,或血小板降低($<50\times10^9/L$)。

(3)无法控制的全身感染或败血症。

(4)严重的碘对比剂过敏。

(5)血管狭窄段较长,或狭窄段有新鲜血栓。

4.术前准备

(1)患者常需禁食禁饮4到8小时(除了抿水吃药)。但在一些医院,直到术前还可允许患者进食少许清液。

(2)术前检查肝功能、肾功能、血常规、凝血功能等,确定其在正常范围内。

(3)行胸片及心电图检查。

(4)术前患者应签手术同意术书,通常医师会当面向患者讲清手术过程及手术风险。

(5)术前患者应排空膀胱,必要时留置导尿管。

(6)根据所用对比剂说明是否做碘过敏试验。

(7)糖尿病患者术前应控制好血糖,手术期间用胰岛素取代二胛双胍。

5.器械

(1)血管造影的X线成像设备、穿刺针、导丝、导管等与经导管血管造影相同。

(2)球囊导管:是一种顶端带有球囊的用于血管成型的细导管,术中将该导管球囊端插至血管病变处,然后将球囊扩张,这样就可以使因动脉粥样硬化斑块所致的动脉狭窄段扩张并恢复到其正常管径,改善相应供血区组织的血氧供应。

(3)支架:某些情况下,在血管病变处放一个金属网状支架以保持血管畅通,放置的过程中支架先是呈压缩状态。支架有多种直径以便据不同的病变血管进行选择。术中,医生常将支架放于导致血管狭窄的动脉粥样斑块处,血管壁的肌肉组织的收缩力就将支架固定于该处,不久,一层新生细胞就会覆盖在支架内壁上,这样支架实际上就变成了血管壁的一部分。在某些情况下,病变动脉的大小和堵塞的部位使支架特别有用。现在,有些血管支架表面还涂有防止血栓形成的药膜,这样有助于使血管长时间保持通畅,延长疗效期。

6. 手术过程

（1）紧张患者可适当给与镇静。

（2）手术穿刺点及附近区域进行消毒。

（3）以消毒区为中心铺无菌巾、无菌单。

（4）对穿刺点进行局部麻醉。

（5）穿刺入路血管（最常用部位为桡动脉、股动脉、股静脉）。

（6）通过穿刺针向血管内引入导引导丝，而后固定导丝退出穿刺针，再沿导引导丝送入导管至靶血管。

（7）经导管向血管内注入对比剂，同时进行一系列的 X 线图象采集，很细小的血管都可在图像上观察到［图 28-4（a）］。

（8）在透视的导引下，将导引导管超选送至目标血管，而后经导引导管插入球囊导管至目标血管的病变段，当球囊到位后将球囊扩张约 30 秒钟而后收缩球囊，有时要这样反复扩张多次（可能的情况下尽量减少扩张次数）。

（9）退出球囊导管，再经导引导管造影以判定血管再通情况［图 28-4（b）］。

（10）拔出导管，对穿刺点进行压迫止血，而后用无菌绷带进行包扎，有时包扎完后还会在穿刺点处放置一个沙袋，以防再发出血，特别是在腹股沟处常用。整个手术过程通常要花 1~2 小时。术后患者卧床 6~8 小时（桡动脉入路可直接下床活动）。

（11）支架放置后，患者需要坚持服用阿司匹林、氢氯吡格雷（波立维）等抗血小板聚集药物一段时间，根据支架不同所需时间从几周至几年不等，静脉内支架需服用抗凝药物。目前绝大多数血管内支架是磁共振兼容的，对于不熟悉的支架注意参考产品说明书。

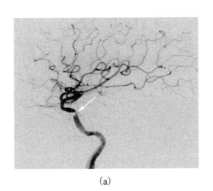 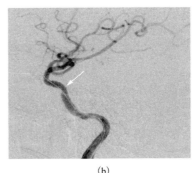

(a)　　　　　　　　　　　　　　(b)

（a）左侧颈内动脉海绵窦段重度狭窄（箭头）；（b）PTA 治疗后狭窄明显改善（箭头）。

图 28-4　左侧颈内动脉海绵窦段重度狭窄 PTA 治疗

7. 并发症

（1）血管阻塞的复发：单行血管成形术后有 1/5~1/3 的患者在术后数天或数周内出现再狭窄。当然，此时仍可考虑球囊血管成形术。对于使用支架的患者，发生再狭窄的概率要低得多，目前的药物洗脱支架进一步降低了再狭窄的发生率。

（2）冠脉成型术后最严重的并发症和外科手术类似，有 1%~3% 的患者术后短期内甚至突然死亡，有 3%~5% 的患者术后出现心肌梗死，约有不超过 3% 患者由于术中血管壁受损伤需急诊行冠状动脉血管傍路移置术。肾动脉和髂动脉血管成形术以及做透析移植手术的患者死亡风险和需要紧急手术的风险大大降低。

（3）过敏反应：由于术中要行血管造影，要用到对比剂及局麻药，所以患者有可能产生过敏反应。特别是有肾脏疾病、糖尿病、哮喘以及既往有对比剂过敏史的患者。

（4）出血：大出血常需要上止血药甚至输血。

(5)冠脉成型术有时可导致心率失常。

(6)脑梗塞:这是由于血管成形术或支架放置术时可能形成血栓阻塞脑血管使脑组织缺血缺氧导致脑梗死。

(7)疼痛:血管成形术或支架放置术后的患者可能感到病变血管附近区域疼痛,比如,冠脉成形术后可感到胸部疼痛、肾血管成形术后可感到背痛、髂动脉成型术后可感到臀部疼痛。

(8)肾功能损害:由于行栓塞术前需行血管造影,所以对比剂可能损伤肾功能或使原有的肾脏疾病加重。

第六节 血栓溶解术

1.概念

多种病因会引起人体血管系统内出现血凝块,即血栓。常见的原因有:①心房纤颤引发心房血栓形成并脱落,栓塞至脑血、肾、肠系膜、下肢等器官的供养动脉;②外伤导致血管内膜损伤诱发急性血栓形成;③动脉粥样硬化狭窄处由于血流缓慢导致急性血栓形成;④由于长时间活动受限、感染、凝血功能异常等导致静脉血栓形成;⑤上述情况下由于血流阻断导致血栓不断增长蔓延。血栓能减缓甚至阻断器官或组织的血流导致器官组织缺乏氧气及营养供应或者阻碍组织液循环。一旦血凝块在血管内形成,就可逐渐增大最后导致血管阻塞,完全切断相应区域的血液循环。四肢血管内血栓形成初期患者可无自觉症状,但不久就会出现肢体疼痛、麻木、温度降低、刺痛、发胀等不适,最后,可损伤组织甚至使其坏死,导致器官功能减退或衰竭如心肌梗塞、脑梗塞等,进而威胁到患者生命。影像引导下血栓溶解术可以用于治疗众多原因导致的动静脉血栓。

血栓溶解术是一种将溶栓药物经过导管注射至血栓局部,通过直接接触将其溶解的治疗方法,是一种安全、高效的治疗血栓重建血液循环的方法。它较传统的外科手术创伤要小的多,尤其是那些位置较深的血管,避免了巨大的创伤性手术。而且出血少、住院时间短、无明显的手术瘢痕。

2.适应证

各部位的动静脉血栓。

3.禁忌证

(1)严重肝、肾或心功能不全。

(2)无法纠正的凝血功能障碍,或血小板降低($<50×10^9/L$)。

(3)无法控制的全身感染或败血症。

(4)严重的碘对比剂过敏。

(5)溶栓治疗禁忌。

4.术前准备

(1)患者常需禁食禁饮4~8小时(除了抿水吃药)。但在一些医院,直到术前还可允许患者进食少许清液。

(2)术前检查肝功能、肾功能、血常规、凝血功能等,确定其在正常范围内。

(3)行胸片及心电图检查。

(4)术前患者应签手术同意术书,通常医生会当面向患者讲清手术过程及手术风险。

(5)排空膀胱,必要时留置导尿管。

(6)根据所用对比剂说明是否做碘过敏试验。

(7)糖尿病患者术前应控制好血糖,手术期间用胰岛素取代二胛双胍。

5.器械

(1)X线成像设备及造影导管、穿刺针、导引导丝和血管造影所用的基本相同。

（2）溶栓剂如尿激酶、链激酶、组织型纤溶酶原激活剂。

（3）破碎血栓的机械装置。

6. 手术过程

（1）术前，患者平卧于检查床上，身上将接上心电监护仪以便术中监测心律、心率、血压、血氧饱和度等。

（2）通过静脉注射镇静药，使患者放松。

（3）选择穿刺点（可选择手臂、颈部，但常选择腹股沟区）并对穿刺点及其附近区域皮肤进行消毒。

（4）以消毒区为中心铺无菌巾、无菌单。

（5）对穿刺点进行局部麻醉。

（6）将较细的穿刺针经穿刺点的小切口插入股动脉。

（7）通过穿刺针向血管内引入导引导丝，而后固定导丝退出穿刺针，再沿导引导丝送入导引导管在透视引导下将导管插至病变区靶血管内。

（8）经导管向血管内注入对比剂，同时进行一系列的X线图象采集，以确定血栓所在的部位［图28-5（a）、（b）］。医生会重复观察所采集到的图象去确定是选择经导管注射溶栓药物溶栓还是选择机械取栓，或两者兼而有之。

（9）如果选择药物溶栓，导管将被留在原处，导管尾部将连接到可以控制溶栓药输注速度的机器上，这样溶栓药就可通过导管不断地输注到血栓处，通常要用24~48小时，有时甚至需要更长的时间才可将血栓彻底溶解。其间，介入科医生会间断地通过造影观察血管再通情况［图28-5（c）、（d）］。

（10）术毕，医生将拔出导管，对穿刺点进行压迫止血，一般要15~20分钟才能止住出血，而后用无菌绷带进行包扎穿刺点。

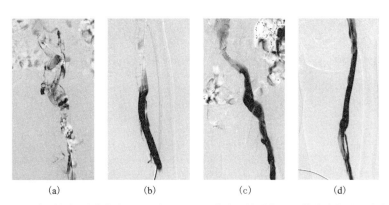

(a)左髂总静脉、髂外静脉血栓形成；(b)左股静脉血栓形成；(c)持续溶栓后左髂总静脉、髂外静脉血栓溶解；(d)持续溶栓后左股静脉血栓溶解。

图28-5　左侧髂总静脉、髂外静脉、股静脉血栓溶栓治疗

7. 并发症

（1）疼痛：疼痛很常见，通常可通过口服或静脉输注止痛药控制。大部分患者可在1-2周内恢复正常的活动。

（2）感染：即使用了抗生素，溶栓后每个患者也还会有感染的风险。

（3）出血：抗凝、抗血小板聚集及溶栓药物均有导致身体的任何部位出血的风险。

（4）过敏反应：由于术中要行血管造影，要用到造影剂，所以患者有可能产生过敏反应。

（5）肾功能损害：由于行栓塞术前需行血管造影，所以对比剂可能损伤肾功能或使原有的肾脏疾病加重。

第七节　经颈静脉肝内门体分流术

1.概念

经颈静脉肝内门体分流术（TIPS）是指在影像引导下，经颈静脉入路从肝静脉穿刺肝内门静脉，在肝静脉与门静脉之间建立门体分流道，以达到降低门静脉高压的介入治疗技术。该技术建立的门体分流道既可有效分流门静脉血流，又能保留部分入肝血流维持生理需要。TIPS 技术最初由 Rosch 等人设想并于 20 世纪 60 年代在动物实验中实施。目前该技术已成为替代外科门体分流术治疗症状性门静脉高压症的有效方法。

2.适应证

（1）无法控制的静脉曲张出血。

（2）接受过内镜治疗的静脉曲张再出血。

（3）顽固性腹水。

（4）门脉高压性胃病。

（5）肝性胸水。

（6）布-加综合征。

（7）肝肾综合征。

（8）门静脉血栓形成。

3.禁忌证

（1）右心或左心压力升高。

（2）心力衰竭或重度心瓣膜功能不全。

（3）快速进展的肝衰竭。

（4）严重或无法控制的肝性脑病。

（5）无法控制的全身感染或败血症。

（6）无法缓解的胆道梗阻。

（7）多囊肝

（8）肝脏弥漫性恶性肿瘤

（9）重度且无法纠正的凝血功能障碍

4.器械

（1）常规穿刺针，5F 血管鞘，5F 导管，150 cm 长、0.035 英寸亲水导丝，260 cm 长、0.035" 硬导丝。

（2）TIPS 套件（如 RUPS-100 TIPS 套件）。

（3）球囊（8 或 10 mm 直径）。

（4）自膨式支架（8 或 10 mm 直径）。

5.患者准备

（1）患者评估。

（2）签署知情同意书。

（3）实验室检查，包括血常规、心功能、肝功能和凝血功能等。

（4）CT 或 MR 检查，用于评估操作技术可行性、是否需要采用改良或拓展 TIPS 技术等。

（5）明确可能的严重全身并发症。

（6）留置导尿管。

（7）根据所用对比剂说明是否做碘过敏试验。

（8）糖尿病患者术前应控制好血糖，手术期间用胰岛素取代二胍双胍。

6.操作步骤

（1）经皮穿刺右侧颈内静脉建立血管入路。

（2）插管至肝静脉，进行肝静脉造影［图28-6(a)］。

（3）引入TIPS穿刺针，从选定的肝静脉穿过肝实质进入门静脉肝内分支［图28-6(b)］。

（4）通过穿刺道，直接测量下腔静脉和门静脉压力。

（5）采用球囊扩张肝静脉-门静脉之间穿刺道。

（6）植入覆膜支架或金属支架，建立门体分流道，以维持分流道通畅［图28-6(c)、(d)］。

（7）测量分流后门静脉和肝静脉之间压力梯度，并造影证实门体分流道建立成功。

（8）必要时栓塞曲张的静脉［图28-6(c)、(d)］。

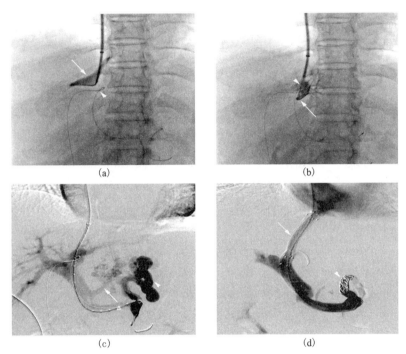

（a）肝右静脉造影显示肝右静脉（箭）通畅。注意预先置入门静脉用于穿刺定位的细导丝（箭头）；（b）采用TIPS穿刺针由肝右静脉（箭头）穿刺进入门静脉左支（箭）；（c）置入导管于脾静脉行门静脉造影显示胃左静脉（箭）和胃短静脉曲张（箭头）；（d）支架植入后门静脉造影显示门体分流道通畅（箭），注意弹簧圈栓塞后的曲张静脉（箭头）。

图28-6　肝硬化门静脉高压食管胃底静脉曲张出血患者的TIPS治疗

7.栓塞后综合征与并发症

（1）操作相关并发症与颈静脉穿刺、楔形肝静脉造影、分流道穿刺和支架植入等操作有关。主要并发症包括腹腔出血、肝动脉损伤、胆汁性腹膜炎、胆道出血、死亡等。TIPS操作并发症的发生率明显低于外科分流术，并且随着操作者经验的增加其并发症可进一步降低。

（2）TIPS术后并发症包括心功能失代偿、肝功能衰竭加速、肝性脑病恶化。心功能失代偿是由于分流后静脉回流增加和右心充盈压升高的共同作用结果；肝功能衰竭和肝性脑病则与门体分流量过大有关。

（梁斌，张利捷，黄炜，王耀恒，熊付，郭栋，肖恩华，张子曙）

Chapter 28

Vascular interventional radiology

According to the area of interventions, IR can be divided into vascular and nonvascular interventional radiology. The basic vascular interventional techniques include diagnostic arteriography, transcatheter arterial embolization, chemoembolization, percutaneous transluminal angioplasty and transcatheter intravascular infusion.

Section 1 Seldinger technique

In 1953, Sven-IvarSeldinger first described percutaneous arterial catheterization using a needle, guidewire, and catheter. This technique, known as Seldinger technique, consists of puncturing an artery using a needle, introducing a guidewire through it, and then using the guidewire to advance an introducer sheath and catheter through the artery. The traditional Seldinger,s technique is used to puncture the anterior and posterior wall of the blood vessel, while the improved Seldinger,s technique only punctures the anterior wall of the blood vessel (Figure 28-1). Seldinger technique eliminates the need for surgical exposure of a blood vessel before catheterization, allowing the transfer of angiography from the operating room to the radiology department. Seldinger technique opens up a totally new medical field and has become the basis of all vascular and many nonvascular interventional procedures.

Section 2 Transcatheter angiography

1. Definition

Transcatheter arteriography is defined as a procedure involving percutaneous passage of a needle and/or catheter into an artery under imaging guidance, followed by injection of contrast media and imaging of the vascular distribution in question. Nowadays transcatheter angiography has been replaced partly by noninvasive imaging techniques such as computed CT angiography and MR angiography. However, transcatheter angiography is still widely used in patients who plan for surgery, angioplasty, or stent placement. Transcatheter angiography provides very clear, accurate and detailed images of the target vessels in real time. The detail displayed by transcatheter angiography can not be available by any other noninvasive imaging modalities. This is especially helpful to diagnose and treat disease, and thus transcatheter angiography remains the gold standard for diagnosing vascular diseases.

By selecting the arteries through which the catheter passes, it is possible to assess vessels in several specific body sites. Unlike CT or MR angiography, the use of a catheter makes it possible to combine diagnosis and treatment in a single procedure.

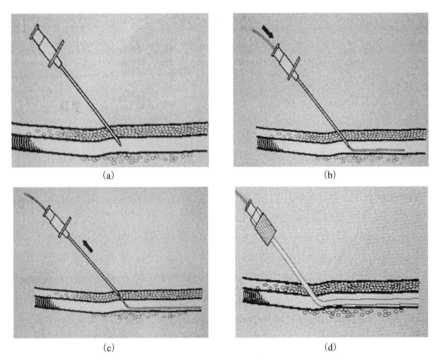

(a) Puncture the artery with a needle; (b) Introduce a guidewire through the needle; (c) Withdraw the needle and leaving the guidewire in place; (d) Using the guidewire to advance an introducer sheath through the artery.

Figure 28-1　The improved Seldinger technique

2. Indications

(2) To diagnose the extent and severity of the blockage or narrowing in a blood vessel that may interfere with the normal flow of blood, including internal carotid artery stenosis.

(2) Aneurysms-an area of a blood vessel that bulges or balloons out, such as abdominal aortic aneurysm.

(3) Cerebral vascular disease, including stroke or bleeding in the brain.

(4) Blood vessel malformations such as arteriovenous fistulas.

(5) Identify a source of bleeding such as a stomach ulcer or tumor.

(6) Identify the nature of a tumor.

(7) Bleeding which could not be detected by other examinations.

3. Contraindications

(1) Severe cardiac, renal, or hepatic dysfunction.

(2) Uncorrectable coagulation dysfunction, or decreased platelets ($<50\times10^9/L$).

(3) Uncontrollable system infection or sepsis.

(4) Severe iodinated contrast allergy.

4. Equipment

(1) Conventional puncture needle, vascular introducer sheath, guidewire.

(2) Catheter: a variety of models and diameters (such as 1. 5F, 1. 8F, 2F, 3F, 4F, 5F, 6F, etc.). Choose the appropriate catheter according to the course and diameter of the target vessel.

(3) Non-ionic iodine contrast agent is commonly used.

5. Patient preparation

(1) Fast within 2 hours or limited to clear liquids within 4 to 8 hours.

（2）Laboratory testing, focusing primarily on hepatic and renal function, hematologic and coagulation parameters, chest radiograph and electrocardiogram.

（3）Establish venous access and place a needle or central venous tube.

（4）Empty the bladder. Indwelling catheter if necessary.

（5）Do iodine allergy test according to the contrast medium used.

（6）Obtain the informed consent.

6. Procedure steps

（1）After entering the interventional operating room, the patient lies on the examination table. Connect vital signs monitoring equipment and inhale oxygen if necessary.

（2）Select the puncture site (mostly the right femoral artery) as needed.

（3）Perform local anesthesia at the puncture point (1% ~ 2% lidocaine is commonly used). The Seldinger technique is used and place the catheter sheath, then catheter is introduced into the target blood vessel.

（4）Inject the contrast into the vessel through the catheter by a high-pressure syringe, and simultaneously perform a series of X-ray image acquisition and processing. Multi-angle imaging or three-dimensional reconstruction can be performed as needed until the diagnostic requirements are met.

（5）After the operation, the patient needs to apply local compression bandaging at the puncture point, and immobilize the limb on the puncture side for 6 to 8 hours.

7. Complications

（1）Allergic Reaction: including a skin reaction, urticaria, severe cases may have blood pressure drop, breathing difficulties and even coma.

（2）Blood Clot: There is a small risk that blood will form a clot around the tip of the catheter, blocking the artery and making it necessary to operate to reopen the vessel. When the guide wire cannot achieve the target vessel after repeated operation in the catheter, it is recommended to withdraw the guide wire, connect the syringe to vigorously draw the blood back, and then inject heparin saline. Then reinsert the guide wire for operation or switch to another shape catheter.

（3）Kidney Injured: The kidneys may be injured when contrast material is eliminated through the urine. If kidney disease is already present, it may become worse. So precautions are taken to reduce this risk. For those who use a large amount of contrast agent during surgery, Post-hydration and diuresis are recommended.

（4）Bleeding: Rarely the catheter dissects the artery, causing internal bleeding.

（5）Pseudoaneurysm formation at the puncture site.

（6）Infection. For those who have potential infections at the operation site and are difficult to avoid, antibiotics can be used preventively.

Section 3 Transcatheter arterial embolization

1. Definition

Transcatheter arterial embolization (TAE) is defined as the intravascular deposition of a device or agent to produce intentional vessel occlusion. The procedure has been widely applied in virtually every vascular territory to arrest hemorrhage, occlude congenital and acquired vascular abnormalities, palliate neoplasms, and infarct tissue. The intravascular occlusion may be performed at any level from capillary beds to large arteries, and it may be temporary or permanent in nature, and curative or palliative in purpose. Based on the indication, partial or complete embolization of the vascular territory may be required, resulting in variable degrees of reduction or cessation of arterial flow of a focal lesion or an entire target organ. Finally, the embolization may be undertaken as an independent procedure or a component of an intervention for regional chemotherapeutic agent, radiation, or other targeted therapy.

2. Indications

(1) Hemorrhage: TAE can be used to treat acute or recurrent hemorrhage, including hemoptysis, gastrointestinal bleeding, posttraumatic and iatrogenic hemorrhage, postpartum hemorrhage, and hemorrhage neoplasms. The embolization achieves hemostasis by directly blocking the blooding artery with embolic materials. It also includes the placement of a covered stent to occlude flow in a pathologic segment of vessel or to slow flow in a branch that is feeding a site of hemorrhage or fistula.

(2) Tumor: TAE can be performed to devascularize benign or malignant tumors for palliation (eg, control tumor growth, relieve pain, or prevent hemorrhage) or to reduce operative blood loss. Common applications include primary and metastatic liver cancers, hepatic hemangioma, renal angiomyolipoma, renal cell carcinoma, nasopharyngeal angiofibroma, uterine fibroids, pelive and other vascular malignancies.

(3) Vascular disorders: TAE can be undertaken to occlude congenital of acquired aneurysm, pseudoaneurysm, vascular malformation, or other vascular abnormalities that have potential to cause adverse health effects.

(4) Devascularization of nonneoplastic tissue: TAE can be used to devascularize nonneoplastic tissue that produces adverse health effects to the body, including hypersplenism, refractory renovascular hypertension, proteinuria in endstage kidney, varicocele, pelvic congestion syndrome, priapism, and ectopic pregnancy.

(5) Flow redistribution: TAE can be performed to redistribute blood flow to protect normal tissue (eg, gastroduodenal artery and right gastric artery embolization in hepatic artery embolization and radioembolization) or to facilitate subsequent other treatments (eg, right portal vein embolization to induce left lobe hypertrophy prior to surgical resection).

(6) Type II endoleaks: The embolization, including direct sac puncture or collateral vessel embolization, can be used to manage type II endoleaks.

3. Contraindications

(1) Severe hepatic, renal, or cardiac dysfunction.

(2) Uncorrectable coagulation dysfunction, or decreased platelets ($< 50 \times 10^9/L$, except partial splenic embolism).

(3) Uncontrollable system infection or sepsis

(4) Severe iodinated contrast allergy

4. Equipment

(1) Conventional puncture needle, vascular introducer sheath, catheter, guidewire, microcatheter system

(2) A large number of embolic agents, with varying physical roperties, methods of delivery, and permanence, are available for TAE treatment. Selection of an embolic agent depends on the clinical factors and the technical aspects of the procedure. The commonly used embolic agents are as follows.

1) Gelfoam (gelatin sponge) was one of the earliest and the most commonly used embolics. This substance is compressible and absorbed over a period of 4~6 weeks. Gelfoam is supplied in small sterile bricks, particles (150 ~2000 μm) or powder (approximately 50 μm). Gelfoam pieces and particles are useful when temporary occlusion is desired. They can be suspended in contrast before injection to aid in fluoroscopic visualization, compressed to fit through a catheter, and then injected into the vessel of interest where it will expand to a large size than when dry. Gelfoam powder frequently leads to permanent occlusion owing to its small size.

2) Polyvinyl alcohol (PVA) is an inexpensive, inert, and permanent embolic agent. The particles are injected

through a catheter and carried to the site of embolization by the arterial flow. PVA is usually supplied as irregular shaped particles, which are more likely to clump and occlude proximally. The size of PVA is critical to prevent blockage of the delivery catheter and to achieve the desired embolization. The particles are delivered by gentle injection during fluoroscopy to prevent reflux into nontarget vessel.

3) Embolic microspheres are uniformly shaped, flow-directed, solid embolic agents. They can be compressed in diameter when injected with catheter. These characteristics of microspheres allows less clumping and more effective embolization than with irregular PVA particles. Some of microspheres have the added capability of controlled delivery of therapeutic agents in addition to block flow.

4) Embolization coils are commercially available in a variety of sizes, lengths, shapes, and materials (usually stainess steel or platinum). Coils occlude vessels by physically obstructing the lumen. Fibers may be attached to the coil to promote platelet aggregation and thrombosis. Coils can be positioned very precisely into a target vessel. Pushable coils can be advanced through a catheter with a guidewire or injected using 1~3 ml syringers. Detachable coils remain conneted to the pusher wire until an electric current is employed to break a bond or until a mechanical technique is used to release the coil.

5) Liquid embolic materials include ethanol, sclerosants, glues and ploymers. The fisrt two permanently destroy the vascular endothelium. When injected into the artery, they can pass the capillary level and achieve distal embolization. Glues and ploymers are very useful flow-directed agents, which can be injected through a small catheter and then solidify to occlude a larger space. This is of particular value in treatment of arteriovenous malformations and varicose veins.

5. Patient preparation

(1) Evaluation of the patient.

(2) Laboratory testing, focusing primarily on renal function, coagulation and hematologic parameters.

(3) Chest radiograph and electrocardiogram examination.

(4) CT or MR imaging, particularly for embolization of tumors.

(5) Antibiotic prophylaxis for splenic artery embolization or especially long cases with multiple catheter exchanges.

(6) Empty the bladder and indwelling catheter if necessary.

(7) Do iodine allergy test according to the contrast medium used.

(8) Obtain the informed consent

6. Procedure steps

(1) Approach through the right common femoral artery and insert a 5F arterial introducer sheath.

(2) Perform arteriography to clarify the nature, location, scope and extent of the disorder [Figure 28-2(a)].

(3) Selective catheterize the target artery with a optimal catheter and/or a coaxial microcatheter.

(4) Select the appropriate embolic agent depending on the nature of the disorder, the purpose of embolization and the condition of the target vessel.

(5) Under the fluoroscopy guidance, accurately deliver the embolic agent through the catheter or microcatheter, control the extent and degree of embolization, and avoid reflux and mis-embolization.

(6) Repeat the arteriography to ensure the efficacy of embolization [Figure 28-2(b)].

(7) Remove the catheter and introducer sheath, and manually compress of the puncture site to achieve hemostasis.

7. Postembolization syndrome and complications

(1) Postembolization syndrome comprises a constellation of symtoms including pain, fever, nausea, vomiting,

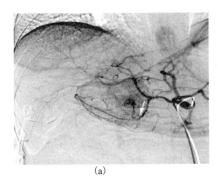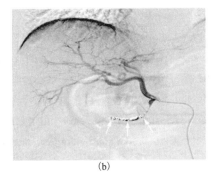

(a)

(b)

（a）Celiac arteriogram shows extravasation of contrast material from the gastroduodenal artery（arrow）；（b）Selective
gastroduodenal arteriogram after embolization shows occlusion of the gastroduodenal artery proximal and distal to the
bleeding site. Note details of the microcoils in place（arrow）.

Figure 28-2 TAE for bleeding after necrosectomy for a patient with necrotizing pancreatitis

and leukocytosis due to ischemia of infarction of the embolized organ or lesion. The postembolization syndrome by
itself should not be considered a complication, but rather an expected outcome of embolization. These symtoms
usually resolved after nominal treatment.

（2）The general complications related to TAE include infection, target ischemia, nontarget embolization,
hemorrhage, spinal infarction, procedure-related mortality. The complication rates are dependent on the clinical
condition of patient, operator experience, vascular territory, the specific disorder addressed, and perioperative
management.

Section 4 Transcatheter arterial chemoembolization

1. Definition

Tanscatheter arterial chemoembolization（TACE）may be performed by using conventional or drug-eluting
embolic approaches. Conventional TACE is defined as the infusion of single or multiple chemotherapeutic agents
with or without ethiodized oil, followed by embolization with particles such as gelatin sponge, polyvinyl alcohol, or
calibrated microspheres. Drug-eluting embolic TACE is defined as the administration of microspheres onto which
chemotherapeutic medication is loaded or adsorbed with the intention of sustained in vivo drug release.

TACE is a well recognized mainstay therapy for unresectable primary and metastatic liver cancer and has
gained wide acceptance over the past 40 years. The rationale for chemoembolization stems from the observation that
normal liver tissue receives most of its blood supply（75%）from the portal vein, whereas hepatic malignant lesions
receive most（90%~100%）of their blood supply from the hepatic artery. It is therefore logical to use the hepatic
artery as an approach to target the tumor while preserving the normal liver. The intraarterial infusion of cytotoxic
agents followed by embolization of the tumor-feeding arteries will induce a strong cytotoxic and ischemic effect,
therefore achieving substantial tumor necrosis. TACE has also been applied to treating several extrahepatic
malignant solid tumors.

2. Indications

（1）Hepatocellular carcinoma：TACE is the most widely used primary treatment for unresectable hepatocellular
carcinoma, and is the recommended first-line therapy for patients with intermediate-stage disease according to the
Barcelona classification.

（2）Intrahepatic cholangiocarcinoma：Intrahepatic cholangiocarcinoma is the second most common primary hepatic malignancy. Patients with unresectable, metastatic, or postsurgical residual local intrahepatic cholangiocarcinoma may benefit from TACE treatment.

(3)Liver metastases: Colon, neuroendocrine, breast, ovarian, sarcomas, uveal melanoma and other hepatic metastases can all be treated with TACE when conventional treatments have failed.

(4)Other malignant solid tumors: TACE has been proven as a palliative treatment for several extrahepatic malignant solid tumors resistant to conventional therapies, such as lung cancer, osteocarcinoma, soft tissue sarcoma, spinal malignancies, renal malignancies, pelvic malignancies, and retroperitoneal malignancies, etc.

3. Contraindications

(1)Severe liver dysfunction (Child~Pugh C).

(2)Complete occlusion of main portal vein.

(3)Tumor burden involving more than 70% of the liver.

(4)Poor performance status (performance status >2).

(5)Uncorrectable coagulation dysfuntion, or decreased platelets ($<50×10^9$/L).

(6)Uncontrollable system infection or sepsis.

(7)Severe renal or cardiac dysfunction.

4. Equipment

(1)Conventional puncture needle, 5-French vascular introducer sheath, 5-French catheter, 0.035 inch guidewire, 2- to 3-French microcatheter system

(2)Chemotherapeutic agents (eg, doxorubicin, cisplatin, 5-fluorouracil, mitomycin, and irinotecan)

(3)Ethiodized oil (eg, Lipiodol)

(4)Embolic agents (eg, gelatin sponge, polyvinyl alcohol, calibrated microspheres, or drug-eluting microspheres)

5. Patient preparation

(1)Evaluation of the patient.

(2)Laboratory testing, focusing primarily on hepatic function, renal function, coagulation and hematologic parameters.

(3)Contrast-enhanced CT or MR imaging of the liver, and additional imaging examinations for assessment of possible extrahepatic spread [Figure 28-3(a), (d)].

(4)Fast for 4-6 hours before procedure.

(5)Antiemetic prophylaxis and antibiotic prophylaxis.

(6)Empty the bladder and indwelling catheter if necessary.

(7)Do iodine allergy test according to the contrast medium used.

(8)Obtain the informed consent.

6. Procedure steps

(1)Approach through the right common femoral artery and insert a 5F arterial introducer sheath.

(2)Introduce a 5F catheter over the guidewire and catheterize the celiac trunk and superior mesenteric artery. Perform selective arteriography to assess the vascular anatomy of the liver, patency of the portal vein, and to detect potential hypervascular lesions [Figure 28-3(b)]. If possible, the inferior phrenic artery, the internal thoracic artery and the intercostal artey should be interrogated to exclude malignant parasitization of blood flow.

(3)Coaxially Introduce a microcatheter through the 5F catheter and superselectively catheterize the branches that supply the tumors.

(4)Infuse single or multiple chemotherapeutic agents with or without ethiodized oil, followed by embolization with embolic particles. When drug-eluting embolic chemoembolization is performed, the microspheres loaded with drug is injected, with or without additional embolization with bland embolic microspheres. The embolization endpoint is complete occlusion or near stasis of the artery directly feeding the tumor.

(5) Perform arteriography to confirm the absence of arterial supply to the tumors [Figure 28-3(c)].

(6) Remove the catheter and introducer sheath, and manually compress of the puncture site to achieve hemostasis.

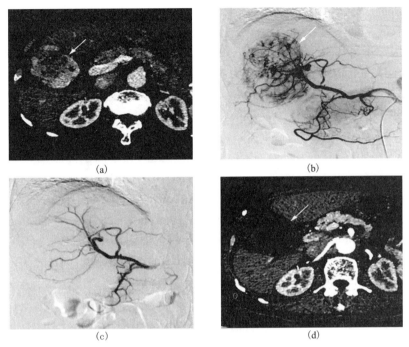

(a) (b)

(c) (d)

(a) This is consistent with hepatocellular carcinoma; (b) Common hepatic arteriogram before chemoembolization confirms the hypervascular tumor (arrow) in the liver; (c) Post-embolization arteriogram shows the absence of arterial supply to the tumor; (d) Contrast-enhanced CT 1 month after chemoembolization shows no enhancement of the tumor (arrow) during the arterial phase, which is suggestive of complete response.

Figure 28-3 TACE for a patient with hepatocellular carcinomas. Contrast-enhanced CT image shows an enhanced mass (arrow) in the liver on arterial phase, with classic washout on portal phase (image not shown)

7. Postembolization syndrome and complications

(1) TACE-induced postembolization syndrome (fever, pain, nausea, and leukocytosis) by itself should not be considered a complication, but rather an expected outcome of embolization. These symptoms are usually self-limited, and more common in cases in whom large tumors are treated.

(2) The complications associated with TACE include liver abscess, biloma, ischemic cholecystitis, gastrointestinal ulceration/hemorrhage, hematologic suppression, pulmonary or cerebral embolization, liver failure, acute renal failure, tumor lysis syndrome, etc.

Section 5 Percutaneoustransluminal angioplasty

1. Definition

Angioplasty is one of the basic techniques of interventional therapy. The specific process is: the balloon part of the balloon catheter is delivered to the obstruction of the diseased vessels (coronary artery, cerebral artery, extremity artery, etc.), and then the balloon is filled to expand the stenosis segment, and then the balloon catheter is withdrawn after contraction. This makes the narrowed vessel recover (or nearly recover) its original shape and blood flowing. The main cause of vascular stenosis or obstruction is atherosclerosis. When lipid deposits on the arterial wall and increases gradually, the vascular lumen will be continuously occupied, resulting in blood flow gradually slowing down. Finally, the organs supplied by the blood vessels will be damaged by ischemia and hypoxia. Angioplasty can make the blood flow of diseased blood vessel return to normal or improve, and block the process of organ function damage.

In many angioplasty procedures, about 70% ~ 90% of the stents are needed to keep the dilated vessels unobstructed. Otherwise, the elastic retraction of thestenosed vessels or the enlargement of atherosclerotic plaques protruding from the arterial lumen will lead to vascular restenosis. Endovascular stents are usually woven with metal wires or carved by laser. When the stent is fixed outside the balloon in the contraction state, it is called balloon-expandable stent. After balloon expansion, the stent will open and cling to the vascular wall, and then shrink the balloon to leave the stent in the diseased vascular area. The stent that expands on its own elasticity is called a self-expanding stent. After the stenosis of the artery is expanded with a balloon, the self-expanding stent will be delivered to the site for release.

Compared with surgery (bypass, embolectomy, endarterectomy, etc.), angioplasty is much less invasive. It only needs to leave a small hole in the skin at the puncture site during the operation, and there is no need to suture the wound after operation. In most cases, the operation can be completed only under local anesthesia. The patients recover quickly and the hospitalization time is short, so it has little effect on life. That is to say, it can improve organ function and quality of life at the cost of minimal physical injury.

2. Indication

(1) The narrowed coronary artery: The patients whose coronary artery is narrowed or blocked can often feel chest pain upon physical effort because part of the heart wall is not getting enough blood. Angioplasty often is used as an alternative to coronary artery bypass surgery, a very major undertaking. It may be done in hope of preventing a heart attack, or afterwards with the goal of preventing another attack.

(2) Peripheral arterial disease: It is often caused by arteriosclerosis too. The most common site of angioplasty in these patients is the iliac arteries of the pelvis. Insufficient blood can keep the leg muscles from working properly and make it very painful to walk. The affected may in time become chair-bound, but angioplasty/stenting can restore their ability to walk. This is especially important for older patients.

(3) The narrowed kidney artery: To control the blood pressure in patients with renal hypertension when disease has narrowed one or both arteries supplying blood to the kidneys.

(4) The narrowed carotid artery: To maintain vital blood flow to the brain by keeping open the carotid artery, the major route of blood and oxygen to the brain. Angioplasty is most helpful to patients who are not good candidates for surgery.

(5) Venous system: angioplasty is also used to ensure the patency of dialysis tubing in patients with renal failure undergoing hemodialysis. Patients with renal failure usually establish a channel between the artery and vein of the arm to facilitate plasma exchange. Generally, this channel remains unobstructed for about 1 year. If stents are placed in it, the patency time can be extended to 3 to 5 years; It can be used to treat the stenosis of inferior vena cava or hepatic vein in patients with Budd-Chiari syndrome; it also can be used to treat intracranial sinus stenosis, etc.

3. Contraindication

(1) Severe hepatic, renal, or cardiac dysfunction.

(2)Uncorrectable coagulation dysfunction, or decreased platelets ($<50\times10^9$/L).

(3)Uncontrollable system infection or sepsis.

(4)Allergy to iodinated contrast.

(5)Very long narrow vessels, or narrow vessels with fresh thrombus.

4. The Preparation for the procedure

(1)The patient may be asked not to eat or drink anything (except sip of water to take pills) for four to eight hours ahead of time. Some hospitals, however, allow clear fluids until shortly before the examination.

(2)Checking liver function, kidney function, blood routine and blood clotting factors are within normal limits.

(3)Checking a chest x-ray and electrocardiogram (ECG).

(4)Before the procedure the patient will have to give his or her consent. This usually involves a face-to-face talk with a physician.

(5)Do iodine allergy test according to the contrast medium used.

(6)The patient has to empty his or her bladder and indwelling catheter if necessary.

(7)If the patient has diabetes, it may be necessary to alter his or her insulin dose on the day of angioplasty. Insulin was used to replace biguanidine during the operation.

5. Equipment

(1)The x-ray equipment, needle, guidewire and catheters of angiography are the same as those used for catheter angiography.

(2)A balloon catheter, a small, thin angioplasty catheter with a balloon at its tip. The catheter is guided into the diseased segment of artery, then the inflatable balloon of the catheter passed to the target vessel and inflated. When plaque is narrowing the artery and limiting the amount of blood that can get through, the inflated balloon will press it against the side of the artery and stretch the artery wall. The result is that the vessel is restored to its initial size and thus allows more blood and oxygen to pass to the body tissues it normally supplies.

(3)Stent: In some cases, a stent is placed in the site of the diseased artery to keep an artery open. A wire mesh stent that is collapsed when passed into the artery. Stents come in varying sizes so that in each case it matches the size of the diseased artery. The radiologist may place a stent that is expanded at the site of plaque. The muscle tissue in the vessel wall holds the stent in place. In time, a layer of cells forms over the stent, which in effect becomes a part of the vessel. In some cases the size of the diseased artery and the site of blockage make a stent especially useful. Some modern stents are covered with a drug preventing its surface from blood clot that helps keep the artery open; they seem to improve the long-term success rate.

6. The procedure

(1)Aa sedative is injected through an intravenous line to relax the patient.

(2)The catheter site (groin or arm) will be cleaned with antiseptic soap.

(3)Sterile towels and a sheet will be placed around this area.

(4)Then a local anesthetic is injected into the skin where the catheter is to be inserted, usually in the groin.

(5)A thin needle is introduced through a very small incision into the femoral artery, a large groin vessel.

(6)A thin guidewire is placed through the needle and the needle is exchanged over the guidewire for a catheter that is advanced up into the blocked artery.

(7)Contrast material then is injected through the catheter and a series of x-rays are taken where even tiny thread-like vessels can be seen[Figure 28-4(a)].

(8)The catheter is guided into the diseased segment of artery while being monitored on a TV screen that shows the artery and the catheter. The balloon-tip catheter, which is thinner, is then inserted through the guide catheter.

When its tip reaches the narrowed part of the artery, the balloon is inflated for about 30 seconds and then deflated. This cycle usually is repeated several times to widen the artery.

(9)The balloon-tip catheter is removed and angiography is repeated to make sure that blood flow has improved [Figure 28-4(b)].

(10)At the end of the procedure, the interventional radiologist removes the catheter and pressure will be applied to the groin area for a short time to prevent bleeding from the site of catheter insertion. Once the physician or assistant is satisfied that bleeding has stopped, a very tight bandage will be placed on the site. A sandbag may be placed on top of the bandage for additional pressure on the site, especially if the site is the groin. This entire process usually takes between one to two hours. The patient can expect to stay in bed for six to eight hours afterwards.

(11)After stent placement, the patients need to insist on taking anti-platelet aggregation drugs such as aspirin, plavix for a period of time. According to different stents, the required time varies from several weeks to several years, intravenous stents need to take anticoagulant drugs. At present, the vast majority of intravascular stents are compatible with MRI. For unfamiliar stents, please refer to the product manual.

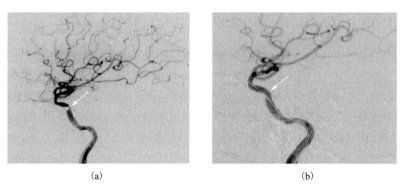

(a)   (b)

(a)Severe stenosis of the cavernous sinus segment of the left internal carotid artery (arrow); (b)The stenosis improved significantly after PTA treatment (arrow).

Figure 28-4   PTA treatment of severe stenosis of the C4 segment of the left internal carotid artery

7. Complication

(1)Recurrence of vascular obstruction: about $1/5-1/3$ patients with single angioplasty developed restenosis within a few days or weeks after operation. Of course, balloon angioplasty can still be considered at this time. For patients with stents, the probability of restenosis is much lower, and the current drug-eluting stent further reduces the incidence of restenosis.

(2)The risk of serious effects from coronary angioplasty is similar to that of surgery. Between one percent and three percent of patients die during or shortly after the procedure. Between three percent and five percent have a heart attack. A small number of patients, fewer than three percent, will require emergency bypass surgery because of damage to the artery wall from balloon inflation. The risk of death and the need for emergency surgery are substantially lower for renal and iliac artery angioplasty and for patients having dialysis graft procedures.

(3)Allergic reaction: Patients may have an allergic reaction to the contrast material injected for angiography. The risk of this happening is greater in patients with kidney disease, diabetes or asthma and those who have had a previous reaction to x-ray contrast material.

(4)Bleeding: Heavy bleeding may call for special medication or blood transfusion.

(5)Coronary angioplasty carries a risk of damaging the heart that could disrupt its normal rhythm.

(6)Stroke: There is a risk of stroke when angioplasty is performed on the carotid artery and a stent is placed.

This is because a blood clot may form and travel to small brain vessels, where it stops blood flow to brain tissue that requires a steady oxygen supply.

(7) Pain: The patient may feel pain briefly in the part of his or her body closest to the site of angioplasty when the balloon is inflated. This could be chest pain for coronary angioplasty, back pain for renal angioplasty, and buttock pain when iliac angioplasty is performed.

(8) Kidney damage: Because angiography is part of the procedure, there is a risk of kidney damage in patients with diabetes or other pre-existing kidney disease.

Section 6 Thrombolysis

1. Definition

A variety of etiologies lead to blood clots in human vascular system, namely thrombosis. The common causes are: (1) Atrial fibrillation causes atrial thrombosis. Once the clot breaks off, it willembolize the feeding arteries of cerebrum, kidney, mesentery, lower extremities and other organs; (2) Trauma leads to vascular intima injury and induces acute thrombosis; (3) Slow blood flow in atherosclerotic stenosis leads to acute thrombosis; (4) Venous thrombosis is caused by long-term activity restriction, infection, abnormal coagulation function, etc; (5) Under the above conditions, blood flow blockage leads to the continuous growth and spread of thrombosis. Thrombosis can slow down or even block the blood flow of organs or tissues, resulting in the lack of oxygen and nutrition supply of organs and tissues, or hindering tissue fluid circulation. Once the blood clot is formed in the blood vessels, it can gradually increase and eventually cause vascular obstruction, and completely cut off the blood circulation in the corresponding area. In the early stage of intravascular thrombosis of extremities, the patients may have no conscious symptoms, but soon there will be limb pain, numbness, temperature drop, tingling, swelling and other discomfort. Finally, tissues can be damaged and even necrosis, leading to organ dysfunction or failure, such as myocardial infarction, cerebral infarction, etc, which will endanger the patient life. Image-guided thrombolysis can be used to treat arteriovenous thrombosis caused by many etiologies.

Thrombolysis is a method of injecting thrombolytic drugs into the thrombus through a catheter and dissolving it directly. It is a safe and effective method to treat thrombus and reconstruct blood circulation (Fig. 16-3). Compared with traditional surgical operation, thrombolysis is much less invasive, especially for those deeper vessels, avoiding huge traumatic operations. It also has less bleeding, shorter hospitalization time and no obvious surgical scar.

2. Indication

Blood clots of vessel.

3. Contradication

(1) Severe hepatic, renal, or cardiac dysfunction.

(2) Uncorrectable coagulation dysfunction, or decreased platelets ($<50 \times 10^9/L$).

(3) Uncontrollable system infection or sepsis.

(4) Severe iodinated contrast allergy.

(5) Contraindications to thrombolysis.

4. The preparation for the procedure

(1) The patient may be asked not to eat or drink anything (except sip of water to take pills) for four to eight hours ahead of time. Some hospitals, however, allow clear fluids until shortly before the examination.

(2) Checking liver function, kidney function, blood routine and blood clotting factors are within normal limits.

(3) Checking a chest x-ray and electrocardiogram (ECG).

(4)Before the procedure the patient will have to give his or her consent. This usually involves a face-to-face talk with an interventional radiologist.

(5)Do iodine allergy test according to the contrast medium used.

(6)The patient has to empty his or her bladder and indwelling catheter if necessary.

(7)If the patient has diabetes, it may be necessary to alter his or her insulin dose on the day of angioplasty. Insulin was used to replace biguanidine during the operation.

5. Equipment

(1)The x-ray equipment, needle, guidewire and catheters of angiography are the same as those used for catheter angiography.

(2)Clot-dissolving medicine such as urokinase, streptokinase, tissue-type plasminogen activator(t-PA).

(3)Mechanical device to break up blood clot.

6. The procedure

(1)At the beginning, the patient will lie on a firm but padded x-ray table and will be connected to equipment that will monitor his or her heart rhythm, the rate of heartbeat, blood pressure, and oxygen levels.

(2)A sedative is injected through an intravenous line to relax the patient.

(3)The interventional radiologist will find an appropriate blood vessel, usually in the groin, arm or neck, then the catheter site (groin or arm)will be cleaned with antiseptic soap.

(4)Sterile towels and a sheet will be placed around this area.

(5)Then a local anesthetic is injected into the skin where the catheter is to be inserted, usually in the groin.

(6)A thin needle is introduced through a very small incision into the femoral artery.

(7)A thin guidewire is placed through the needle and the needle is exchanged over the guidewire for a catheter that is guided by x-rays and maneuvered to the area of poor circulation.

(8)Contrast material then is injected and a series of x-rays are taken to pinpoint the location of the clot[Figure 28-5(a), (b)]. The radiologist will review the images to determine whether the clot would be best treated by a clot-dissolving medication, by breaking it up with a mechanical device, or both.

(9)If the clot will be treated with medication, the catheter is left in place, connected to a special machine that delivers the medication at a precise rate. The clot-dissolving medications are delivered through the catheter. It usually takes 24-48 hours for the clot to dissolve. During that time, the interventional radiologist monitors the progress of the treatment using additional imaging scans[Figure 28-5(c), (d)].

(10)After the procedure, the catheter will be removed and the radiologist will hold pressure on the insertion site for about 15-20 minutes, so that the blood can begin to form a clot at the site and stop bleeding. After that, a very tight bandage will be placed on the site.

7. Complication

(1)Pain: Pain is the most common effects. But it can completely be controlled by oral or intravenous medication. Most patients can resume their normal activities within a week or two.

(2)Infection: Everyone has a risk of infection after thrombolysis, even if an antibiotic has been given.

(3)Bleeding: Whatever anticoagulant or thrombolytic agents are used, there is a risk that bleeding will occur elsewhere in the body.

(4)Allergic reaction: Because angiography is part of the procedure, there is the same as a risk of an allergic reaction to contrast material with angiography.

(5)Because angiography is part of the procedure, there is a risk of kidney damage in patients with diabetes or other pre-existing kidney disease.

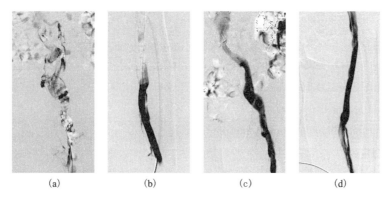

(a) Thrombosis of left common iliac vein and external iliac vein; (b) Left femoral vein thrombosis; (c) Thrombolysis in left common iliac vein and external iliac vein after continuous thrombolysis; (d) Left femoral vein thrombolysis after continuous thrombolysis.

Figure 28-5　Thrombolysis treatment of left common iliac vein, external iliac vein, and femoral vein thrombolysis

Section 7　Transjugular intrahepatic portosystemic shunt

1. Definition

Transjugular intrahepatic portosystemic shunt (TIPS) is a percutaneous image-guided procedure in which a decompressive channel is created between a hepatic vein and an intrahepatic branch of the portal vein to reduce portal hypertension. The procedure is a side to side shunt of a determined diameter designed to function as a partial shunt that preserves a portion of portal flow to the liver. TIPS was conceived and its technique developed in animal experiments in the late 1960s by Rosch et al, and it has currently been extablished as percutaneous alternative to surgical portosystemic shunts for decompression of symptomatic portal hypertension.

2. Indications

(1) Uncontrollable varicral hemorrhage.

(2) Recurrent variceal hemorrhage despite endoscopic therapy.

(3) Refractory ascites.

(4) Portal hypertensive gastropathy.

(5) Hepatic hydrothorax.

(6) Budd-Chiari syndrome.

(7) Hepatorenal syndrome.

(8) Portal vein thrombosis.

3. Contraindications

(1) Elevated right or left heart pressures.

(2) Heart failure or severe cardiac valvular insufficiency.

(3) Rapidly progressive liver failure.

(4) Severe or uncontrolled hepatic encephalopathy.

(5) Uncontrolled systemic infection or sepsis.

(6) Unrelieved biliary obstruction.

(7) Polycystic liver disease.

(8) Extensive primary or metastatic hepatic malignancy.

(9) Severe, uncorrectable coagulopathy.

4. Equipment

(1)Conventional puncture needle, 5-French vascular introducer sheath, 5-French catheter, 150 cm long 0. 035 inch hydrophilic guidewire, 260 cm long 0. 035 inch stiff guidewire.

(2)TIPS set (eg, RUPS-100 TIPS set).

(3)Balloon (8- or 10-mm diameter).

(4)Stent (8- or 10-mm diameter self-expanding).

5. Patient preparation

(1)Evaluation of the patient.

(2)Obtain the informed consent.

(3) Laboratory testing, including complete blood count, heart function tests, liver function tests, and coagulation profile.

(4)Obtain CT or MR imaging to assess candidacy for the procedure, technical feasibility, and need for modified or advanced techniques.

(5)Identify possible significant systemic comorbidities

(6)Indwelling catheter.

(7)Do iodine allergy test according to the contrast medium used.

(8)If the patient has diabetes, it may be necessary to alter his or her insulin dose on the day of angioplasty. Insulin was used to replace biguanidine during the operation.

6. Procedure steps

(1)Approach through the right internal jugular vein.

(2)Catheterize a hepatic veins and perform the hepatic venography [Figure 28-6(a)].

(3)Advance a long curved transjugular needle from the chosen hepatic vein through the liver parenchyma into an intrahepatic brance of the portal vein[Figure 28-6(b)].

(4)Directly measure the systemic and portal vein pressures through the transjugular access.

(5)Dilate the tract between the hepatic and portal veins with a balloon.

(6)Deploy a covered stent/stent graft or metallic stent within the tract to maintain its patency[Figure 28-6 (c), (d)]

(7)Measure the gradient between invasive portal pressure and hepatic vein pressure and obtain a portogram to confirm the result of the procedure

(8)Embolize varices when indicated [Figure 28-6(c), (d)]

7. Complications

(1) The procedure-related complications are related to venous access, wedged hepatic venography, transhepatic needle puncture and stent placement. The major procedural complications include hemoperitoneum, hepatic artery injury, biliary peritonitis, hemobilia, death, etc. The complication rate are much lower than for conventional surgical shunts and can be reduced with increased operator experience.

(2) Postprocedural complications of TIPS include cardiac decompensation, acceleration of liver failure, worsening hepatic encephalopathy. The cardiac decompensation results from a combination of increased venous return through the shunt and elevation of right heart filling pressure. Liver failure and hepatic encephalopathy are considered to be related to excessive shunting.

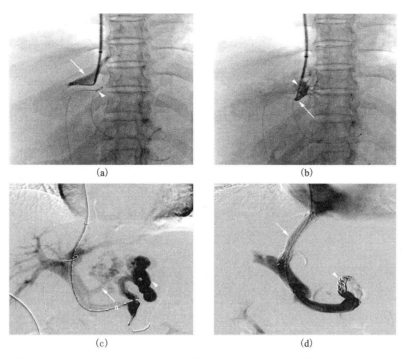

(a) Right hepatic venography shows a patent right hepatic vein (arrow). Note the micro-guidewire positioned in advance in the portal vein for targeted puncture (arrowhead); (b) Accessing the left portal vein (arrow) from the right hepatic vein (arrowhead) with a TIPS needle; (c) Subtracted portography with a catheter positioned in splenic vein shows varicose dilation of the left gastric vein (arrow) and the short gastric vein (arrowhead); (d). Subtracted portography after stenting shows patent portosystemic shunt (arrow). Note the varices embolized with coils (arrowhead).

Figure 28-6　TIPS for a patient with uncontrollable varicral hemorrhage

(Bin Liang, Lijie Zhang, Wei Huang, Yaoheng Wang, Fu Xiong, Dong Guo, Enhua Xiao, Zixu Zhang)

第二十九章

非血管介入技术

活检应用疾病定性诊断已有百余年历史。近 20 年来，放射学引导的经皮穿刺活检术已成为放射学的一种重要方法，该技术几乎适应全身各处的可疑肿块的确诊。早期的经皮穿刺活检术为了尽可能的安全，多选用 21~22G 细针对病灶进行穿刺抽吸后行细胞学活检，但有时存在抽吸的材料不足以提供组织学诊断的情况。近年来，采用较粗管径的切割式活检针(16~19G)穿刺进行组织学诊断已成为一种常规的安全的可靠的穿刺活检手段。

1. 适应证

穿刺刺活检的主要目的是明确可疑恶性肿瘤的性质。穿刺活检的适应症包括但不限于以下情况：

(1)需明确结节/肿块良恶性或某些弥漫性疾病具体类型。

(2)经内镜检查、细胞学检查或菌落培养无法明确性质的病变。

(3)评估恶性病变的组织学类型或者分子病理学类型以指导治疗。

(4)疾病进展或复发后组织学或分子病理学类型再评估。

放射学引导的活检术常见部位有胸部、肝脏、肾脏、胰腺、腹膜后，肾上腺、骨盆、骨骼、四肢和颈部软组织肿块等。

2. 禁忌证

穿刺活检存在一些相对禁忌证：

(1)严重心肺功能不全(如肺动脉高压)。

(2)不可纠正的凝血功能障碍。

(3)缺乏安全的活检路径。

(4)不合作的患者。

(5)需要避免电离辐射的人群如孕妇。

3. 放射学导引系统

选择超声、CT、MRI 或透视作为引导，主要依赖于个人习惯和经验，原则是只要使用者熟悉所用方法的优缺点，则都可改善活检的精确性。另外还有医生的偏好，肿块的可见度、大小和位置，患者的体型和相对费用等。

4. 活检针选择

活检针主要包括两种，其一为管径较小的抽吸式活检针(FNA)，为 20~25G，活检用于细胞学检查，现应用已明显减少；其二管径较大的切割式活检针(CNB)，通常为 14~20G，活检用于组织学检查，现应用较多。对于恶性病变，FNA 与 CNB 敏感性类似，特异性有差异，对良性病变，不推荐 FNA。另外，FNA 并发症如气胸及出血发生率明显较低。目前同轴穿刺活检系统已得到广泛应用。同轴穿刺活检技术指是以穿刺针外套针套进行穿刺，穿刺后活检针亦通过该针套，此技术有以下几个优点：①只需一次穿刺组织，减少了反复穿刺引起出血的可能性和患者的不适；②可获得充足的组织样本；③精确的穿刺定位只需一次，这点对于深部或较难到达的部位的肿块尤为重要；④活检针不接触肿瘤外其他脏器组织，减少了肿瘤细胞沿针道转移的风险。

5. 术前准备

(1)术前评估患者心肺功能、凝血功能及配合能力。

(2)完善穿刺部位增强 CT。

(3)检查胸片及心电图。

(4)术前停用抗凝和抗血小板药物。

(5)除少数过度紧张者，一般不需术前注射镇静或镇痛药物。

(6)向患者及家属交待活检术的步骤、风险及心理疏导，并取得知情同意。

(7)绝大部分放射学引导穿刺活检术可在门诊患者进行且仅在局麻下施行。

6. 操作方法

(1)大部分操作位置是仰卧位或俯卧位，但根据取样部位，有时也选择斜位、侧卧位等。目的是避开骨骼、血管、气管等重要解剖结构、采用最短的进针路径，有利活检针的准确定位并减少并发症的发生。通常建议自然呼吸状态下穿刺，避免深呼吸与剧烈咳嗽；必要时训练患者呼吸。

(2)采用栅形定位贴纸或者自制标记物固定于病灶相应体表，采用 1~3 mm 薄层扫描定位来确定进针层面、位置、角度与深度并进行标记。

(3)常规消毒、铺无菌单。

(4)1%~2%利多卡因溶液逐层浸润麻醉。

(5)采用分步进针法将穿刺针置于病变组织内，再次扫描确认。

(6)需根据病灶的性质来选择活检取材的部位，病灶体积较大时，应避开中央缺血坏死区域；空洞性病变应在实性组织部位取材。

7. 效果

穿刺活检的成功率取决于穿刺器官、病变大小及位置、病变良恶性、活检针管径、穿刺医生及病理医师的经验，整体成功率为 70%~90%左右。

8. 并发症

经皮穿刺活检的并发症发生率低且轻微，可分为一般并发症和器官特异性并发症。

(1)一般并发症是指所有部位或脏器活检都可发生的并发症，主要包括出血、感染、穿孔和意外器官损伤等。临床实践中大出血罕见，但出血风险随着活检针管径增加、切割针的使用及活检器官/病变的血管性而增加。活检造成的感染罕见，脏器损伤可能发生于穿刺针通过相应脏器时的意外损伤，较为严重时需要进一步干预。

(2)脏器特异性并发症是指与特定脏器活检相关的唯一或最常见的相关并发症。例如气胸最常与肺活检有关，但也可发生于其他邻近脏器活检如椎体、肝脏、乳房等，另外如血尿多发生于肾或前列腺活检后，咯血发生于肺活检后，其他罕见的严重并发症如肾上腺活检后的高血压危象、肺活检后的空气栓塞等。穿刺活检导致死亡极为罕见，有学者估计约 0.05%或更低。

第二节 食管狭窄支架术

治疗食管良性、恶性疾病引起的狭窄有许多方法。良性狭窄可用扩张探条或球囊进行扩张治疗，一部分贲门失驰缓症可用肉毒杆菌毒素注射治疗或球囊扩张治疗,覆膜支架亦被应用于良性狭窄的治疗。对于不能切除的食管恶性病变可置入金属支架改善进食症状,对于早期癌症,手术切除仍是主要方法。目前有多种金属支架用于临床:包括普通的和特殊定制的,覆膜支架和裸支架及放射性粒子支架等。

1. 适应证

(1)支架治疗主要适用于恶性食管狭窄。

(2)手术吻合口的肿瘤复发。

(3)原发性或继发性纵隔肿瘤压迫食管狭窄。

(4)食管气管瘘。

(5)医源性食管穿孔。

(6)食管胃吻合口瘘。

(7)良性食管狭窄。

2. 禁忌证

(1)患者失去自主吞咽功能或吞咽会造成误吸(双侧喉返神经损伤)者。

(2)自发食管破裂的破裂口太长(超过 10 cm),放 2 个重叠的支架虽能封住破口,但支架外面无食管壁,不能自行愈合者。

(3)上段食管穿孔,高于第 1 胸椎平面者。

(4)自发食管破裂同时伴有食管静脉曲张者。

(5)患者生命体征不稳定,随时可能发生心跳骤停者。

3. 支架置入技术

(1)术前通过食管钡餐评估食管狭窄的位置、程度和长度。

(2)用喷雾器进行咽部表面麻醉。

(3)嘱患者吞咽少许(约 10 mL)碘对比剂以确定狭窄的食管腔。

(4)用 0.035" 的加硬导丝及导管经口通过狭窄段进入食管远段或胃内。

(5)再次经导管测量食管狭窄位置及长度。

(6)如果支架不能经导丝引导通过狭窄,可以用球囊导管进行预扩张(最大直径 10 mm)[图 29-1(a)]。

(7)超硬导丝保留在食管内。

(8)准备支架,其长度应比狭窄段长 4 cm,因支架上下端须各超过狭窄部 1~2 cm 长。在透视引导下用直径 8 mm 的输送系统(导管鞘)将支架精确释放在狭窄段[图 29-1(b)]。

(9)最后复查食道造影以验证支架的位置和膨开程度。

4. 效果

覆膜或裸式自膨式金属支架已被证明是一种简单、安全、有效的治疗食管恶性梗阻和食管呼吸瘘的方法。随着新型抗反流支架,防移位支架,可回收支架,内覆膜支架等的开发运用,食管支架置入治疗术也在不断完善。大部分患者(70%~90%)可恢复几乎正常的饮食,结合化疗、放疗将增加患者的生存期,尽管这可能会导致更多的支架相关并发症。该领域仍需进一步研究。

5. 并发症

几乎 100% 患者有短暂胸痛,大约 13% 的患者胸痛时间较长,如果狭窄严重或使用了较大直径的支架可能引起较重的胸痛。较大的并发症如出血、穿孔、返流、发热或瘘等,发生率约 10%,覆膜支架移位发生率较高,约 25%,尤其当支架靠近贲门时。

再狭窄比较常见(8%~35%),这主要是由于肿瘤向未覆膜的支架内生长造成。肿瘤内生长在覆膜型支架则极少见,其他后期并发症还有出血(3%~10%),食管溃疡(7%),食管穿孔或瘘(5%),支架扭转

(5%)，支架移位(5%)和支架断裂(2%)。

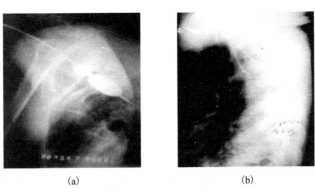

(a)扩张球囊显示食管狭窄段；(b)支架植入后。

图 29-1　食管癌支架治疗

第三节　经皮胃造口术

20世纪80年代初期，成功地开展了经皮内镜下胃造口术。基于同样的概念，1983年几个作者首次独立报导透视下经皮胃造口术(PG)的方法。此后，随着技术的不断改进，透视下经皮胃造口技术逐渐积累了许多临床经验，经皮胃造口术已成为一种被广泛接受的手术，并不断扩大适应证。X线透视下的经皮胃空肠造口、空肠造口及及盲肠造口目前也有应用。

1.适应证

(1)具有功能性胃肠道且需要营养支持的患者。

(2)需要行胃肠减压的患者。

(3)由于头颈部肿瘤或吞咽功能失调引起吞咽困难的患者，需要营养支持。

(4)难治型糖尿病性胃瘫也适合经皮胃造口向小肠中喂食。

(5)需要营养支持的重症监护室患者(如创伤患者)也适合经皮胃造口来进行营养支持。

(6)厌食症患者，如神经食欲缺乏、抑郁性精神病或晚期恶性肿瘤患者也适合胃造口术，该技术对于婴幼儿也是安全有效的。

2.禁忌证

(1)无经腹壁穿刺窗口。

(2)大量腹水。

(3)胃切除术后。

(4)凝血功能障碍。

(5)胃恶性肿瘤。

(6)腹膜炎患者。

(7)门静脉高压导致胃静脉曲张。

(8)胃食管返流。

3.术前准备

(1)患者术前应该检查其凝血功能，如有异常，应予纠正。

(2)术前空腹4小时，并停止鼻饲喂食。

(3)放置鼻饲管于胃内，抽出残留胃液。

(4)术前静脉给 0.5~1 mg 胰高血糖素或 20 mg 丁溴东莨菪碱,减少胃蠕动。

4.手术过程

(1)在前后位及侧位透视下用空气(200~800 mL)充填胃腔,使胃前壁与腹前壁相贴。并使用前后位和侧位透视,通过将镊子的尖端放在上腹的拟皮肤进入部位,确认前胃壁与前腹壁的贴合。

(2)穿刺部位最好在腹直肌外侧或中线,以避免损伤上腹上动脉。

(3)确定好穿刺点后局部注射少量麻药。

(4)用刀切一小口。

(5)可选择 22~18G 穿刺针,一般常选用 18G 套管针向下迅速推进穿刺胃体,进入胃腔后有明显落空感,注入少量对比剂,透视下证实已位于胃腔内。

(6)插入导丝拔去穿刺针,再沿导丝置入扩张器,扩张创道,达胃造口管外径大小。在扩张过程中可以使用胃固定术,如 T 形锚钩等固定法固定胃壁。

(7)然后沿导丝插入胃造口管。胃造口管有多种形态,管径大小 10F-18F,建议先使用 12F 造口管,经 12F 扩张后造口管较易插入,扩张器旋转插入必须穿透胃壁(图 29-2)。在插入扩张器和随后插入胃造口导管时,也应通过鼻胃管进一步充气来维持胃部扩张。

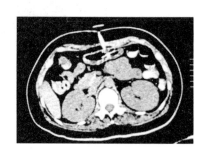

图 29-2 经皮胃造口术

(8)胃壁固定术:标准的经皮胃造口术中,胃前壁未与前腹壁固定,当胃回缩后可在腹膜腔内留下一个潜在性腔隙,理论上说可能会有造口管脱落或胃内容物瘘入此腔。为预防这个问题,经皮置入锚钩将胃壁腹壁紧密固定在一起即可。

5.术后处理中

术后 4~8 小时注意监测生命体征,腹膜体征,建议保留鼻饲管 24 小时以利胃肠减压,24 小时后可开始经胃造口管喂食。

6.效果

PG 技术成功率接近 100%

7.并发症

并发症率约 5%。主要并发症,特别是造瘘口外漏和伤口感染,多发生在外科手术患者,这主要由于技术上的差异所致,PG 中胃造口管与胃壁紧密封口,而外科造口管是在胃壁切开后围绕造口管荷包缝合。

第四节 经皮肝穿刺胆管引流术

直接穿刺肝脏行胆管置管应用于术前临时性外部减压已有多年。近年来,改进的操作技术上的可将穿刺肝脏引入的导管通过阻塞病变进入十二指肠。导管通过阻塞病变的上段和下段都带有侧孔时,就可建立起引流通道将胆汁顺行引流到十二指肠。

1.适应证

(1)手术前减压:肝穿胆管引流一经建立,与黄疸直接有关的症状很快消失,患者的营养状况常常也有明显改善。

(2)永久性导管引流:肝穿导管引流对于减轻胆管梗阻的长期效果,又与永久引流外科手术相媲美,不管阻塞病变的部位与性质如何,此法可很快达到减压,且病死率极低。

(3)恶性疾病(胆管癌,肝门转移癌,胰腺癌):大多数恶性疾病中,如果胆管梗阻得到充分缓解,则能延长生存期，因为放置引流导管后，患者的状况可有明显改善，使之能接受全面的化疗和放疗。

（4）良性疾病：①手术后良性狭窄；②硬化性胆管炎；③胆总管结石；④胰腺炎。

2.禁忌证

肝穿胆管引流临床上没有绝对的禁忌证，只有相对禁忌证：

（1）严重凝血机能障碍者。

（2）严重心、肝、肾功能衰竭者。

（3）大量腹水者。

（4）对碘过敏者。

（5）症状轻微的临终患者。

（6）败血症。

（7）肝内胆管被肿瘤分隔成多腔，不能引流整个胆管系统者。

（8）超声检查证实肝内有大液平面，Casoni 试验阳性，疑为肝包虫病者。

3.术前准备

（1）做生化检查，如延长凝血酶原时应给维生素 K 以纠正。

（2）做超声、CT 和 MRI 检查，以判断病变性质，鉴别是肝细胞性黄疸还是阻塞性黄疸。

（3）造影前一日晚清洁灌肠，并给镇静药。

（4）造影前一小时给镇静剂，但禁用吗啡，以免引起俄狄括约肌痉挛而混淆诊断。

（5）造影前腹部透视，观察肝下有无充气肠管，以免穿刺时误伤。

（6）根据所用对比剂说明是否做碘过敏试验。

4.手术过程

（1）细针穿刺胆管造影：在引流之前，一律先作细针穿刺胆管造影，它可以证实诊断，并明确梗阻的解剖方位以及确定导管插入的位置。

（2）插入带套管的针：细针穿刺胆管造影完成后、摄一张仰卧水平侧位 X 线影像。根据侧位影像选择第二穿刺点。第二穿刺点比细针穿刺的位置偏向腹侧或偏向背侧。在透视引导下将 16 号带套管的针插入肝脏，以水平方向插入确定的胆管。

（3）操纵导管进入胆管：胆管置管要进行一系列更换步骤，先不断地操控导丝通过胆管和鞘管并前进一小段，旋转导丝的外段并施加轻微的推力使导丝进入到梗阻部位以上的胆管树。

（4）通过梗阻位置：经皮穿刺胆管引流的最关键一步就是推送导丝通过梗塞部位［图 29~3（a）］。显然，若这一步不能完成，顺行引流也就不可能。幸运的是，置管通常能通过梗阻处。

（5）插入引流管［图 29-3（b）］：用于长期顺行胆道引流的导管必须有足够大的内径以通过每日的胆汁流量，而外径必须足够小以通过肝实质和梗阻部位。

5.术后处理

一旦导管留置在适当的位置，在皮肤入口周围盖上敷料，在导管尾部接头接上一封闭式引流袋，建立外引流。在 48 小时内要注意观察胆汁引流的量和性质。顺行性引流一般在置管后 1~2 天内建立，拆下引流袋，并在导管尾端盖上封闭帽。

6.结果

肝穿胆道引流满意与否，取决于梗阻平面以上胆管之间的连续性和相互沟通。术后全身瘙痒明显好转，血清胆红素大幅度下降。

7.并发症

（1）导管入口处的局部感染。处理：每天热敷 2 次，局部涂以抗生素软膏。

（2）导管入口处肉芽肿形成。处理：用硝酸银烧灼。

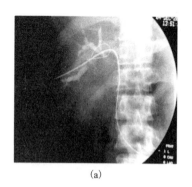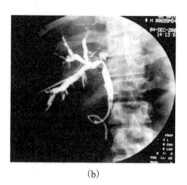

（a）导丝成功穿过梗阻段；（b）成功送入引流管。

图 29-3　胆管梗阻行 PDCT

（3）导管闭塞，胆汁外渗，粪尿颜色的改变，黄疸或发热。处理：更换导管。

第五节　经皮肾盂穿刺造口术

经皮肾盂穿刺造口术（简称 PCN）：在影像引导下将导管置入肾集合系统，其是作为多种上尿路疾病的治疗手段之一，特点是进入肾集合系统快速、可靠，成功率高，并发症和病死率远远低于开放性手术。

1.适应证

短期尿流改道适应证：

（1）良性病变（最常见是结石）引起上尿路梗阻。

（2）严重的细菌或真菌感染（肾盂积腔）。

（3）输尿管损伤（外伤或医源性）。

（4）尿瘘（腹膜后尿管瘘）。

（5）新生儿肾积水（术前）。

（6）高血压继发性肾积水。

（7）出血性膀胱炎。

（8）为其他介入手术和内镜手术建立通道。

（9）肾盂输尿管异物取出。

长期尿流改道适应证：

（1）恶性输尿管梗阻。

（2）晚期膀胱癌。

（3）尿瘘（常见于妇科癌症）。

（4）输尿管梗阻（腹膜后纤维化或放射性纤维化）。

2.禁忌证

绝对禁忌证：在某些情况下应避免或延迟使用 PCN，但没有绝对禁忌证。

相对禁忌证：

（1）无法纠正的严重凝血功能障碍（如肝或多系统衰竭患者）。

（2）患者病情危重、即将死亡。

3.方法步骤

PCN 留置导管最常用超声或 X 光透视作为引导，透视最便于引导、跟踪导丝、扩张通道、放置引流管和顺行性肾盂造影术。

（1）渐近性扩张通道：通常选择超声、透视或两者联合引导下穿刺，首选肾后盏作为穿刺目标。用22G针穿刺肾盂，然后通过内芯引入柔软的 φ0.018吋导丝进入肾收集系统，导丝加强部分进入3~4 cm后方可退出穿刺针，用同轴系统沿 φ0.018吋导丝行预扩张，然后用 φ0.035吋导丝交换。用18G针穿刺确定进入肾盂后，可直接将 φ0.035吋硬导丝推进肾盂内，进一步将通道扩张至引流管大小。

（2）放置引流管（图29-4）：引流管应选用8-10F带多个侧孔的猪尾导管，有较大的侧孔导管适合于含有碎屑的黏稠脓液引流，大部分引流套装配有较硬的塑料套管和金属内芯。放置的引流管外侧可连接外引流袋。

（3）导管的作用：①当不需要外引流时，可关闭阀门做内引流使尿液进入膀胱；②需要时可行肾盂盏造影；③每3个月更换一次导管；④可起到双J型内支架的相同作用；⑤不容易脱落；⑥患者容易接受。

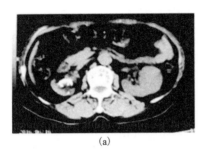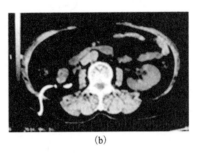

（a）　　　　　　　　　　　　　　（b）

图 29-4　右输尿管结石致右肾重度积水行经皮右肾盂穿刺造口术，积水解除

4. 并发症

（1）轻微并发症：发生轻微并发症占10.84%，发热、输尿管狭窄、短暂出血或血尿、引流管脱出、肾盂、输尿管穿孔、尿瘤、腹水、末段输尿管梗阻等。

（2）较大的并发症：发生较大的并发症占2.77%（病死率0.05%），感染（感染休克）、出血并发症（穿刺通道出血，大量血尿，动脉损伤，动静脉瘘肾被膜下血肿、肾破裂、腹膜后出血）、内脏损伤（结肠或脾脏）、胸部并发症（大量胸水、血胸、脓胸、气胸）、肾静脉血栓等。

总之，PCN后造成肾脏形态学变化远小于开放式外科手术，并发症发生率也随经验的增加而减少。

第六节　经皮椎体形术

经皮椎体成形术（PVP）是一项用于治疗疼痛性压缩性骨折及椎体肿瘤性疾病的微创新技术，1984年由法国放射学家Galibert首次实施。该技术是在透视引导下经皮将骨穿刺针插入椎体内，注入骨水泥（PMMA）。通常的治疗目的是缓解疼痛，但该技术同时也提高了压缩椎体的机械强度。骨水泥的聚合作用和固化作用使椎体的稳固性和强度得以提高。机械效应可使疼痛缓解，并避免椎体进一步塌陷。骨水泥的甲基丙烯酸甲酯体释放，以及聚合反应释放的热能可以破坏痛觉神经末梢感受器从而达到缓解疼痛的作用。PVP作为一项较新的技术，有待进一步评估和完善。

1. 适应证

（1）骨质疏松性压缩性骨折。

（2）转移瘤和多发性骨髓瘤。

（3）椎体血管瘤：椎体血管瘤可因为椎体压缩、椎管和（或）椎间孔的占位效应而引发剧痛而需治疗。

2. 禁忌证

（1）无症状的骨质疏松性压缩骨折。

（2）没有压缩的骨质疏松椎体。

(3)药物疗法已改善症状的骨质疏松性压缩骨折。

(4)正常椎体的急性损伤性骨折。

(5)完全性椎体塌陷。

(6)完全性椎体破坏，硬膜外或椎间肿瘤，神经根或脊髓压迫等。

(7)难以纠正的凝血障碍。

(8)局部感染。

3. 患者的选择和评估

欲获得良好的 PVP 临床疗效，仔细筛选合适的患者至关重要，首先必须确认患者背痛的原因是症状性椎体压缩性骨折，还是其他原因(如椎间小关节病变、椎间盘病变，椎间盘突出或骶髂关节炎等)，因为后者不适合 PVP 治疗，当然，全面评估需要相关病史、体检和适当的影像资料如 X 线平片，MRI 及骨扫描等。

4. 操作步骤

(1)首先是选择好进针的位置，最好使用双球管 X 线机透视定位，便单 C 臂 X 线机透视定位也完全可行。

(2)一般腰椎穿刺可选用 11G 骨穿针，胸椎部选用 13G 骨穿针，在侧位透视下缓慢地将针插入椎体至前三分之一的理想位置[图 29-5(a)、(b)]。

(3)再慢慢地注入少量骨水泥混合物[图 29-5(c)]，在注射过程中间歇地前后位观察有无侧面渗漏。

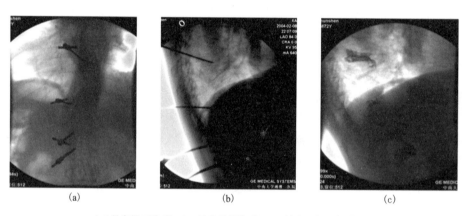

(a)骨穿针正位观；(b)骨穿针侧位观；(c)骨水泥沉积侧位观。

图 29-5　多发骨质疏松性压缩性骨折行经皮椎体成形术

5. 并发症

约 50%的椎体成形术患者出现并发症，但其中约 95%无临床症状。部分 PVP 术后可以有短暂的疼痛或发热加重，通常用几天的非甾体抗炎药或类固醇有效缓解。在骨质疏松椎体压缩骨折患者偶可出现肋骨骨折，严重并发症包括骨水泥肺栓塞，神经根病或脊髓压迫。

6. 展望

具有成骨效应和骨支架作用的新型非 PMMA 骨水泥，既有强化作用又能传递化疗药物的骨水泥都在积极研究之中，目前，PVP 对于转移性椎体破坏和骨质疏松椎体的预防性治疗也在逐步扩大应用。在椎体恶性肿瘤的治疗中，椎体成形术联合射频消融、血管栓塞等微创方法发挥着越来越重要的作用。

第七节　肿瘤消融术

对于不能切除的肿瘤，肿瘤消融是局部肿瘤控制的一种选择。消融治疗包括物理消融、化学消融和不可逆电穿孔等。物理消融包括低温消融和热消融。热消融包括射频消融(RFA)、微波消融(MWA)。还有一些其他的消融，如高强度聚焦超声、激光热消融等。乙醇和冰醋酸则常用于化学消融。

热消融技术包括高温消融，如射频消融和微波消融，以及低温消融，如冷冻消融。射频消融利用组织内振荡离子传递的摩擦能量加热和治疗肿瘤。当细胞被加热到超过54°超过1秒时，细胞会发生凝固性坏死。治疗性射频消融术将组织温度控制在60℃到100℃之间。MWA导致细胞死亡的机制与RFA相似。微波治疗时，连续振荡的微波场以极性分子（主要是水）为目标，极性分子与该场对准，导致动能和组织温度增加。冷冻消融通过细胞内和细胞外冰晶的形成和随后细胞内物质的释放而导致细胞死亡。气体（通常是氩气）通过内部进料管线在高压下输送到低温探头的膨胀室；当气体膨胀时，会产生一个吸热作用，冷却探头和周围的组织。

1.肺肿瘤

消融技术已被证明是治疗肺癌的可行而有效的手段，已被用于治疗原发性肺癌、肺转移癌，以及胸壁恶性肿瘤（止痛）治疗。

（1）适应证：

1）早期原发性肺癌：活检证实；不能手术/拒绝手术；放疗、化疗后复发。

2）局限性转移瘤及挽救疗法：放疗后局部复发；术后局部复发；缓解症状如疼痛。

（2）禁忌证：

1）未纠正的凝血功能异常：血小板小于50000/μL且INR>1.5。

2）菌血症或活动性感染。

3）主要脏器严重功能障碍。

4）弥漫性肺癌或肿瘤过大，需要消融范围达1/3肺脏体积。

5）大量胸水。

6）晚期恶液质。预计生存小于3个月。

（3）术前准备：

1）影像检查：2周内胸片、增强肺CT扫描、必要时PET/CT检查。

2）心、肺功能检查及凝血肝肾功能等实验室检查。

3）支气管镜活检或CT引导下活检明确病理细胞学或组织学诊断。

4）手术设备及抢救设备与药品的准备。

5）患者局麻术前6小时禁食和水、建立静脉通道。

6）患者及被委托人签署手术知情同意书。

（4）手术流程：

1）麻醉：可使用中度镇静或全身麻醉。

2）定位和进入部位（类似于肺活检），见图29-6a：穿刺路线应减少穿小叶间裂隙数目，避免肺大泡和肺气肿，避开纵隔结构和大血管。当使用多个消融针时，有协同效应，消融覆盖范围增大。

3）消融针定位：理想的消融针定位应该使消融区覆盖肿瘤[图29-6(b)]。与外科手术相似，有效地消融区域应覆盖肿瘤边界外0.5~1cm。

4）消融能量的选择（射频消融、微波或冷冻消融）：①病灶距胸膜表面<1~2cm时应避免微波。邻近胸膜表面的微波消融容易发生支气管胸膜瘘；②当使用冷冻消融时，预处理短周期的冻融（3分钟冻融，3分钟解冻）可以使冰球更好的形成；③在清醒镇静状态下接受冷冻消融治疗耐受较高温消融好。

5）术中监控：患者体温、脉搏、呼吸、血压、氧饱和度；消融区域温度分布、阻抗、肿瘤区域和周围正常肺组织的变化。

（5）术后处理：广人稀术毕缓慢拔出消融针，再次CT扫描观察有无出血及气胸；术后常规止血、抗菌治疗3天；术后1个月、3个月、6个月常规肺部增强CT检查观察肿瘤变化。

（6）疗效：治疗成功率超过90%；肿瘤直径<5cm1次治疗灭活率达90%，残余病灶第2次追加治疗可完全灭活。可明显改善生存质量、延长生存期。

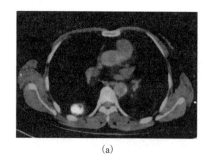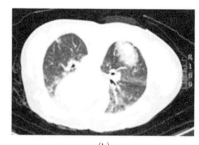

(a)术前 CT 显示肺癌;(b)术后 CT 显示消融区覆盖肿瘤。

图 29-6　肺癌冷冻消融

(7)并发症

1)气胸:发生气的胸者占 9%~13%。

2)咯血:发生咯血者占 3%,大部分咯血是自限性的。

3)神经病变:纵隔旁肿块治疗致膈神经损伤已有报道。虽常自限,仍应避免。

4)疼痛:患者自控镇痛(PCAs)或麻醉药可以在手术的晚上使用,绝大多数疼痛在手术后几天内消失或明显改善。

5)发热、感染和支气管胸膜瘘。

2. 肝肿瘤

当肝移植或手术切除不合适时,消融治疗被认为是极早期和早期肝细胞癌(HCC)的最佳治疗选择。此外,对于肝转移性疾病,特别是结直肠癌(CRC)的不能手术的患者,消融治疗被认为是一种可行的替代手术。

(1)适应证:

1)根据巴塞罗那临床肝癌(BCLC)分类的极早期和早期 HCC,当患者不能肝脏切除或移植时。要求单个肿瘤小于 5 cm 或最多 3 个结节小于 3 cm,无血管侵犯或肝外扩散的证据,Child-Pugh A 级或 B 级。

2)结直肠癌肝内寡转移的非手术患者,且无外科指征。预计肝外疾病可以治愈。

3)其他原发性癌症的肝转移。有报导称乳腺肿瘤肝转移和肝内分泌肿瘤的消融治疗有较好疗效。

(2)禁忌证:

1)绝对禁忌证:

①肿瘤位于距主胆管<1cm 处,因其可以引起胆管延迟性狭窄

②无法治疗/纠正的凝血异常

2)相对禁忌证:

①大于 5 个病灶。如果所有转移性灶都有可能得到成功的治疗,那么病变的数目不应被视为射频消融的绝对禁忌症。但多数中心优先治疗 5 个或更少病变的患者。

②肿瘤在最长轴上的大小不应超过 3 厘米,因目前大多数可用设备的最佳完全消融范围为 3cm。

③胆肠吻合术或 PTCD 内外引流,因有肝脓肿的危险。

④浅表病变,因为并发症的风险更高。

⑤由于胃或肠壁热损伤的风险,靠近胃肠道任何部分的浅表病变(考虑人工腹水/人工气胸分离组织再消融治疗)。

⑥肿瘤位于胆囊附近,有医源性胆囊炎的风险。

⑦铁磁性假肢,RFA 进可能起到散热作用,导致皮肤烧伤。

⑧起搏器/除颤器患者不宜用 RFA。

(3)术前准备:

1)影像学和血清学检查:影像学检查确定肿瘤位置、大小,消融手术可行性;心脏功能的超声,检查了解心脏的情况;血清学检查,如血红蛋白、血小板、凝血功能,评估手术风险。

2）胸片与心电图检查。

3）术前评估：医生对患者肿瘤位置进行评估，确定消融相关器械的型号等。

4）患者准备：穿刺部位的皮肤毛发的处理；患者术前应配合医生进行行呼吸训练、抗炎治疗和饮食控制，防止术后严重感染，术中恶心呕吐等并发症；如肿瘤挨近胆囊，要求患者术前进食高脂饮食，促进胆囊排空，以便暴露病变部位；预计手术时间比较长，患者在手术之前不要过量的饮水、必要时导尿技术。

（4）手术程序：

1）定位：主要是手术前根据影像学表现，选择最佳治疗体位以及进针位点、路径，然后进针路径必须经过部分正常的肝组织，避开大血管、胆管以及胃肠道这些重要的脏器，从而可以有效地降低并发症的发生。

2）麻醉：目前最常用的麻醉方式是穿刺点局部麻醉，然后联合手术中静脉使用一定量的镇静和镇痛药物进行麻醉。必要时在全身麻醉下进行。

3）常规消毒，麻醉以后在皮肤上做 2~3 mm 切口。

4）影像引导/监测包括 US、CT 或 MR 成像。在影像学引导下，根据术前定位、图像以及设计好的路线，将消融针分布进针，精准的穿刺到肿瘤靶区，通过再次扫描确定消融针的位置和肿瘤关系，确定位置关系比较好以后固定消融针[图 29-7（a）、（b）]。

5）启动消融的冷循环系统和消融系统，一般从低功率逐渐开始，患者耐受的情况下可以适当提高功率，增大消融范围，提高治疗疗效，而且还可以缩短手术时间，降低手术并发症。

6）热消融是肝脏肿瘤最常见的消融治疗方法。射频或微波加热引起的热损伤取决于所获得的组织温度和加热时间。在 50℃到 55℃的温度下加热组织 4~6 分钟会产生不可逆的细胞损伤。在 60℃到 100℃的温度下，组织几乎立即凝固，细胞的线粒体和胞浆酶受到不可逆的损害。因此，消融治疗的一个基本目标是在整个靶体积内达到并维持 50℃到 100℃的温度至少 4 到 6 分钟。然而，当使用 RFA 时，组织加热相对缓慢，故 RFA 应用时间延长到 10~20 分钟。

微波消融是射频消融治疗肝癌的替代方法。电磁微波通过诱导超高速（900 兆赫至 2450 兆赫）交变电场加热物质，引起水分子旋转。与现有的热消融技术相比，微波技术的主要特点包括持续较高的瘤内温度、更大的肿瘤消融体积、更快的消融时间和更少的热沉降，获得好的消融效果[图 29-7（d）、（e）]。与射频消融术相比，MWA 的优点是治疗结果受肿瘤附近血管的影响较小（二者在手术结束时，可进行针道凝固以防止肿瘤种植）。

（5）术后处理：

1）术后用无菌纱布覆盖穿刺部位。

2）24 小时心电监护，必要时延长监护时间。

3）术后常规禁食 4 小时，邻近胃肠道病变消融后，适当延长禁食时间。

4）术后 3 天内进行血常规、肝肾功能、尿常规检查。

5）根据情况补液、保肝、护胃、利尿、对症处理。

（6）疗效评估：术后 4-6 周复查增强 CT 或增强 MRI 检查和抽血检测肿瘤标志物及肝功能。肿瘤完全消融：肿瘤及消融边缘无强化，伴或不伴同心、匀称、光滑的环形强化带；肿瘤残余或复发：消融区存在散在、结节状、不规则偏心强化。

（7）并发症：

1）主要并发症（占 2.2%~3.1%）：腹腔出血（占 1%）；肝脓肿（占 0.3%）；肠穿孔（占 0.3%）；气胸/血胸（占 0.1%）；胆管狭窄（占 0.1%）；沿针道种植肿瘤（占 0.5%）；皮肤烧伤（占 0.1%）。

2）轻微并发症（占 5%~8.9%）：疼痛、发热；无症状性胸腔积液；无症状自限性腹腔内出血。

3）病死率（占 0.1%~0.5%）。最常见的死亡原因是败血症，肝衰竭，结肠穿孔，门静脉血栓形成。

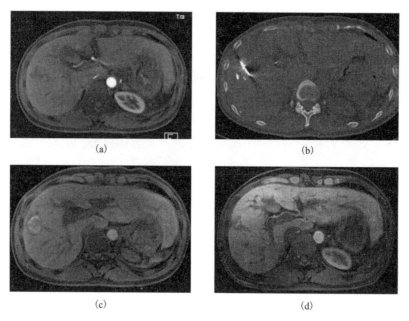

(a)术前 MR;(b)消融术中;(c)术后 1 个月;(d)术后 6 年。

图 29-7 肝癌微波消融

(马聪,王福安,胡李男,王天明,肖恩华,张子曙)

Chapter 29

Non-vascular interventional radiology

Biopsy has been used for qualitative diagnosis of diseases for more than a hundred years. Radiologically guided percutaneous needle biopsy has emerged as one of the significant advances in radiology during the past two decades. It is now a widely accepted technique to establish the identity of masses detected in almost any location in the body. In the early years of radiologically guided needle biopsy, almost all biopsies were performed with thin-caliber (21 ~ 22 G) needles, although the material was sometimes insufficient for a specific histologic diagnosis. In recent years, the use of larger diameter cutting biopsy needles (16 ~ 19 G) for histological diagnosis has become a routine, safe and reliable method of biopsy.

1. Indications

In most cases, the main purpose of needle biopsy is to clarify the nature of suspicious malignant tumors. The indications for needle biopsy include but are not limited to the following conditions:

(1) To clarify the pathogen of infectious lesions or the characterization of some diffuse diseases.

(2) To evaluate the lesions whose nature cannot be determined by endoscopy, cytological examination or colony culture.

(3) To obtain tissue and assess the histologic or molecular pathological types of malignant lesions to guide therapy.

(4) To re-evaluate local histology or molecular pathology after disease progression or recurrence.

The most common sites ofradiologically guided biopsy include the chest, liver, pancreas, retroperitoneum, adrenal, pelvis, bone, extremity, and cervical soft-tissue masses.

2. Contraindications

(1) Thereis no abdominal puncture window.

(2) A lot of ascites.

(3) After gastrectomy.

(4) Coagulation dysfunction.

(5) Gastric cancer.

(6) Patients with peritonitis.

(7) Portal hypertension leads to gastric varices.

(8)Gastroesophageal reflux.

3. Radiologic guidance systems

The choice among ultrasound, computed tomography (CT), magnetic resonance imaging, and fluoroscopic imaging guidance largely depends on the personal preference and previous experience of the radiologist performing the procedure. In general, the accuracy of these imaging methods forneedle biopsy improves if one is familiar with the method and understands the strengths and limitations of each method. In addition, there are physician preference, the visibility, size and location of the mass, the patient's body habitus, and relative cost.

4. Needle selection

There are two main types of biopsy needles. One is thefine-needle aspiration (FNA) with a smaller diameter (20-25G) used for cytological examination, whose application has been significantly reduced. Another biopsy needle is core-needle biopsy (CNB) with a larger diameter (usually 14-20G), which used for histological examination and is widely used currently. FNA and CNB are similar in diagnostic sensitivity and different in diagnostic specificity for malignant lesions. FNA is not recommended for benign lesions. In addition, the incidence of FNA complications such as pneumothorax and bleeding is significantly lower. At present, the coaxial puncture system have been widely used. There are several advantages in coaxial technology: (1) It only needs to puncture the tissue once, which reduces the possibility of bleeding and the discomfort of the patient. (2) It can obtain sufficient tissue samples. (3) The precise needle positioning only needs one time. This is particularly important for lesions in deep or hard-to-reach areas. (4) The biopsy needle does not touch the organ tissues other than the tumor, which reduces the risk of tumor cell metastasis along the needle tract.

5. Preoperative preparation

(1) The patient's cardiopulmonary function coagulation function and coordination ability are assessed before the biopsy operation.

(2) The patient needs to complete the contrast-enhanced CT of the diseased organs.

(3) To check chest radiograph and electrocardiogram.

(4) Anticoagulant and antiplatelet drugs are stopped before the biopsy.

(5) Premedication with parenteral sedatives or analgesics generally is not required unless the patient is unduly apprehensive.

(6) The doctor explained the steps, risks and psychological counseling of the biopsy to the patient and family members, and obtained informed consent.

(7) Most radiologically guided needle biopsies are performed with local anesthetic on an outpatient basis.

6. Operating procedures

(1) Most procedures can be done with the patient in a comfortable supine position, but oblique, decubitus, or prone positions are occasionally necessary. The purpose is to avoid important anatomical structures such as bones, blood vessels, and trachea, and to adopt the shortest puncture path, which facilitates the accurate positioning of the biopsy needle and reduces the occurrence of complications. It is usually recommended to puncture under natural breathing to avoid deep breathing and severe coughing, and train the patient to breathe if necessary.

(2) The grid-shaped positioning stickers or self-made markers are used to fix the corresponding body surface of the lesion. Thin-slice CT scan (1~3 mm) is used to locate and mark the needle level, position, puncture angle and depth.

(3) Routinely disinfect and spread sterile sheets.

(4) 1% to 2% lidocaine solution was use to inject layer by layer infiltration anesthesia.

(5) The puncture needle is pushed into the diseased tissue by the stepping needle method, and then the CT

scan was performed again to confirm the position of the puncture needle tip.

(6)The location for biopsy should be selected according to the nature of the lesion. When the size of the lesion is large, the central avascular necrosis area should be avoided. For hollow lesions, the material should be taken from the solid tissue site.

7. Results

The success rate of radiologically guided biopsy depends on the puncture organ, the size and location of the lesion, the benign and malignant lesion, the diameter of the biopsy needle, the experience of the puncture physician and the pathologist. The overall success rate is about 70%~90%.

8. Complications

The complication rate of percutaneous needle biopsy is rare and mild, and can be divided into general complications and organ-specific complications.

(1)General complications refer to complications that can occur in biopsy of all body organs, mainly including bleeding, infection, perforation, and accidental organ damage. Major bleeding is rare in clinical practice. But the risk of bleeding increases with the increase in the diameter of the biopsy needle, the use of the cutting needle, and the vascularity of the biopsy organ/lesion. Infections caused by biopsy are rare. Organ damage may occur when the puncture needle passes through the corresponding organ. Further intervention is required when it is more serious.

(2)Organ-specific complications refer to the only or most common complications related to specific organ biopsy. For example, pneumothorax is most often related to lung biopsy, but it can also occur in biopsy of other nearby organs such as vertebral body, liver, breast, etc. In addition, hematuria usually occurs after kidney or prostate biopsy, hemoptysis occurs after lung biopsy. Other rare and serious complications such as hypertensive crisis after adrenal gland biopsy, air embolism after lung biopsy, etc. Death due to needle biopsy is extremely rare, and some scholars estimate that its incidence is about 0.05% or less.

Section 2　Stenting for esophageal stricture

There are many approaches to treat esophageal obstruction secondary to benign or malignant disease. Solid dilators or balloon dilatationare useful with benign strictures. Injection of the gastroesophageal junction with Botulinum toxin has had some success in primary achalasia, as has balloon dilatation. Covered stents are also used in the treatment of benign stenosis. The use of self-expanding metallic stents has recently become popular in the literature for the palliation of unresectable malignant disease. Surgery is the mainstay in definitive treatment for cancer of low stage. There are many types of metallic stents, both generic and custom made. They come uncovered or covered, being embedded in a thin layer of sterile plastic or biosynthetic material and radioactive particle stent.

1. Indications

(1)Stents are used primarily in patients with malignant oesophagealobstruction.

(2)Anastamotic tumour recurrencefollowing surgery.

(3)Primary or secondary tumourswithin the mediastinum causingextrinsic oesophageal compression.

(4)Tracheo-oesophageal fistulae.

(5)Oesophagealperforation, which is usually iatrogenic, from directendoscopictrauma or following stricture dilatation.

(6)Treatment of symptomaticmalignant gastro-oesophageal anastomoticleaks.

(7)Benignoesophageal strictures.

2．Contraindications

(1)The patient loses the function of swallowing autonomously or swallowing may cause aspiration (bilateral recurrent laryngeal nerve injury).

(2)The rupture orifice of spontaneous esophageal rupture is too long (more than 10 cm). Two overlapping stents can seal the rupture, but there is no esophageal wall outside the stents, which can not heal spontaneously.

(3)Upper esophageal perforation, higher than the first thoracic level.

(4)Spontaneous rupture of esophagus accompanied by esophageal varices.

(5)The patient's vital signs are unstable and cardiac arrest may occur at any time.

3. Stent placement technology

(1)Site, severity, and length of the stricture were evaluated with barium esophagography before stent placement.

(2)Topical anesthesia of the pharynx was achieved with an aerosol sprey routinely before the procedure. Agents for sedation or general anesthesia were not used.

(3)The patient swallowed a small amount of contrast agent (approximately 10 ml, iodine contrast agent)for opacification or the narrowed esophageal lumen.

(4)A 0.035-inch stiff glide wire with catheter was inserted through the mouth across the stricture into the distal portion of the esophagus or stomach.

(5)The position and length of esophageal stenosis were measured again.

(6)If the stent cannot be guided through the stenosis by the guide wire, the balloon catheter can be used for pre expansion (the maximum diameter is 10 mm)[Figure 29-1(a)].

(7)The guide wire remained in the esophagus.

(8)A stent at least 4 cm longer than the stricture was then placed so that the proximal and distal parts (approximately 2 cm of each part)of the stent rested on the upper and lower margins of the stricture, respectively. The stent was placed under fluoroscopic guidance with a 8 mm introducing system in the sane way as described previously[Figure 29-1(b)].

(9)Esophagography was performed to verify the position and patency of the stent.

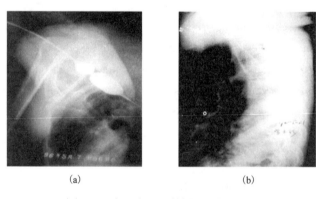

(a)   (b)

(a)strictured esophagus; (b)Stent placement.

Figure 29-1   Stent placement in esophagal cancer. Inflated balloon showed

4. Results

Covered or uncovered self-expanding metallic stents have been proved to be an easy, safe, and effective device for palliation of esophageal malignant obstruction and esophagorespiratory fistula. Stenting of malignant oesophageal obstruction and refractory benign strictures continues to evolve with the introduction of newer anti-reflux, anti-migration stents with an internal plastic coating and with retrievable stents. Most patients (75%~90%) resume a near normal diet after stent placement, with a mean reduction in dysphagia score of around 1. 8. Survival may be increased by the use of adjuvant chemoradiotherapy or endoluminal brachytherapy either before or after stent placement, although this may result in more stent-related complications. Further studies are needed in this area.

5. Complications

Early chest pain occurs in up to 100% of patients, but prolongedchest pain occurs in less than 13% of patients. Chest pain maybe more severe in patients with high strictures and when usinglarge diameter stents. Major complications such as bleeding, perforation, aspiration, fever and fistula occur in 10% of patients. A higher rate of stent migration, about 25%, is reported for placement of covered stents, especially when positioned across the cardia.

Re-intervention following stent placement is common. This is predominantly due to tumour in-growth with uncovered stents (8% ~ 35% of cases). However, tumour in-growth is rare with covered stents. Other late complications include haemorrhage (3%~10%), oesophageal ulceration (7%), perforation or fistula (5%), stent torsion (5%), stent migration (5%) and stent fracture (2%).

Section 3 Perctaneous fluoroscopically guided gastrostomy

Percutaneous endoscopic gastrostomy was successfully introduced by the endoscopists in the early 1980s. Based on a similar concept, the technique of percutaneous fluoroscopically guided gastrostomy was first described by several workers independently in 1983. Since then, much clinical experience has accumulated with many technical refinements to technique, and these are well reported in the literature. Consequently, percutaneous gastrostomy and transgastric jejunostomy has become a well-accepted procedure with continually expanding indications. Percutaneous gastrojejunostomy, jejunostomy and cecostomy under fluoroscopy are also used.

1. Indications AND CONTRAINDICATIONS

(1) Percutaneous gastrostomy and transgastric jejunostomy can be performed in patients who require nutritional support and have a functioning gastrointestinal tract.

(2) In those who require gastric or small bowel decompression.

(3) Patients requiring nutritional support by far account for the larger group. Most of these patients have dysphagia usually due to disabling neurologic disorders or head and neck tumors.

(4) Patients with intractable diabetic gastroparesis also benefit from percutaneous gastrostomy for feeding to the small bowel.

(5) Patients in Intensive Care Units requiring nutritional support (e. g. trauma patients) are also suitable candidates.

(6) Gastrostomies have also been placed in anorexic patients such as those with anorexia nervosa, psychiatric depression, or advanced malignancies. The procedure can also be safely and effectively performed in infants and children.

2. Contraindications

(1) Percutaneous gastrostomy can only be performed if the anterior stomach wall and anterior abdominal wall are in close apposition. Interposition of the liver, colon, or small bowel thus constitutes a contraindication to gastrostomy.

(2) Gross ascites is also a relative contraindication although the procedure can be successfully performed with

fluoroscopically guided gastropexy (vide infra).

(3)Partial gastrectomy per se is not an absolute contraindication.

(4)Other contraindications to the procedure include an increased risk of hemorrhage.

3. Preoperative preparation

(1)Theassessment of the patients coagulation profile, which should be corrected if abnormal.

(2)The patient should have an empty stomach for at least 4 hours, and thus any nasogastric feeding should be stopped prior to the procedure.

(3)A nasogastric tube should be placed in the stomach, and residual gastric fluid aspirated.

(4)Before puncture, intravenous administration of 0.5~1 mg glucagon or 20mg scopolamine Butyl bromide was given to reduce gastric peristalsis.

4. Operation process

(1)The stomach is fully distended with air (200 ~ 800 mL). Using anteroposterior position and lateral fluoroscopy, apposition of the anterior stomach wall to the anterior abdominal wall is confirmed by placing the tip of forceps at the proposed skin entry site in the epigastrium.

(2)A puncture site lateral to the rectus muscle or midline is preferable to avoid injury to the superior epigastric artery.

(3)Once the skin entry site is chosen, the skin is infiltrated with local anesthetic.

(4)The entry site cuts with a scalpel.

(5)Various needles ranging from 22 G to 18 G have been used to enter the stomach. We prefer the use of an 18 G trocar needle, and this is inserted into the stomach with a sharp downward thrust. Entry into the stomach lumen is evident from the free movement of the needle tip when the needle shaft is moved from side to side. Contrast can also be injected to confirm intragastric placement.

(6)A guidewire is inserted through the needle and the tract dilated to the required size. In the process of expansion, gastric fixation, such as T-shaped anchor hook, can be used to fix the gastric wall on the anterior abdominal wall.

(7)The gastrostomy catheter is then inserted. Various purpose-made gastrostomy catheter types, varying from 10 to 18 Fr in size have been described. We recommend the use of 12 Fr catheters for the initial placement. These can be easily introduced into the stomach after a single 12 Fr dilation. Dilation is performed using a short sharp twisting action. This is necessary to penetrate the muscular stomach wall (Figure 29-2). Stomach distension should also be maintained by insufflating further air through the nasogastric tubeduring insertion of the dilator and also during subsequent insertion of the gastrostomy catheter.

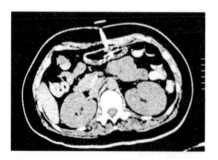

Figure 29-2　Percutaneous gastrostomy

(8)Percutaneous gastropexy: In the standard percutaneous gastrostomy, the anterior stomach wall is not fixed to the anterior abdominal wall of the stomach. Retraction of the stomach from the anterior abdominal wall can thus occur leaving a potential space in the peritoneal cavity theoretically permitting gastric contents to leak or allow displacement of the gastrostomy catheter into the peritoneal cavity. To combat this problem of poor stomach, anterior abdominal wall apposition, percutaneously placed suture anchor have been developed that allow fixing of the stomach to the abdominal wall.

5. Postoperative management

Regular vital signs assessment is suggested for 4-8 hours after the procedure. Development of peritoneal signs should be watched for. We recommend the nasogastric tube remain for 24 hours to allow gastric decompression. Feeding through thegastrostomy tube may commence in 24 hours after stomach placement and 4 hours after jejunostomy placement.

6. Results

Technical success rate forpercutaneous gastrostomy insertions are reported to approach 100%.

7. Complications

Complication rates of approximated 5%. Major complications, particularly peristomal leakage and wound infection, were more frequent in surgical patients. This is thought to be due to the difference in techniques since in a percutaneous gastrostomy the stomach wall is dilated to fit the gastrostomy tube maintaining a tight seal, whereas in surgical placement, the stomach wall is cut and a purse-string suture placed around the gastrostomy tube.

Section 4 Percutaneous transhepactic biliary drainage

Direct transhepatic catheterization of the biliary tree has used for many years for temporary external decompression prior to surgery. Recent improvements in manipulation techniques now make it possible to consistently advance transhepatic cathetersacross obstructing lesions into the duodenum. When sideholes are positioned in the segements of cather above and below an obstructing lesion, a conduct is created that permits antegrade drainage of bile into the duodenum.

1. Indications

(1)Preoperative decompression: Once transhepatic biliary drainage has been established, symptoms directly related to jaundice rapidly disappear and there is usually significant improvement in the patient's nutritional stat

(2) Permanent catheter drainage: Transhepatic catheters provide long-term palliation of biliary obstruction comparable to permanently implanted surgical drainage tubes. Decompression is rapidly achieved with minimal mortality regardless of the nature or location of the obstructing lesion.

(3)Malignant diseases (Cholangiocarcinoma, Metastasis to the porta hepatis, Carcinoma of the pancreas): Prolonged survival can be expected in most cases if the biliary obstruction is relieved adequately. Because of, after the drainage catheter has been placed, the patient's condition may improve sufficiently to permit extensive chemotherapy or radiation therapy.

(4)Benign disease: 1)Postoperative benign stricture; 2)Sclerosing cholangitis; 3)Common-duct stones; 4) Pancreatitis.

2. Contraindications

There are no absolute clinical contraindications to transhepatic biliary drainage. There are relative contraindications:

(1)Severe coagulation dysfunction.

(2) Severe heart, liver and kidney failure.

(3) Large amount of ascites.

(4) Those who are allergic to iodine.

(5) Terminal patients with mild symptoms.

(6) Septicemia.

(7) The intrahepatic bile duct is divided into multiple cavities by the tumor and cannot drain the whole bile duct system.

(8) Ultrasound examination confirmed that there was a large fluid level in the liver, Casoni test was positive, suspected of hepatic echinococcosis.

3. Preoperative preparation

(1) Do biochemical examination, such as prolonged prothrombin, vitamin K should be given to correct.

(2) Ultrasound, CT and MRIare performed to determine the nature of the lesion and to identify whether it was hepatocellular jaundice or obstructive jaundice.

(3) The enemais cleaned and sedated the night before the contrast.

(4) Sedationis given one hour before the contrast, but morphine was forbidden to avoid causing spasm of the sphincter of Oddi and confusing the diagnosis.

(5) Abdominal fluoroscopy was performed before the contrast to observe whether there is an inflatable intestinal tube under the liver, so as to avoid accidental injury during puncture.

(6) Do iodine allergy test according to the contrast medium used.

4. Operation process

(1) Performing a thin-needle cholangiogram: A thin-needle cholangiogram is always done before the actual drainage procedure is begun. It is done to confirm the diagnosis, determine the anatomical position of the obstruction, and provide a visible target to guide the subsequent catherization.

(2) Introducing the stylet/sheath: The drainage procedure begins after the thin-needle cholangiogram has completed and across table lateral radiograph obtained. Based on the lateral film, a second puncture site may be chosen that is either more dorsal or more ventral than the original thin-needle puncture site. Under fluoroscopic guidance, a 16-gauge stylet/sheath is introduced into the liver and directed horizontally toward a specific duct.

(3) Manipulating the catheter into the biliary tract: Biliary catheterization consist of a series of alternating steps. The guidewire is actively manipulated a short distance through the ducts and the sheath is then advanced over it. The guidewire is advanced through the biliary tree up to the site of obstruction by rotating the external segment and applying gentle forward pressure.

(4) Crossing the obstruction [Figure 29-3(a)]: The most critical step is percutaneous biliary drainage is advancing the guidewire across the obstruction. Obviously if this stepcannot be carried out, antegrade drainage is impossible. Fortunately catheterization through an obstruction is almost always feasible.

(5) Introducing the drainage catheter [Figure 29-3(b)]: The catheter used for long-term antegrade biliary drainage must have an inner diameter large enough to carry daily bile flow and an outer diameter small enough to pass through the liver parenchyma and the site of the obstruction.

5. Postoperative management

Once the catheter is in satisfactory position, a dressing is applied around the skin entry site and external drainage is established. An adaptor allows attachment from the hub of the Luer lock catheter to a closed-system drainage bag. The volume and character of the bile drainage is monitored for 48 hours. Antegrade drainage is usually established 1 to 2 days after the initial procedure. The collecting bag is detached and a cap is placed over

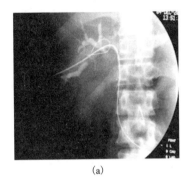
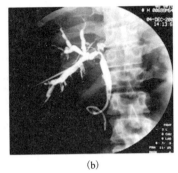

(a)   (b)

(a) Advancing guidewire across the obstruction; (b) Introducing the drainage catheter. .

Figure 29-3   PTCD in biliary obstruction

the catheter hub.

6. Results

The satisfaction of transhepatic biliary drainage depends on the continuity and communication between bile ducts above the obstruction plane. After the operation, the pruritus of the whole bodyis obviously improved, and the serum bilirubin is significantly decreased.

7. Complications

(1) Local infection at the entry site which is treated with hot soaks twice daily and a topical antibiotic ointment.

(2) Granuloma formation at the entry site which is treated with silver nitrate cauterization.

(3) Obstruction of the tube with leakage of bile, change in the color of the stool and urine, jaundice, or fewer which are treated by catheter replacement.

Section 5   Precutaneous nephrostomy

Percutaneous Nephrostomy (PCN): Image guided placement of a catheter into the renal collecting system. PCN allows rapid and reliable access to the renal collecting system for urinary diversion and for the management of a number of diverse upper urinary tract lesions. The access can be created successfully in most of the patients and with significantly less morbidity and mortality than open operative techniques.

1. Indications

Indications for short-term urinary diversion:

(1) Supravesical obstruction from benign lesions (most commonly calculi).

(2) Severe bacterial and fungal infection (pyonephrosis).

(3) Ureteral injuries (traumatic and iatrogenic).

(4) Urinary fistulas, retroperitoneal leaks with urinoma.

(5) Neonatal hydronephrosis (preoperative).

(6) Hypertension secondary to hydronephrosis.

(7) Hemorrhagic cystitis.

(8) Access for other interventional procedures and for endoscopic procedures.

(9) Removal of ureteropelvic foreign body.

Indications for long-term urinary diversion：

（1）Malignant ureteral obstruction.

（2）Advanced bladder cancer.

（3）Urinary fistula（commonly from gynecologic cancer）.

（4）Ureteral obstruction（from retroperitoneal fibrosis or postradiation fibrosis）.

2. Contraindications

Absolute contraindications：PCN should be avoided or delayed in certain circumstances but there are no absolute contraindications. Relative contraindications：

（1）Uncorrectable severe coagulopathy（eg, patients with liver or multisystem failure）.

（2）Terminal illness, imminent death.

3. Procedure

A combined US-fluoroscopy—guided access procedure is the most commonly used method for the PCN catheter placement. Fluoroscopy is convenient for guide wire tracking, tract dilation, drainage catheter placement, and antegrade pyelography.

（1）Progressivedilation of the tract：A target calyx is selected using either ultrasound or fluoroscopic guidance or both. A posterior calyx is usually preferred for entry. A guide wire is then advanced into the collecting system. The thin-wall 22-gauge needle accepts a 0.018 cope mandril wire. The soft end of the guide wire is allowed to coil in the renal pelvis or manipulated into the ureter whenever possible. The stiff segment of the guide wire should be at least 3 to 4 cm inside the renal pelvis before the needle is taken out. The track is initially dilated over the 0.018 guide wire with a hockey stick of a cope set or by the coaxial dilator of neff set. The 0.018 guide wire is then exchanged with a stiff 0.035 guide wire. When an 18-gauge needle is used for the definitive puncture, a stiff 0.035 guide wire can be directly advanced into the renal pelvis. Further dilation of the tract to the size of the drainage catheter is performed with tapered teflon fascial dilators over the 0.035 wire. Progressive dilation of the tract to the size of the drainage catheter to be introduced is performed in 2-Fr increments.

（2）Placement of adrainage catheter（Figure 29-4）：Drainage catheters of 8- to 10-Fr in diameter with a pigtail tip and multiple side holes in the pigtail portion are adequate for most indications. Larger catheters or catheters with a larger end hole are preferable for drainage of thick pus and debris. Most drainage catheter kits come with lockable metal and plastic stiffening cannulas. The catheters are connected to a closed system bag to allow external drainage.

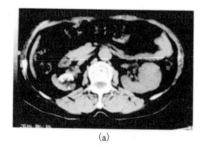
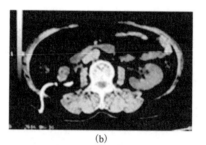

(a)　　　　　　　　　　(b)

Figure 29-4　Severe hydronephrosis due to right ureteral calculi was removed by percutaneous right pyelostomy

（3）The catheter does the followings：①It allows internal drainage of urine into the bladder when the hub of the catheter is capped and eliminates the need for an external bag. ②It allows access to the collecting system and nephrostogram when needed. ③It allows exchange of the catheter every 3 months. ④It acts as a stent that serves the same purpose as an indwelling double-J stent. ⑤It is less likely to be dislodged. ⑥Patient acceptance is high.

4. Complications

(1) Minor: 10. 84%, Fever, Ureteral and infundibular strictures, transient hemorrhage and hematuria, catheter dislodgment, perforation of the pelvis and ureter, urinoma, ascites, distal ureteral obstruction.

(2) Major: 2. 77% (mortality rate 0. 05%), infection (septic shock), bleeding complications (hemorrhage through the track, hematuria requiring transfusion, arterial injury, arteriovenous fistula, subcapsular hematoma, ruptured kidney, retroperitoneal hemorrhage), visceral injury (colon or spleen), thoracic complications (massive hydrothorax, hemothorax, pyothorax, and pneumothorax), renal vein thrombosis.

The morphologic alterations in the kidney from PCN are minimal and considerably less than those associated with open surgery. The complication rate tends to fall as the radiologic and urologic teams gain experience.

Section 6 Percutaneous vertebroplasty

Percutaneous vertebroplasty (PVP) is a relatively new and promising minimally invasive technique to treat painful vertebral compression fractures (VCFs) and vertebral neoplastic lesions, which was firstly performed in France in 1984. The procedure consists of the percutaneous insertion of a relatively large-gauge bone needle into a vertebral body and the instillation of a viscous liquid mixture of polymethylmethacrylate cement (PMMA) under fluoroscopic guidance. Although the usual therapeutic goal is symptomatic pain relief, the procedure may also be performed to mechanically reinforce the pathologically weakened vertebra. Polymerization and solidification of the injected PMMA strengthens and stabilizes the vertebral body. The mechanical effects are thought to provide pain relief and prevent further vertebral collapse. Neurotoxic effects from the methylmethacrylate monomer and heat from the exothermic polymerization reaction may also contribute to pain relief by destroying nociceptive receptors and nerves. As a relatively new medical procedure, PVP is undergoing continual assessment and refinement.

1. Indications

(1) Osteoporotic vertebral compression fractures(VCF).

(2) Metastases and muliple myeloma.

(3) Vertebral hemangioma: Vertebral hemangiomas may cause pain by compression fracture or by spinal canal and/or neural foraminal mass effect.

2. Contraindications

(1) Asymptomatic osteoporotic VCF.

(2) There is no compressed osteoporotic vertebral body.

(3) Drug therapy has improved the symptoms of osteoporotic compression fractures.

(4) Acute traumatic fracture of a previously normal vertebra.

(5) Complete vertebral collapse.

(6) Complete vertebral destruction, epidural or foraminal tumor, nerve root or spinal cord compression.

(7) Uncorrectable coagulopathy.

(8) Local infection.

3. Patient selection and evaluation

Careful patient selection is crucial for good clinical results from PVP. There should be convincing evidence that the patient's back pain is caused by a symptomatic VCF. Back pain from other causes such as facet arthropathy, degenerative disc disease, herniated discs, and sacroiliac disease will not respond to PVP. Complete evaluation requires a relative history and physical examination and review of the appropriate imaging studies, including serial plain films, magnetic resonance imaging (MRI) scans, and bone scans.

4. Procedure

(1) The first procedural step is the needle placement for the PMMA injection. This procedure can be performed with one C-arm transitioning between anteroposterior AP and lateral images. Or with two C-arms, one positioned for AP and the other for lateral images.

(2) The 11-gauge osteo-site needle in the lumbar spine and 13-gauge osteo-site needle in the smaller pedicles of the thoracic spine are used. The ideal needle tip position is near the midline in the anterior third of the vertebral body[Figure 29-5(a), (b)].

(3) The PMMA mixture is slowly injected during continuous fluoroscopic observation in the lateral view. During the injection the AP view is intermittently evaluated for lateral extravasation [Figure 29-5(c)].

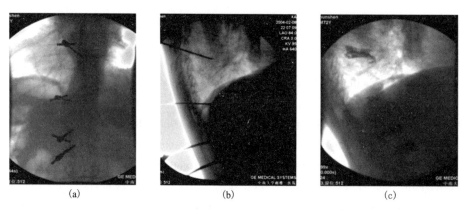

(a) | (b) | (c)

(a) The anteroposterior view; (b) The lateral view; (c) The lateral view shows adequate filling with PMMA.

Figure 29-5　Percutaneous vertebroplasty for multiple osteoporotic compression fractures

5. Complications

Complications occur in about 50% of the patients who undergo vertebroplasty, but about 95% of them are clinically asymptomatic. Transient worsening of pain or fever may occur immediately after the PVP and is usually effectively treated with a several-day course of nonsteroidal anti-inflammatory drugs or steroids. Nondisplaced rib fractures in osteoporotic patients have been reported. More serious complications have included symptomatic cement pulmonary embolism, radiculopathy, and spinal cord compression.

6. Future directions

New non-PMMA bone cements with osteoinductive andosteoconductive properties, and also cements delivering chemotherapy along with strength augmentation, are under active investigation. These may expand PVP applications for malignant vertebral lesions and possibly for prophylactic treatment of osteoporotic vertebral bodies.

Restoration of vertebral body height with apercutaneously placed inflatable bone tamp followed by PMMA strength augmentation has been described (kyphoplasty). A comparison of the efficacy and safety of PV and kyphoplasty for various indications will be necessary. In the treatment of malignant vertebral tumors, PVP combined with other minimally invasive methods, such as radiofrequency ablation, vascular embolization and so on, plays an increasingly important role.

Section 7　Tumor ablation

Ablation of tumors is an option for local tumor control for unresectable tumors.

Ablation includes physical ablation, chemical ablation and electroablation (irreversible electroporation). Physical ablation includes cryoablation, and thermal ablation. Thermal ablation includes radiofrequency thermal ablation (RFA), microwave ablation (MWA). There are some other ablations, such as high-intensity focused ultrasound, laser interstitial thermal therapy, and so on. Alcohol and glacial acetic acid were used for chemical ablation.

Thermal ablative techniques include heat-based modalities such as RFA and microwave ablation in addition to cold-based techniques such as cryoablation. RFA utilizes frictional energy imparted by oscillating ions within tissue to heat and treat tumors. Cells undergo coagulation necrosis when heated to more than 54℃ for more than 1 second. Therapeutic RFA strives to bring tissue temperatures to the range of 60℃ to 100℃. The mechanism of cell death caused by MWA is similar to RFA. With microwave, a continuously oscillating microwave field targets polar molecules (predominately water), which align with this field resulting in increased kinetic energy and tissue temperatures. Cryoablation causes cell death through cell membrane disruption from both intra and extracellular ice crystal formation and subsequent release of intracellular material. Gases (typically argon) are delivered at high pressures through an internal feed line into an expansion chamber in the cryoprobe; as the gas expands, a heat sink is created cooling the probe and surrounding tissues.

1. Pulmonary tumor

Ablative techniques has been proven to be both feasible and efficacious in the treatment of lung cancers. These techniques have been used to treat primary lung cancers, metastatic disease to the lungs, and in palliation for painful chest wallmasses.

(1) Indications

1) Early-stage primary lung cancer: Biopsy-proven, medically inoperable/refusing surgery, recurrence after surgery, radiation, or chemotherapy.

2) Limited metastatic disease and salvage therapy: Local recurrence in postradiation bed, local recurrence in postsurgical bed, symptom palliation such as usually pain.

(2) Contraindications

1) Uncorrected coagulopathy: Platelets less than 50, 000 /μL and INR>1. 5.

2) Bacteremia or active infection.

3) Major organ dysfunction.

4) Diffuse lung cancer or tumor is too large, which needs ablation range up to 1/3 of lung volume.

5) A lot of hydrothorax.

6) Late cachexia. The expected survival is less than 3 months.

(3) Preoperative preparation

1) Imaging examination: Chest X-ray, enhanced CT scan, PET / CT examination if necessary within 2 weeks.

2) Heart and lung function test, coagulation, liver and kidney function and other laboratory tests.

3) Bronchoscopic biopsy or CT guided biopsyare performed to confirm the pathological cytological or histological diagnosis.

4) Preparation of surgical equipment and rescue equipment and drugs.

5) The patientis fasted and watered 6 hours before local anesthesia.

6) The patient and the client signed the informed consent for the operation.

(4) Procedure

1) Anesthesia: Moderate sedation or general anesthesia can be used.

2) Positioning and access sites (similar to lung biopsies) [Figure 29-6(a)]: Trajectory should limit number of interlobular fissures traversed, avoid bullae and cysts, and avoid mediastinal structures and large vessels. When

multiple probes are combined, synergistic effects can be seen, which means more optimal ablation coverage.

3)Probe positioning: Ideal probe positioning allows for post-ablative zone to cover tumor [Figure 29-6(b)]. Similar to surgery, the effective ablation zone should ideally cover 0.5 to 1 cm beyond the boundaries of the tumor.

4)Choice of ablation energy (RFA, microwave, or cryoablation): ① Microwave should be avoided with lesions <1 to 2 cm from the pleural surface. Microwave ablation zones abutting pleural surfaces are prone to bronchopleural fistula. ②A pretreatment short cycle of freeze and thaw (3-minute freeze, 3-minute thaw) may allow better ice ball formation when cryoablation is used secondary to enhanced conductivity of hemorrhage versus air. ③ Cryoablation is often better tolerated than hyperthermia in the patient who is undergoing the procedure under conscious sedation versus general anesthesia.

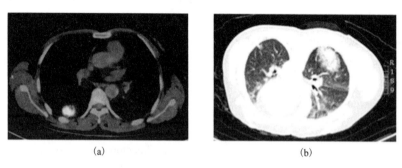

(a)Preoperative CT showed lung cancer; (b)Postoperative CT showed that the ablation area covered the tumor.

Figure 29-6　Lung cancer cryoablation

5)Intraoperative monitoring: Patient's temperature, pulse, respiration, blood pressure, oxygen saturation, changes of temperature distribution, impedance, tumor area and surrounding normal lung tissue in ablation area.

(5)Postoperative management

The ablation needle is pulled out slowly after the operation. The CT scan is performed again to observe whether there is bleeding and pneumothorax. The routine hemostasis and antibacterial treatment are performed for 3 days after the operation. The routine lung enhanced CT examination is performed to observe the changes of tumor at 1 month, 3 months and 6 months after the operation.

(6)Resluts

The success rate of treatmentis more than 90%. The inactivation rate of tumor diameter less than 5 cm is 90%, and the residual lesions can be completely inactivated by the second additional treatment. It can significantly improve the quality of life and prolong the survival period.

(7)Complications

1)Pneumothorax (9%~13%).

2)Hemoptysis: 3%, Most hemoptysis are self-limiting.

3)Neuropathy: Phrenic nerve injury from treatment of para mediastinal masses has been reported. Though it is usually self-limiting, avoidance is preferred.

4)Pain: Patient-controlled analgesias (PCAs)or narcotics can be used the night of the procedure with the vast majority of pain either resolving or becoming significantly improved by the days after the procedure.

5)Fever, infection and bronchopleural fistula.

2. Hepatic tumors

Ablation is accepted as the best therapeutic choice for patients with very early and early stage hepatocellular carcinoma (HCC)when liver transplantation or surgical resection is not a suitable option. In addition, ablation is considered as a viable alternative to surgery for inoperable patients with limited hepatic metastatic disease, especially from colorectal cancer (CRC).

(1) Indications

1) Very early and early stage HCC according to the Barcelona Clinic Liver Cancer (BCLC) classification when patients are not candidates for either liver resection or transplantation. Patients are required to have a single tumor smaller than 5 cm or as many as three nodules smaller than 3 cm each, no evidence of vascular invasion or extrahepatic spread, Child-Pugh class A or B.

2) Nonsurgical patients with CRC oligometastases isolated to the liver. Selected patients with limited hepatic and pulmonary CRC metastatic disease may qualify provided that extrahepatic disease is deemed curable.

3) Hepatic metastases from other primary cancers. Promising initial results have been reported in the treatment of breast and endocrine tumors.

(2) Contraindications

1) Absolute contraindications

① Tumor locates <1 cm from a major biliary duct due to risk of delayed stenosis.

② Untreatable/unmanageable coagulopathy.

2) Relative contraindications

① Greater than five lesions. The number of lesions should not be considered an absolute contraindication to RF ablation if successful treatment of all metastatic deposits can be accomplished. Nevertheless, most centers preferentially treat patients with five or fewer lesions.

② Tumor size should not exceed 3 cm in longest axis to achieve best rates of complete ablation with most of the currently available devices.

③ Bilioenteric anastomosis or PTCD internal and external drainage, because of the risk of hepatic abscesses.

④ Superficial lesions, because of a higher risk of complications.

⑤ Superficial lesions that are adjacent to any part of the gastrointestinal tract, because of the risk of thermal injury of the gastric or bowel wall (consider hydro/gas dissection).

⑥ Tumors located in the vicinity of the gallbladder, due to the risk of iatrogenic cholecystitis.

⑦ Ferromagnetic prostheses that may act as heat sinks and cause skin burns.

⑧ RFA is not suitable for pacemaker/defibrillator patients.

(3) Preoperative preparation

1) Imaging and serological examination: Imaging examination is needed to determine the location and size of the tumor, the feasibility of ablation surgery. Ultrasound examination of cardiac function is needed to understand the heart. Serological examination such as hemoglobin, platelet, coagulation function is needed to assess the risk of surgery.

2) Chest X-ray and ECG examination.

3) Preoperative evaluation: Doctors evaluate the location of the tumor and determine the type of ablation related equipment.

4) Patient preparation: Treatment of skin and hair is needed at puncture site. Patients should cooperate with doctors for respiratory training, anti-inflammatory treatment and diet control before operation to prevent postoperative severe infection, intraoperative nausea and vomiting and other complications. If the tumor is close to the gallbladder, patients are required to eat high-fat diet before operation to promote gallbladder emptying, so as to expose the lesion site. It is expected that the operation time is relatively long, and the patients don't drink too much water before the operation and catheterize if necessary.

(4) Procedure

1)Positioning: It is mainly to select the best treatment position, needle entry site and path according to the imaging findings before operation. Then the needle entry path must pass through some normal liver tissues. It is needed to avoid the major vessels, bile ducts and gastrointestinal tract these important organs, which can effectively reduce the incidence of complications.

2)Anesthesia: At present, the most common way of anesthesia is local anesthesia at the puncture point, and then which combines with intravenous use of a certain amount of sedative and analgesic drugs for anesthesia. If necessary, it should be performed under general anesthesia.

3)Routine disinfection is carried. The 2~3 mm incision on the skin is carried after anesthesia.

4)Imaging guidance/monitoring includes US, CT, or MR imaging. Under the guidance of imaging, the ablation needle is distributed into and punctured accurately to the tumor target area according to the preoperative positioning, image and the designed route. The position of the ablation needle and the relationship between the needle and tumor are determined by scanning again. The ablation needle is fixed after the position relationship is better [Figure 29-7(a), (b)].

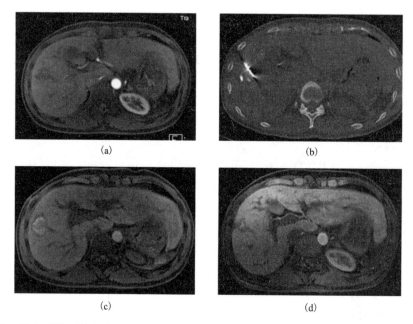

(a)   (b)

(c)   (d)

(a)Pre-ablation MR; (b)In the middle of ablation; (c)One month post-ablation; (d)Six year post-ablation.

Figure 29-7　Microwave ablation of liver cancer

5)The cold circulation system and ablation system start from low power gradually. Whenthe patient tolerates it, it is appropriately that increases the power to increase the ablation range, improve the therapeutic effect, shorten the operation time and reduce the complications.

6)Thermal ablation is the most common way of ablative therapy of liver tumor. The thermal damage caused by RF or MWA heating is dependent on both the tissue temperature achieved and the duration of heating. Heating of tissue at 50℃ to 55℃ for 4 to 6 minutes produces irreversible cellular damage. At temperatures between 60℃ and 100℃, near immediate coagulation of tissue is induced, with irreversible damage to mitochondrial and cytosolic enzymes of the cells. Thus, an essential objective of ablative therapy is the achievement and maintenance of 50℃ to 100℃ temperature throughout the entire target volume for at least 4 to 6 minutes. However, when RFA is used, the relatively slow thermal conduction from the electrode surface through the tissues increases the duration of application to 10 to 20 minutes.

MWA is emerging as a valuable alternative to RF ablation for thermal ablation of HCC. Electromagnetic microwaves heat matter by inducing an ultra-high-speed (between 900 MHz and 2,450 MHz) alternating electric field, causing the rotation of water molecules. The main features of MW technology include consistently higher intratumoral temperatures, larger tumor ablation volumes, faster ablation times, and an improved convection profile when it is compared with existing thermoablative technologies[Figure 29-7(d)]. As a result, the advantage of MWA over RF ablation is that treatment outcome is less affected by vessels located in the proximity of the tumor (At the end of the procedure, coagulation of the needle track is performed to prevent tumor seeding.

(5)Postoperative management

1)The puncture siteis covered with sterile gauze after operation.

2)24h ECG monitoring is needed. If necessary, it is needed to extend the monitoring time.

3)Fastingis performed for 4 hours after operation. The time of fasting is prolonged after ablation of the lesion which is adjacent to the gastrointestinal tract.

4)Blood routine examination, liver and kidney function and urine routine examinationare performed within 3 days after operation.

5) According to the situation, rehydration, liver protection, stomach protection, diuresis, symptomatic treatment are carried out.

(6)Complications

1)Major complications (2.2% to 3.1%): Intraperitoneal bleeding (1%); Liver abscess (0.3%); Intestinal perforation (0.3%); Pneumothorax/hemothorax (0.1%); Bile duct stenosis (0.1%); Tumor seeding along the needle tract (0.5%); Skin burns (0.1%).

2)Minor complications (5% to 8.9%): Pain; Fever; Asymptomatic pleural effusion; Asymptomatic self-limiting intraperitoneal bleeding.

3) Mortality (0.1% to 0.5%). The most common causes of death are sepsis, hepatic failure, colon perforation, and portal vein thrombosis.

(Cong Ma, Fuan Wang, Linan Hu, Tianmin Wang, Enhua Xiao, Zixu Zhang)